OXFORD MEDICAL PUBLICATIONS

Oxford Handbook of
Palliative Care

Published and forthcoming Oxford Handbooks

Oxford Handbook of Clinical Medicine 7/e (also available for PDAs)
Oxford Handbook of Clinical Specialties 7/e
Oxford Handbook of Acute Medicine 2/e
Oxford Handbook of Anaesthesia 2/e
Oxford Handbook of Applied Dental Sciences
Oxford Handbook of Cardiology
Oxford Handbook of Clinical Dentistry 4/e
Oxford Handbook of Clinical and Laboratory Investigation 2/e
Oxford Handbook of Clinical Diagnosis
Oxford Handbook of Clinical Haematology 2/e
Oxford Handbook of Clinical Immunology and Allergy 2/e
Oxford Handbook of Clinical Pharmacy
Oxford Handbook of Clinical Surgery 3/e
Oxford Handbook of Critical Care 2/e
Oxford Handbook of Dental Patient Care 2/e
Oxford Handbook of Dialysis 2/e
Oxford Handbook of Emergency Medicine 3/e
Oxford Handbook of Endocrinology and Diabetes
Oxford Handbook of ENT and Head and Neck Surgery
Oxford Handbook for the Foundation Programme   2/e
Oxford Handbook of Gastroenterology and Hepatology
Oxford Handbook of General Practice 2/e
Oxford Handbook of Genitourinary Medicine, HIV and AIDS
Oxford Handbook of Geriatric Medicine
Oxford Handbook of Medical Sciences
Oxford Handbook of Nephrology and Hypertension
Oxford Handbook of Nutrition and Dietetics
Oxford Handbook of Neurology
Oxford Handbook of Occupational Health
Oxford Handbook of Obstetrics and Gynaecology
Oxford Handbook of Oncology 2/e
Oxford Handbook of Ophthalmology
Oxford Handbook of Palliative Care 2/e
Oxford Handbook of Practical Drug Therapy
Oxford Handbook of Pre-Hospital Care
Oxford Handbook of Psychiatry
Oxford Handbook of Public Health Practice 2/e
Oxford Handbook of Rehabilitation Medicine
Oxford Handbook of Respiratory Medicine
Oxford Handbook of Rheumatology 2/e
Oxford Handbook of Sport and Exercise Medicine
Oxford Handbook of Tropical Medicine 2/e
Oxford Handbook of Urology

Oxford Handbook of
Palliative Care

SECOND EDITION

Max Watson

Consultant in Palliative Medicine, Northern Ireland
Hospice, Belfast; Lecturer in Palliative Care,
University of Ulster, Belfast; Special Adviser,
Hospice Friendly Hospitals Programme, Dublin;
Honorary Consultant in Palliative Medicine,
The Princess Alice Hospice, Esher

Caroline Lucas

Deputy Medical Director, The Princess Alice Hospice, Esher;
Consultant in Palliative Medicine, Surrey Primary Care
Trust; Honorary Consultant in Palliative Medicine, Ashford
and St. Peter's Hospital NHS Trust

Andrew Hoy

Medical Director, The Princess Alice Hospice, Esher;
Consultant in Palliative Medicine, Epsom and St Helier
NHS Trust

Jo Wells

Support Service Coordinator, The Leukaemia Foundation,
South Australia; Formerly Nurse Consultant in Palliative Care,
The Princess Alice Hospice, Esher

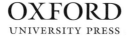

OXFORD
UNIVERSITY PRESS

OXFORD
UNIVERSITY PRESS

Great Clarendon Street, Oxford OX2 6DP

Oxford University Press is a department of the University of Oxford.
It furthers the University's objective of excellence in research, scholarship,
and education by publishing worldwide in

Oxford New York

Auckland Cape Town Dar es Salaam Hong Kong Karachi
Kuala Lumpur Madrid Melbourne Mexico City Nairobi
New Delhi Shanghai Taipei Toronto

With offices in

Argentina Austria Brazil Chile Czech Republic France Greece
Guatemala Hungary Italy Japan Poland Portugal Singapore
South Korea Switzerland Thailand Turkey Ukraine Vietnam

Oxford is a registered trade mark of Oxford University Press
in the UK and in certain other countries

Published in the United States
by Oxford University Press Inc., New York

First edition published 2005

Second edition published 2009, reprinted 2010

British Library Cataloguing in Publication Data
Data available

Library of Congress Cataloging in Publication Data
Oxford handbook of Palliative Care

Typeset by Cepha Imaging Private Ltd., Bangalore, India
Printed in China
on acid-free paper through
Asia Pacific Offset

ISBN 978-0-19-923435-6

10 9 8 7 6 5 4 3

Foreword

When a book rapidly goes to a second edition, it is a mark of esteem of the first edition. And this book is no exception—it is a handbook for anyone providing care for those approaching the end-of-life.

It covers, concisely, all aspects of palliative care, tackling difficult subjects such as ethical issues, communication and breaking bad news, up front at the beginning of the book. The section on the principles of drug use in palliative care specifically addresses the problems of drugs prescribed beyond licence and drug interactions, making this book one of those essential handbooks that will be taken off the shelf time and time again.

Many books are being replaced by internet publications; not this one. This book will be on the desk or in the pocket of many doctors and nurses around the globe. It is equally applicable in countries which are resource-rich and those that are resource-poor.

While providing the theoretical background and evidence base, the book remains eminently practical, for example in its step by step guide on the use of intravenous analgesics in pain emergencies and how to deal with cancer pain that appears to be resistant to opioids. It also elegantly gives the indications for referring across to others such as radiotherapy and outlines different types of chemotherapy that a patient might be having. Few reference books are quite this packed with information.

Paediatric palliative care has recently emerged as a specialty in its own right in the UK is also included in this book; the needs of dying children have been neglected for far too long; here again, the book is up to date, practical and helpful.

This book does not shy away from controversy; it has a balanced critique of complementary therapies, their benefits and their place in the delivery of care overall.

The authors provide objective evidence and their enormous experience shines through the text. The specific resources and further reading given at the end of every chapter complements the 'no nonsense' layout of each chapter throughout the book.

As a guide to modern palliative care, this book will serve patients well.

Professor Ilora Finlay FRCP FRCGP
(Baroness Finlay of Llandaff)

Preface to the second edition

I am always willing to learn, however I do not always like to be taught.
Winston Churchill

The first edition of the *Oxford Handbook of Palliative Care* has been warmly received. We have been encouraged by colleagues to make the material presented here more relevant to non-medical readers. We therefore welcome to our team, Jo Wells, who is a nurse consultant in palliative care. We have added new sections on antibiotics, increased emphasis on non-malignant disease, learning disabilities, palliative care in developing countries and communication. All the chapters of the first edition have been reviewed and many have been completely rewritten.

We hope that the result will be a Handbook which is useful to the whole of the multiprofessional team and will achieve a better balance than its predecessor. Although the Handbook is somewhat larger than the first edition, we feel that this is a reflection of the rapid changes and progress of this field of clinical practice in a relatively short period.

The aim of the Handbook remains as originally stated. We would like to provide a readily accessible source of help to all those who care for people who cannot be cured. This will include generalists and those whose specialty is not palliative care. We hope that the Handbook may also be a useful ready reference for those engaged in full-time palliative, hospice or end-of-life care. We remain proud to be associated with the Oxford University Press Handbook series, and are well aware of the heavy responsibility which this confers.

We regard the *Oxford Textbook of Palliative Medicine* as the parent text for much of the material in this Handbook. There are various references throughout to the current, third edition. However, readers may need to be aware that a new fourth edition is in preparation, and should be available later in 2009.

MW
CL
AH
JW

Preface to the first edition

Most clinical professionals have been affected by caring for patients with palliative care needs. Such patients may challenge us at both a professional and at a personal level in areas where we feel our confidence or competence is challenged.

> I wanted to help her, but I just didn't know what to do or say

As in every other branch of medicine, knowledge and training can help us extend our comfort zone, so that we can better respond to such patients in a caring and professional manner. However, in picking up this Handbook and reading thus far you have already demonstrated a motivation that is just as important as a thirst for knowledge, the central desire to improve the care of your patients.

It was out of just such a motivation that the modern hospice movement began 40 years ago, and it is that same motivation that has fuelled the spread of the principles of palliative care—in fact the principles of ALL good care—across the globe: respect for the person, attention to detail, scrupulous honesty and integrity, holistic care, team caring and consummate communications (often more about listening than telling and talking).

> I knew we couldn't cure him, but didn't know when or how to start palliative care

Increasingly it is being recognized that every person has the right to receive high-quality palliative care whatever the illness, whatever its stage, regardless of whether potentially curable or not. The artificial distinction between curative and palliative treatments has rightly been recognized as an unnecessary divide, with a consequent loss of the border crossings that previously signified a complete change in clinical emphasis and tempo.

Medical knowledge is developing rapidly, with ever more opportunities for and emphasis on curative treatment, to the point when any talk of palliative care can sometimes be interpreted as 'defeatist'.

Today the principles of palliative care interventions may be employed from the first when a patient's illness is diagnosed. Conversely, a patient with predominantly palliative care needs, late in their disease journey, may benefit from energetic treatments more usually regarded as 'curative'.

> I just felt so helpless watching him die. Surely it could have been better?

Governments and professional bodies now recognize that every nurse and doctor has a duty to provide palliative care and, increasingly, the public and the media have come to expect—as of right—high-quality palliative care from their healthcare professionals irrespective of the clinical setting.

Many of these palliative care demands can best be met, as in the past, by the healthcare professionals who already know their patients and families well. This Handbook is aimed at such hospital- or community-based professionals, and recognizes that the great majority of patients with palliative needs are looked after by doctors and nurses who have not been trained in specialist palliative care but who are often specialist in the knowledge of their patients.

> Even though I knew she had had every treatment possible, still, when she died I really felt that we had failed her and let her family down.

Junior healthcare staff members throughout the world have used the Oxford Handbook series as their own specialist pocket companion through the lonely hours of on-call life. The format, concise (topic-a-page), complete and sensible, teaches not just clinical facts but a way of thinking. Yet for all the preoccupation with cure, no healthcare professional will ever experience greater satisfaction or confirmation of their choice of profession, than by bringing comfort and dignity to someone at the end-of-life.

> I had never seen anyone with that type of pain before and just wished I could get advice from someone who knew what to do.

The demands on inexperienced and hard-pressed doctors or nurses in looking after patients with palliative care needs can be particularly stressful. It is our hope that this text, ideally complemented by the support and teaching of specialist palliative care teams, will reduce the often expressed sense of helplessness, a sense of helplessness made all the more poignant by the disproportionate gratitude expressed by patients and families for any attempts at trying to listen, understand and care.

> It was strange, but I felt he was helping me much more than I was helping him

While it is our hope that the Handbook will help the reader access important information quickly and succinctly, we hope it will not replace the main source of palliative care knowledge: the bedside contact with the patient.

It is easier to learn from books than patients, yet what our patients teach us is often of more abiding significance: empathy, listening, caring, existential questions of our own belief systems and the limitations of medicine. It is at the bedside that we learn to be of practical help to people who are struggling to come to terms with their own mortality and face our own mortality in the process.

Readers may notice some repetition of topics in the Handbook. This is not due to weariness or oversight on the part of the editors, but is an attempt to keep relevant material grouped together—to make it easier for those needing to look up information quickly.

It is inevitable that in a text of this size some will be disappointed at the way we have left out, or skimped on, a favourite area of palliative care interest. To these readers we offer our apologies and two routes of redress: almost 200 blank pages to correct the imbalances; and the OUP website, http://www.oup.co.uk/isbn/0-19-850897-2, where your suggestions for how the next edition could be improved would be gratefully received.

Acknowledgements

We must acknowledge and thank many people, without whom this edition of the Oxford University Handbook of Palliative Care would not have been possible. Our colleagues in Ireland and Surrey have been endlessly tolerant of our absence both physical and psychological. They have kept the patient care show on the road when we were chasing references, new procedures, novel drugs or faulty syntax. They have also been asked to provide new review material for inclusion or been required to comment on our initial efforts. We hope that all these expert witnesses have been included in the updated list of contributors. Particular mention and thanks must go to the consultant staff at the North Ireland Hospice and the Princess Alice, the eager specialist registrars, the ward staff and clinical nurse specialists and the allied health care professiobals. All have given time and expertise with unstinting generosity.

We would be lost without the invaluable backup of our secretaries, Liz Huckle, and Susan Lockwood. Jan Brooman has unfailingly checked every single reference. Gill Eyers and Margaret Gibbs have provided invaluable pharmacy advice. The staff at OUP have been both expert and also infinitely patient, especially Beth Womack and Kate Wilson.

We continue to be indebted to Dr. Ian Back for the excellence of his http://www.pallcare.info website as an invaluable palliative resource. We are also grateful to Baroness Finlay for her willingness to write the foreword to this edition on top of her many commitments

Our greatest thanks, however, are reserved for the many contributors and reviewers who so generously gave of their time to allow this edition to be completed. We realise that this work was often carried out in the "small hours", after the completion of clinical responsibilities. Without such collaboration this handbook would not have been possible.

Finally, we must acknowledge and thank our respective spouses who have patiently kept us both fed and watered but also tried to supply a sense of proportion and humour.

We are also indebted for permission to reproduce material within the handbook from the following sources:

Bruera E., Higginson I. (1996) *Cachexia–Anorexia in Cancer Patients*. Oxford: Oxford University Press.

Doyle D., et al (eds) (2004) *Oxford Textbook of Palliative Medicine* (3rd edn). Oxford: Oxford University Press.

Ramsay J.-H. R. (1994) A King, a doctor and a convenient death. *British Medical Journal*, **308**: 1445.

The South West London and the Surrey, West Sussex and Hampshire, Mount Vernon and Sussex Cancer Networks. M. Watson, C. Lucas, A. Hoy (2006) *Adult Palliative Care Guidance* (2nd edn).

Thomas K. (2003) *Caring for the Dying at Home: Companions on the Journey*. Oxford: Radcliffe Medical Press.

Twycross R., Wilcock A. (2007) *Palliative Care Formulary* (3rd edn). palliativedrugs.com

Winston's Wish: supporting bereaved children and young people. www.winstonswish.org.uk.

www.rch.org.au/rch_palliative

MW
CL
AH
JW

Contents

Contributors

Owen Barr
Head of School,
School of Nursing,
University of Ulster,
N. Ireland

Pauline Beldon
Nurse Consultant in Tissue
Viability, Epsom and St Helier NHS
Trust, UK

Barbara Biggerstaff
Senior Occupational Therapist,
The Princess Alice Hospice, Esher,
UK

Kathy Birch
Physiotherapist, The Princess Alice
Hospice, Esher, UK

Maggie Breen
Macmillan Clinical Nurse Specialist,
Oncology Outreach and Symptom
Care Nurse Specialist Team, Royal
Marsden Hospital, Surrey, UK

Michael Burgess
H.M.Coroner for Surrey, Coroner
of The Queen's Household, UK

David Cameron
Associate Professor in the
Department of Family Medicine,
University of Pretoria, South Africa

Robin Cole
Consultant Urological Surgeon,
Ashford and St Peter's Hospital
NHS Trust, UK

Simon Coulter
Specialist Registrar in Palliative
Medicine, Marie Curie Hospice,
Belfast, UK

Melaine Coward
Deputy Head of Programmes,
Division of Health and Social Care,
Faculty of Health and Medical
Sciences, University of Surrey, UK

Kay de Vries
Research Fellow at Surrey
University, and Senior lecturer at
The Princess Alice Hospice, Esher,
UK

Judith Delaney
Haematology/Oncology Senior
Pharmacist, Great Ormond Street
Hospital for Children NHS Trust,
London, UK

Gill Eyers
Senior Principal Pharmacist,
Princess Alice Hospice, Esher,
Kingston Hospitals NHS Trust, UK

Craig Gannon
Consultant in Palliative Medicine,
Princess Alice Hospice, Esher, UK

Rebecca Goody
Specialty Registrar in Clinical
Oncology at the Northern Ireland
Cancer Centre, Belfast City
Hospital, Belfast, UK

Patricia Grocott
Reader in Palliative Wound Care
Technology Transfer, Division of
Health and Social Care Research,
King's College London, UK

David Hill
Consultant in Pain Medicine,
Ulster Hospital, Belfast,UK

Jenny Hynson
Consultant Paediatrician,
Victorian Paediatric Palliative
Care Program, Royal Children's
Hospital, Victoria, Australia

Jean Kerr
Specialist Speech & Language Therapist, The Princess Alice Hospice, Esher, and Head of Speech & Language Therapy, Kingston Hospital NHS Trust, UK

Lulu Kreeger
Consultant in Palliative Medicine, The Princess Alice Hospice, Esher, Kingston Hospitals NHS Trust, UK

Victoria Lidstone
Consultant in Palliative Medicine, Cwm Taff NHS Trust, Wales, UK

Mari Lloyd-Williams
Professor / Director of Academic Palliative and Supportive Care, School of Population, Community and Behavioural Sciences, University of Liverpool, UK

Stefan Lorenzl
Associate Professor of Neurology and Consultant in Palliative Medicine, University Hospital Grosshadern, Munich, Germany

Farida Malik
Clinical Research Training Fellow, Cicely Saunders International, London, UK

James McAleer
Senior Lecturer and Consultant in Clinical Oncology, Queen's University, Belfast, UK

Joan McCarthy
Lecturer in Healthcare Ethics, School of Nursing and Midwifery, Brookfield Health Sciences Complex, University College Cork, Ireland

Linda McEnhill
Founder of the National Network of Palliative Care for People with Learning Disabilities and Widening Access Manager, Help the Hospices, London, UK

Dorry McLaughlin
Lecturer in Palliative Care, Northern Ireland Hospice Care, Belfast, UK

Caroline McLoughlin
Specialist Registrar in Palliative Medicine, Northern Ireland Deanery, UK

Alan McPhearson
Specialist Registrar in Palliative Medicine, Northern Ireland Hospice, Belfast, UK

Teresa Merino
Consultant in Palliative Medicine, Royal Surrey County Hospital, Guildford, UK

Caroline Moore
Specialist Registrar in Urology, Frimley Park NHS Trust, UK

Barbara Monroe
Chief Executive St Christopher's Hospice, London, UK

Simon Noble
Clinical Senior Lecturer in Palliative Medicine, Cardiff University, Cardiff, Wales, UK

Steve Nolan
Chaplain, The Princess Alice Hospice, Esher, UK

Ciaran O'Boyle
Professor of Psychology and Chairman, International School of Healthcare Management, Royal College of Surgeons in Ireland, Dublin, Ireland

Julian O'Kelly
Day Hospice Manager / Music Therapist, The Princess Alice Hospice, Esher, UK

David Oliviere
Director of Education and Training, Education Centre, St Christopher's Hospice, London, UK

Victor Pace
Consultant in Palliative Medicine, St Christopher's Hospice, London, UK

Malcolm Payne
Director, Psycho-social and Spiritual Care, St Christopher's Hospice, London, UK

Sheila Payne
Help the Hospices Chair in Hospice Studies, Institute for Health Research, Lancaster University, UK

Max Pittler
Senior Research Fellow in Complementary Medicine, Peninsula Medical School, Universities of Exeter and Plymouth, UK

Mandy Pratt
Art Psychotherapist, Creative Response - Professional Association of Art Therapists in Palliative Care, AIDS, Cancer & Loss Affiliated to St Helena Hospice, Colchester, UK

Sue Read
Reader in Learning Disability Nursing, Keele University, Staffordshire, UK

Joan Regan
Consultant in Palliative Medicine, Marie Curie Hospice & Belfast NHS Trust, UK

Margaret Reith
Social Work Manager, The Princess Alice Hospice, Esher, UK

Karen Ryan
Consultant in Palliative Medicine, St Francis Hospice, Mater Misericordiae University Hospital and Connolly Hospital, Dublin, Ireland

Nigel Sage
Consultant Clinical Psychologist, The Beacon Community Cancer & Palliative Care Centre, Guildford, Surrey, UK

Libby Sallnow
Specialty Trainee in Medicine, Brighton and Sussex University Hospitals Trust, UK

Paula Scullin
Locum Consultant in Medical Oncology, Cancer Centre, Belfast City Hospital, Belfast, UK

Kathy Stephenson
Macmillan Palliative Care Community Liaison Pharmacist, Craigavon Area Hospital, Southern Health and Social Care Trust, N.Ireland, UK

Nigel Sykes
Medical Director and Consultant in Palliative Medicine, St Christopher's Hospice, London, UK

Keri Thomas
National Clinical Lead for the Gold Standards Framework Centre, Walsall PCT, UK, Hon Senior Lecturer, University of Birmingham, UK, and Chair Omega, the National Association for End of Life Care

Jo Venables
Consultant in Community Child Health, Abertawe Bro Morgannwg University Trust, Wales, UK

Barbara Wider
Research Fellow in Complementary Medicine, Peninsula Medical School, Universities of Exeter and Plymouth, Exeter, UK

Meg Williams
Specialist Registrar in Palliative Medicine, All Wales Higher Training Programme, Cardiff, UK

Abbreviations

ADLs	activities of daily living
AF	atrial fibrillation
AIDS	acquired immune deficiency syndrome
Amp.	ampoule
ARV	anti-retroviral
b.d.	twice daily
BNF	British National Formulary
BP	blood pressure
Caps	capsules
CD	controlled drug
CHF	congestive heart failure
CMV	cytomegalovirus
CNS	central nervous system
CO_2	carbon dioxide
COPD	chronic obstructive pulmonary disease
COX	cyclo-oxygenase
CSCI	continuous subcutaneous infusion
C/T	chemotherapy
CT	computed tomography
CTPA	computed tomography pulmonary arteriogram
CTZ	chemoreceptor trigger zone
CVA	cerebrovascular accident
DIC	disseminated intravascular coagulation
DN	district nurse
DVT	deep vein thrombosis
ECG	electrocardiogram
ECOG	Eastern Cooperative Oncology Group
EDDM	equivalent daily dose of morphine
FBC	full blood count
FEV_1	forced expiratory volume in one second
FNA	fine needle aspiration
g	gram
GERD	gastro-oesophageal reflux disease
GI	gastrointestinal
GMC	General Medical Council
GP	general practitioner
Gy	Gray(s): a measure of radiation

h	hour or hourly
HAART	highly active anti-retroviral therapy
HIV	human immunodeficiency virus
HNSCC	head and neck squamous-cell carcinoma
ICP	intracranial pressure
IM	intramuscular
Inj.	injection
i/r	immediate release
i/t	intrathecal
IV	intravenous
IVI	intravenous infusion
IVU	intravenous urogram
KS	Kaposi's sarcoma
kV	kilovolt
L	litre
L/A	local anaesthetic
LFT	liver function tests
LVF	left ventricular failure
MAI	Mycobacterium avium intracellulare
MAOI	monoamine oxidase inhibitor(s)
max.	maximum
MeV	mega electronvolt
mcg	microgram
MND	motor neurone disease
m/r	modified release
MRI	magnetic resonance imaging
MUPS	multiple unit pellet system
MV	megavolt
m/w	mouthwash
NaSSA	noradrenergic and specific serotoninergic antidepressant
neb	nebulizer
NG	nasogastric
NMDA	N-methyl-D-aspartate
nocte	at night
NSAID	non-steroidal anti-inflammatory drug
NSCLC	non small-cell lung carcinoma
NYHA	New York Heart Association
o.d.	once daily
o.m.	in the morning
OTFC	oral transmucosal fentanyl citrate
PCA	Patient controlled analgesia

PCF	Palliative Care Formulary
PCT	palliative care team
PE	pulmonary embolism
PEG	percutaneous endoscopic gastrostomy
PET	positron emission tomography
PHCT	primary healthcare team
p.o.	by mouth
PPI	proton pump inhibitor
p.r./PR	per rectum/progesterone receptor
p.r.n.	when required
PSA	prostate-specific antigen
PTH	parathyroid hormone
p.v.	per vaginam
PVS	persistent vegetative state
q.d.s.	four times daily
QoL	quality of life
RBL	renal bone liver (investigations)
RCT	randomized controlled trial
RIG	radiologically inserted gastrostomy
RT	radiotherapy
SALT	speech and language therapy
SC	subcutaneous
SCLC	small-cell lung carcinoma
S/D	syringe driver (CSCI)
SE	side-effects
SERMs	selective oestrogen-receptor modulators
SL	sublingual
soln	solution
SPC	specialist palliative care
SR	slow or modified release
SSRI	selective serotonin-reuptake inhibitor
Stat	immediately
Supps	suppositories
Susp.	suspension
SVC	superior vena cava
SVCO	superior vena cava obstruction
Tabs	tablets
TB	tuberculosis
TBM	tubercular meningitis
t.d.s.	three times daily
TENS	transcutaneous electrical nerve stimulation

Introduction

Palliative care definitions

Palliative care is an approach that improves the quality of life of patients and their families facing the problems associated with life-threatening illness, through the prevention and relief of suffering by means of early identification and impeccable assessment and treatment of pain and other problems, physical, psychological and spiritual.[1, 2]

Palliative care:
- Provides relief from pain and other distressing symptoms
- Affirms life and regards dying as a normal process
- Intends neither to hasten nor postpone death
- Integrates the psychological and spiritual aspects of patient care
- Offers a support system to help patients live as actively as possible until death
- Offers a support system to help the family cope during the patient's illness and in their own bereavement
- Uses a team approach to address the needs of patients and their families, including bereavement counselling, if indicated
- Will enhance quality of life, and may also positively influence the course of illness
- Is applicable early in the course of illness, in conjunction with other therapies that are intended to prolong life, such as chemotherapy or radiation therapy, and includes those investigations needed to better understand and manage distressing clinical complications

1 World Health Organization (1990) *Cancer Pain Relief and Palliative Care*. Geneva: WHO: 11 (World Health Organization technical report series: 804)

2 www.who.int/cancer/palliative/definitionen

Principles of palliative care

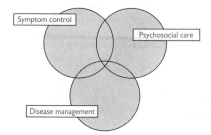

Symptom control

Psychosocial care

Disease management

No single sphere of concern is adequate without considering the relationship with the other two. This usually requires genuine interdisciplinary collaboration.[3]

General palliative care is provided by the usual professional carers of the patient and family with low to moderate complexity of palliative care need. Palliative care is a vital and integral part of their routine clinical practice which is underpinned by the following principles:

- Focus on quality of life, which includes good symptom control
- Whole person approach, taking into account the person's past life experience and current situation
- Care, which encompasses both the person with life-threatening illness and those who matter to the person
- Respect for patient autonomy and choice (e.g. over place of care, treatment options)
- Emphasis on open and sensitive communication, which extends to patients, informal carers and professional colleagues

Specialist palliative care

These services are provided for patients and their families with moderate to high complexity of palliative care need. The core service components are provided by a range of NHS, voluntary and independent providers staffed by a multidisciplinary team whose core work is palliative care.[2]

3 National Council for Hospice and Specialist Palliative Care Services (2002) *Definitions of Supportive and Palliative Care.* London: NCHSPCS (Briefing Bulletin 11)

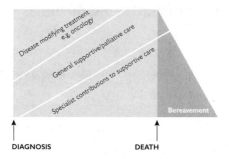

DIAGNOSIS   **DEATH**

Supportive care for cancer is that which helps the patient and their family to cope with the disease and its treatment—from pre-diagnosis, through the process of diagnosis and treatment, to cure, continuing illness or death and into bereavement. It helps the patient to maximize the benefits of treatment and to live as well as possible with the effects of the disease. It is given equal priority alongside diagnosis and treatment. This definition can be applied equally to non-cancer diagnoses.

The principles that underpin supportive and palliative care are broadly the same.

Hospice and hospice care refer to a philosophy of care rather than a specific building or service, and may encompass a programme of care and array of skills deliverable in a wide range of settings.

Terminal care or end-of-life care

This is an important part of palliative care and usually refers to the management of patients during their last few days, weeks or months of life from a point at which it becomes clear that the patient is in a progressive state of decline. However, end-of-life care may require consideration much nearer the beginning of the illness trajectory of many chronic, incurable non-cancer diseases.

History of palliative medicine as a specialty

The specialty of palliative medicine as a specific entity dates from the mid-1980s. However, medical activity related to terminal care, care of the dying, hospice care and end-stage cancer is, of course, as old as medical practice itself.[4] Palliative medicine is the medical component of what has become known as palliative care.

The history of the hospice movement during the nineteenth and twentieth centuries demonstrates the innovations of several charismatic leaders. These practitioners were enthusiasts for their own particular contribution to care of the dying, and they were also the teachers of the next generation of palliative physicians. Although they were products of their original background and training, they all shared the vision of regarding patients who happened to be dying as 'whole people'. They naturally brought their own approaches from specific disciplines of pharmacology, oncology, surgery, anaesthetics or general practice. This whole person attitude has been labelled as 'holistic care'. Comfort and freedom from pain and distress were of equal importance to diagnostic acumen and cure. However, rather than being a completely new philosophy of care, palliative medicine can be regarded more as a codification of existing practices from past generations.

Histories of the development of palliative medicine illustrate the thread of ideas from figures such as Snow, who developed the Brompton Cocktail in the 1890s, to Barrett who developed the regular giving of oral morphine to the dying at St Luke's, West London, to Saunders who expanded these ideas at St Joseph's and St Christopher's Hospices. Worcester, in Boston, was promoting the multidisciplinary care of whole patients in lectures to medical students at a time when intense disease specialization was very much the fashion as it was yielding great therapeutic advances.[5] Winner and Amulree, in the UK in the 1960s, were promoting whole person care particularly for the elderly, first challenging and then re-establishing the ethical basis for palliative medicine.

The early hospice movement was primarily concerned with the care of patients with cancer who, in the surge of post-war medical innovation, had missed out on the windfall of the new confident and increasingly optimistic medical world.

That this movement was responding to a need perceived across the world, has been evidenced by the exponential growth in palliative care services throughout the UK and across the globe since the opening of St Christopher's Hospice in south-east London in 1967.

---

4 Saunders C. (1993) Introduction—history and challenge. In *The Management of Terminal Malignant Disease* (3rd edn) (ed. C. Saunders, N. Sykes), pp. 1–14. London: Edward Arnold.

5 Worcester A. (1935) *The Care of the Aged, the Dying and the Dead.* London: Bailliere & Co.

The expansion is set to increase further, as the point has now been reached where patients, doctors and governments alike are calling for the same level of care to be made available to patients suffering from non-malignant conditions as for those with cancer.

If this new challenge is to be met, healthcare professionals from early in their training will need to be exposed to palliative care learning, which can be applied across the range of medical specialties.

The essence of such palliative medicine learning both for generalists and specialists remains that of clinical apprenticeship. Alfred Worcester, in the preface to his lectures, notes that:

> The younger members of the profession, although having enormously greater knowledge of the science of medicine, have less acquaintance than many of their elders with the art of medical practice. This like every other art can of course be learned only by imitation, that is, by practice under masters of the art. Primarily, it depends upon devotion to the patient rather than to his disease.[5]

Hope

A pessimist sees the difficulty

Winston Churchill

The ways in which hope is spoken about suggests that it is understood to be a fragile but dynamic state. For example, hope:
- Is intended—we hope in…or for…or of…or to…someone or something
- Is associated with longing, as in 'hopes and dreams'
- Is usually passive: hope is brought, given, revived, restored, inspired, provided, maintained, offered, injected, developed, pinned or lost; it can be kept alive or it can be crushed
- Can be hoped against
- Can be false, mistaken for wishfulness, optimism, desire or expectation
- Can be new, fresh, big, strong

Hope is closely linked with wants and desires. The phrase 'Freud had hoped to revisit Paris' says something about a future oriented desire Freud nurtured when he left Vienna en route to London. The phrase implies an expectation that the desired thing might be achieved. This expectation may itself be realistic or unrealistic, but assessment of what might or might not be realistic depends on one's perception of reality.

Because hope is future orientated, the question posed by terminal illness may become: 'What hope can there be if death is this patient's only and impending future?'

Hope has long been associated with belief.

> Now faith is being sure of what we hope for and certain of what we do not see.
>
> The New Testament, Hebrews 11:1

Hope nurtures within it the belief that that which is hoped for has the potential to be realized: a trip to Paris. The dilemma for healthcare professionals is: How can I work with a terminally ill patient in a way that avoids collusion and yet sustains hope? Addressing this question locates healthcare professionals firmly on the terrain of psychospiritual care.

> Hope is a dynamic inner power that enables transcendence of the present situation and fosters a positive new awareness of being.[6]

But part of the difficulty in answering this question is in understanding:
- *What* hope is
- *How* it differs from wishfulness, and
- *Why* it can remain hope even when if it sounds like despair

The development of hope: Rumbold's three orders

Building on a psychiatric description of the defences deployed by patients to shield themselves from the knowledge of imminent death, Rumbold (1986) describes hope developing through 'three orders'.[7]

First order: Denial of symptoms → Hope for recovery
Diagnosis of a terminal illness is often met with denial. Symptoms are ignored or interpreted as something other than what they are said to be. Denial serves to protect the person from the reality of their condition, but it also prevents them from accepting treatment. However, as symptoms progress the fantasy sustaining denial breaks down, and acceptance generates hope, that either recovery may be possible, or that at least death may be long delayed. Rumbold suggests hope may emerge:
- From a straightforward transition from admitting the reality of their illness to affirming a hope for recovery; or
- From a period of despair following the breakdown of denial.

(The transition is delicate, and admitting illness may actually plunge patients into a despair and resignation from which they do not emerge.)

Second order: Denial of non-recovery → Hope beyond recovery
Hope for recovery, paradoxically, supports a higher level of denial, which is actively supported by medical staff and by family and friends. Whereas denial of symptoms keeps the person from becoming a patient, the denial of possibilities other than recovery 'gives medical access to the symptoms while suppressing fear of death and the difficult questions which attend that fear'.

---

6 Herth K. (1993) Hope in the family caregiver of terminally ill people. *Journal of Advanced Nursing*, **18**: 538–48.

7 Rumbold B. D. (1986) *Helplessness & Hope: Pastoral Care in Terminal Illness*, pp. 59–75. London: SCM Press

Yet, for hope to continue developing and become hope beyond mere insistence on recovery, patients need to face and explore the possibilities for dying. The social support that once buoyed hope of recovery now works against patients contemplating dying as part of their hope. And lack of support at this point can mean that the acceptance emerging in the patient as this denial breaks down results in resignation and despair; 'for the withdrawal of community is particularly destructive of hope.'

The breakdown of this denial of non-recovery is a critical transition: 'If all our hope has been invested in recovery, then that hope may virtually be destroyed by the new perception of second-order acceptance.'

Hope beyond recovery is a more varied hope than the single-minded hope for recovery, the patient may simply hope:

- To die with dignity;
- For the continuing success of children;
- That a partner will find the support they need;
- That their life's contribution will continue and be found useful.

Most terminally-ill people do seem to reach this second stage where such a hope becomes possible; but those who can find a meaningful hope which they are allowed to affirm are distressingly few.

Bruce Rumbold, 1986

Development of hope in terminal illness

third-order
hope that faces existential extinction

Denial	breakdown of denial	acceptance	hope
refuses to contemplate the possibility of extinction in death	leads on to crucial question of meaning	choosing a stance concerning the ultimate meaning of life	affirms stance; supported and validated by memory not denial examines all possibilities, chooses what will be hoped for

second-order
denial of non-recovery → hope beyond recovery

denial	breakdown of denial	acceptance	hope
excludes possibilities other than recovery; gives medical access to symptoms; generally encouraged; supported by hospitals; suppresses fear of death	critical transition: patient open to possibilities inherent in dying; but if those around the patient unable to accept patient's wishes as a legitimate hope patient may be unable to explore and appropriate possibilities for dying as part of hope	coming to accept that illness may be terminal; withdrawal of community is destructive of hope	patient needs to hope going beyond mere insistence on recovery; patient may realistically choose hope for death above life at any price

second-order acceptance emerging from breakdown commonly issues in resignation and despair

first-order
denial of symptoms → hope for recovery

denial	breakdown of denial	acceptance	hope
people often deny early symptoms of their illness; denial is confronted by experience; keeps the person from becoming a patient	denial only maintained by retreating into phantasy	recognition of symptoms and of need for help	for recovery

(Based on Rumbold, 1986[7])

Third order: Hope that faces existential extinction

Hope beyond recovery has the capacity for yet further development:

- Hope for recovery (which supported denial of the terminal reality of their illness) develops into the higher level hope beyond recovery;
- Hope beyond recovery (which realistically accepts death 'rather than crave life at any price') may develop into a higher level yet of hope that accepts the existential possibility of extinction at death, but nevertheless finds a sense of ultimate meaning in the life that has been lived.

Such hope may hold to a belief in a life after death, but recognizes this belief as a contingency of faith.

Prior to her first hospice admission, Elaine had been very angry about her illness (second-order denial). Her realization that she didn't want to die angry broke down her denial, opening new possibilities to her.

Elaine: *I was angry...very angry—angry at the world; and that's not me. I'm not like that. I'm usually very calm. That's not the way I want to be. I think that's a quite natural reaction, but I don't want to be angry; I don't want to die angry...actually, I feel as if I'm moving on from that now. I feel as if I'm moving into trying to make sense of what is ahead.*

By allowing her to say and think what she needed to, those around Elaine supported her to explore the possibilities for her dying. When she returned for terminal care she was in a different place spiritually.

Elaine: *It's that the anger has gone. I've worked through a lot of stuff while I was at home. We talked about a lot of things. This is the way it is going to be and there's no use fighting it. We'd rather things were going to be different, but they're not. There's no point in being angry; it takes up so much energy. I know I'm going to be on a gradual, slow decline now, so I have to get on with it. My body is getting weaker, but I feel emotionally stronger. I hope I will.*

Hope and the psychospiritual value of denial

When healthcare professionals deny the legitimacy of patients' hopes, they are likely to be expressing their own fears about death and dying.

- Healthcare professionals need to validate patients' exploration to allow patients the possibilities of their dying.
- Patients should not be pressured to confront their denying—denial should be respected as a legitimate psychological defence strategy.
- Health carers should not think that challenging denial will help patients to explore their dying—only the patient can determine the right time to open to their dying.

To attempt to steal 'denial' from another is an act of righteousness and separatism.[8]

8 Levine S. (1986) *Who Dies? An Investigation of Conscious Living and Conscious Dying.* Dublin: Gateway.

Dignity

'Dignity' as defined by the *Oxford English Dictionary* is 'the state of being worthy of honour or respect' or 'high regard or estimation'. The 1984 Universal Declaration of Human Rights and Article 1 of the Charter of Fundamental Rights of the European Union recognize dignity as a human right. The Department of Health in England launched a policy in 2007 to 'create a zero tolerance of lack of dignity in the care of older people in any setting'. Upholding the dignity of patients within a palliative care setting is essential not only for the patient him/herself but also for the family, particularly in their bereavement.

Patients approaching the end of life fluctuate in their will to live, a situation closely associated with dignity. The meaning and experience of human dignity relates to:

- The presence of symptoms
- Loss of independence
- Fear of becoming a burden
- Not being involved in decision-making
- Lack of access to care
- Lack of adequate communication between patients, families and professionals
- Some attitudes of staff
- Spiritual matters, especially when people feel vulnerable

Patients with a terminal illness become vulnerable to a loss of dignity if they begin to feel that they are no longer respected and the person that they once were. As they become increasingly dependent patients often feel that professionals no longer see them as an individual, which can compound a sense of loss of self. Patients may suffer the ultimate indignity of feeling that their life has no worth, meaning or purpose.

A core framework of dignity conserving care has been developed by Chochinov,[9] with the aim of reminding practitioners about the importance of caring for, as well as caring about, their patients. The mnemonic ABCD stands for Attitude, Behaviour, Compassion and Dialogue.

Attitude

Professionals need to be respectful in their attitudes towards patients, acknowledging the patient as an individual with cognisance of many issues including culture and ethics. Professionals unwittingly make incorrect assumptions: seeing a patient who has difficulty in communicating does not mean that he/she is not competent to have an opinion about his/her care. The attitude of the professionals to a patient plays a large part in determining the patient's ongoing sense of worth, a factor which is often underestimated.

9 Chochinov H. (2007) Dignity and the essence of medicine: the A,B,C, and D of dignity conserving care. *British Medical Journal*, **335**: 184–7.

Behaviour

An awareness of one's attitude may lead to a more positive behaviour towards patients. Small acts of kindness and respect boost a patient's sense of worth. Taking a little time to explain to patients what is happening dispels fear. Practising open and honest communication and giving patients full attention allows them to develop trust, thereby enabling more personal and appropriate care.

Compassion

Compassion refers to a deep awareness of the suffering of another coupled with the wish to relieve it. Compassion is felt beyond simply intellectual appreciation. Compassion may be inherent in the healthcare provider and hopefully develops over time with both professional and life experience. Demonstrating compassion does not need to take time and can be both verbal and non-verbal.

Dialogue

Healthcare professionals speak to patients about their illness but may fail to touch on the issues that are most important to the patient, such as the emotional impact of the illness and the importance of being recognised as an individual and not another sick person. Healthcare decisions need to be taken considering not only the medical facts but also the life context of the patient. Psychotherapeutic approaches, such as life review or reminiscence, can be used to support patients to regain or retain a sense of meaning, purpose and dignity.

These four facets compromise a framework for upholding, protecting and restoring dignity which embraces the very essence of medicine.

Further reading

Charon R. (2001) Narrative medicine: a model for empathy, reflection, profession and trust. *Journal of the American Medical Association*, **286**: 1897–1902.

Chochinov H. (2006) Dying, dignity and new horizons in palliative end-of-life care. *CA: A Cancer Journal for Clinicians*, **56**: 84–103.

Downman TH (2008) Hope and hopelessness: theory and reality. *Journal Royal Society Medicine*, **101**: 428–430

Higginson I. (2007) Rediscovering dignity at the bedside. *British Medical Journal*, **335**: 167–8.

Resilience

Hercules himself must yield

3 Henry VI (2.1.54–6)

Strengths exist in everyone. Any strength is a pathway to resilience. Even people facing the end of their lives or bereavement can be resilient. The concept of resilience is an approach, philosophy or mind-set which is consistent with the holistic model in palliative care.

Resilience is the ability to thrive in the face of adversity and stress. 'The capacity to withstand exceptional stress and demands without developing stress-related problems'.[10] People demonstrate resilience when they cope with, adjust to or overcome adversities in ways that promote their functioning. It is a process that allows for some kind of psychological, social, cultural and spiritual development despite demanding circumstances. It is, therefore, important that those involved in delivering palliative care appreciate the nature of resilience and how to enhance it. We should promote methods of enhancing and supporting coping mechanisms with the same vigour applied to assessing risk and defining problems.

Resilience has been described as a 'universal capacity which allows a person, group or community to prevent, minimise or overcome damaging effects of adversity'.[11] It is not just about re-forming but about the possibility of growth. The concept of resilience is important to the future delivery of end-of-life care and the significant challenges it faces. It offers a unifying concept to both retain and sustain some of the most significant understandings of the last four decades of palliative care and to incorporate more effective investment in a community approach and a public health focus, in addition to the direct care of patients and families. This integration is vital if we are to resolve the ever-increasing tension between the rhetoric of choice and equity coupled with the demands of rising healthcare expectations in ageing populations, and the inevitably limited availability of informal and professional carers and financial resources.[12]

'The capacity of an individual person or a social system to grow or to develop in the face of very difficult circumstances'.[13] Resilience can be promoted at different levels in:

• Individuals
• Families and carers
• Groups
• Communities
• Staff, teams and organizations

Each of these components has strengths and resources that can be encouraged and reinforced. It is important to remember that resilience is a dynamic process, not a static state or a quality that people do or do not possess. It can change over time and is a combination of internal and external characteristics in the individual and their social, cultural and physical environment.

10 Carr A. (2004) *Positive Psychology. The Science of Happiness and Human Strengths*, p. 300. London: Routledge.

11 Newman T. (2004) *What Works in Building Resilience*. Ilford: Barnardo's.

12 Monroe B., Oliviere D. (2007) *Resilience in Palliative Care. Achievement in Adversity*. Oxford: Oxford University Press.

13 Vanistendael S. (2002) *Resilience and Spirituality*, p. 10. Geneva: BICE.

Everyone needs opportunities to develop coping skills and it is important that individuals are not excessively sheltered from the situations that provide such challenges. Some of the characteristics of resilience that health professionals can recognize and use to encourage it include:

- Secure attachments
- Self-esteem
- Belief in one's own self-efficacy
- Realistic hope, whether or not mediated by faith
- Use of 'healthy' defence mechanisms including humour and denial
- Capacity to recognize achievements in the present
- Ability to find positive meaning in stressors
- Good memories
- Community support
- One supportive person

Even the existence of just one of these features can promote resilience and growth.

Various interventions and tools can promote the process of resilience in clinical practice:

Intervention	Resilience and growth
Accurate and timely information	knowledge is power and can promote control
Use of stories and narratives, e.g. life review	assists the integration and surmounting of difficult events
Brief, short-term, focused interventions	maximize opportunities for change and boost confidence
Cognitive restructuring, e.g. cognitive behavioural therapy	develops coping and self-confidence
Creative activities	provide opportunities for expression of thoughts and emotions, affirmation and opportunities to learn new skills
Family systems' approach	harnesses the potential of those involved to find their own solutions
User involvement	invites users and carers to give back and to leave a legacy of better services
Self-help groups	promote mutual exchange and peer support, reducing isolation
Public education and social marketing	share some of the lessons with users, carers and the public, including children, remembering that the values and attitudes of society affect the ways in which people cope with loss
Empowered communities	engage with communities to minimize harm and maximize care, potentiating social capital so that communities themselves respond sensitively and supportively to the dying and bereaved
Robust management/organizations	provide structure for empowered staff to achieve objectives

Prognostication in end-of-life care

The natural history of disease has been documented over many years. This has become increasingly less relevant as successful therapies have developed. In present day palliative care, prognosis frequently relates to chronic progressive disease in patients with multiple co-morbidities, and not to the recovery prediction of a young adult with an acute illness, as was more common in the nineteenth century.

The reasons for making an attempt at predicting how long a patient with incurable disease might live include:

- Providing information about the future to patients and families so that they can set goals, priorities and expectations of care
- Helping patients develop insight into their dying
- Assisting clinicians in decision-making
- Comparing like patients with regard to outcomes
- Establishing the patient's eligibility for care programmes (e.g. hospice) and for recruitment to research trials
- Policy-making regarding appropriate use and allocation of resources and support services
- Providing a common language for healthcare professionals involved in end-of-life care

Prognostic factors in cancer

There is a good literature on the probability of cure for the different cancers.

- Although individual cancers behave differently, as a generalization, predictions relate to tumour size, grade and stage
- Other factors include hormonal status (for hormone-dependent tumours such as cancer of the breast and prostate)
- Age
- Biochemical or other tumour markers
- The length of time taken for the disease to recur.

In palliative care such prognostic indices may not be so relevant.

Factors such as physical dependency (due to e.g. weakness, low blood pressure), cognitive dysfunction, paraneoplastic phenomena (e.g. anorexia–cachexia, cytokine production), certain symptoms (weight loss, anorexia, dysphagia, breathlessness), lymphopenia, poor quality of life and existential factors (either 'giving up' or 'hanging on' for symbolically important times) may be more important.

Some patients may survive for a long time (months and years) with a seemingly high tumour load, while others succumb within a short time (days) for no obviously identifiable reasons.

Several scores have been developed to aid prediction of survival. The Palliative Prognostic (PaP) score is predictive of short-term survival and summarizes scores for dyspnoea, anorexia, Karnovsky performance status, the clinician's estimate of survival (in weeks), total white count and percentage of lymphocytes.

Oncologists rely on prognostic assessments in order to predict which patients are likely to benefit from oncological interventions. Many of their decisions are based on the patient's functional status.

Patients with an ECOG score greater than two are usually deemed unsuitable for most chemotherapy interventions.

Eastern Co-operative Oncology Group (ECOG) Oken MM et al (1982)
Toxicity and response criteria of the Eastern Cooperate Oncology Group.
Am J Clin Oncol **5: 649–655**

ECOG	Grade
Fully active; able to carry on all activities without restriction	0
Restricted in physically strenuous activity but ambulatory and able to carry out work of a light or sedentary nature	1
Ambulatory and capable of all self-care but unable to carry out any work activities. Up and about more than 50% of walking hours	2
Capable of only limited self-care; confined to bed or chair 50% or more of waking hours	3
Completely disabled; cannot carry on any self-care; totally confined to bed or chair	4
Dead	5

Prognostic factors in non-malignant disease

Predicting prognosis in patients with a non-cancer diagnosis is very diffi-cult. These patients often remain relatively stable, albeit at a low level, only to deteriorate acutely and unpredictably. They are usually then treated acutely in hospital, and the disease course may consist of acute exacerba-tions from which recovery may take place.

One study showed that even during the last 2–3 days of life patients with congestive heart failure (CHF) or COPD were given an 80% and 50% chance, respectively, of living six months.

There are, however, general and specific indicators of the terminal stage approaching.

General predictors

Those predicting poorer prognosis include reduced performance status, impaired nutritional status (greater than 10% weight loss over six months) and a low albumin.

Specific predictors

Congestive heart failure (CHF)

- More than 64 years old
- Left ventricular ejection fraction less than 20%
- Dilated cardiomyopathy
- Uncontrolled arrhythmias
- Systolic hypotension
- CXR signs of left heart failure
- A prognosis of less than six months is associated with NYHA Class IV (chest pain and/or breathless at rest/minimal exertion) and already optimally treated with diuretics and vasodilators

Chronic obstructive pulmonary disease (COPD)

- Advanced age
- FEV_1 less than 30% of predicted

- Pulmonary hypertension with cor pulmonale/right heart failure
- Short of breath at rest
- On 24-hour home O_2 with pO_2 less than 50mmHg (6.7kPa) and/or pCO_2 more than 55mmHg (7.3kPa) and documented evidence of cor pulmonale

Cortical dementias (Alzheimer's disease)
- Functional status—the onset of being unable to walk unaided
- Unable to swallow
- Unable to hold a meaningful conversation
- Increasing frequency of medical complications, e.g. aspiration pneumonia, urinary tract infections, decubitus ulcers

Stroke
- Impaired consciousness
- Lack of improvement within three months of onset
- Age
- Incontinence
- Cognitive impairment
- Dense paralysis

Communicating prognosis

Prognostication is a notoriously difficult task to perform accurately. The world abounds with stories of patients who have been told by their physicians that they have only a matter of months to live who twenty years later can recount in vivid detail the day they were given the news.

One of the reasons that prognostication is so difficult is that it is fraught with uncertainty and also with opportunities for misunderstandings between doctors and patients, who often have very different agendas as to what they want to get out of the interview.

> Mr. Jones listened carefully as the consultant went into great detail about the nature and the extensive spread of his metastatic prostate tumour. The explanations were detailed and scientific and long. Eventually the consultant stopped. 'Now Mr. Jones, do you have any more questions?'
> 'Well, I didn't like to interrupt you but I was only asking how long I had before I needed to go down to get my X-ray.'

Over the past 20 years there has been a huge shift in attitudes regarding disclosure of information to patients, and a culture of complete disclosure has now become the norm. Yet prognostication does not just involve passing on clinical details and predictions of disease progression; it also involves assessing:
- What does the patient actually want to know? (Giving too much information to a patient who does not want to have the exact details spelt out is as unprofessional as the patronizing attitudes of 'best not to trouble the patient'.)
- How is the patient dealing with the information that is being given?
- How can the patient be helped to deal with the implications of the news?

To pass on facts without regard for the implications of those facts is to increase the risk of dysfunctional communication taking place. (📖 see Chapter 2.)

Risk and chance

While doctors are used to describing risk in terms of percentages, when such percentages are measuring out your own longevity it is hard to translate the mathematical chances into personal experience.

A doctor may feel that he has provided the patient with the clear facts when he states that in 100 patients with the particular malignancy, 36 will be alive after five years following treatment. Such sentences can be easily misunderstood, and the patient may hear something very different from what the doctor is saying.

Professional discomfort

Doctors are also particularly vulnerable to miscommunication at the time of passing on prognostic information.

- Society in the West is now death-denying, and if the prognosis is poor it can be uncomfortable for the doctor to pass on the information and confront the patient with their imminent death
- There is increasing fear of litigation, particularly if disease is not responsive to treatment, and any admission of failure may come across as an admission of guilt
- Doctors may feel uncomfortable in dealing with the emotional impact that their news may have on the patient, and develop techniques to protect themselves from this discomfort

Prognostic information can be extremely important to patients as it allows them to focus on tasks and goals which they want to achieve before their disease takes over: communicating such information effectively is a skill which all healthcare professionals should covet.

Further reading

Gold Standards Framework/RCGP (2006) *Prognostic Indicator Guidance.*

Ethical issues

- Respect for autonomy (self-determination)
- Beneficence (do good)
- Non-maleficence (do no harm)
- Justice (fairness)

The exploration of ethical issues that arise at the end of life is inherent to the work of palliative care. This is because the process of dying and death raises profound ethical questions about the meaning and value of human life. These questions are negotiated every day by the individuals who are dying, by their loved ones and by those who are caring for them. With good communication and trust in the patient/professional relationship, patients' attitudes and concerns can be discussed sensitively, confusion unravelled and fears dispelled. For example, in practice, when some patients ask for euthanasia there may be areas of 'unfinished business', fear, guilt or other issues that need to be explored. After sensitive and open communication, most patients feel a sense of relief and their need to press for a deliberate ending of their life diminishes.

We live in a world which has become increasingly complex. Ethical issues that arise towards the end of life are often fraught with difficulty in an increasingly technological age in which the process of dying may be prolonged. In many healthcare situations, it is often difficult, sometimes impossible, to be certain about what is the right thing to do; at best we try to reach a consensus that is based on sound and sensitive ethical reasoning and evidence. The most widely used ethical framework in healthcare decision-making in the West obliges health professionals to respect four basic principles:

- **Autonomy** (respect patients' values and inform and involve them in decision-making)
- **Beneficence** (do good)
- **Non-maleficence** (do no harm)
- **Justice** (treat patients fairly and balance the needs of individuals with those of society)

In the abstract, these principles can seem straightforward; in the heat of a clinical situation their application can be anything but clear. It is, however, very useful to have a framework with which to deal with ethical crises.

The following clinical scenarios are examples which occur commonly. Applying the principles of ethics in order to reach a balanced compromise can help provide a path through uncertainty.

Example 1: 'My father is not drinking adequately. Why are you not giving him extra fluids?'

Ethical issues

- **Beneficence**: Will artificial fluids help the patient?
- **Non-maleficence**: Will giving or not giving artificial fluids cause the patient harm?
- **Autonomy**: Does the patient want a drip?

It is instilled in all of us, from childhood years onwards, that food and drink are essential for life. There are clinical situations in palliative care when extra systemic fluids might be useful, for instance in hypercalcaemia or profuse diarrhoea and vomiting. These may be salvageable clinical situations where we are expecting the patient to return to his 'normal', albeit generally deteriorating, state of health.

Artificial hydration

- A blanket policy of artificial hydration, or of no artificial hydration, is ethically indefensible
- If dehydration is thought to be due to a potentially correctable cause, the option of artificial hydration should be considered
- The appropriateness of artificial hydration should be weighed up in terms of harm and benefit on a day-to-day basis

When someone is considered to be dying irreversibly, however, the routine of giving systemic fluids may not be in the patient's best interests.

Background information

A few studies address this issue, but there is no proof that either the giving or withholding of fluids interferes with the length of remaining life or affects comfort.

- Biochemical parameters show that only 50% of patients have any evidence of dehydration within the final 48h of life and, even then, only in mild to moderate degree
- There is no evidence that thirst or dry mouth (particularly) improve with artificial hydration
- The extensive experience of nurses working in hospices suggests that systemic fluids, at best, make no difference and, at worst, may actually contribute to suffering at the end of life
- The more fluid available, the more likely it is that it will gather in the lungs and dependent parts of the body, particularly in the presence of hypoalbuminaemia, which is common in advanced malignancy
- Artificially increasing fluids at the end of life, when the body physiology is winding down, may lead to worsening respiratory secretions, increased vomiting, increase in volume of ascites, raised intracranial pressure in the presence of intracerebral disease and an uncomfortable urinary output

EXAMPLE 1   3

- Families can spend precious time worrying about intravenous infusions running out or plastic cannulae being displaced and causing discomfort, instead of concentrating on quality time with the patient.

Discussion

Withholding systemic fluids is inevitably a very emotive issue signifying finally and clearly, perhaps for the first time to the family, that their loved one is now entering the final stage of his/her life. In practice, patients are often able to take small amounts of fluids until shortly before death. It should be explained to families that the body is gradually shutting down and is unable to handle an extra fluid load. They need to be aware that the patient will not be allowed to suffer from pain or other discomfort and they will need explanations of the measures that will be taken to avoid discomfort. These will include medication where necessary and, most importantly, meticulous mouthcare to prevent the common symptom of a dry mouth.

Palliative care is neither about shortening life nor prolonging the dying period.

Occasionally, families cannot bring themselves to accept the inevitability of death and insist on artificial hydration. Although healthcare professionals must act only in the best interests of the patient, it would be unwise to ignore the views of the family, who have to go on surviving with vivid memories of the dying phase. On occasion, if it is felt that extra fluids will not adversely affect comfort, it is sometimes helpful to have a contract with the family for a relatively small volume of fluid to be used subcutaneously or intravenously for a defined short period, on the understanding that it would be discontinued at any time if it was thought to be causing the patient distress.

As in most ethical crises, a balance has to be made—in this situation, between the harm caused by withholding or giving artificial hydration:

- Acknowledge family distress
- Explore concerns
- Discuss the above points
- Reassure the family that the patient will be looked after and kept comfortable whether or not fluids are given artificially

Example 2: 'How long have I got left?'

Ethical issue

- **Autonomy**: Is every attempt being made to inform the patient adequately?

This type of question usually relates to prognosis. As ever, however, it is always important to make sure that the question has been entirely understood, since to enter into a conversation about how long a patient has to live when all they want to know is when they are leaving hospital can cause unnecessary distress.[1]

When it is certain that the patient is talking about prognosis, first find out what they already know, how they see the situation, why they are asking the question and how much they really want to know.

The following questions can be useful:
- 'What have the doctors told you so far?'
- 'What has prompted you to ask this question now?'
- 'How do you see the situation?'
- 'Are there other specific issues, related to how long there is left, on your mind that you would like to talk about?'
- 'Are you the kind of person who likes to know everything?'

In practice, patients often say they have not been told anything by the doctors: this may be true, or they may have inadvertently used denial mechanisms to 'forget' the bad news. The patient may also deny knowledge in an attempt to find out more information. It is important to explore what they understand accurately thus far. Patients often want to achieve goals such as writing a will, attending a family wedding, reaching a wedding anniversary, being reunited with old friends and family who they have not seen for a long time or seeing their religious adviser. Some patients like to consider writing a formal Advance Directive or 'living will', which should give a more formative, clearly defined record of their wishes in order to facilitate more informed decision-making. Patients may not find it easy to discuss these issues, even with close family members, and may need help to facilitate discussions. They may need help in setting realistic and achievable goals while planning their limited future.

1 Launer J. (2005) Breaking the news. *Quarterly Journal of Medicine*, **98**: 385–6.

EXAMPLE 2   5

Before addressing prognosis directly, it is important to be aware of the full medical history and to build up a picture of the pace of clinical deterioration. Comments such as 'I believe you have not been feeling so well recently' or 'the doctors/your medical notes tell me that you feel that life has become more difficult over the past few weeks' open up these issues, giving you and the patient a chance to estimate prognosis. Remember that studies show that health professionals tend to overestimate prognosis.

> Centuries of systematic insensitive deception cannot be instantly remedied by a new routine of systematic insensitive truth telling.
>
> Buckman

Background

Literature on determining prognosis is available, especially for patients with cancer. For a population presenting with a defined stage, grade, cancer type and histology, five-year survival rates are available and often quoted to families. Many other factors have been studied singly and in combination in an attempt to categorize patients into prognostic groups, and this can be helpful in broad terms. In practice, however, it is not possible to predict prognosis for an individual accurately, because there are so many different influencing factors—including psychosocial, emotional and existential issues—all of which defy measurement of any kind.

- Make sure that you are answering what the patient wants to know
- Stress that you are not evading the question but that it is difficult to answer
- Find out specific issues that should be addressed, e.g. weddings, wills, etc.
- Do not be specific, but use days/weeks or weeks/months, etc.

Despite all these pitfalls, it is still important to answer the patient's question. It is still relatively common for a precise prognosis, for example 'six months', to be given and this is invariably inaccurate. If the patient dies before the due date, the family feel cheated of time that they would otherwise have spent differently had they known that time was so short. If the patient survives longer than the due date, both patient and family may feel proud that they have defeated the odds and take comfort from this; on the other hand, if the family have altered their lifestyles including giving up work (and salary) to look after a patient who has not significantly deteriorated by the due date, family tensions inevitably build up alongside all the normal feelings of guilt and anger.

It is not helpful to give a precise date, which patients and families often take literally, but to talk in terms of days/weeks, weeks/months and months/years. It is also important to say that even within these broad terms we may still be inaccurate.

It is also useful to talk about the pace of deterioration and to say that the pace may continue at the same rate but it may also either stabilize for a while or accelerate.

Example 3: 'Don't tell my mother the diagnosis. I know her better than you.'

Ethical issues

- **Autonomy**: Does this patient not need to be told regardless of what the family think?
- **Beneficence**: Would it help this patient to know her diagnosis?
- **Non-maleficence**: Would it harm this patient to know her diagnosis?

It is common to be caught in the hospital or health practice corridor by anxious relatives who (possibly wrongly) have been told that their relative has cancer, before this information has been given to the patient. There is increasing evidence that patients want to know what is wrong with them and to be involved in decisions. Generally speaking, we have moved away from a paternalistic approach in truth-telling whereby doctors often avoided telling patients they had cancer, to a more open approach, respecting the principle of autonomy.

However, family members have known the patient over many years and are aware of how he/she has responded to bad news in the past. They may feel that there is no point in discussing the diagnosis, particularly if the patient is very elderly and there is no available treatment.

- For understandable reasons the family want to protect the patient from bad news, but very often they want to protect themselves from further hurt and the reality that the patient may now be entering the last stages of life
- It needs to be acknowledged with the family that this is a difficult area but that the patient may have important things to say or do (financial, wills, gifts, etc.) or opinions to voice (regarding both medical and after-death decisions)
- The family also need to know that patients pick up non-verbal clues from professionals and relatives; they are often aware of the diagnosis and are not unduly surprised if it is confirmed
- Patients often want to protect the family, by denying that they know anything
- The family need to be aware that patients are often comforted by a 'label' to their illness, even if it is cancer, because it explains why they have been feeling so unwell. This gives them a genuine reason for feeling so wretched
- Families need to know that it becomes more difficult to conceal the truth from the patient as time goes on and as more professionals, family members and friends share the secret. There are increasing opportunities for the truth to slip out and for the patient to lose trust in and be angry with the family for not having been more honest in the first place
- Families also need to know that patients are not always frightened of death but of the process leading up to it, over which they may want some control
- It is very important not to lie to the patient as this breaks all communication, confidence and trust

EXAMPLE 3   7

- Acknowledge family anxiety
- Inform family of the issues as above
- Stress that it is important for neither professionals nor family to lie if the patient starts asking direct questions

If there are no particular decisions to be made, the patient has dealt with his or her affairs and is living with the family, there may be no pressing need to try to discuss the issue and invite family disquiet. However, if the patient begins to ask direct questions, the family should be advised not to lie. The family also needs to be aware that family tensions reduce considerably when there are open discussions about diagnosis.

The professional is able to override family views if it is clearly in the interests of the patient to do so, but it is also always advisable and prudent to listen to and take account of the views of the family. If it is felt important to discuss the diagnosis with the patient, it is usually acceptable to families to say that we will try to find out what the patient understands by their illness and whether or not they would like more information.

Example 4: 'I want full resuscitation if my heart or lungs fail.'[2]

Ethical issues

- **Autonomy**: Does the patient have the right to demand treatments from nursing and medical staff?
- **Beneficence**: Would it be in the patient's best interests to initiate resuscitation?
- **Non-maleficence**: Would it do the patient any harm to initiate resuscitation?
- **Justice**: Would it be an appropriate use of resources to initiate resuscitation measures and allocate a bed in an intensive care unit

Background

Patients and families are increasingly aware of the many ethical issues surrounding cardiopulmonary resuscitation. These have been highlighted recently with 'DNR' (Do Not Resuscitate) notices being recorded in patients' notes without the patients being aware that they had been thus assigned. This has caused much concern, particularly among the weakest and most vulnerable sections of the community.

The issues have caused marked unease within hospices where, until very recently, resuscitation was regarded as an unacceptable practice. Patients with non-malignant disease and patients with cancer in the early stages, who may have a less predictable and possibly more favourable prognosis however, are increasingly requiring specialist palliative care. Such patients may feel very strongly that, in the event of a sudden cardiac or respiratory collapse, they want full resuscitation.

Litigation anxiety can cause a dilemma and increase the strain on staff to make the right decision. The need to document the resuscitation status of patients, following full discussion, can of itself lead to increased anxiety for all involved in handling what can be a very distressing issue.

- Patients have the right to ask for whatever treatment they choose. Medical and nursing staff are not obliged to comply with such expressed wishes if:
  - they feel it would not be in the patient's best interests
  - the intervention is deemed to be futile

2 Willard C. (2000) Cardiopulmonary resuscitation for palliative care patients: a discussion of ethical issues. *Palliative Medicine*, **14**: 308–12.

EXAMPLE 4   9

Good practice would dictate that such matters are addressed by the whole multiprofessional team, although the senior doctor has ultimate responsibility for the decision.[3]

Approximate achievement of success from CPR in any setting:

In hospital	15%
In community	5%
In hospices	1%

A king, a doctor, and a convenient death

Lord Dawson of Penn was the most admired and respected doctor of his generation. The skill with which he managed King George V's respiratory illness in 1928 undoubtedly saved the King's life and made Dawson a national celebrity. He was also respected within the medical profession. He was president of the Royal College of Physicians, elected twice president of the BMA, and honoured with a viscountcy.

His reputation would have been considerably diminished, however, had it been known that when the King was suffering from cardiorespiratory failure in January 1936 he administered a lethal combination of morphine and cocaine at a time when the King was already comatose and close to death. His action remained a well kept secret and the truth came to light only 50 years later when his private diary was opened, Dawson having died in 1945.

The King had been in failing health for several weeks when Queen Mary summoned Dawson to Sandringham on 17 January. Contemporary accounts of the King's last days given by the Archbishop of Canterbury and others tell of days that were tranquil and pain free with the King sitting in an armchair before a log fire for much of the time but becoming steadily weaker and with consciousness gradually slipping away.

At 9:25 pm on 20 January Dawson issued the memorable bulletin stating that the King's life was moving peacefully towards its close. The action which he took one and a half hours later is described in his diary thus:

'At about 11 o'clock it was evident that the last stage might endure for many hours, unknown to the patient but little comporting with the dignity and serenity which he so richly merited and which demanded a brief final scene. Hours of waiting just for the mechanical end when all that is really life has departed only exhausts the onlookers and keeps them so strained that they cannot avail themselves of the solace of

3 National Council for Palliative Care. (2002) *Ethical Decision-Making in Palliative Care. Cardiopulmonary Resuscitation (CPR) for people who are terminally ill.* London: NCPC. See also: Decisions Relating to Cardiopulmonary Resuscitation: a joint statement from the British Medical Association, the Resuscitation Council (UK) and the Royal College of Nursing (2001). *Journal of Medical Ethics*, **27**: 310–16.

thought, communion or prayer. I therefore decided to determine the end and injected (myself) morphia gr.3/4 and shortly afterwards cocaine gr. 1 into the distended jugular vein.'

Dawson did not consult the other two doctors in the case, and his diary indicated that he was acting entirely on his own. To her credit, Sister Catherine Black of the London Hospital, who was present and who had nursed the King since the 1928 illness, refused to give the lethal injection, which is why Dawson had to give it himself. Nevertheless, faced with conflicting loyalties, she kept quiet about what had been done and her autobiography published in 1939 made no mention of what must have been the most poignant and unforgettable episode in her long and distinguished career.

The reason for his action, which Dawson frankly admits in his diary, was to ensure that the announcement of the King's death should appear first in the morning edition of The Times and not in some lesser publication later in the day. To make doubly sure that this would happen Dawson telephoned his wife in London asking her to let The Times know when the announcement was imminent.

Nevertheless, it was surely special pleading to claim that he also acted to reduce the strain on the royal family. Apart from the Prince of Wales, who was unhappy at being separated from his mistress Mrs Wallis Simpson, there was no evidence of such strain and in particular, as Dawson noted in his diary, Queen Mary remained calm and kindly throughout. The earlier death suited Dawson. Having issued his famous bulletin he had a vested interest in ensuring that death occurred sooner rather than later. At the same time it allowed him to get back to his busy private practice in London.

Although Dawson spoke against euthanasia when it was debated in the House of Lords in December 1936, he clearly felt that it or something similar might sometimes be appropriate for his own patients and there is no reason to think that King George V was the only patient he treated in this way. He described his management of the King's final illness as 'a facet of euthanasia or so called mercy killing.' But even the most ardent supporter of euthanasia would hesitate to describe the killing of an unconscious patient, without the patient's prior knowledge or consent, as mercy killing. Indeed, when examined closely this and almost all similar cases turn out in the end to be examples, not of mercy killing but of convenience killing. This was so in this case and the person most convenienced was Dawson.

The ethical line which separates acceptable from unacceptable conduct is sometimes a narrow one. What caused Dawson to stray across the line is a matter of speculation but the likely answer is that he was guilty of the besetting sin of doctors and that is of arrogance. Although in daily contact with the great and good of the land, including the Archbishop of Canterbury who was living at Sandringham at the time, he arrogantly assumed that he, and he alone, had the special insight to appreciate the importance of the timing of the King's death. It was also unfeeling of

EXAMPLE 4   **11**

Dawson to involve Sister Black in his plan and arrogant to assume that her conscience was as elastic as his own.

This whole episode seems a piece of pointless folly which Dawson was wise to conceal at the time. The emergence of the truth 50 years later did nothing to enhance his reputation nor did his half-hearted espousal of euthanasia do anything to diminish the opprobrium which rightly attaches to doctors who break the sixth commandment.

J H R Ramsay

British Medical Journal (1994); **308**: 1445, with permission from the BMJ Publishing Group.

Consent and competence

A patient is able to give *valid consent* to a procedure if he is *informed*, *uncoerced* and *competent*.

'Informed' means that a patient has all the relevant information, given in an appropriate form, with which to make a decision.

'Uncoerced' means that the person is free to make decisions without any undue influence or pressure from any other person.

To be considered 'competent' (the medical term) or to be deemed to have 'capacity' (the legal term) the patient must be able to:
1 Understand the issue in question
2 Retain the information in memory for long enough to use it in making a decision
3 *Believe* the information given
4 Weigh the information in the balance and evaluate arguments for and against in order to reach a decision
5 Express the decision in some form

The requirement for the consent of individuals for treatment protects patients from harm (non-maleficence); benefits them (beneficence); and respects their autonomy.
- **Non-maleficence**: This is viewed as a means of respecting a patient's privacy and dignity and protecting him/her from bodily invasion, assault, deception or coercion
- **Beneficence**: Therapeutic benefit ensues because it encourages patients' adherence with treatment and care procedures, and enables them to communicate a more complete picture of their concerns in relation to proposed treatments
- **Autonomy**: Having information about the potential advantages and disadvantages of any proposed treatment enables patients to reflect and deliberate on whether or not to accept or refuse the treatment that is offered. In consenting to the treatment that a health professional plans for them, they make the aims and objectives of the health professional part of their own

If a patient is not competent to be involved in discussions regarding medical care, in the UK a medical decision should be taken in the 'best interests' of the patient. It is best practice for the multidisciplinary team and the family to be involved in these discussions. The family cannot make decisions for incompetent patients in the absence of appropriate legal documentation but, where possible, they should be consulted to find out what the patient would have wanted. It often focuses the minds of a distressed family to ask questions such as 'What do you think your mother would want, given this situation?'

Points to consider:
- It is perfectly in order to provide all measures to enhance competence by managing the environment, e.g. optimize the senses (glasses/hearing aids), ensure a comfortable familiar environment with good lighting and heating, bring an advocate to the meeting, provide writing materials, and an interpreter, etc.

- Patients are entitled to make seemingly illogical decisions provided they are made with competence
- Patients may be competent even if they are mentally ill
- Patients may have lucid intervals

Specific situations

In palliative medicine we may be asked to assess competence in order that a patient can, for instance, make a will, change a codicil to a will, execute a Lasting Power of Attorney or document Advance Decisions to refuse treatment. All the above points apply.

Making a will

Clinical staff members are generally advised not to witness the signing of a will for fear of legal complications. In palliative care, however, we are endeavouring to support patients and their families through a very difficult time and it may be helpful for us to assist. In this situation, a senior doctor, if witnessing a signature, would be advised to do this only if they have assessed competency. The competency then needs to be documented.

Lasting Power of Attorney

As above, doctors witnessing the signing of these documents should ensure and document that the patient is fully competent. (📖 See also Chapter 19A.)

Advance Decisions to refuse treatment

Again, doctors need to assess and document competency. (📖 See also Chapter 19A.)[4]

4 Perkins H. S. (2007) Controlling death: the false promise of advance directives. *Annals of Internal Medicine*, **147**(1): 51–9.

Euthanasia

He jests at scars, that never felt a wound.

Shakespeare, *Romeo and Juliet*

Etymologically, the term 'euthanasia' derives from the ancient Greek, '*eu*', meaning good and '*thanatos*', meaning death, thus a 'good death'. Today, the term 'euthanasia' refers to the administration of death, the active intentional ending of life. It is a final and irreversible step and the subject of great debate engendering, on the one hand, strong feelings about the right to demand death and, on the other, strong feelings that life is so precious that we have a duty to preserve it at all costs. It must not be forgotten that patients are often making decisions regarding euthanasia on the basis of inadequate prognostic information, since medical advances will never be able to identify accurately when an individual patient will die naturally.

Proponents of euthanasia feel that:

Euthanasia is the only alternative to avoiding a painful death
Comment: Although the control of pain is not perfect, patients can usually achieve a degree of relief acceptable to them. Public education has started to erode the myth that all patients with cancer inevitably die in considerable pain, although this fear is still held strongly by some.

In practice, even patients with distressing symptoms and an apparent high level of suffering rarely request euthanasia consistently.

Euthanasia is the only answer to the fear of being kept alive at all costs
Comment: Extraordinary advances in medicine over the last few centuries have pushed forward the frontiers, extending the quantity of life and potentially, therefore, the extension of an 'unacceptable' poor quality of life. Medical ethics, however, has also advanced, allowing competent patients to refuse treatment and supporting the concept that burdensome, futile treatment is bad medicine. Assuming that healthcare professionals act with multidisciplinary support within an ethical framework, the fear of being kept alive at all costs should be minimized.

Euthanasia is the only way to die with dignity
Comment: Families are torn between not wanting to see their loved ones deteriorate and wanting them to survive as long as possible to nurture precious time. A natural death and all the potential healing and strengthening of family unity that so often occurs during the final days is often worthwhile and dignified, a sentiment supported by most healthcare professionals experienced in the care of the dying. Furthermore, the efficacy of drugs used to carry out euthanasia is unpredictable. There are literature reports of failure to achieve coma and patients re-wakening in considerable discomfort, which cannot be described as dignified.

'My dear Schur, you remember our first talk. You promised to help me when I could no longer carry on. It is only torture now, and it has no longer any sense'.

Sigmund Freud

(After years of suffering from cancer of the jaw, Freud convinced his personal physician to give him several large doses of morphine, for the pain. He fell into a coma and died the next day.)

Euthanasia should be legalized to uphold the principle of autonomy

Comment: In the West, individual rights are viewed as key to a democratic society, implying that the individual has the right to control his/her own destiny.

In society, however, others also have rights and the concept of a healthcare professional delivering euthanasia as a technical act may not be in the best interests of individuals or society.

Euthanasia, if carried out, should rightly occur only when the patient is fully competent and consistently requests it. However, patients who are ill, often bed-bound, unable to care for themselves and wholly reliant on others for care may feel a burden and under pressure to acquiesce.

A diagnosis of a reversible clinical depression may be missed if families and healthcare professionals are slow to recognize it. The concept of the 'slippery slope' argument, in which patients may be subjected to euthanasia without their expressed consent and within a short time of having had the discussions, has already been reported in the literature.

Whatever the arguments, the fundamental principles are that life is infinitely precious and that the vulnerable deserve protection. We should always consider the views of our competent patients and act in the best interests of those who are unable to give consent.

It is also fundamentally important to recognize what is *not* euthanasia, which includes the following, where the primary intention is to prevent suffering:

Euthanasia is not

- Withholding or withdrawing futile, burdensome treatment including nutrition and hydration if the patient is dying and is unable to swallow
- Giving opioids, or any other medications, to control symptoms including pain, fear and overwhelming distress
- Sedating a patient in the terminal stages if all other practical methods of controlling symptoms have failed
- Issuing a *Do Not Resuscitate* order

The Royal Dutch Medical Association has formulated five requirements that must be fulfilled for euthanasia to be acceptable or legally excusable. These are:

1 There is voluntary, competent and durable request on the part of the patient
2 The request is based on full information
3 The patient is in a situation of intolerable and hopeless suffering (physical or mental)

4 There are no acceptable alternatives
5 The physician has consulted another physician before performing euthanasia

The physician has to notify the local medical examiner and complete an extensive questionnaire. It is then reported to the public prosecutor who decides if prosecution is necessary. This notification procedure has formal legal status and also covers cases involving euthanasia without the patient's explicit request.

In some American states, physicians are allowed to prescribe medication to hasten death in terminally ill adults.

Further reading

Books

Bass M. (2006) *Palliative Care Resuscitation*. Chichester: John Wiley.

British Medical Association (2007) *Withholding and Withdrawing Life-Prolonging Medical Treatment: Guidance for Decision Making* (3rd edn). Oxford: Blackwell Publishing.

Campbell C., Partridge R. (2007) *Artificial Nutrition and Hydration: Guidance in End of Life Care for Adults*. London: NCPC.

Have H ten., David C. (2002) *The Ethics of Palliative Care, European Perspectives*. Maidenhead: Open University Press.

Jeffrey D. (2006) *Patient-centred Ethics and Communication at the End of Life*. Oxford: Radcliffe.

Woods S. (2007) *Death's Dominion: Ethics at the End of Life*. Maidenhead: Open University Press.

Worthington R. (ed.) (2005) *Ethics and Palliative Care: A Case-based Manual*. Abingdon: Radcliffe.

Articles

Hancock K., et al. (2007) Truth telling in discussing prognosis in advanced life-limiting illnesses: a systematic review. *Palliative Medicine*, **21**(6): 507–17.'

Hoflenberg R. (2006) Assisted dying. *Clinical Medicine*, **6**: 72–4.

Hoffer L. (2006) Tube feeding in advanced dementia: the metabolic perspective. *British Medical Journal*, **333**(7580): 1214–15.

Jennings B., et al. (eds.) (2005) Improving end of life care: Why has it been so difficult? *A Hastings Center Special Report*, November–December.

Johnston C. (2007) The Mental Capacity Act 2005 and advance decisions. *Clinical Ethics*, **2**(2): 80–4.

Mann T., Cornock M. (2007) Decision making in palliative care: the Mental Capacity Act 2005. *International Journal of Palliative Nursing*, **13**(8): 402–7.

Morita T., et al. (2006) Artificial hydration therapy, laboratory findings and fluid balance in terminally ill patients with abdominal malignancies. *Journal of Pain and Symptom Management*, **31**(2): 130–8.

Pereira J. et al (2008) The response of a Swiss university hospital's palliative care consult team to assisted suicide within the institution. *Palliative Medicine*, **22**: 659–67.

Sokol D. (2007) Can deceiving patients be morally acceptable? *British Medical Journal*, **334**(7601): 984–6.

Stone P., Lund S. (2007) Predicting prognosis in patients with advanced cancer. *Annals of Oncology*, **18**: 971–6.

Stone P. (2008) Development and Validation of a prognosticscale for use in patients with advanced cancer. *Palliative Medicine*, **22**: 6: 711–18.

Van Delden J. (2007) Terminal sedation: a source of a restless ethical debate. *Journal of Medical Ethics*, **33**(4): 187–8.

Ziegler S., Bosshard G. (2007) Role of non-govermental organizations in physician assisted suicide. *British Medical Journal*, **334**: 295–8.

Communication: Breaking bad news

Introduction

Effective communication is essential in all clinical interactions. Although some clinicians have innate communication skills, most of us can improve our ability to give and receive information. There is good evidence that unlike many clinical skills that improve with experience, communication ability does not reliably improve unless specific educational effort is made.

> Effective symptom control is impossible without effective communication
> Buckman, 2000[1]

Communication is fundamental to good palliative care, but difficulties can arise that need to be understood and addressed. It is always a two-way activity, requiring sensitivity, empathy and 'active listening'.

Society's attitudes towards death and dying can hinder open communication. Health professionals may be uneasy with issues of death and dying: they may wish to protect themselves and others, and feel a sense of discomfort with strong emotions.

It is easy for the busy health professional to use a variety of blocking tactics which inhibit communication, such as hiding behind task-focused practice. An additional hazard may arise if the setting is not conducive to privacy with space and time to listen.

Information giving can take the place of hearing the underlying feelings and emotions. The essence of good communication is not what we say, but how we listen. The quality of listening empathically to patients should not be underestimated if patients are to feel understood and cared for.

Communication in palliative care is necessary to achieve an accurate assessment of patients' physical, emotional and psychosocial needs. If we are to be able to find ways of supporting patients and families facing change and uncertainty, we as health professionals need to find out about the patients' expectations and goals.

1 Buckman, R. (2000) Communication in palliative care: a practical guide *Neurologic Clinics*, **19**(4) 989–1004.

Enabling people to make informed choices and to make future plans involves careful listening and sensitive responses. Attending to cultural and language issues and helping people face some of the strong emotions aroused by their situation, such as anger, denial, depression and fear, are essential in providing holistic PALLIATIVE CARE.

- Communication is not just 'being nice' but produces a more effective consultation for both patient and healthcare professional
- Effective communication significantly improves:
  - accuracy, efficiency and supportiveness
  - health outcomes for patients
  - satisfaction for both patient and HCP
  - the therapeutic relationship
- Communication bridges the gap between evidence-based medicine and working with individual patients

Adapted from Silverman J., Kurtz S., Draper J. (2005) *Skills for Communicating with Patients* (2nd edn). Oxford: Radcliffe Press.

Barriers to effective communication

There are various barriers which prevent or inhibit communication.

Healthcare professional-led barriers

Four factors are known to impact on communication behaviour: fears, beliefs, inadequate skills and lack of support.

Fears
- Of unleashing strong emotions
- Of upsetting the patient
- Of causing more harm than good
- Of being asked unanswerable and difficult questions (e.g. why me?)
- Of saying the wrong thing and getting into trouble with the HCP hierarchy
- Of taking up too much time
- Of dealing with patients' emotional reactions

Beliefs
- That emotional problems are inevitable in patients with serious disease and that nothing can be done about them
- That it is not my role to discuss certain things. These should be discussed with senior team members
- That there is no point talking about fears when we have no answers
- Talking about concerns that cannot be resolved falsely raises expectations

Inadequate skills
- Not knowing how to assess knowledge and perceptions
- Not being able to integrate medical, psychological, social and spiritual agendas
- Not knowing how to move both into and out of feelings safely
- Being uncertain how to handle specific communication situations such as breaking bad news, difficult questions, collusion, handling anger, denial

Lack of Support
- Feeling that there was no support for the patient if problems were identified
- Feeling no support would be available for the HCP
- Conflict within the team

Patient-led barriers

There is evidence that patients disclose as few as 40% of their concerns,[2] and that those who are most anxious or most distressed, disclose least.

Reasons for non-disclosure by patients reflect the professional-led barriers: fears, beliefs and other difficulties.

Fears

- Of admitting inability to cope
- Of breaking down/losing control in front of strangers
- Of stigmatisation by admitting psychological problems
- Of having their worst fears confirmed
- Trying to protect staff from their distress

Beliefs

- Healthcare professionals perceived as being too busy
- That HCP is only concerned with certain aspects of care, e.g. nurses with physical care, doctors with disease and treatment related worries.
- That talking concerns will increase the burden for the HCP
- That life depends on treatment and complaining about treatment will lead to its withdrawal. "I mustn't alienate or upset the doctor"
- That their worries are insignificant

Difficulties

- Unable to express how they feel. They may be overawed by the consultation and forgot to mention their foremost concern
- Unable to find the right words. They may be unfamiliar with both the technical language but also the concepts of disease evolution and spread.
- When they have tried to express their concerns to healthcare professionals, cues are met with distancing
- Does not have a good enough command of the language and no independent or any interpreter is available to help.
- The relevant questions are not asked by the professional

2 Heaven C., Maguire P. (2003) Communication issues. In *Psychosocial Issues in Palliative Care* (ed. M. Lloyd Williams), pp. 13–34. Oxford: Oxford University Press.

Specific communication issues

Here are various examples of communication issues which frequently require careful thought and handling.

> I have received two wonderful graces. First, I have been given time to prepare for a new future. Secondly, I find myself—uncharacteristically—calm and at peace.
>
> Cardinal Basil Hume, breaking the news of his imminent death from cancer to the priests of the Westminster diocese, 16 April, 1999.

Breaking bad news

Breaking bad news is such a fundamental aspect of communication in palliative care because it requires an understanding of so many other aspects of the healthcare professional/patient relationship. It is unusual for patients not to voice difficult or awkward questions, and strong emotions are likely to be elicited. The steps required for the successful breaking of bad news can act as a template for most other communication problems encountered.

Patients and relatives need time to absorb information and to adapt to bad news. Breaking bad news takes time, and issues often need to be discussed further and clarified as more information is imparted.

There is increasing evidence that most patients want to know about their illness. Many patients who have been denied this knowledge have difficulty in understanding why they are becoming weaker and are then relieved and grateful to be told the truth. They may be angry with the family who has known about the illness all along and have not thought it right to tell them.

Professionals often become involved unwittingly in a potential conspiracy of silence when the family demand information before the patient has been appraised of the situation. The family might say, 'Do not tell him the diagnosis/prognosis because he will not be able to cope with it. We know him better than you do.' The family needs to know that their concerns, of not wanting to cause any more hurt to the patient, have been heard. They also need to be aware that the bad news may be more painful for themselves than for the patient. The family also needs to know that it would be unwise for clinical staff to be untruthful if the patient appeared to want to know the truth and was asking direct questions, because of the inevitable breakdown in trust that this could cause.

Advising patients and families with regard to prognosis is important since they may want (and often need) to organize their affairs and plan for the time that is left. However, it is *not possible to be accurate with prognosis*. Overestimating or underestimating the time that someone has to live can cause untold anguish. It is therefore more sensible to talk in terms of days/weeks, weeks/months and months/years as appropriate.

There is a balance to be made between fully informing the patient about their disease and prognosis, completely overwhelming them with facts and figures, or providing only minimal and inadequate information.

While it is important to avoid being patronizing, it is also important not to cause distress by 'information overload'.

It is important to be aware that people have divergent attitudes to receiving bad news and that this needs sensitive handling. Patients and families respond badly to being told bad news in a hurried, brusque and unsympathetic manner with no time to collect their thoughts and ask questions. However sensitively bad news is imparted, patients and families are naturally devastated and the impact of the news can obliterate a great deal of the communication that took place. Patients may either not remember or misinterpret what has been said, particularly if they use denial as a coping technique.

A strategy for breaking bad news

Nothing in all the world is more dangerous than sincere ignorance and conscientious stupidity.
                    Martin Luther King 1929–68: *Strength to Love (1963).*

Outlining a strategy for breaking bad news is difficult because it turns a process which should be natural and unforced into something which seems constrained and awkward. The following advice encompasses the techniques that health professionals have found, through trial and error, to be helpful. It can be used as a guide to develop an individual's personal confidence and skills in breaking bad news.

The goals of breaking bad news

The process of breaking bad news needs to be specifically tailored to the needs of the individual concerned, for every human being will have a different history and collection of fears and concerns. The goal of breaking bad news is to do so in a way that facilitates acceptance and understanding and reduces the risk of destructive responses.

The ability to break bad news well involves skills which need to be coveted and trained for, audited and kept up to date with as much objective determination as that shown by a surgeon in acquiring and maintaining surgical skills. The consequences of performing the process badly may have immediate and long-term damaging effects for all involved, every bit as catastrophic as surgery going wrong. For example, patients and families may lose trust. Having awareness of strategies to complete the process well is vital, but breaking bad news must never become so routine that patients, or their families, detect little individual caring compassion.

Break bad news well and you will always be remembered, break bad news badly and you will never be forgotten.

Prepare to tell bad news

Acquire all the information possible about the patient and their family. (A genogram is particularly useful in quickly assimilating the important people in the patient's life, and the web of relationships within the family.)

Read the patient's notes
For:
- Diagnostic information
- Test results
- An understanding of the patient's clinical history
- The support system for the individual
- Background knowledge of the patient's life—making basic mistakes will undermine the patient's confidence
- The patient's understanding of spoken language, e.g. English. If not, arrange for an interpreter to be present

Discuss with other members of the team, and then select the most appropriate team member to break the bad news. Decide which other member of the team should be present during the interview. Ensure there is an interpreter or advocate present for those with special needs or language difficulties.

Check
That you have:
- A place of privacy where there will be no interruptions. Unplug the telephone and switch off the mobile phone, etc.
- Tissues, a jug of water and drinking glasses
- Time to carry out the process
- Your own emotional energy to do so—this job is better done earlier in the day than late
- Pressing tasks are completed so that there will be minimal interruptions

Plan

Prepare a rough plan in your mind of what you want to achieve in the communication, and what you want to avoid communicating. Having a rough goal will bring structure to the communication, though it is important to avoid imposing your agenda on that of the patient.

Set the context
- Invite the patient to the place of privacy
- Introduce yourself clearly
- Let the patient know that they have your attention and how long you have got
- Ensure that the patient is comfortable and not distracted by pain or a full bladder, etc.
- Give a 'warning shot' indication that this is not a social or routine encounter
- Sit at the same eye level as each other and within easy reach

A *warning shot* is concerned with preparing a patient that bad news is coming. This allows them to be more receptive than if it comes 'out of the blue'. An example would be, 'I'm sorry to say that the results were not as good as we had hoped.'

Assess
- How much the patient knows already
- How much the patient wants to know
- How the patient expresses him/herself and what words and ways he/she uses to understand the situation

'Are you the sort of person that likes to know everything?'

Acquire empathy with the patient
- What would it be like to be the patient?
- How is the patient feeling?
- Is there anything that is concerning the patient which he or she is not verbalizing?
- What mechanisms has the patient used in the past to deal with bad news?
- Does the patient have a particular outlook on life or cultural understanding which underpins his or her approach to dealing with the situation?
- Who are the important people in the patient's life?

Respond to *non-verbal* as well as *verbal* clues.

Encourage the patient to speak by listening carefully and responding appropriately.

Share information
- Having spent time listening, use the patient's words to recap the story of the journey so far, checking regularly with the patient that you have heard the story correctly

'Would you mind if I repeated back to you what I have heard you tell me to make sure I have understood things correctly?'

- Slowly and gradually draw out the information from the patient while regularly checking that they are not misunderstanding what you are saying
- Use the 'warning shot' technique to preface bad news to help the patient prepare themself
- Use diagrams to help understanding and retention of information if appropriate and acceptable to the patient
- Avoid jargon and acronyms which are easily misunderstood
- Do not bluff. It is acceptable to say 'I do not know, and I will try to get an answer for you for our next meeting'

Remember

Ensure that:
- The patient understands the implications of what you are saying
- The patient is in control of the speed at which information is being imparted
- The patient can see that you are being empathic to their emotional response. It can be very appropriate to say something like 'Being told something like this can seem overwhelming'
- You address the patient's real concerns, which may be very different from what you expect them to be
- You offer a record of the consultation, for example a tape recording or short written notes if appropriate

Response
- You should respond to the patient's feelings and response to the news
- You should acknowledge the patient's feelings
- You should be prepared to work through the patient's emotional response to the bad news with them

It can be very distressing to get such news, and it is not unusual to feel very angry, or lonely or sad on hearing such news.

Let the patient speak first

Use open questions, such as:
How are you feeling today?
Can you tell me how this all came about?
How do you see things going from here?

Make concrete plans for the next step

Your appointment to see Dr Brown the oncologist is provisionally booked for next Thursday at 2 o'clock. How would that fit in with your other arrangements?

Immediate plans

'What are you doing now?' 'How are you getting home?' 'Who will you tell?' 'How will you tell them?' 'What will you say?' 'How will they cope?'
Such questions can help the patient to start formulating the answers that they will need for their family or friends.

Summarize

For the patient
- Try to get the patient to repeat the key points to ensure they have understood

For other healthcare professionals
- Record details of the conversation in the patient's notes clearly
- Convey information quickly to those who need to know, most importantly the patient's GP

Deception is not as creative as truth. We do best in life if we look at it with clear eyes, and I think that applies to coming up to death as well.

Cicely Saunders, in *Time* 5 September, 1988

Deal with questions
- 'Are there any questions which you would like me to deal with at this point?'

Contract for the future

I know the news today was not what you were hoping for but you are not going to go through this on your own. We are there for you, your family is there for you and we are going to go through this together. Dr Brown will be seeing you next Thursday and I'll see you back here on Monday morning.

- Closing remarks should identify support networks, including contact telephone numbers and times of easy access. Be fairly concrete about the next meeting but also allow the patient the option to postpone if they do not feel able to attend.

Handling difficult questions

e.g. Is it cancer? Am I dying? What is going to happen to me?

Key points

- Find out the patient's perceptions as to what makes them ask the question: *'What makes you feel it may be cancer or you are dying?'*
- After obtaining a response, repeat the question if necessary by asking if there are any other reasons for the patient feeling this way.

• If the patient gives no other reason or changes the subject

You might say: *'You asked about the diagnosis, is that something you would like to talk about?'* If the patient says *'no'* – leave it there; they are probably not ready to have the truth confirmed.

• If the patient gives other reasons

Confirm the patient's thoughts if they are correct. You should invite the patient to express their emotions and provide support if appropriate. Pause to see if the patient spontaneously raises any concerns. If not, invite the patient to voice their concerns. It is sensible to address only the concerns that the patient raises. However, you should answer realistically and avoid rushing in with premature or false reassurances:

- invite further questions
- offer to provide information (written or verbal) that may be relevant. Drawings are sometimes helpful if conceptualization is difficult. Just the name of the disease or complication written legibly is useful for patients to take away with them. They are likely to consult friends and the internet
- assure continuity of care. This will include the offer of further access for discussion, as when breaking bad news. It may also include a contingency plan for the near future

Collusion

This may occur when a healthcare professional is approached and pressurized by, for example, a relative to withhold medical information from the patient. The HCP is being invited to collude with the relative in constructing or maintaining a conspiracy of either silence or falsehood concerning the seriousness of the patient's illness. The stated rationale is often that the relative knows the patient extremely well and that 'they would just turn their face to the wall'. Alternatively, they would be unable to cope with the truth about the situation, and that there is no reason in the view of the relative for the patient to be bothered or alarmed by unpleasant news.

Key points

Focus on:
- The relative's feelings
- The relative's reasons for not wanting to be truthful
- Acknowledging the relative's motives, e.g. protecting the patient from distress
- The strain placed on the relative/patient relationship by not being truthful with someone who they are usually very close to emotionally
- The relative's perception of the patient's understanding. Seek to identify any evidence that the patient might already suspect the truth.

Then:
- Offer to assess the patient's understanding of their illness directly
- Reassure the relative that information will not be forced onto the patient if such information is not explicitly requested or wanted

Such a strategy often results in the patient disclosing to the HCP that they are fully or partially aware of the true nature of the situation. In the majority of instances, this information will be seen as a great relief to both the relative and the patient. Communication is thereby considerably enhanced by resisting the initial pressure to withhold the truth. There are occasions, however, when a relative has invested so much energy over a long period in fostering a false picture of the true nature of the patient's diagnosis and prognosis that they are quite unable to contemplate dismantling the barrier created by the collusion. In this case, the HCP must think very carefully about what action on their part is in the best interests of the patient, or alternately how the patient's confidence and trust in their relative and the HCP might be compromised by unrequested and unexpected disclosure.

Dealing with anger

Key points

The following strategies help to diffuse anger:

- Acknowledge the anger – 'You seem to be very angry' which may have the effect of increasing the person's anger temporarily. This is especially the case if their anger is displaced onto you. However, the anger will not subside if there has been no chance to articulate it
- Invite the patient/relative to explain the cause of the anger – 'Can you help me understand what is making you so angry?'
- Listen to their story to get as much information as possible
- Try not to be defensive, even if the anger seems to be misdirected. Once anger has been expressed the angry person often realizes that displacement was unjust
- Focus on the individual's stress/feelings
- Apologize if appropriate, but there is no point in apologizing for something which is clearly not your fault or responsibility
- Clarify the situation if appropriate, e.g. 'It must be very difficult for you to see your husband in pain'
- If possible, negotiate a mutually acceptable solution. This may include agreement that a particular situation is quite unacceptable and helping the person to look to the correct place to register a complaint

Exploration of feelings (e.g. anxiety)

Key points

- Recognition — Non-verbal/verbal evidence
- Acknowledgement — 'I can see you are anxious'
- Permission — 'It's OK to be anxious'
- Understanding — 'I want to find out what is making you anxious'
- Empathic acceptance — 'You are anxious because…'
- Assessment — Severity and effects of anxiety
- Alteration (if appropriate) — Removal of stress, cognitive challenge, boosting coping strategies, medication

The above steps will usually need to be taken before the most appropriate intervention can be suggested. The short-cut of prescribing sedative medication is likely to fail to relieve the anxiety unless there has been some understanding and insight on the part of the patient. Medication is nearly always going to be an adjunct to discussion and alteration in coping strategies with the stress of a difficult set of problems.

Patients who do not want to talk

The key task is to assess what is making the patient reluctant to talk. This can include:
- Denial – of the facts or of unacceptable feelings
- Ignorance – low IQ/incorrect information
- Depression
- Dementia
- Disengagement
- Talking to someone else
- Previously dealt with – 'wanting to forget'

Handling denial

Denial occurs when a patient maintains a positive outlook on their illness/prognosis in spite of medical information given to the contrary. Denial is a coping mechanism, its function is to protect oneself against distress that could be intolerable and lead to psychological disorganization. Health professionals may explore the denial to determine if it is an absolute barrier to understanding, but forcing through it could lead to severe psychological problems.

Key points in exploring denial

Look for any evidence that denial is not absolute (a window), e.g.:
- **Now**: 'How do you feel things are going at the moment?'
- **Past**: 'Has there ever been a moment when you think things aren't going to work out?'
- **Future**: 'How do you see your illness affecting your future?'

If there is no evidence of awareness – leave the situation as it is. However, you should ensure regular follow-up to reassess the denial. It may well become much less absolute, especially in light of the changing clinical situation and increasingly unpleasant symptoms.

Unrealistic expectations

When patients or relatives appear to be unrealistic in their beliefs about the possible outcomes of the illness or treatment or length of prognosis there may be several reasons why this is the case:

- They have never been properly informed
- They have misunderstood the meaning of the information they have been given. Explanations may have been over-technical, or incomprehensible because of jargon. There may have been ambiguous or conflicting information given resulting from an uncertain clinical situation
- Clarification may not have been sought because no real opportunities were offered
- They are clinging onto false hope, which may have been the result of false reassurance at the time of breaking bad news
- They are in true denial. As mentioned above, this is usually an effective defence mechanism

The key to dealing with unrealistic expectations is to establish WHY patients believe what they do.

Key points

- Use the patient's cues to **explore** their perception of their situation – *'You say you have had quite a bit more pain recently? What do you think is causing the problem?'*
- Using negotiation, test out whether they **really believe** what they are saying, or whether they are simply trying to cling onto false hope
- Gently **challenge unrealistic beliefs** about outcomes, by confronting any inconsistencies in the story
- Look for windows of worry by asking if the patient ever worries about the possible outcomes. Worry usually indicates that denial is not absolute and that the patient has allowed themselves to look at realistic scenarios on occasions
- Establish whether the patient is ill-informed and needs to be told bad news, or is in absolute denial

It is important that all healthcare professionals work to elicit accurately patients' problems and concerns, but at the same time are able to recognize their professional limitations. They need to be able to identify when patients or carers have needs that are best met by other people (e.g. counsellors or mental healthcare professionals with specialist skills in 'speaking to children', psychologists, psychiatrists, etc.). In such instances, healthcare professionals need to be aware of the specialists/services that exist locally, and how they can refer to these services.

Working with ethnic diversity patients

Useful strategies

Greeting
- Check with the patient that you are pronouncing his or her name properly. Our names are very important to our sense of self
- Welcome the patient in a friendly manner, in terms of verbal and non-verbal communication. If patients are unwell *and* worried about understanding you *and* unsure they can make themselves understood, they will already feel under pressure and anything which makes them feel more relaxed can only help the interaction

Language style
- Speak in short, clear and grammatical sentences
- Deal with one point at a time
- Do not ask more than one question before waiting for an answer
- Avoid clinical terms unless you are going to explain them. (Some explanation of key terms can be empowering for patients)
- Beware of using idioms – these are words and phrases that can be puzzling to a non-native speaker, for example, *'Have you been feeling down in the dumps?'*
- Try not to use euphemisms, for example, 'passing away' for 'dying'
- Do not use local dialect terms unless you know the patient understands them
- Break down instructions into short, clear steps
- Summarize important points at the end of the interaction

Paralinguistic features (tone, pitch, etc.)
- Speak loudly enough but don't shout. Non-native speakers often find that people shout as if it was their hearing that was a problem
- Speak in an unhurried way, but not so slowly that it interferes with the flow
- Emphasize important words and phrases
- Look at the patient when you are talking

Understanding the patient
- Give adequate time for answers. These may take longer to formulate if English is not the patient's first language
- Ask the patient to explain any words or phrases of which you are unsure
- Double-check with the patient that you have understood them correctly

Checking the patient understands you
- Check understanding at regular intervals throughout the interaction
- For important points, ask the patient to tell you what they understand of what you have said
- Do not assume that a nod or a 'yes' indicates understanding – these gestures are sometimes just to show politeness or deference. Some Asian cultures use shaking of the head to mean 'yes', whereas this would indicate the opposite to a native English speaker

- If understanding seems poor, ask whether they would prefer an interpreter to be present and explain how you can organize this (otherwise they might think *they* have to both organize and pay for one)

Backing up
- Use pictures or diagrams where they will clarify meaning
- Write down important points for the patient to take away with them. Even if their English reading ability is limited, someone else in the family might be able to help
- In some cases where there is important information to transmit, an audio recording can be made and given to the patient

Strategies for working with an interpreter
- Check the interpreter and the patient speak the same language and the same dialect
- Allow time for pre-interview discussion with the interpreter in order to talk about the contents of the interview and the way in which you will work together
- Ask the interpreter to teach you how to pronounce the patient's name correctly
- Allow time for the interpreter to introduce himself/herself to the patient and explain his/her role
- Explain that the interview will be kept confidential
- Check whether she/he as an interpreter is acceptable to the patient
- Introduce yourself and your role to the patient
- Encourage the interpreter to interrupt and intervene during the consultation as necessary
- Use straightforward language and avoid jargon
- Actively listen to the interpreter and the patient
- Allow enough time for the consultation (*perhaps double the time used for an English speaking patient*)
- At the end of the interview check that the patient has understood everything or whether she/he wants to ask anything else
- Have a post-interview discussion with the interpreter

Things to remember
- The pressure is on the interpreter
- The responsibility for the interview is yours as the health professional
- Your power as a healthcare professional - as perceived by the interpreter and the patient
- To show patience and compassion in a demanding situation
- To be aware of your own attitudes towards those who are different from you, including awareness of racism
- To be aware of your own shortcomings, for example not being able to speak the patient's language
- To show respect for the interpreter and his/her skills

Points to check if things seem to be going wrong in the consultation
- Does the interpreter speak English and the patient's language fluently?
- Is the interpreter acceptable to the patient (same sex and similar age, for example)?

- Is the patient prevented from telling you things because of his/her relationship to the interpreter? An interpreter who is a family member, especially if she/he is a child of the patient is likely to act as a barrier to effective communication
- Are you creating as good a relationship as possible with your patient?
- Is the interpreter translating exactly what you and your patient are saying or is she/he advancing his/her own views and opinion?
- Does the interpreter understand the purpose of the interview and his/her role?
- Have you given the interpreter time to meet the patient and explain what is going on?
- Does the interpreter feel free to interrupt you as necessary to indicate problems or seek clarification?
- Are you using simple jargon-free English?
- Is the interpreter ashamed or embarrassed by the patient or the subject of the consultation?
- Are you allowing the interpreter enough time?
- Are you maintaining as good a relationship as you can with the interpreter (for example by showing respect for his/her skills and maintaining an awareness that the interpreter is probably under pressure)?

Adapted from PROCEED: Professionals responding to ethnic diversity and cancer (ed. J. Kai): Cancer Research UK, 2005. Copyright © University of Nottingham.

Further reading

Books

Bacon F. (1912) Of death. In *Essays*. London: Black.

Dickenson D., Johnson M., Katz J. (eds.) (2000) *Death, Dying and Bereavement* (2nd edn). Maidenhead: Open University Press.

Kaye P. (1996) *Breaking Bad News. A 10 Step Approach.* Northampton: EPL Publications.

London Strategic Health Authority on behalf of the Cancer Action Team (2007) *Advanced Communication in Cancer Care.*

Macdonald E. (ed) (2004) *Difficult conversations in medicine.* Oxford: OUP

Silverman J., Kurtz S., Draper J. (2005) *Skills for Communicating with Patients* (2nd edn). Oxford: Radcliffe.

Wilkes E. (1982) *The Dying Patient: The Medical Management of Incurable and Terminal Illness.* Lancaster: MTP Press.

Worden J. W. (2002) *Grief Counselling and Grief Therapy* (3rd edn). London: Routledge.

Articles

Charlton R., Dolamn E. (1995) Bereavement: a protocol for primary care. *British Journal of General Practice*, **45**: 427–30.

Jewell D. (1999) Commentary: Use of personal experience should be legitimized. *British Medical Journal*, **319**: 296.

Raphael B. (1977) Preventive intervention with the recently bereaved. *Archives of General Psychiatry*, **34**: 1450–4.

Saunderson E. M., Ridsdale L. (1999) General practitioners' beliefs and attitudes about how to respond to death and bereavement: qualitative study. *British Medical Journal*, **319**: 293–6.

Scott J.T. et al (2003) Interventions for improving communication with children and adolescents about their cancer. *Cochrane Database of Systematic Reviews*, Issue 3.

Research in palliative care

The origins of palliative care research in the modern UK Hospice movement date from the founding of St Christopher's Hospice in 1967. Dame Cicely Saunders advocated scientific observation and systematic research as an essential component of the specialty.

To ensure that patients are managed in the most appropriate way a solid body of knowledge must be developed. However, this can only be done on the basis of good research, which some would say is an absolute moral imperative.

Many treatments widely used in the palliative care setting have never been proven to be effective and their use is based on anecdotal evidence and doctor preference. For instance, nebulized morphine was in vogue for many years within the palliative care setting but it has since been shown to be only as effective as normal saline in helping with breathlessness. However, it would be unethical and impractical to generate doubt in nearly all palliative medicine treatments purely on the basis that they had not been submitted to quantitative trials.

Some of the evidence cited to support the use of medication in palliative care comes from populations of patients who do not traditionally fall within the remit of palliative care. This is particularly relevant for drugs used for neuropathic pain, where the research has largely been focused on patients with post-herpetic neuralgia or diabetic neuropathy and not those with complex mixed pains seen in palliative care.

The overarching difficulty in palliative care research is the balance between the needs of the individual patient—who, due to the advanced nature of their disease, may not have a 'second chance' of another treatment—with those of future patients for whom their treatment should be improved and based on research evidence.

The Declaration of Helsinki was drawn up by the World Medical Association in 1964 in response to the need for a code of ethics on human experimentation. This is particularly pertinent in the field of palliative care where the core practice is looking after the dying and the clear need for guidance for the physician caught in the conflict between patients' own best interests and the necessity to advance knowledge for society as a whole.

Some people feel that palliative care research in dying patients is always inappropriate, an affront to dignity and an expression of profound disrespect for the emotional and physical state of those people who are terminally ill. Others feel that precious time, which is limited by disease and growing physical incapacity, should not be wasted or taken from patients or their families by conducting 'research', particularly when patients may be emotionally vulnerable and may feel easily coerced into studies in order to maintain the level of care that they need from staff.

Research has shown, however, that patients are not always adverse to participating even when it is clear that such research will have no immediate benefit for them. They may not share the concerns of ethicists about the difficulties and hazards of research with the terminally ill.

Patient-identified reasons for being involved in research:
- Altruism
- Enhancement of a sense of personal value
- Autonomy
- Supporting the commitment of doctors in optimizing care

Thus the methodological, ethical and practical difficulties encountered in conducting palliative care studies need to be looked at clearly, and strategies devised which are both sensitive to the needs of this particular group of patients as well as to the need of similar patients in the future to have access to improved care.

Methodological difficulties

Evidence-based practice

Evidence based practice is the conscientious, explicit and judicious use of current best evidence in making decisions about the care of individual patients

Sackett *et al.*, 1996

Evidence-based practice is graded according to a system which attributes high evidence to the 'gold standard' research method of the randomized controlled trial (RCT) and lower evidence to studies of a more descriptive nature (Table 3a.1).

Table 3a.1 The five strengths of research evidence

Type	Strength of evidence
I	Strong evidence from at least one systematic review of multiple well-designed RCTs
II	Strong evidence from at least one properly designed RCT of appropriate size
III	Evidence for well-designed trials without randomization, single group pre-post, cohort, time series or matched case-control studies
IV	Evidence from well-designed non-experimental studies from more than one centre or research group
V	Opinions of respected authorities, based on clinical evidence, descriptive studies or reports of expert committees

The Agency for Health Care Policy and Research (AHCPR) 1997

RCTs have not been used a great deal within the field of palliative care. There are different possible explanations for this, but the nature of palliative care itself may sometimes fit more readily with research methodologies such as qualitative and descriptive studies. Although tools are available to investigate issues such as quality of life and emotional distress as part of quantitative trials, qualitative research may better assess patient experience (Table 3a.2).

Table 3a.2 Differences between quantitative and qualitative research

Quantitative research	Qualitative research
Tests theories	Develops theories
Rigid methods	Flexible methods
Experiments	In depth interviews
Surveys	Observation
Large samples	Small samples
Numbers	Words
Statistics	Meaning

Qualitative research

Qualitative research techniques, which are often more suited to palliative care, incorporate the subjective experience that cannot be measured so easily within a mathematical framework. Evidence from qualitative research studies have not been bestowed with the weight of evidence attributed to quantitative research, although the techniques can be as rigorous and are gradually becoming more accepted. Specific aims (generic goals) and objectives (specific ends or outcomes) and precision and clarity are important whether or not the methodology, data collection and analysis are qualitative or quantitative.

Qualitative research takes account of ways in which the research subject makes sense of his/her individual experience. Ideas and concepts develop as the research progresses, which may then be redirected back to further inform the research findings. Words are used as opposed to numerical data. The method is inductive, to discover new knowledge and to 'ground' it into the subjective experience. Although hotly challenged by enthusiasts of quantitative methodology, qualitative research—which often uses the imaginative expression of language—may have the power to disrupt existing assumptions and to challenge what has been considered as reliable, factual material.

Qualitative and quantitative research methods can be combined to bring a different perspective and to enhance knowledge in a more holistic way.

A range of techniques, guided by set principles, exist. Techniques include:
1 **Observation**: Researchers are involved in a fieldwork setting within, for instance a ward, recording conversations, encounters, non-verbal communication, spatial arrangements and physical environment. Aspects such as the quality of care of patients can be explored in this way.
2 **Participant observation**: Researchers become an active subject within the study group. For instance, they may join in with practical tasks in a ward or day hospice setting with the sole purpose of observing and not influencing.
3 **Interviews**: This is the most widely adopted method within qualitative research. Interviews may be interactive, with opportunities to develop or deepen the discussion according to the subject in question. Bereavement research may usefully be conducted in this way.

4 **Focus groups**: Group interviews have the capacity to generate large amounts of data. Tape-recorded transcripts may be analysed. A number of computer packages exist to sort and code items for analysis which facilitates the handling of large volumes of data. The researcher acts as the facilitator, usually for a group of about eight people. Ideas and experiences can be explored. For instance, a multidisciplinary group of healthcare professionals might explore issues surrounding attitudes to such issues as organ donation at the end of life.

Difficulties in defining study populations

Palliative care covers a very wide range of patients with different morbidities. Such patients may include patients with slow growing metastatic cancer who may have many months or even years to live to others with end-stage heart failure and only a few days to live.

For clinical research to be clinically applicable it is important that the research is carried out in relevant patient groups rather than extrapolated from studies, which, although superficially similar, may include patients with widely varying characteristics.

Further, many patients with palliative care needs will have significant co-morbidities in addition to their primary illness, which can make defining a uniform palliative study population very difficult.

Levels of morbidity

A significant proportion of patients with palliative care needs will be unable to adequately report their symptoms or complete questionnaires, either because they are too ill, too fatigued or have a cognitive impairment. This raises issues of the validity of consent to participate in research. Will consent for today cover consent in a week's time when the patient's condition deteriorates and they are no longer able to communicate clearly? Setting appropriate eligibility criteria is crucial and trial design needs to take account of these issues at the outset.

Endpoints and outcomes

Setting appropriate endpoints in palliative care studies can be very difficult. If these endpoints are not specific enough then outcomes will be hard to evaluate. If the endpoints are too specific then the trial will be at risk of irrelevance to the complexity of the clinical situation encountered by patients at the end of life. It is very difficult to isolate a single variable and monitor its changes over time, particularly in the palliative care population which is commonly frail and elderly. Furthermore, patients are often receiving multiple interventions for several co-morbid conditions and facing the emotional and spiritual demands of confronting mortality. A more complex approach is necessary to take account of these different factors and to view interventions in the context of the patient's overall disease journey.

Recruitment, attrition and compliance

Recruiting patients to trials is difficult for many reasons. They are often 'protected' by their families and also by clinical staff, who see them as being vulnerable and in need of protection against unnecessary burdens.

There may be only limited opportunities to approach such patients to discuss trial involvement since rapidly changing clinical and emotional situations may make recruitment inappropriate. The recruitment to trials is therefore often much slower than anticipated.

Once patients are enrolled into studies, sample attrition rates up to 60% have been recorded due to rapidly changing physical and emotional conditions, or even death, during the course of the study.

Compliance can become a particular issue as the disease progresses in terms, for instance, of completing questionnaires. In designing trials which extend into the last weeks of life this needs to be anticipated and other simpler methods of evaluation built into the study from the outset.

Research, audit or service evaluation

There is often much confusion on the differences between research, audit or service evaluation (Table 3a.3) and in particular whether ethical approval is required.

For example, questions are often raised if palliative care patients are interviewed as part of a service evaluation and whether ethical approval is required.

Many clinicians will often approach an ethics committee for clarification.

Ethical difficulties

The need for equipoise in studies

Palliative care patients are considered a vulnerable group and include those with dementia, learning difficulties and children. This makes it difficult to allocate such patients to any form of care that could be deemed in any way less optimal than another.

Thus, randomized trials, which are understood by many to offer the best opportunity to minimize bias, should only involve patients with palliative care needs if there is a high degree of demonstrable equipoise between the interventions being studied. No possibility of disadvantage or morbidity associated with trial participation can be tolerated.

European Trials Directive

The European Trials Directive, introduced in 2004, brought with it increased protection for vulnerable patient groups. It has brought increased scrutiny from ethical and sponsorship committees.

With the implementation of the directive the length of time required to bring a trial through the process has increased considerably, adversely affecting cost and the practical administrative process. This difficulty has been addressed, in part, with the setting up of two National Palliative Care support collaboratives, SuPaC and COMPASS, and through organizations like the National Cancer Research Institute and other Supportive and Palliative Care initiatives to promote appropriately funded and supported multicentre studies.

Funding for palliative care research is limited, especially in comparison with cancer research. The necessary infrastructure to conduct palliative care research and to gather the teams of people together who have the necessary skills and knowledge is therefore difficult.

Consent

As previously discussed, matters of competence and consent are particularly important issues in relation to running studies in patients with palliative care needs, especially when their physical and emotional condition is deteriorating. Researchers are currently devising methods of consenting patients to enable recruitment into a specific study in the future should the patient become incompetent in the meantime.

Practical difficulties

Finance

In the UK, government funding for hospice services is still less than 50% of the total running costs. Given a choice between a research programme and clinical services, most hospice directors will be obliged to maintain the latter. There are however, many examples of small unfunded studies taking place in hospices. However, larger more comprehensive and time-consuming studies need funding either from industry, e.g. pharmaceutical, or other sources such as research charities.

The need for sponsorship and trial insurance is a major issue for palliative care units in the UK, two-thirds of which are charities without access to NHS research governance.

Lack of research centres

Most of those involved in palliative care research are heavily involved in clinical work without specific time dedicated to research. The need to collaborate with other research teams, with logistical and administrative support, therefore becomes very important.

The difficulties in conducting palliative care research are therefore many, but this must not reduce its importance nor its potential to make a real difference to the lives of the growing number of patients who will need palliative care in the years to come. Collaboration, finance, new methodologies, new research tools and ways of studying clinically complex patients will make future palliative care research more robust.

The models of research inherited from oncology may not all be appropriate, and as the specialty becomes more involved with patients who do not have cancer, new and distinctive ways of conducting clinical trials amongst the palliative care population are needed. Studies must be of the highest standard and yet practical with the promise to produce significant outcomes. Examples, include N of 1 studies, which are trials in which patients are repeatedly treated with the same treatment in order to compare their usefulness on an individual basis.

Differentiating audit, service evaluation and research (Table 3a.3)

Differentiating audit, service evaluation and research

Research	Clinical audit	Service evaluation
The attempt to derive generalisable new knowledge, including studies that aim to generate hypotheses, as well as studies that aim to test them.	Designed and conducted to produce information to inform delivery of best care.	Designed and conducted solely to define or judge current care.
Quantitative research – designed to test a hypothesis. Qualitative research – identifies/ explores themes following established methodology.	Designed to answer the question: "Does this service reach a predetermined standard?"	Designed to answer the question: "What standard does this service achieve?"
Addresses clearly defined questions, aims and objectives.	Measures against a standard.	Measures current service without reference to a standard.
Quantitative research – may involve evaluating or comparing interventions, particularly new ones. Qualitative research – usually involves studying how interventions and relationships are experienced.	Involves an intervention in use ONLY (the choice of treatment is that of the clinician and patient according to guidance, professional standards and/or patient preference).	Involves an intervention in use ONLY (the choice of treatment is that of the clinician and patient according to guidance, professional standards and/or patient preference).
Usually involves collecting data that are additional to those for routine care, but may include data collected routinely. May involve treatments, samples or investigations additional to routine care.	Usually involves analysis of existing data, but may include administration of simple interview or questionnaire.	Usually involves analysis of existing data, but may include administration of simple interview or questionnaire.
Quantitative research – study design may involve allocating patients to intervention groups. Qualitative research uses a clearly defined sampling framework underpinned by conceptual or theoretical justifications.	No allocation to intervention groups: the healthcare professional and patient have chosen intervention before clinical audit.	No allocation to intervention groups: the healthcare professional and patient have chosen intervention before service evaluation.
May involve randomisation.	No randomisation.	No randomisation.
ALTHOUGH ANY OF THESE THREE MAY RAISE ETHICAL ISSUES, UNDER CURRENT GUIDANCE:-		
RESEARCH REQUIRES REC REVIEW	**AUDIT DOES NOT REQUIRE REC REVIEW**	**SERVICE EVALUATION DOES NOT REQUIRE REC REVIEW**

national research ethics service (2008).

Further reading

Book

Webb P. (2005) *Ethical Issues in Palliative Care*. Oxford: Radcliffe Publishing.

Articles

de Raeve L. (1994) Ethical issues in palliative care research. *Palliative Medicine*, **8**(4): 298–305.

Hardy J. R. (1997) Placebo-controlled trials in palliative care: the argument for. *Palliative Medicine*, **11**(5): 415–18.

Jordhoy M. S., *et al.* (1999) Challenges in palliative care research; recruitment, attrition and compliance: experience from a randomized controlled trial. *Palliative Medicine*, **13**(4): 299–310.

Keeley P. W. (2008) Improving the evidence base in palliative medicine: a moral imperative. *Journal of Medical Ethics*, **34**: 757–60.

Kirkham S. R., Abel J. (1997) Placebo-controlled trials in palliative care: the argument against. *Palliative Medicine* **11**(6): 489–92.

Kuper A. *et al.* (2008) An Introduction to reading and appraising qualitative research. *British Medical Journal*, **337**: 404–7.

Payne S. A. (2008) Research methodologies in palliative care: a bibliometric analysis. *Palliative Medicine*, **22**: 4: 336–43.

Sackett D. L., *et al.* (1996) Evidence based medicine: what it is and what it isn't. *British Medical Journal*, **312**(7023): 71–2.

Terry W., *et al.* (2006) Hospice patients' views on research in palliative care. *Internal Medicine Journal*, **36**(7): 406–13.

White C. (2008) Gatekeeping from palliative care research trials. *Progress in Palliative Care*, **16**: 4: 167–7.

Williams C. J., *et al.* (2006) Interest in research participation among hospice patients, caregivers, and ambulatory senior citizens: practical barriers or ethical constraints? *Journal of Palliative Medicine*, **9**(4): 968–74.

Leaflet

National research Ethics Service (2008)

Defining research (Issue 3). Available at www.nres.npsa.nns.uk

Quality of life

If you really want to help somebody, first you must find out where he is. This is the secret of caring. If you cannot do that, it is only an illusion if you think you can help another human being. Helping someone implies your understanding more than he does, but first of all you must understand what he understands

Quality of life assessment in healthcare

Over the past 30 years, there has been a rapid growth in research on the impact of disease and treatment on the quality of life of patients. A search of PubMed reveals that in 1976, 229 articles were listed under the term 'quality of life'. The corresponding totals in 1986, 1996 and 2006 were 676, 3130 and 10116, respectively. Pressure to improve the cost-effectiveness of care, as well as an epidemiological shift from dealing with predominantly acute to predominantly chronic conditions, has highlighted the need to supplement traditional outcomes such as morbidity and mortality with subjective measures that focus on patients' experiences. A further factor has been the emergence of a post-modern society in which the values of equality, empowerment and autonomy have challenged the traditional paternalism of professions.

Researchers and clinicians have developed and tested hundreds of measures of patient experiences across a wide variety of conditions. These measures are known variously as 'Health status measures', 'Health-related quality of life (HRQoL) measures' or simply 'Quality of life measures'. Increasingly, the term 'Patient reported outcomes' (PROs) is used to refer to all subjective measures generated from patients. These measures occupy a continuum from highly standardized econometric methods, such as time-trade off and standard gamble, to individualized global measures. Each has it supporters, each involves different assumptions about the nature and interpretation of HRQoL and each has advantages and disadvantages. The research literature is now so vast and the available measures so numerous that it can be very confusing for anyone new to the field.

HRQoL measures

The development of HRQoL measures has been influenced by the World Health Organization (WHO) definition of health as: 'a state of complete physical, mental and social well-being and not merely the absence of disease or infirmity.' Most researchers (but not all), accept that there is a subcomponent of quality of life that is influenced by health and it is this we should concern ourselves with in healthcare. One widely used definition is that of Patrick and Erickson who defined HRQoL as: 'the value assigned to the duration of life as modified by the social opportunities, perceptions, functional states, and impairments that are influenced by disease, injuries, treatments, or policy'.

Most HRQoL measures are multidimensional and usually assess symptoms, physical functioning, psychological well-being and social functioning (Table 3b.1). The most common elements include:
- Physical symptoms such as nausea, vomiting, fatigue and pain
- Functional ability
- Sexuality, intimacy and bodily perception
- Emotional symptoms such as worry, anxiety and depression
- Social functioning
- Work life
- Family situation
- Hope for the future, future planning
- General life satisfaction

Rigorously designed questionnaires such as the EORTC measures or the SF36 are available that meet the requirements of reliability, validity, sensitivity and applicability. The aim is to collect standardized information often for use in clinical trials or epidemiological studies. However, the routine use of such scales in clinical practice, especially in palliative care, presents a number of problems. Much of the confusion in the HRQoL literature arises from the failure to distinguish between levels of care. The *micro* level is concerned with individual patients in clinical situations, the *meso* level is concerned with groups of patients as, for example, in a clinical trial or an institutional policy and the *macro* level is the level of decision-making that affects large communities. Selecting an appropriate measure of HRQoL depends on the level of analysis.

Table 3b.1 Uses of HRQoL assessments in oncology

1	To measure the impact of specific cancers and to describe the nature and extent of functional and psychosocial problems at various stages of the disease trajectory
2	To establish norms for psychological and social complications in specific patient populations
3	To screen individual patients for possible behavioural and/or pharmacological interventions
4	To monitor the quality of care in order to improve delivery
5	To evaluate the efficacy of competing medical, surgical or psychological interventions

Quality of life and palliative care

It is widely accepted that the essence of palliative care is maintaining and improving the quality of life of patients and their families. The WHO defines palliative care precisely in these terms. Therefore, the best strategy for dealing with patients in palliative care settings is simply to measure their quality of life and make sure that they receive integrated care to maximize it. However, that is easier said than done. Much of the research on quality of life in healthcare has been driven by experts in measurement and scale construction, and many of the studies have had an epidemiological or clinical trials focus rather than focusing on day to day clinical applications.

Challenges in measuring quality of life in palliative care

- What is the definition of quality of life and how does it differ from health-related quality of life or health status?
- How should informed consent be obtained?
- To what extent is it acceptable to burden the patient and the family?
- Given the need for research in palliative medicine, how should a doctor balance being overly protective (paternalistic) with being overly demanding?
- Given multisystem problems, limited survival and polypharmacy, what outcome measures, timing and study design should be used and how can compliance be maximized?
- How can studies deal with patient attrition?
- How can measures be designed to cope with 'floor' and 'ceiling' effects?
- What is the clinical significance of changes in the measures?

Quality of life measures in palliative care

There are many good measures now available for measuring health-related quality of life in cancer patients, but most of these have been developed for assessing the impact of the disease and its treatment in the 'pre-palliative' phases of the illness.

> ## Health-related quality-of-life scales commonly used in oncology and palliative care research
>
> **Instrument**
> *Generic health status measures*
> Short Form Health Survey (SF-36)
> Sickness Impact Profile
> Spitzer Quality of Life Index (QLI)
> Visual Analogue Scales
>
> *Cancer-specific measures*
> EORTC—QLQ-C30
> EORTC—Site-specific modules
> Functional Assessment of Cancer Therapy (FACT-G)
> Cancer Rehabilitation Evaluation System (CARES)
> Functional Living Index Cancer (FLIC)
> Quality of Life Index-Cancer
>
> *Palliative measures*
> EORTC QLQ-C15-PAL
> McGill Quality of Life Questionnaire (MQOL)
> Missoula-VITAS Quality of Life Index
> Edmonton Symptom Assessment Schedule
> Hospice Quality of Life Index (HQLI)

A number of measures have been designed specifically for palliative care settings, some of which are discussed below.

EORTC QLQ-C15-PAL

The EORTC QLQ-C30 was developed by the European Organization for Research and Treatment of Cancer Quality of Life for assessing HRQoL in clinical trials. It consists of 30 questions organized into 5 scales measuring function, 1 global health/overall quality-of-life scale, 3 scales measuring symptoms (fatigue, nausea, vomiting and pain) and 6 single questions on symptoms and financial difficulties. A shortened version of the measure, the EORTC QLQ-C15-PAL has recently been developed for use in palliative care.[1] Derived from interviews with 41 patients and 66 healthcare

1 Groenvold M., *et al.* for the EORTC Quality of Life Group (2006) The development of the EORTC QLQ-C15-PAL: A shortened questionnaire for cancer patients in palliative care. *European Journal of Cancer*, **42**: 55–64.

professionals in palliative care, the measure consists of scales measuring pain, physical function, emotional function, fatigue, global health status/quality of life, nausea/vomiting, appetite, dyspnoea, constipation and sleep.

The McGill Quality of Life Questionnaire (MQOL)

This scale was developed at McGill University specifically for use in all phases of the disease trajectory for people with a life-threatening illness. The questionnaire differs from most others in three ways: the existential domain is measured; the physical domain is important but not predominant; positive contributions to quality of life are measured. The scale generates scores on four subscales: physical symptoms, psychological symptoms, outlook on life and meaningful existence.

Missoula-VITAS Quality of Life Index

This is a 25-item scale for seriously ill patients aimed at measuring adaptation to and integration of their physical decline, as well as attainment of life tasks and life closure. The measure addresses five quality-of-life domains that are relevant to end-of-life care: symptom control, function, interpersonal issues, well-being and transcendence.

Individualized measures of quality of life

Questionnaire approaches to the measurement of quality of life provide important information. However, such measures have one particularly important limitation. They impose a predetermined external value system on the respondent. Someone other than the respondent has decided which questions to ask, which areas of life should be explored and what weights should be assigned to the respondent's answers to obtain a summary score. The weights are standardized and fixed and are generally derived from grouped data. Although these measures may be reliable, they may not be relevant to an individual's present life situation. Apparently similar behaviours do not have the same relevance or importance for all individuals. Furthermore, the relevance or importance of particular behaviours or events is unlikely to remain static for a given individual with the passage of time or over the course of an illness.

In assessing quality of life in a clinical situation, one needs to know, at a given time, what particular issues are of most concern to the patient. Individuals, even when seriously ill, are active agents, engaged in an unfolding life-cycle, involved in a continuous search for meaning and constantly striving towards the goal of self-actualization. Only individuals can judge their own experiences and they do so in the context of their own expectations, hopes, fears, values and beliefs. To quote the psychotherapist Karl Rogers, 'the best vantage point for understanding behaviour is from the internal frame of reference of the individual himself'. In order to obtain a valid measurement of quality of life, as opposed to health status, a measure is needed that evaluates each individual on the basis of the areas of life that he or she considers to be most important, quantifies current functioning in each of these personally nominated life areas, and weights their relative importance for that individual at that particular time. A life area that is going badly for an individual but is of little importance to him or her clearly has less implication for that individual's quality of life than a life area that is going badly but is of great importance. HRQoL measures can be supplemented by individualized QoL measures. Much is to be gained in the clinical situation from finding out what areas of life are important to the patient, the relative importance of each and the level of functioning or satisfaction with each.

Individualized measures of QoL

Schedule for Evaluation of Individual Quality of Life (SEIQoL)

The SEIQoL was developed based on the argument that quality of life can be defined only by the individual whose life is being assessed. In a semi-structured interview, respondents are asked to nominate the five areas (cues) of their lives most important to their overall quality of life. They then rate their level of satisfaction with each on a 100 mm visual analogue scale. Finally, they are asked to judge the overall quality of life they would associate with 30 scenarios incorporating their own cues. This provides a measure of the relative importance or weight of each cue.

SEIQoL DW

The elicitation of cues and levels of satisfaction is the same as that used in the full SEIQoL. The direct weighting instrument is a simple apparatus consisting of five interlocking, coloured circular disks that can be rotated around a central point to form a type of pie chart. The disks are mounted on a larger backing disk, which displays a scale from 0 to 100, and from which the relative size of each coloured segment can be read. Each segment is labelled with one cue and the respondent adjusts the disks until the size of each coloured segment corresponds to the relative importance of the cue represented by that segment.

Patient Generated Index (PGI)

The PGI presents patients with either a list of quality-of life-areas (ingredients) that are most frequently mentioned by patients with the particular disease, or asks them to generate the ingredients themselves. After selecting the five most important areas, patients are asked to rate how badly affected by their condition each is. Patients are then asked to prioritize, using a fixed number of hypothetical points, the areas they would like most to improve.

Anamnestic Comparative Self Assessment (ACSA)

This is a single scale in which the respondents rate their overall well-being on a scale ranging from +5 to −5. The anchors are defined by respondents' memories of the best and the worst period in their lives.

Proxy ratings of HRQoL

Early attempts to measure HRQoL in patients with advanced incurable disease relied heavily on proxy ratings, the underlying assumption being that those patients would not be able to make such assessments themselves. It is now well established that HRQoL is subjective and the ratings provided by healthcare personnel and even by close family often do not tally with the ratings of patients. The consensus, based on research findings, is that:

1 Health professionals and significant others underestimate patients' quality of life to a significant and comparable degree
2 Healthcare providers tend to underestimate pain intensity
3 Proxy ratings appear to be more accurate when the information sought is concrete and observable

4 While the ratings of significant others tend to be more accurate when they live in close proximity to the patients, ratings can be biased by the caregiving function of the rater

These findings are hardly surprising. Health professionals evaluate patients using their own particular paradigm and this is different from that used by the patient who is experiencing the condition. Even carers who know the patient very well may be applying a particular paradigm that, again, does not tally with that of the patient. Furthermore, patients are not passive in the face of their changing circumstances but use a wide range of coping processes. Findings such as the above, highlight the importance of maintaining ongoing and excellent communication between patients, carers and health professionals.

Adaptation and response shift

The Greek philosopher Heraclitus famously said 'You cannot step in the same river twice...all is flux....all is becoming...both you and the river are changed.' There is now considerable interest in HRQoL research in exploring the psychological mechanisms by which patients adapt to their illness. Patients' judgements of their health may stay relatively stable despite large changes in objective measures of health, or their judgement of health may change in a situation where there is little or no objective change. This phenomenon, which is increasingly known as 'response shift', is due to the fact that patients may change the criteria they use to make their judgements. For example, a patient's judgement of his or her health might remain stable despite objective evidence of worsening cancer because, in the course of treatment, they may have seen others who are far worse off. Response shift can help to explain apparently paradoxical findings in the health literature such as:

- Patients with chronic diseases often rate their quality of life at a level similar to that of non-patients
- Patients tend to rate their quality of life higher than do health professionals or carers
- There are usually marked discrepancies between objective measures of health and self-rated health or quality of life

The important thing to remember is that patients are actively engaged in trying to cope with their condition and that they will use a variety of coping mechanisms to make their journey more meaningful and more bearable. Health professionals who have the motivation and the communication skills to share the patient's world view by focusing, not only on the objective indicators of disease, but also on the quality of life of the individual patient can have the privilege of walking part of that journey with the patient. In Kierkegaard's words they will have discovered the 'secret of caring'.

Further reading

Books

Fayers P., Hays R. (eds) (2005) *Assessing Quality of Life in Clinical Trials*. Oxford: Oxford University Press.

Joyce C. R. B., McGee H. M., O'Boyle C. A. (eds) (1999) *Individualised Quality of Life: Approaches to Conceptualisation and Assessment*. Amsterdam: Harwood Academic Publishers.

Schwartz C. E., Sprangers M. A. G. (2000) *Adaptation to Changing Health: Response Shift in Quality-of-Life Research*. Washington: American Psychological Association.

Articles

Cohen S. R., *et al.* (1995) The McGill Quality of Life Questionnaire: a measure of quality of life appropriate for people with advanced disease. A preliminary study of validity and acceptability. *Palliative Medicine*, **9**: 207–19.

Kaasa S., Loge J. H. (2002) Quality of life assessment in palliative care. *Lancet Oncology*, **3**: 175–82.

Osoba D. (2002) A taxonomy of the uses of health-related quality-of-life instruments in cancer care and the clinical meaningfulness of the results. *Medical Care*, **40**, (6): Suppl. III-31–III-38.

Rees J., O'Boyle C. A., McDonagh R. (2001) Quality of life; impact of chronic illness on the partner. *Journal of the Royal Society of Medicine*, **94**(11): 563–6.

Schwartz C. E., Sprangers M. A. G. (2002) An introduction to quality of life assessment in oncology: the value of measuring patient-reported outcomes. *American Journal of Managed Care*, **8**(18): S550–S559.

Principles of drug use in palliative care[1]

> We can no more hope to end drug abuse by eliminating heroin and cocaine than we could alter the suicide rate by outlawing high buildings or the sale of rope.
>
> Ben Whittaker, *The Global Fix*, 1987

Introduction

Drugs are not the total answer for the relief of pain and other symptoms. For many symptoms, the concurrent use of non-drug measures is equally important, and sometimes more so. Further, drugs must always be used within the context of a systematic approach to symptom management, namely:

- Evaluation
- Explanation
- Individualized treatment
- Attention to detail

In palliative care, the axiom 'diagnosis before treatment' still holds true. A particular symptom may have different causes, e.g. in lung cancer vomiting may be caused by hypercalcaemia or by raised intracranial pressure. Clearly, treatment will vary according to the cause.

Attention to detail includes *precision in taking a drug history*. It is important to ascertain, as precisely as possible, the drug being taken, the dose and the frequency and to confirm that the drug alleviates the symptom throughout the day and night. It is very common for patients to be non-compliant with medication for many different reasons. In palliative care, patients may not have understood the reason for taking medication regularly to prevent symptoms. The medication (e.g. analgesic) consequently may not help adequately, leaving him/her either to suffer in pain, thinking that the drug does not work, or to take inappropriately large extra doses which cause side-effects. Patients may also stop taking the drugs because of the side-effects. Vicious circles may develop, adding to patient and family despair. As the patient becomes weaker and less well they may become less able to swallow large numbers of tablets, leading again to less than optimal symptom control.

---

[1] General guidance about the use of drugs in palliative care (www.palliativedrugs.com).

Attention to detail also means *providing clear instructions for drug regimens*. 'Take as much as you like, as often as you like', is a recipe for anxiety and poor symptom relief. The drug regimen should be written out in full for the patient and his family to work from (Fig. 4.1). This should be in an ordered and logical way, e.g. analgesics, antiemetics, laxatives, followed by other drugs. The drug name, times to be taken, reason for use ('for pain', 'for bowels', etc.) and dose (x mL, y tablets) should all be stated. The patient should also be advised how to obtain further supplies, e.g. from their GP.

When prescribing an additional drug, it is important to ask:
- What is the treatment goal?
- How can it be monitored?
- What is the risk of adverse effects?
- What is the risk of drug interactions?
- Is it possible to stop any of the current medications?

Good prescribing is a skill, and makes the difference between poor and excellent symptom control. It extends to considering the size, shape and taste of tablets and solutions; and avoiding awkward doses which force:
- Patients to take more tablets than would be the case if doses were 'rounded up' to a more convenient tablet size. For example, it is better to prescribe m/r morphine 60mg (a single tablet) rather than 50mg (3 tablets: 30mg + 10mg + 10mg)
- Nurses to spend more time refilling syringes for 24h infusions. For example, in the UK, it might be appropriate to prescribe diamorphine 100mg (a single 100mg ampoule) instead of 95mg (3 × 30mg ampoule + 5mg ampoule)

It is necessary to be equally thorough when re-evaluating a patient and supervising treatment, because it is often difficult to predict the optimum dose of a symptom relief drug, particularly opioids, laxatives and psycho-tropic drugs. Some drugs, e.g. steroids, may be given as a trial only and continued or stopped as appropriate after a certain time. Arrangements must be made, therefore, for continuing supervision and adjustment of medication.

Finally, it may be necessary to compromise on complete symptom relief in order to avoid unacceptable adverse effects. For example, the sedative side-effects of levomepromazine or the dry mouth caused by octreotide may limit dose escalation in inoperable bowel obstruction. The patient may prefer to reduce the frequency of nausea or vomiting to an accept-able level (i.e. vomit once a day) rather than to tolerate side-effects of higher doses of effective medication.

The drugs mentioned in this text are listed alphabetically in the Formulary and are based on as robust evidence as is currently available. Many of these drugs are used outside their current product licences.

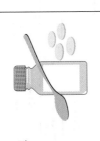

Medication
Information
Chart

Patient details/Identification label

Mr Albert Brown

1 Park Road

Anytown AB1 2CD

General Advice

- Keep this chart with you so that you can show your doctor or nurse a list of your medications.
- If you need a further supply, give your GP at least *48h* notice.
- If your chemist has difficulty in obtaining your medicines, please ask him to contact the palliative care pharmacist, on tel:.............. or in the evening/at weekends contact the on-call pharmacist at............ Hospital via the switchboard on tel:.............
- Occasionally your medication may be supplied in different strengths or presentations. If you have any concerns about this, check with your local pharmacist or district nurse.
- If you need to see a doctor, telephone your GP first unless advised otherwise.
- If you, or your family doctor, need any advice, please ring tel:............... and ask to speak to the Hospice Community *Team nurse.*

Regular Medication	STRENGTH	REASON	WHEN TO TAKE				
Description (Trade Name)			ON WAKING	LUNCH 2pm	TEA 6pm	BED TIME	
Morphine Sulphate MR (MST) Purple tablet	30mg	Pain Relief * take 12 h apart *	1			1	
Diclofenac Round brown tablet	50mg	Bone Pain	1		1	1	
Sodium Valproate (Epilim) Lilac tablet	200mg	Nerve Pain				2	
Co-danthramer Orange liquid	5 rows	Gas Bowels			TWO 5ml spoons		
Domperidone (Motilium) Small white tablet	10mg	Stop Sickness	2	2	2	2	
As Needed							
Morphine Solution (Oramorph) Clear liquid	10mg in 5ml	Breakthrough Pain	Take ONE 5ml spoon every 2–4 h if needed				
Asilone suspension White liquid		Indigestion	Take TWO 5ml spoonfuls FOUR times a day				

Completed by: *S Thorp*   Nurse/Pharmacist   Checked by *M Smith*   On: *24.2.05*

Fig. 4.1 Sample Medication Information Chart. Adapted with permission from HAYWARD HOUSE Macmillan Specialist Palliative Care Cancer Unit, Nottingham, UK.

The use of drugs beyond licence

If a lot of cures are suggested for a disease, it means that the disease is incurable.

Anton Chekhov, *The Cherry Orchard*, 1904

The Medicines and Healthcare Products Regulatory Agency in the UK grants a product licence for a medical drug. The purpose of the drug licence is to regulate the activity of the pharmaceutical company when marketing the drug. The licence does not restrict the prescription of the drug by properly qualified medical practitioners. Licensed drugs can be used legally in clinical situations that fall outside the remit of the licence (referred to as 'off-label'), for example a different age group, a different indication, a different dose or route or method of administration. Use of unlicensed drugs refers to those products that have no licence for any clinical situation or may be in the process of evaluation leading to such a licence.

A recent audit in palliative care found that 'off-label' use is common (around 25% of prescriptions affecting 66% of patients in one specialist palliative care unit), but the use of unlicensed drugs is rare. Recommendations from bodies such as the General Medical Council and the medical defence organizations place a duty on doctors to act responsibly and to provide information to patients on the nature and associated risks of any treatment, including 'off-label' and unlicensed drugs.

Guidance also recommends that such drugs are prescribed by a consultant or GP, following informed consent by the patient, and that this decision is recorded in the patient's notes. This may not be practical in palliative care where the use of 'off-label' medication is routine.

Prescribing outside the licence

In the UK, a doctor may legally:
- Prescribe unlicensed medicines
- In a named patient, use unlicensed products specially prepared, imported, or supplied
- Supply another doctor with an unlicensed medicine
- With appropriate safeguards, use unlicensed drugs in clinical trials
- Use or advise the use of licensed medicines for indications or in doses or by routes of administration outside the licensed recommendations
- Override the warnings and precautions given in the licence

The responsibility for the consequences of these actions lies with the prescribing doctor[1,2] or non-medical prescriber.

It has been recommended that when prescribing a drug outside its licence, a doctor or non-medical prescriber should:[3,4]

- Record in the patient's notes the reasons for the decision to prescribe outside the licensed indications
- Where possible explain the position to the patient (and family as appropriate) in sufficient detail to allow them to give informed consent (the Patient Information Leaflet obviously does not contain information about off label indications)
- Inform other professionals, e.g. pharmacist, nurses, GP, involved in the care of the patient to avoid misunderstandings

In addition to clinical trials, prescriptions beyond licence may be justified:

- When prescribing generic formulations (for which indications are not described)
- With established drugs for proven but unlicensed indications
- With drugs for conditions for which there are no other treatments (even in the absence of strong evidence)
- When using drugs in individuals not covered by licensed indications, e.g. children

1 Anonymous (1992) Prescribing unlicensed drugs or using drugs for unlicensed applications. *Drug and Therapeutics Bulletin*, **30**: 97–9.

2 Cohen P. J. (1997) Off-label use of prescription drugs: legal, clinical and policy considerations. *European Journal of Anaesthesiology*, **14**: 231–50.

3 Atkinson C. V., Kirkham S. R. (1999) Unlicensed uses for medication in a palliative care unit. *Palliative Medicine*, **13**: 145–52.

4 The Association of Palliative Medicine, The Pain Society (2002) *The Use of Drugs Beyond Licence in Palliative Care and Pain Management*. Southampton and London: APM and Pain Society.

Drug interactions in palliative care

> It may seem a strange principle to enunciate as the very first require-
> ment in a hospital that it should do the sick no harm.
>
> Florence Nightingale, *Notes on Hospitals*, 1863

The potential for drug interactions is high in palliative care due to polypharmacy.

Cytochrome P450 isoenzymes

Metabolism of drugs in the liver principally involves oxidation or conjuga-
tion. There are several types of oxidation reactions, each catalysed by a
group of enzymes called cytochrome P450. The most important isoenzymes are CYP3A4 and CYP2D6. Most drugs that are metabolized by
the liver are metabolized via several pathways, usually including the cytochrome P450 isoenzyme 3A4. Some drugs such as erythromycin and
clarithromycin, some SSRIs, cimetidine, grapefruit juice, amiodarone and
itraconazole inhibit CYP3A4 and therefore slow down the metabolism of
any other drugs that are metabolized by CYP3A4, which can increase the
effects of these other drugs. Drugs that may be affected because they are
metabolized by cytochrome 3A4 include warfarin, the dose of which may
need to be reduced when these drugs are started in combination with
the drugs outlined above. Other drugs metabolized by cytochrome 3A4
include phenytoin, carbamazepine, benzodiazepines and St John's Wort.

The following are some selected drug interactions which are pertinent to
palliative care prescribing:

Warfarin

The anticoagulation effect of warfarin can be affected by many drugs. Some
drugs such as amitriptyline may increase or reduce the anticoagulant effect
of warfarin. The anticoagulation effect may be reduced by St John's Wort.

Anticoagulation may increase with:

- amiodarone
- cimetidine, omeprazole
- erythromycin, clarithromycin,
  ciprofloxacin, metronidazole
- NSAIDs, aspirin
- cranberry juice
- paracetamol
- fluconazole, itraconazole,
  miconazole, ketoconazole
- clopidogrel
- possible effect with SSRIs,
  venlafaxine, mirtazepine
- tramadol

Amiodarone

Amiodarone has a long half-life. There is a potential for drug interactions to occur for several weeks (or even months) after treatment with it has been stopped. Drugs that interact with amiodarone may increase the risk of ventricular arrhythmias and the advice is to avoid them:

- tricyclic antidepressants (amitriptyline etc.)
- phenothiazines, haloperidol
- grapefruit juice
- flecainide
- quinine
- erythromycin (parenteral), co-trimoxazole

The low doses of haloperidol used as an antiemetic, and tricyclic antidepressants for neuropathic pain, used in palliative care, probably carry a reduced risk, but one that cannot be completely dismissed.

Anticonvulsants

Carbamazepine levels are increased (risk of toxicity) with e.g. clarithromycin, erythromycin, fluoxetine and cimetidine. There is also an increased risk of toxicity with hyponatraemia due for instance to diuretics. Carbamazepine reduces the plasma concentration of clonazepam and accelerates the metabolism of steroids. Anticonvulsant effects of carbamazepine are antagonized by antipsychotics.

Phenytoin levels are reduced by St John's Wort and may be increased or decreased by benzodiazepines. Phenytoin reduces the plasma concentration of mirtazepine and clonazepam and accelerates the metabolism of methadone, corticosteroids and ondansetron. The anticonvulsant effects of phenytoin may be antagonized by tricyclic antidepressants, SSRIs and antipsychotics. Absorption is reduced by antacids.
Phenytoin levels are increased (toxicity) by:

- amiodarone
- clarithromycin
- fluconazole, miconazole
- fluoxetine
- metronidazole
- cimetidine
- omeprazole
- trimethoprim

The management of patients with cerebral tumours may be affected since carbamazepine, phenytoin and phenobarbital can reduce the efficacy of corticosteroids.

Antifungal drugs

- Fluconazole increases phenytoin levels
- Fluconazole increases the effect of sulphonylureas, e.g. gliclazide, glibenclamide (risk of hypoglycaemia)
- Fluconazole inhibits the metabolism of alfentanil (watch opioid side-effects)
- Itraconazole and fluconazole increase sedation with midazolam
- Fluconazole and itraconazole enhance the anticoagulation effect of warfarin

Proton pump inhibitors (PPIs)
- Omeprazole may increase blood diazepam levels (increase in sedation)
- Omeprazole may enhance anticoagulation effect of warfarin

Metronidazole
- Disulfiram-like reaction with alcohol
- Enhances anticoagulation with warfarin
- Increases phenytoin blood levels (toxicity)

SSRI antidepressants
- Antagonize anticonvulsant effects of common antiepileptics and lower seizure threshold
- Care with drugs that can stimulate the CNS, e.g. selegeline, tramadol
- Interact with cytochrome P450 enzymes
- Serious reaction with MAOIs, selegiline (serotonin syndrome)
- Increased serotonergic effects with St John's Wort (avoid)

St John's Wort
- Increased serotonergic effects with SSRIs (avoid)
- Reduced plasma concentration of amitriptyline
- Reduced anticoagulant effect of warfarin
- Reduced plasma levels of carbamazepine, phenytoin, phenobarbital (risk of fits)
- Reduced plasma levels of digoxin

Torsades de pointes
An increasing number of drugs (such as haloperidol, ondansetron, SSRIs, erythromycin, ciprofloxacin) have been recognized to prolong the QT interval and potentially cause torsades de pointes, a serious ventricular tachycardia. A register of drugs that cause QT prolongation is available on the internet at http://www.torsades.org

Corticosteroids
The use of corticosteroids in palliative care varies considerably from unit to unit and physician to physician. Traditionally they have been used to reduce oedema, to promote appetite and well-being; and for their specific use in disease processes such as asthma, or chronic lymphatic leukaemia, or in emergency situations where their use can buy time until a more definitive treatment can be instituted.

Corticosteroids are produced by the adrenal gland and have a number of physiological roles, including catabolic effects on protein, carbohydrate and fat metabolism, and anti-inflammatory effects. They influence water and electrolyte balance and suppress immunity.

Dexamethasone is the corticosteroid of choice in palliative care (Table 4b.1).

Table 4b.1 Indications and daily doses of dexamethasone

Indication for use	Daily dose of dexamethasone
Anorexia	2–4mg
Weakness	
Pain (where caused by tumoral oedema)	
Improvement in well-being/mood	
Nerve compression pain	4–8mg
Liver capsule pain	
Nausea	
Bowel obstruction	
Post-radiation inflammation	
Raised intracranial pressure	12–16mg
Superior vena caval obstruction	
Carcinomatosa lymphangitis	
Malignant spinal cord compression	

Side-effects of corticosteroids include a rise in blood glucose, increased susceptibility to infection (especially oral thrush), fluid retention and additive insult to the gastrointestinal mucosa with NSAIDs. Insomnia and agitation sometimes lead to a disturbed mental state.

Corticosteroids may also give rise to proximal myopathy, often manifesting as difficulty in standing from a sitting position. Classical cushingoid effects may develop, including a very frail skin which bleeds easily on contact. If patients are expected to be on long-term steroids (longer than 6 months or so), consideration may need to be given to prophylaxis for osteoporosis.

Equivalent anti-inflammatory effects of steroids:
• Prednisolone   5mg
• Hydrocortisone   20mg
• Methylprednisolone   4mg
• Dexamethasone   750mcg
• Cortisone acetate   25mg
• Betamethasone   750mcg
• Triamcinolone   4mg

Consider:
• Increasing the dose for patients on phenytoin, carbamazepine or phenobarbital
• Giving steroids before midday since they may disturb sleep
• Prophylactic gastric mucosal protection if also taking NSAIDs
• Switching from dexamethasone to prednisolone if myopathy develops
• The possibility that steroids may be masking the clinical signs of perforation of an abdominal viscus or sepsis

- Carefully weighing up the burden/benefit of continuing steroids subcutaneously should the patient become unable to swallow
- Checking blood glucose if any relevant symptoms occur

Always:
- Reduce dose of steroids to the minimum possible
- Review treatment every week, stopping after one week if no benefit
- Reduce dose slowly every few days if the patient has taken steroids for longer than two weeks or has been taking a relatively large dose

In the terminal care situation the patient's inability to swallow oral medication is often the provoking factor which leads to stopping steroids. Continuation of steroids by injection (usually SC) should be considered on an individual basis.

Side-effect risks of steroids

- Doses of dexamethasone >4mg o.d. are likely to lead to significant side-effects after several weeks
- Doses <4mg o.d. are often tolerated in patients with a prognosis of months
- Doses <4mg can be stopped abruptly IF used for less than three weeks

Reducing steroids

- Dexamethasone above 2mg daily—reduce by 2mg every 5–7 days (and check for symptoms before the next dose reduction), until reaching 2mg
- Dexamethasone doses of 2mg or less—reduce by 0.5mg every 5–7 days or on alternate days for a more conservative approach

Liver disease

Liver disease may alter drug metabolism and drug prescribing should therefore be kept to a minimum. The main problems occur in patients with jaundice, ascites or hepatic encephalopathy. Hepatic metabolism is the main route of elimination for many drugs, but the hepatic reserve is large and liver disease has to be severe before important changes in drug metabolism occur. Routine liver function tests are a poor guide to the capacity of the liver to metabolize drugs. Hypoalbuminaemia is associated with reduced protein binding and increased toxicity of some highly protein-bound drugs such as phenytoin and may also complicate the interpretation of plasma phenytoin levels. Reduced hepatic synthesis of blood-clotting factors increases the sensitivity to oral anticoagulants such as warfarin. All sedative drugs, diuretics that cause hypokalaemia (NB. use potassium-sparing diuretics), and opioid analgesics may further impair cerebral function and precipitate encephalopathy. Oedema and ascites may be exacerbated by drugs such as NSAIDs and corticosteroids which cause fluid retention. Biliary obstruction may prevent the excretion of some drugs, e.g. rifampicin, and the action of others, e.g. colestyramine.

Other drugs affected by liver dysfunction

Anxiolytics and hypnotics can precipitate coma. A small dose of oxazepam or temazepam is probably safest. The dose of zopiclone should be reduced and avoided in patients with severe liver disease. Clonazepam should be reduced in mild to moderate liver impairment and avoided if severe.

Antipsychotics can precipitate coma and phenothiazines are hepatotoxic.

Antidepressant drugs such as SSRIs should be dose-reduced or avoided. The sedative effects of tricyclic drugs are increased and should be avoided in severe liver disease.

Antiemetics such as cyclizine and domperidone should be avoided and metoclopramide used in reduced dose. Ondansetron should be used at a dose of not more than 8mg daily in moderate or severe liver failure.

Opioids; the liver is the major site of biotransformation for most opioids. The major metabolic pathway for most opioids including fentanyl/alfentanil is oxidation, although morphine and buprenorphine primarily undergo glucuronidation. Glucuronidation is rarely impaired in liver failure—which reflects clinical experience. Morphine is well tolerated in most patients with impaired hepatic function. There is evidence, however, that the plasma half-life of morphine may be significantly prolonged in patients with cirrhosis and liver failure. The bioavailability may be considerably higher and caution with oral morphine is needed.

Fentanyl/alfentanil should be titrated with care in severe liver disease. Modified release preparations of tramadol should be avoided in cirrhosis and smaller doses used.

Renal disease (📖 See Chapter 8d, p. 697)

Formulary

Drugs in **bold** can be given in a syringe driver 📖 See Table 4c.1, p.102

Drug	Route	Dose	Frequency	Indications/Side-effects/Remarks
Aprepitant	p.o.	80mg	o.d.	Neurokinin receptor antagonist used as adjunct to dexamethasone and ondansetron to prevent chemotherapy induced N&V
Alfentanil	**CSCI**	**Titrate**	**24h**	Synthetic opioid working on similar opioid receptors to fentanyl. Alternative CSCI-delivered opioid for patients unable to tolerate morphine. e.g. in renal failure. Half-life short so only provides effect for around an hour. Alfentanil spray 5mg/5mL is available for nasal or buccal use. Morphine 30mg **CSCI** ≡ alfentanil 2mg **CSCI**
Aminophylline m/r	p.o.	225–450mg	b.d.	Theophylline Reversible airways obstruction Theophylline concentration for optimal response is 55–110micromol/L Narrow therapeutic/toxicity margin Half-life increased in heart failure, the elderly, and with drugs such as erythromycin and ciprofloxacin. SE: Tachycardia, palpitations, nausea, CNS stimulation.
Amitriptyline	p.o.	10–50mg	nocte	Neuropathic pain. Start at 10–25mg. Faster effect at lower doses than for depression. Salivary dribbling (e.g. in MND). SE: Blurred vision, dry mouth, hypotension, sedation. Caution if cardiac disease, frail elderly or history of urinary retention
Artificial saliva	Spray, gel, pastilles		As required	Some products may contain mucin, an animal product not suitable for some religions
Arthotec (see also diclofenac)	p.o. p.o. (m/r)	50mg 75mg	t.d.s. b.d.	Contains diclofenac + misoprostol (for prophylaxis against NSAID induced gastro-duodenal ulceration). SE: Diarrhoea. May enhance the anticoagulation effect of warfarin

Baclofen	p.o.	5–10mg max. 100mg/day	t.d.s.	Spasticity i.e. in MND, MS. Increase dose slowly SE: sedation and weakness
Benzydamine	0.15% oral mouth wash/spray	15mL 4–8 sprays	1.5–3h	Local analgesic. Dilute with water if stings
Bethanechol	p.o..	25mg	t.d.s.	Dry mouth
Bicalutamide (Casodex)	p.o.	150mg	o.d.	Anti-androgen for prostate cancer With orchidectomy or gonadorelin therapy, start three days beforehand SE:, nausea, vomiting, depression, loss of libido, hot flushes
Bisacodyl	p.o. p.r.	5–10mg 10mg	nocte o.d.	Stimulant laxative. 5mg tabs—action 6–12h. 10mg Supps.—action 20–60 min Avoid in bowel obstruction
Bupivacaine	neb.	5mL 0.25%	6h	Useful for persistent dry cough, not breathlessness. Beware reflex bronchospasm. (Pretreat with nebulized salbutamol.) No food for one hour after treatment because of pharyngeal anaesthesia
Buprenorphine	SL	0.2–0.4mg	t.d.s.	0.4mg t.d.s. equivalent to 10–15mg morphine 4h Beware use in palliative care as it is a partial agonist, i.e. it can displace more effective opioids from their receptor sites
Buprenorphine (Transtec)	Transdermal matrix patch	35, 52.5, 70 mcg/n	96h	Maximum dose = 140mcg/h For breakthrough, buprenorphine SL, or other opioids can be used
Buprenorphine (Butrans)	Transdermal Matrix patch	5, 10, 20 mcg/n	Every seven days	20mcg/h equivalent to codeine 120–180mg/24h p.o.
Buscopan see Hyoscine butylbromide				

(Continued)

Drug	Route	Dose	Frequency	Indications/Side-effects/Remarks
Capsaicin	topical	0.075% cream	t.d.s.–q.d.s.	Neuropathic pain/post herpetic neuralgia. May cause stinging. Wear gloves to administer. Avoid contact with eyes and broken skin
Carbamazepine	p.o.	100–200mg	o.d.–b.d.	Generalized tonic–clonic seizures; neuropathic pain. Build up dose slowly. Check serum levels. Watch drug interactions. Tabs/chewtab/Supps. SE: Ataxia and blood, hepatic and skin disorders
Carbocisteine	p.o.	750mg	t.d.s.	Reduces sputum viscosity and increases expectoration. SE: Gastric irritant. Avoid if peptic ulceration
Chlorphenamine	p.o.	4mg	4–6h	Antihistamine. SE: Sedation.
Chlorpromazine	p.o. p.r.	25–50mg 100mg	o.d.–t.d.s. t.d.s.–q.d.s.	Severe agitation. Tenesmus (low dose). Hiccup (low dose). SE: sedative/hypotensive. Half dose in elderly. Supps. available by special order 100mg p.r ≡ 20–25mg IM ≡ 40–50mg p.o.
Citalopram	p.o.	20mg	o.d.	SSRI for depression, panic disorder Caution in epilepsy, cardiac disease and GI bleeding 10mg tab ≡ 8mg oral drops

Clonazepam	p.o.	0.5–2mg	nocte or b.d.	Neuropathic pain, anticonvulsant.
	csci	1–4mg	24h	May stick to plastic of syringe making titration difficult SE. Sedation
Co-codamol Weak 8/500 or 15/500 (Not recommended for palliative care patients)	p.o.	1–2 tabs	4–6h Max 8 in 24h	Codeine phosphate 8mg/15mg + paracetamol 500mg. Soluble preparations available. There is no evidence that 'weak co-codamol' is anymore efficacious in pain control than paracetamol alone.[6]
Co- codamol Strong 30/500	p.o.	1–2 tabs	4–6h Max 8 in 24h	Codeine phosphate 30mg + paracetamol 500mg e.g. Tylex, Solpadol. Soluble preparations available
Co-danthramer	p.o.	5–10mL 1–2 caps	nocte nocte	Stimulant (dantron) + softener (poloxamer) Useful for drug induced constipation. 'Strong' capsules and Susp. also available. SE: May colour urine red. Do not use if incontinent as is associated with burning of perineal skin and excoriation Not licensed for patients with non-malignant disease as dantron is a potential carcinogen.
Co-danthrusate	p.o.	5–15mL 1–3 caps	nocte nocte	Stimulant (dantron) + softener (docusate) See co-danthramer
Co-dydramol	p.o.	1–2	4–6h Max 8 in 24h	Dihydrocodeine 10mg + paracetamol 500mg. There are also combined preparations containing dihydrocodeine 20mg and 30mg

(Continued)

Drug	Route	Dose	Frequency	Indications/Side-effects/Remarks
Celecoxib	p.o	100mg	b.d.	NSAID- Cox-2 inhibitor Increased risk of myocardial infarction/stroke Lower risk of serious upper GI side effects than with non-selective NSAIDs
Colestyramine	p.o.	4–8g	o.d.	Anion-exchange resin, binding bile acids preventing their reabsorption Pruritus associated with biliary obstruction (not likely to be effective in complete biliary obstruction), diarrhoea associated with ileal resection/radiation SE: Constipation and nausea
Cyproterone Acetate	p.o.	300mg/24h	Divided doses	Anti-androgen Covers flare of initial gonadorelin therapy Watch for hepatotoxicity
Cyclizine	p.o. SC **CSCI**	25–50mg 25–50mg **100–150mg**	t.d.s. t.d.s. **24h**	Antihistamine. Useful for vomiting of GI cause, or raised intracranial pressure. SC route may cause skin reaction.
Dalteparin	SC SC	5000 units 200 units/kg	o.d. o.d.	Prophylaxis for DVT ** Low molecular weight heparin** Treatment of DVT and PE
Dexamethasone	p.o. IM/SC IV **CSCI**	Up to 16mg Up to 16mg Up to 16mg **Up to 16mg**	24h 24h 24h **24h**	2–4mg o.d. for appetite 8–16mg daily for raised intracranial pressure, SVCO, spinal cord compression. 2–6mg for prevention of chemotherapy emesis. Give a.m. to avoid excitation. Reduce dose ASAP. Watch glucose and proximal myopathy. Consider PPI prophylaxis in patients at risk of peptic ulceration or on NSAID or with additional risk factor Prescribe PPI if taking NSAID. Separate syringe driver.

Diamorphine	SC	Titrated	Strong opioid analgesic. More soluble than morphine.
	CSCI	**Titrated**	SC diamorphine is three times as potent as oral morphine.
	Topical	10mg	Modify dose in elderly patients and in patients with renal failure.
			SE: see pain section
			Mix in lidocaine gel or intrasite gel
Diazepam	p.o.	2–10mg	Anxiety; agitation; night sedation; breathlessness; convulsions. Alternative is SC midazolam
	p.r.	5–10mg	which is shorter acting.
		o.d.–t.d.s.	Caution in chronic respiratory disease
		p.r.n.	SE: Drowsiness, confusion, paradoxical increase in agitation
		(Supps. or	
		soln.)	
Diclofenac	p.o.	25–50mg	Bone pain and other inflammatory conditions if paracetamol and weak
	p.o.	75mg (m/r)	opioids found to be ineffective. May enhance the anticoagulant effect
	IM	75mg	of warfarin and caution required in patients with asthma. Increased risk of
	p.r.	100mg	thrombotic events
	CSCI	**up to 150mg**	If ineffective, try another NSAID. Contra-indicated with active peptic ulcer, GI bleeding
		t.d.s.	or renal failure. Consider PPI prophylaxis in patients at risk of peptic ulceration.
		b.d.	Use separate syringe driver. SE: Local irritation
		stat	
		o.d.	
		24h	
Digoxin	p.o.	62.5–500mcg	Supraventricular tachycardia especially atrial fibrillation
		(maintenance)	Reduce dose in elderly, and if reduced renal function.
		o.d.	Avoid if hypokalaemic
			SE: Anorexia, nausea, vomiting, diarrhoea, visual disturbance, abdominal pain, confusion.
			Do not give if ventricular rate is <60 beats per minute

(Continued)

Drug	Route	Dose	Frequency	Indications/Side-effects/Remarks
Dihydrocodeine	p.o. p.o. (m/r)	30–60mg 60–120mg	4–6h b.d.	Moderate pain. Similar efficacy to codeine orally—one tenth as potent as morphine. Increased risk of toxicity in renal failure, requires dose reduction to 8h. Anticipate constipation.
Disodium pamidronate	IV	30–90mg	In minimum 500mL sodium chloride 0.9% over 2–4h	Hypercalcaemia. Rehydrate first. max. dose rate 1mg/min. Dose according to corrected plasma calcium concentration. Repeat after one week if poor initial response. Bone pain (especially breast cancer and multiple myeloma). Takes 7 days to produce maximal effect which lasts 2–3 weeks. Repeat every 3–4 weeks as long as benefit maintained. Meticulous attention to dental care. Avoid teeth extractions after treatment commenced.
Docusate sodium	p.o.	100–200mg	b.d.	Softens stool. May help constipation in presence of partial bowel obstruction. Acts in 12–72h.
Domperidone	p.o. p.r.	10–20mg 30–60mg	6–8h 6–8h	Antiemetic, bowel motility stimulant. Beware intestinal obstruction as may cause colic. b.d. dosing may be adequate, 30mg PR = 10mg p.o., less extrapyramidal problems than with metoclopramide
Dosulepin	p.o.	50–150mg	o.d.	Tricyclic antidepressant Neuropathic pain: Use Lower doses starting at 10mg nocte. Depression: Use Higher doses from 50mg initially SE: lowers convulsion threshold, dry mouth, urine retention, constipation, blurred vision
Duloxetine	p.o	60mg	o.d.	Neuropathic Pain
Epoetin	SC	Seek specialist advice	Weekly	Recombinant human erythropoietin Anaemia associated with erythropoietin deficiency in chronic renal failure, cancer chemotherapy Aim to elevate haemoglobin at a rate not exceeding 2g/dL/month. Target Hb no more than 12g/dL: dose withheld if Hb ≥2g/dL in 1 month SE: Hypertension

Etamsylate	p.o.	500mg	q.d.s.	Useful for capillary bleeding in presence of normal platelet numbers.
Fentanyl	transdermal	12, 25, 50, 75, 100mcg/h	72h	Strong opioid for severe pain.

Due to slow onset of action, patients may need extra analgesia for up to 24h after fentanyl patch is started. Laxatives may be reduced, as causes less constipation than other opioids. On removal of patch it may take 17h or more for plasma levels to drop by 50%.

Unsuitable for unstable pain due to slow onset of action.

Conversion:

Daily oral morphine mg	Fentanyl patch delivery mcg/h
50–130	25
135–224	50
225–314	75
315–404	100
405–494	125

Caution: when changing from transdermal fentanyl to morphine; use lower morphine dose.

Beware different bioavailability of generic fentanyl patches. It may be safer to prescribe a proprietary product

Some evidence that patients on anticonvulsants may need increased doses.

(Continued)

Drug	Route	Dose	Frequency	Indications/Side-effects/Remarks
Fentanyl	OTFC Lozenge	200, 400, 600, 800, 1200 mcg	For breakthrough pain	Dose of breakthrough analgesia with OTFC is not related to background analgesic dose so start with 200mcg. Mouth needs to be moist (See page 253–254)
Fluconazole	p.o.	50mg	o.d.	Oral Candidiasis. Give 7–14 day course
Fludrocortisone	p.o.	50–300mcg	o.d.	Mineralocorticoid Postural hypotension Adrenal replacement with hydrocortisone
Fluoxetine	p.o.	20mg	mane	Enervating antidepressant. Long half-life (5 weeks) SE: anxiety. GI symptoms usually settle within a few days
Gabapentin	p.o.	Starting dose 100–300mg Doses above 1800mg/24h need specialist attention.	Initially nocte then t.d.s.	Neuropathic pain. Anticonvulsant. Higher benefit/side-effect ratio than most other agents used for neuropathic pain. Use lower dosing in elderly and if renal failure present. Avoid in psychotic illness BNF recommends 300mg day 1, 300mg b.d. day 2, 300mg t.d.s. day 3, then titrate according to response in 300mg steps to max. of 1.8mg/day. Slower titration over several weeks is advisable in debilitated, elderly patients and those with renal impairment or receiving CNS depressant drugs Avoid abrupt withdrawal. (Withdraw over 1 week.) SE: drowsiness, fatigue, ataxia
Gliclazide i/r ml/r	p.o. p.o.	40–80mg 30mg (equivalent to 80mg i/r)	o.d. o.d. max 120mg/24h	Sulphonylurea SE: Weight gain, hypoglycaemia, GI upset.
Glycopyrronium	p.o. cscı SC	0.2–0.4mg **0.6–1.2mg** 0.2–0.4mg	t.d.s. **24h** t.d.s.	Dries secretions. Used for drooling, death rattle and antispasmodic/inoperable bowel obstruction. Probably less central and/or cardiac side-effects than atropine or hyoscine hydrobromide.

Goserelin (Zoladex, Zoladex LA)	Implant (long acting)	10.8mg	Every 12 weeks	Gonadorelin analogue used in prostate breast cancer. Implant in anterior abdominal wall. 'Flare' of androgen release when starting therapy can lead to increased activity of disease. Symptoms such as back pain need to be taken very seriously if there are known spinal metastases, since spinal cord compression can be precipitated. (Flare can be minimized with an anti-androgen, such as cyproterone acetate)
	implant	3.6mg	Every 4 weeks	
Granisetron	p.o.	1–2mg	o.d.	Serotonin (5HT3) antagonist. Nausea/vomiting especially post RT or C/T patch available soon. SE: Constipation
Haloperidol	p.o.	0.5–10mg	o.n.	Antiemetic. Small doses (e.g. 1.5mg–3mg o.n.) for nausea, particularly drug or metabolic induced.
	SC	2.5–10mg	o.d.–b.d.	Higher doses in psychosis and agitation. The management of delirium or psychosis should be distinguished from the long-term treatment of behavioural disturbance in dementia for which antipsychotics should be regarded as the last resort.
	CSCI	**3–10mg**	**24h**	Beware extrapyramidal side-effects and avoid in Parkinson's disease
Hydromorphone i/r	p.o.	Titrated	4h	Alternative strong opioid. Caps. i/r 1.3, 2.6mg x 7.5 potency of morphine; i.e. 1.3mg hydromorphone = 10mg morphine
Hydromorphone m/r	p.o.	Titrated	b.d.	Caps. m/r 2, 4, 8, 16, 24mg (12h)

hydromorphone (mg)   morphine (mg)

hydromorphone (mg)	morphine (mg)
2	15
4	30
8	60
16	120
24	180

(Continued)

Drug	Route	Dose	Frequency	Indications/Side-effects/Remarks
Hydromorphone inj	CSCI	Titrated	24h	10mg/mL, 20mg/mL, 50mg/mL
	SC		4h	× 7.5 the potency of morphine Conversion factors from oral hydromorphone to SC hydromorphone. Reported range from equipotent to 3:1 Available as a 'special' from Martindale Pharmaceuticals
Hyoscine butylbromide (*Buscopan*)	CSCI	60–120mg (Intestinal obstruction) 20–60mg (reduce bronchial secretions)	24h	Antimuscarinic, anticholinergic. Less sedating than hyoscine hydrobromide as does not cross blood brain barrier. Uses: intestinal colic, reduces GI and bronchial secretions Very short half-life **Poor oral bioavailability**
	SC	10–20mg	4h p.r.n.	
Hyoscine hydrobromide	SC	0.4mg	4–8h	Antimuscarinic, anticholinergic
	CSCI	1.2–2.4mg	24h	Antiemetic for refractory nausea
	SL patch	0.3mg 1 patch (1mg)	6h p.r.n. Change every 72h	Dries respiratory and GI secretions, second line to glycopyrronium SE: sedation, confusion, paradoxical agitation
Ibandronic acid	p.o.	50mg	o.d.	Bisphosphonate. Reduction of bone resorption in bone metastases in breast cancer and myeloma. Avoid dental extraction during treatment. Monitor calcium and renal function.
	IV	2–6mg		
Ibuprofen	p.o.	200–600mg	t.d.s.	First line NSAID. Lower risk of side-effects than with other commonly used NSAIDs. Topical preparations available. See diclofenac for contra-indications. SE: Oesophageal irritation with oral preparation.

Ipratropium bromide	Neb.	0.25–0.5mg	6h	Reversible airways obstruction, particularly if COPD present. Drying effect on secretions. Avoid solution reaching the eyes
Ketamine	p.o.	10–100mg	t.d.s./q.d.s.	Under specialist supervision only. Neuropathic pain; build up dose slowly. May need prophylactic oral haloperidol 3mg nocte or a benzodiazepine to cover psychotomimetic side-effects.
	CSCI	75–300mg (Higher doses have been reported)	24h	Oral solution available. May need to reduce opioids by 50%. Use separate syringe driver. Caution: epilepsy, BP↑, heart disease
Ketorolac	p.o.	10mg	4–6h (elderly 6–8h)	Bone pain and other inflammatory conditions. Max 40mg p.o. daily. Max 90mg sc daily. See diclofenac warnings and cautions. Beware gastric bleeding. Use separate syringe driver
	sc	10–30mg	4–6h	
	CSCI	60–90mg	24h	High risk of Gastric side effects; Use gastric protection (PPI)
Lactulose	p.o.	15–30mL	b.d.	Osmotic laxative. May cause abdominal bloating and wind. Requires a good fluid intake May take 48h for full effect.
Lansoprazole	p.o.	30mg	o.d.	Proton pump inhibitor. Gastric and duodenal ulcer and oesophagitis Prophylaxis with NSAIDs and corticosteroids. Orodispersible tablet available.

(Continued)

Drug	Route	Dose	Frequency	Indications/Side-effects/Remarks
Levomepromazine	p.o.	6.25–25mg (6.25mg = 1/4 Tab.)	o.d.–b.d.	**Nausea and vomiting.** Broad-spectrum 'second line' antiemetic. 25mg tabs; 6mg tabs available on a named patient basis SE: Sedation
	sc	6.25–25mg	4–8 h	sc route may cause skin reaction
	CSCI	**6.25–25mg**	**24h**	Dilute with sodium chloride 0.9% There is a 2:1 oral: sc conversion ratio
Levomepromazine	p.o.	6.25–200mg	o.d.–b.d.	**Psychosis or severe agitation.** Used occasionally in terminal phase to help reduce distress and agitation. SE: May cause anticholinergic side-effects, hypotension and extrapyramidal symptoms. Can reduce the fit threshold
	CSCI	**25–150mg**	**24h**	sc route may cause skin reaction. Dilute with sodium chloride 0.9%. Avoid in Parkinson's disease
Lidocaine (lignocaine)	Topical	5% ointment 5% plaster		Topical analgesia Apply no more than three to cover painful area once a day for up to 12 h within each 24 h
Lithium (Carbonate/citrate)	p.o.	Dose adjusted to individual patient		Treatment and prophylaxis of mania, bipolar disorder, recurrent depression. Narrow therapeutic/toxic window. Target serum lithium concentration 0.4–1mmol/L, 12h after a dose. Requires regular monitoring. SE: GI upsets, tremor, renal impairment, oedema, blurred vision, drowsiness. Worse if sodium depleted, so beware if using diuretics. Drug interactions: Numerous—check each medicine.

Lofepramine	p.o.	140–210mg	Divided doses	Antidepressant Lower incidence of antimuscarinic side-effects than amitriptyline
Loperamide	p.o.	2–4mg max. 16mg/24h	t.d.s. or with each loose stool	Useful for diarrhoea and the pain of bowel colic. May need to increase to twice recommended dose (32mg) No CNS effects. Ensure diarrhoea not secondary to faecal impaction
Loratadine	p.o.	10mg	o.d.	Non-sedating antihistamine
Lorazepam	p.o./SL	0.5–2mg	b.d.	Anxiety/panic attacks. Shorter duration of action than diazepam. Useful sublingually in acute anxiety and breathlessness.
Macrogols (polyethylene glycols) (Movicol)	p.o.	Dissolve sachet in 125mL water	1–3 sachets/day up to 8 sachets/day for faecal impaction	Licensed for faecal impaction.
Medroxyprogesterone acetate	p.o.	400mg	o.d.–b.d.	**Appetite stimulation in anorexia.** Effect enhanced with concurrent NSAID Takes 2–3 weeks to produce maximal effect. **Hot flushes** after surgical or chemical castration SE Weight gain, DVT, male impotance
	p.o.	5–20mg	b.d.–q.d.s.	
Megestrol acetate	p.o.	80–160mg	o.m.	See Medroxyprogesterone acetate

(Continued)

Drug	Route	Dose	Frequency	Indications/Side-effects/Remarks
Methadone	p.o.	Titrated	b.d.–t.d.s	May be used for nociceptive and possibly neuropathic pain if no longer responsive to/tolerant of morphine.
	s.c.	Titrated	b.d.–t.d.s	Long half-life.
	CSCI	**Titrated**	**24h**	Subcutaneously, use 50–70% oral dose. Can be used in renal failure. Prescribed differently from morphine, see pain chapter: SE: Long 1/2 life can lead to overdosing
Methotrimeprazine, see levomepromazine				
Methylnaltrexone	s.c.	8–12mg depending on weight		Opioid antagonist for reversal of GI tract effects only. Bowel action 30–60mins after dose. 🕮 See p. 320
Methylphenidate	p.o.	5mg	o.d.–b.d.	Similar to dexamfetamine but less potent and shorter half life. Uses: Opioid-induced drowsiness, depression in terminal illness SE: restlessness, confusion, sleep disturbance
Metoclopramide	p.o.	10–20mg	q.d.s.	Antiemetic,
	p.o.(m/r)	15mg	b.d.	Increases gut motility and gastric emptying.
	SC	10–20mg	q.d.s.	Use cautiously in GI obstruction. Stop if makes GI cramps or diarrhoea worse.
	CSCI	**30–90mg**	**24h**	SE: Extrapyramidal side-effects, (reversible with procyclidine)
Metronidazole	p.o.	400mg	t.d.s.	Antibiotic for anaerobic infections.
	topical		t.d.s.	Topically useful for fungating, odorous wounds
	p.r.	500mg	t.d.s.	200mg tablet crushed in lubricating gel SE: Nausea
Midazolam	SC	2.5–5mg	p.r.n.	Benzodiazepine. Shorter duration of action than diazepam. Buccal liquid available
	Buccal	10mg		Single doses useful for quick, uncomfortable procedures, anxiety and agitation.
	intranasal			Used in the management of terminal agitation. A dose of 20–30mg/24h needed to
	CSCI	**10–60mg**	**24h**	replace oral antiepileptics.

Mirtazepine	p.o.	15–45mg titrate	Nocte	Noradrenergic and specific serotoninergic antidepressant (NaSSA). Some evidence of faster onset of action and promotion of appetite and sleep than other newer antidepressants. (Lower doses more sedating than higher, enervating doses)
Morphine (i/r)	p.o. p.r. Topical	Titrated Titrated	4h 4h	Pain/breathlessness. Oramorph 10mg/5mL, 100mg/5mL. Sevredol tabs; 10mg, 20mg, 50mg. Supps. 10, 15, 20, 30mg 10mg in 10mL intrasite gel SE:constipation, N&V, drowsiness, jerks etc.
Morphine (m/r)	p.o.	Titrated	12h	MST continus 5, 10, 15, 30, 60, 100, 200mg. (b.d.) MST Susp. 20, 30, 60, 100, 200mg (sachets). (b.d.) Zomorph 10, 30, 60, 100, 200mg. (b.d.)
Morphine (m/r)	p.o.	Titrated	24h	MXL 30, 60, 90, 120, 150, 200mg.(o.d.)
Morphine inj	SC **CSCI**	Titrated **Titrated**	4h **24h**	Conversion: p.o. to sc 2:1.
Nabilone	p.o.	1mg	b.d.	Cannabinoid for Breathlessness, nausea, spasticity and paraneoplastic night sweats. Oral solution can be made up SE: Sedation/dysphoria may occur with higher doses. Unsuitable in atrial fibrillation, heart failure & psychosis
Naloxone	IV IM/SC	0.1–0.2mg 0.1–0.2mg	every 2min every 2min	Reversal of opioid-induced respiratory depression. Beware return of severe pain. If resp. rate < 8/min and hard to rouse, mix Ampoule of 400mcg naloxone with 10mL of 0.9% NaCl and give 0.5mL iv every 2 minutes titrating response. Beware that treating opioid-induced respiratory depression may require repeated dosing and close monitoring for several hours.

(Continued)

Drug	Route	Dose	Frequency	Indications/Side-effects/Remarks
Naproxen	p.o.	250–500mg	b.d.	Bone pain and other inflammatory conditions. If ineffective, try another NSAID. Beware with warfarin and in patients who are asthmatic. Contra-indicated with active peptic ulcer or GI bleeding See diclofenac for warnings and cautions. No increase in thrombotic events compared with other commonly used NSAIDs
Nifedipine	p.o. SL	5–10mg 5mg	t.d.s. t.d.s.	Smooth muscle relaxant; useful for hiccups, oesophageal spasm and tenesmus. SE: Hypotension, peripheral oedema, headache. Patients with angina should not bite into or use a normal release capsule
Nystatin	p.o.	1–5mL 100,000 u/mL	q.d.s.	Oral Candidiasis Encourage coating of whole mouth including dentures if present.
Octreotide	SC **csci**	0.1–0.2mg **300–1000mcg**	t.d.s. **24h**	Somatostatin analogue. Very short duration of action. Carcinoid symptom control, Reduces GI secretions and motility.
Sandostatin LAR	Depot injection	20mg/month		Useful in intestinal obstruction, enterocutaneous fistulae and intractable diarrhoea. Not sedative.
Lanreotide	Depot injection	30mg/2 weeks		Expensive; use when other treatments have failed. Use with caution if patient has diabetes mellitus
Olanzapine	p.o.	5–10mg	o.d.	New generation antipsychotic Moderate to severe mania and nausea (off-label). Starting dose for nausea 1.25mg SE: less than with older antipsychotic. QT interval prolongation Caution: Parkinson's disease, hyperglycaemia, elderly stroke patients with dementia.
Omeprazole	p.o.	10–20mg	o.d.	Proton pump inhibitor (PPI). Gastric and duodenal ulcer and reflux oesophagitis. Dispersible tabs available

Ondansetron	p.o./sc/iv p.r. **CSCI**	8mg 16mg **8–24mg**	b.d.–t.d.s. o.d. **24h**	Serotonin (5HT$_3$) antagonist. Uses: Vomiting caused by RT or C/T, intestinal obstruction, hepatic cholestatic itch. Max. 8mg daily in severe hepatic failure. SE: Constipation, headache Melt forms available
Oxybutynin	p.o.	2.5–5mg	b.d.–t.d.s.	Antispasmodic on detrusor muscle of bladder. Detrusor instability Urinary incontinence (urge) SE: Antimuscarinic effects
Oxcarbazepine	p.o.	300mg	b.d.	Neuropathic pain Caution: hypersensitivity to carbamazepine; hyponatraemia; heart failure; cardiac conduction disorders.
Oxycodone m/r	p.o.	Titrated	12h	Modified release tabs 5mg,10mg, 20mg, 40mg, 80mg 12h. 20mg oral morphine equivalent to 10mg oral oxycodone
Oxycodone i/r	p.o. p.r.	Titrated Titrated	4–6h 8h	Moderate to severe pain. 5mg, 10mg, 20mg caps. Liquid 5mg/5mL, 10mg/mL 20mg Oral morphine equivalent to 10mg oxycodone Oxycodone 30mg Supps. available. (Longer acting than morphine Supps.)
Oxycodone inj	SC **CSCI**	5–10mg **Titrated**	4h **24h**	10mg/mL 1mL and 2mL amps Twice as potent as oral oxycodone e.g. 20mg of oral oxycodone is equivalent to 10mg of injectable oxycodone.

(Continued)

Drug	Route	Dose	Frequency	Indications/Side-effects/Remarks
Pamidronate (see Disodium pamidronate)				
Pancreatin (Creon 10,000)	p.o.	1–2 caps with meals		For fat malabsorption e.g. Creon 1–2 sachets with meals Preparations containing higher doses of lipase and amylase available.
Paracetamol	p.o.	0.5–1g	4–6h	Analgesic. Antipyretic.
	p.r.	0.5–1g	4–6h Max. 4g in 24h	Available as tabs, caps, caplets, Susp. dispersible and 125 and 500mg Supps.
Parecoxib	sc/iv	40mg initially then 20–40mg	12 h	Cox-2 NSAID injection SE: as per other NSAID drugs
	csci	**40mg**	**24h**	
Paroxetine	p.o.	20mg	o.m.	SSRI antidepressant/anxiolytic. Short half-life. Used for itch and sweating. Withdraw slowly SE: Beware serotonin syndrome.
Phenobarbital	p.o.	60–180mg	Nocte	Anticonvulsant. Useful as replacement oral anticonvulsant and in terminal agitation.
	csci	**200–1600mg**	**24h**	Use separate syringe driver. Max. 1600mg daily (extreme terminal agitation)
Pilocarpine	p.o.	5mg	t.d.s.	Parasympathomimetic
		4% eye drops (4 drops in 5mL water)	t.d.s.	Sialagogue for dry mouth

Piroxicam	p.o.	20mg	o.d.	NSAID
	melt	20mg	o.d.	Inflammatory pain. Not given as first-line treatment. Consider PPI
				Melt useful when swallowing not possible.
				SE: as per diclofenac

Pregabalin — p.o. — 75mg max. — b.d. — Neuropathic pain. Similar mode of action to Gabapentin
300mg — b.d. — Dose regime:

Normal Kidney Function

Time	Breakfast	Supper
Step 1	75mg	75mg
Step 2	150mg	150mg
Step 3	300mg	300mg

Impaired Kidney Function

Time	Breakfast	Supper
Step 1	25–50mg	25–50mg
Step 2	100mg	100mg
Step 3	75mg	75mg

If necessary step 2 can be started after 3–4 days, and step 3 after a further 7 days
Common side-effects are sedation, dizziness, and headaches.
Potentiated by alcohol and oxycodone.

Prochlorperazine	p.o.	5–10mg	t.d.s.	Neuroleptic antiemetic.
	IM	12.5mg	t.d.s.	May be useful for metabolic/drug induced nausea.
	buccal	3–6mg	b.d.	Too irritant to be given subcutaneously.

| Procyclidine | p.o. | 2.5–5mg | t.d.s. | For management of extrapyramidal side-effects of neuroleptic drugs or dopamine |
| | IM/iv | 5–10mg | p.r.n. | antagonists. (max. 30mg daily) |

| Promazine | p.o. | 25–50mg | q.d.s. | Typical antipsychotic. |
| | | | | Useful for agitation and restlessnes in the elderly |

Quetiapine	p.o.	25mg	b.d	Atypical antipsychotic
				Used in delirium
				Sedative

(Continued)

Drug	Route	Dose	Frequency	Indications/Side-effects/Remarks
Ranitidine	p.o.	300mg 150mg	nocte b.d.	Peptic ulceration and gastric reflux. Less evidence of protection against NSAID induced gastric ulceration than PPIs.
Riluzole	p.o.	50mg	b.d.	Used to extend life or the time to mechanical ventilation in patients with Motor Neurone Disease. SE: Nausea, vomiting, abdominal pain, circumoral paraesthesia, altered liver function tests
Risperidone	p.o.	0.25–2mg	b.d.	'Atypical antipsychotic' useful for psychoses in which both positive and negative symptoms are prominent. Extrapyramidal symptoms are less common than with traditional antipsychotics. Increased risk of stroke in elderly patients with dementia. Caution in presence of cardiovascular disease or epilepsy. In elderly start at 0.25 or 0.5mg
Salbutamol	neb	2.5–5mg	2–6h	β₂ agonist for bronchospasm SE:tachycardia and multiple doses can lead to agitation and tremor.
Senna	p.o.	2–4 tabs	nocte	Stimulant laxative. Acts in 8–12h Avoid in bowel obstruction.
Sertraline	p.o.	50mg	o.d.	SSRI antidepressant. Recent concerns about effectiveness in mild depression Caution in epilepsy as reduces fit threshold. SE: GI upset (avoid if gastric bleeding) As effective as amitriptyline in treating depression with anxiety. Relieves diabetic neuropathic pain. Benefit in cholestatic pruritus
Sodium valproate	p.o.	100–300mg	b.d.	Anticonvulsant Start at 100mg b.d. for neuropathic pain; 300mg b.d. for convulsions. Tabs, m/r tabs, Supps. available by special order. SE: Nausea, blood dyscrasia, liver dysfunction, pancreatitis

Spironolactone	p.o.	100–200mg Max. 400mg for ascites	o.d.	Potassium-sparing diuretic. Potentiates thiazide or loop diuretics Ind: Oedema, and ascites in cirrhosis of the liver, malignant ascites, CCF. (Ascites dose regimes vary considerably). Trial with furosemide for few days. Avoid with ACE inhibitors, potassium supplements and potassium sparing diuretics as could cause hyperkalaemia. SE: Gynaecomastia, GI disturbance
Sucralfate	p.o.	2g	b.d.	Protects mucosa from acid-pepsin attack in gastric and duodenal ulcers (suspension) and also protects oral mucosa (paste) SE: Constipation, bezoar formation with enteral feeds
Tinzaparin	sc	175u/kg (units)	o.d.	Low molecular weight heparin (LMWH). **Treatment.** pulmonary embolus (PE) and deep venous thrombosis (DVT)
	sc	50u/kg (units)	o.d.	**Prophylaxis** In cancer patients LMWH is now the treatment of choice if anticoagulation is required
Tizanidine	p.o.	2mg titrate 3-day intervals, 2mg steps Max. 36mg/day	o.d.	Muscle relaxant for spasticity associated with multiple sclerosis or spinal cord disease. Regular LFT monitoring for first four months SE:Drowsiness
Tramadol i/r m/r	p.o. p.o.	50–100mg 100–200mg (max 400mg/24h)	q.d.s. b.d.	May be useful for nociceptive and neuropathic pain. Tramadol 50mg equivalent to morphine 5–10mg Less constipating than codeine

(Continued)

Drug	Route	Dose	Frequency	Indications/Side-effects/Remarks
Tranexamic acid	p.o.	1g	b.d.–q.d.s.	Inhibits fibrinolysis. Useful for capillary bleeding e.g. surface bleeding from ulcerated tumours. Cauties if: Haematuria, as may encourage clot formation and ureteric obstruction. Contraindicated: History of thromboembolism, DIC
Trazodone	p.o.	25–150mg	nocte	Tricyclic-related antidepressant Insomnia, anxiety, depression. May be safer than atypical antipsychotics for behavioural problems in patients with dementia Avoid following MI. SE: Drowsiness Insomnia 25–50mg o.n. Anxiety 75mg o.n. Depression 150mg o.n.
Venlafaxine	p.o.	37.5–75mg	b.d.	Serotonin and noradrenaline re-uptake inhibitor (SNRI) antidepressant - useful in anxiety Used also for hot flushes and neuropathic pain Caution: Cardiac arrythmia, bleeding disorders, BP↑
Warfarin See p.504	p.o.	As per INR	o.d.	Coumarin anticoagulant Takes 48–72h to be fully effective Used to treat DVT and PE Used for prophylaxis with indwelling iv lines and atrial fibrillation. Usual adult induction *10mg o.d. for 2 days then depending on INR target daily maintenance. * Lower dose if abnormal liver function, renal failure. Caution: Paracetamol, NSAIDs, cranberry juice.
Zoledronic acid	IV 15 minutes	4mg	3–4 weeks	Bisphosphonate Bone pain and hypercalcaemia Monitor calcium levels in bone pain, as may require Vit D and calcium

Syringe drivers

Syringe drivers are used to aid drug delivery when the oral route is no longe feasible

Indications for use
- Intractable vomiting
- Severe dysphagia
- Patient too weak to swallow oral drugs
- Decreased conscious level
- Poor alimentary absorption (rare)
- Poor patient concordance

Drugs that may be mixed with morphine or diamorphine

- cyclizine
- haloperidol
- hyoscine hydrobromide
- metoclopramide
- octreotide
- granisetron
- glycopyrronium
- hyoscine butylbromide
- levomepromazine
- midazolam
- ondansetron

Drugs not suitable for subcutaneous usage
- Diazepam
- Chlorpromazine
- Prochlorperazine

Use separate syringe driver

For:
- Dexamethasone
- Phenobarbital
- Diclofenac
- Ketamine
- Ketorolac

Conversion of oral morphine (or oral morphine equivalent) to parenteral morphine

morphine 10mg p.o.   =   morphine 5mg SC

Method: add the total daily oral dose of morphine (or oral morphine equivalent) and divide by two.

e.g. morphine 10mg p.o. 4h
    or
MST 30mg b.d.   } = morphine 60mg p.o. 24h
    or
MXL 60mg o.d.

morphine 60mg p.o. 24h = morphine 30mg SC 24h

Morphine conversion

Diamorphine can be administered subcutaneously in a smaller volume than morphine, and in countries where diamorphine is available is the preparation of first choice.

	Oral morphine	Subcutaneous morphine	Subcutaneous diamorphine
Ratio	3	1.5	1

When converting from opioids other than morphine, calculate the equivalent dose of oral morphine over 24h and continue as above.

General principles

- Care should be taken when mixing more than two drugs in a syringe and ensuring that the diluent used is compatible with the drugs. Water for injection or 0.9% sodium chloride can be used, but water for injection **must** be used with cyclizine or diamorphine =/>40mg/mL
- If more than three drugs are required in one syringe driver, treatment aims need to be re-assessed
- With combinations of two or three drugs in one syringe, a larger volume of diluent may be needed, e.g. 20mL or 30mL syringe

Preparation of syringe driver

Important—check the type of portable syringe driver. At present Graseby syringe drivers are most commonly used in palliative care but other models such as the McKinley T_3 which delivers at a rate setting of mL/h are available. There are two commonly available Graseby models, MS26 and MS16A.

The following is an example using Graseby syringe drivers. The example is only used to illustrate the principle since local practices may differ. Training is essential. Always consult local guidelines.

We strongly encourage the use of only the green Graseby MS 26, mm per 24h, syringe driver as having two different types can cause dangerous dose errors.

1 Draw up the prescribed 24h medication mixed with the appropriate diluent
2 Prime the line
3 Set the rate on the syringe driver

The rate of delivery is based on a length of fluid in mm per unit time; for example:

MS 26—Green (mm per 24h, a **daily** rate)

$$\text{rate} = \frac{\text{measured 'length of volume' in mm}}{\text{delivery time in days}}$$

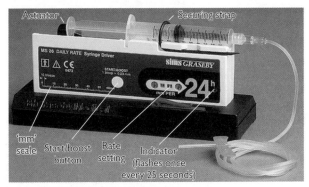

Fig. 4c.1 A GRASEBY MS26 syringe driver.

e.g.:

> 48mm = 48mm per day—rate on dial is 48

MS 16 A—Blue (mm per h, an **hourly** rate)

> rate = measured 'length of volume' in mm
>   ───────────────────────────────────
>   delivery time in hours

e.g.:

> 48mm/24h = 2mm per hour—rate on dial is 02

Skin areas to avoid when siting CSCI
Oedematons areas
Skin folds
Breast
Broken, inflamed or infected skin
Recently irradiated sites
Cutaneous tumour sites

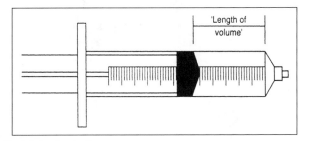

Fig. 4c.2 A primed syringe.

Bony prominences
Near a joint
Anterior chest wall in cachectic patients
Scarring

Problems

Infusion running too fast:	Check the rate setting and recalculate.
Infusion running too slow:	Check start button, battery, syringe driver, cannula and make sure injection site is not inflamed or that the solution is cloudy.
Site reaction:	Cyclizine and levomepromazine cause site reactions most commonly. Firmness or swelling is not necessarily a problem, but the needle site should be changed if there is pain or obvious inflammation. If there is no alternative to sc administration of drugs it may be helpful to add dexamethasone 1mg to the mixture.
	A plastic/Teflon needle may reduce local irritation if there is a nickel allergy
Precipitation:	Check compatibility of drugs. Check solution regularly for precipitation and discoloration and discard if it occurs. Cyclizine may precipitate at high doses, particularly in combination with high doses of diamorphine. Other combinations may also cause cloudiness in the syringe. On rare occasions a patient may need two or three separate syringe drivers to separate the drugs.
Light flashing	This is normal. The light flashes: Blue—Once per sec.; Green—Once per 25 sec.
	Flashing will stop when the battery needs changing or is running low. The syringe driver will continue to operate for 24h after the light has stopped flashing.
Alarm	This always sounds when the battery is inserted. The alarm also sounds for 15 sec. when the syringe driver stops. It can be silenced by pressing the Start/Test button. Check for—empty syringe—kinked tube—blocked needle/tubing—jammed plunger.

Table 4c.1 Common drugs, doses and ranges for palliative care use with a 24h syringe driver

The following is a guide to drugs that may be used in a 24h subcutaneous syringe driver. They may be used alone or in combinations. Advice should be sought when combining drugs or in exceptional circumstances

All drugs should be mixed with WATER for injection unless otherwise indicated.

Drug class of drug/ (Amp. size)	Indications	Compatibility	Contra-indications	Possible side-effects	p.r.n. dose onset of action	24h infusion dose ranges
Alfentanil opioid analgesic 500mcg/mL 2ml amp 10ml amp 5mg/1mL	Pain in presence of renal failure	Mixes with most commonly used drugs, may be incompatible with cyclizine	As for other opioids Levels increased by CYP 3A4 inhibitors e.g. Fluconazole	As for other opioids	SL and spray preparation available but very short acting	Variable depending on total oral intake of opioid Diamorphine 10 mg sc ≡ Morphine 15 mg sc ≡ Alfentanil 1.0 mg sc ≡
Cyclizine Antihistaminic, antimuscarinic antiemetic (50mg/1mL)	Nausea and vomiting associated with motion sickness, Anticipatory nausea, Pharyngeal stimulation, Mechanical bowel obstruction, Raised intracranial pressure	Can precipitate with dexamethasone, diamorphine, metoclopramide, (in higher doses), alfentanil, oxycodone and 0.9% sodium chloride	No absolute ones in patients with advanced cancer Do not give with metoclopramide Do not give with levomepromazine Do not give with buscopan	Drowsiness, dry mouth, blurred vision, hypotension Injection can be painful Can be sedating If syringe driver site is irritated try to dilute further	50mg IM/SC every 8h Within 2h	100–150mg usual dose
Dexamethasone Corticosteroid (4mg/mL)	Antiemetic Pain relief Raised Intracranial pressure	Mixes with metoclopramide Precipitates with	Diabetes—may need supervision	Gastro intestinal side effects, Impaired healing,	Discuss with oncology/ palliative care team	4–16mg usual dose

Diamorphine Opioid analgesic (5mg, 10mg, 30mg, 100mg, 500mg)	Pain Dyspnoea Cough Diarrhoea	cyclizine, glycopyrronium midazolam, haloperidol, levomepromazine, Advisable to put in separate driver but can mix with diamorphine	weight gain, hirsutism, increased appetite	Not usually needed
	Spinal cord compression intestinal obstruction	With most drugs	None if titrated carefully, caution with cyclizine or haloperidol at higher concentrations Modify dose in renal failure	Variable depending on total oral intake of morphine Conversion of oral morphine to subcutaneous diamorphine is 3:1
			Nausea Drowsiness Dry mouth Constipation Confusion Twitching	One sixth of total 24h infusion dose Within 10–30min
Diclofenac NSAID Non-opioid analgesic (75mg/3mL)	Pain (particularly associated with tissue inflammation or bone pain/movement related pain)	Incompatible with most drugs. Give in a separate syringe driver Use sodium chloride 0.9% for dilution	Active peptic ulceration Urticaria Rhinitis Asthma Angioedema	75mg sc every 12h (do not give as well as the infusion) Within 20–30min
			Skin ulceration especially with prolonged use	75–150mg usual dose

(Continued)

Table 4c.1 Common drugs, doses and ranges for palliative care use with a 24h syringe driver (Continued)

Drug class of drug/(Amp. size)	Indications	Compatibility	Contra-indications	Possible side-effects	p.r.n. dose onset of action	24h infusion dose ranges
Glycopyrronium bromide Quaternary ammonium antimuscarinic (0.2mg/mL, 0.6mg/3mL)	Death rattle Colic in inoperable bowel obstruction, Reduction of secretions May be effective if no response to hyoscine Does not cross the blood brain barrier so does not cause drowsiness	With most drugs	2–5 times more potent than hyoscine hydrobromide	Tachycardia Dry mouth	0.2mg sc every 6–8h Within 20–40min	0.6–1.2mg usual dose
Haloperidol Butyrophenone Antipsychotic (5mg/mL)	Nausea and vomiting Psychotic symptoms Agitated delirium Intractable hiccup	With most drugs	Parkinson's disease Possible CNS depression with anxiolytics & alcohol	Extra-pyramidal symptoms, dry mouth, sedation, drowsiness, difficulty in micturition, hypotension, blurred vision	1.5–3mg sc daily upto every 8h Within 10–15min	2.5–5mg usual dose for nausea and vomiting

						Bowel obstruction with colic: 60–120mg usual dose
Hyoscine butylbromide Antimuscarinic antispasmodic antisecretory (20mg/mL)	Obstructive symptoms with colic and antisecretory effects, Death rattle	With most drugs, except cyclizine	Narrow angle glaucoma Myasthenia gravis	Does not cross blood brain barrier so does not cause drowsiness	10–20mg SC every 8h Within 3–5min	
Hyoscine hydrobromide 0.4mg/1mL or 0.6mg/mL	Death rattle Colic Reduce salivation Some antiemetic action	as above	as above	Sedation	0.4mg	1.2–2.4mg
Levomepromazine Antiemetic phenothiazine antipsychotic (25mg/mL)	Nausea and vomiting Insomnia Terminal agitation Intractable pain Useful as antiemetic and sedation Can be very sedating	Precipitates with dexamethasone	Parkinson's disease, Postural hypotension, Antihypertensive therapy, Epilepsy, Hypothyroidism Myasthenia gravis	Sedation, dose dependent postural hypotension	6.25–12.5mg IM/SC every 4–6h usual dose within 30minutes	6.25–25mg usual dose for nausea & vomiting 25–150mg usual dose for terminal agitation
Metoclopramide Prokinetic anti-emetic (10mg/2mL)	Nausea and vomiting caused by gastric irritation Delayed gastric emptying Obstructive bowel symptoms without colic Non-sedating	With most drugs	Concurrent administration with antimuscarinic drugs, Concurrent iv administration of $5\text{-}HT_3$ receptor antagonists Do not give in bowel obstruction if colic present	Dizziness Diarrhoea Depression Extra-pyramidal effects	10–20mg t.d.s.	30–100mg

(Continued)

Table 4c.1 Common drugs, doses and ranges for palliative care use with a 24h syringe driver (*Continued*)

The following is a guide to drugs that may be used in a 24h subcutaneous syringe driver. They may be used alone or in combinations. Advice should be sought when combining drugs or in exceptional circumstances

All drugs should be mixed with WATER unless otherwise indicated

Drug class of drug/(Amp. size)	Indications	Compatibility	Contra-indications	Possible side-effects	p.r.n. dose onset of action	24h infusion dose ranges
Midazolam Benzodiazepine (10mg/2mL) Anxiolytic	Sedation for terminal agitation, Multifocal myoclonus Epilepsy Intractable hiccup Muscle spasm	With most drugs	Drowsiness, Hypotension	Dizziness, drowsiness	2.5–5mg sc every 4h Within 5–10min	10–60mg usual dose
Morphine opioid analgesic 10mg, 15mg, 20mg, 30mg/1mL 1mL amp, 2mL amp	Pain Dyspnoea Cough Diarrhoea	Incompatible with ketorolac caution with higher concentrations of haloperidol or midazolam	None if titrated carefully. Modify dose in renal failure	General opioid SEs	One sixth of total 24h infusion dose within 10–30 min	Variable depending on total oral intake of morphine oral morphine to sc morphine is 2:1

Octreotide Somatostatin analogue FOR SPECIALIST USE ONLY 50mcg/mL 100mcg/mL 200mcg/mL 500mcg/mL	Intestinal obstruction associated with vomiting intractable diarrhoea Symptoms associated with hormone secreting tumours Bowel fistulae Injection can be painful (gently hand warm the vial)	Precipitates with dexamethasone	May alter glucose tolerance	Dry mouth, nausea, vomiting anorexia abdominal pain, flatulence	50–100mcg sc every 8h Within 30min	Intestinal obstruction: 300–1000mcg usual dose
Oxycodone opioid analgesic 10mg/mL 1mL amp. 2mL amp	Pain	Incompatibility may occur with cyclizine at concentrations >3mg/mL	Titrate carefully In renal failure plasma concentrations increase by 50% Inhibitors of CYP 3A4 can inhibit metabolism	Same as morphine, constipation may be more common but vomiting and hallucinations less common	One sixth of total 24h infusion	Variable depending on total oral intake of opioid oral oxycodone to sc oxycodone is 2:1

Further reading

Book

Dickman A., Schneider J., Varga J. (2005) *The Syringe Driver: Continuous Subcutaneous Infusions in Palliative Care*, 2nd edn. Oxford: Oxford University Press.

Articles

Pickard J. (2008) Syringe driver site reactions: a review of the literature. *European Journal of Palliative Care*, **15**: 3: 125–31.

Scottish Intercollegiate Guidelines Network, (2000) *Control of Pain in Patients with Cancer* a National Clinical Guideline. Edinburgh: SIGN.

Antibiotics in palliative care

There are three questions that should be answered when starting empirical antibiotics in palliative patients.
- Does the patient have an infection?
- Is it clinically appropriate to either start or withhold antibiotic therapy?
  The physician needs to weigh the benefits of antibiotics against the risk of prolonging dying
- Which antibiotic will be the most effective while minimizing any burden to the patient?

The first two questions are difficult and complex, and may challenge physicians. Decisions need to be made on an individual basis. The third question should be the easiest to answer, however often it is not.

To look for information to help answer question three, we have reviewed the literature on the use of antibiotics in palliative care.

On quick review of these articles common themes emerge:
- Infections are very common in palliative patients who may have been immunosuppressed either by the disease or treatment
- The commonest site for bacterial infection seems to vary between chest and urinary tract in different studies. Soft tissue infections are less common
- Antibiotics seem, at best, to offer small improvements in symptom control, with urinary symptoms the most likely to improve

In order to produce this guidance we have looked at the published antibiotic policies for other specialties and tried to tailor them to the needs of palliative care patients. It has also been necessary to liaise closely with the local microbiology expert.

These suggestions have been developed in a particular context; microbial profiles and microbiological opinion may vary in different regions.

The aim of antibiotic guidance
- To inform the choice of empirical antibiotics for hospice patients so that the most effective regimens are used producing the least burden
- They will not deal with the ethics of commencing, withdrawing or withholding treatment
- They will not discuss the difficulties of making a diagnosis of infection in the palliative population

The decision regarding the transfer of patients from the hospice setting to an acute unit for treatment of an infection is not included here but should always be considered.

Importance of guidelines/ance
- To help make the right antibiotic choice
- To limit the number of antibiotics that need to be stocked
- To reduce the risk of the emergence of multiresistant organisms
- To allow audit

Aim of antibiotic therapy within the hospice
- Life prolongation without prolonging dying
- Symptom control (pyrexia, pain, bleeding, delirium, dyspnoea, reduce odour)

Generic severity considerations

The severity of an infection is of critical importance when planning the appropriate management. In all patients infection severity may determine the antibiotic choice, the route of administration and the safety of outpatient management. Hospice patients will invariably have multiple problems, placing them at risk of more severe infections. However, these risk factors do not allow for accurate prognostication and should be seen as an aide to clinical judgement only.

Risk factors for more severe infections include:
- Advanced age
- Advanced disease
- Steroids
- Immunosuppression from disease or treatment
- ECOG status 3 and 4
- Evidence of organ dysfunction, e.g. biochemical derangement, delirium
- Clinical findings of infection severity, e.g. rigors, peripheral hypo-perfusion
- Change in vital observations, e.g. hypotension
- Anatomical distortion in the affected organ system, e.g. chronic obstructive pulmonary disease, bladder tumour

Cultures

- If antibiotic treatment is deemed necessary, then it is necessary to culture samples. Directed antibiotic therapy gives better outcomes, with fewer adverse effects
- Cultures and swabs should always be taken prior to starting antibiotics
- There is no point in taking samples for microbiological culture and leaving them sitting at room temprature overnight for a morning collection. This will increase the chance of having false-positive and false-negative results
- Swabs and urine samples can be stored overnight at 4°C. Investing in a fridge for this purpose seems most appropriate
- Blood cultures must be kept at body temperature
- Swabs will pick up commensals as well as pathogens so only treat a positive swab result if symptomatic
- Bacteriuria is common so a positive MSU/CSU should only be treated if symptomatic
- Positive blood cultures should be treated unless there is a good reason not to. Discussion with the microbiology department would help to assess clinical significance

Other important considerations

- It is important to know if the patient has a history of drug allergies
- Antibiotic courses can be assumed to be for 5 days unless specifically stated
- If the infection is severe then the first 24 hours of antibiotics should be given intravenously (IV)
- Parenteral antibiotics IV or IM may need to be used for a prolonged course if the patient cannot swallow tablets or absorb them from the gastrointestinal tract. In this case the reason should be clearly documented in the medical notes
- After 48 hours, if the patient's condition has not improved discuss with microbiology regarding changing antibiotics
- Direct antibiotic therapy once culture results are known
- Cross-reaction in 15–20% of people between penicillin and the cephalosporins, carbapenems and monobactam.
- Remember to consider boosting steroids if necessary
- If in doubt—liaise with the local microbiology service

Non-medical prescribing

Non-medical prescribing was first suggested in 1986 in the Cumberledge Report. It took 13 years for the vision to be realized and for nurse prescribing to be piloted in the community setting using a very limited formulary. Following a successful pilot, non-medical prescribing became a national initiative in 1998. Initially, it was aimed at health visitors and district nurses. Then in 2002 this was extended to enable nurses in other clinical areas, including palliative care, to train as non-medical prescribers using a limited formulary. In 2006 the decision was made to allow nurses, who had completed relevant training, to prescribe independently within their professional scope of practice, from the whole *British National Formulary* (with the exception of certain controlled drugs).

Evaluations of non-medical prescribing have been favourable, with patients and doctors being generally positive about the concept.[1] The majority of nurse prescribers feel strongly that prescribing has had a positive impact on quality of patient care and improved access to medicines. Nurses have also reported that the training to be a non-medical prescriber has enhanced their knowledge about medication and increased their confidence to engage in prescribing decisions.[2]

With end of life care and choice of place of care being key principles of palliative care, nurse prescribing could play an important role in developing and meeting these challenges in the future. We repeatedly hear how there have been delays in gaining a prescription for a patient in the community, causing them to have to wait to commence new medication, or in the extreme case needing to be admitted to hospital. Non-medical prescribing is an option to be considered to assist in meeting these issues as community palliative care nurses will often advise GPs on medication options. Community palliative care nurses who have become non-medical prescribers suggest that patients receive medicines more quickly which they have interpreted as improving patient care.[3]

It is not only community palliative care nurses who should consider non-medical prescribing as part of their role. Hospital palliative care nurses and hospice nurses need to consider whether there is a place for non-medical prescribing within their role, asking the question would it improve the care I provide for patients?

1 Latter S., *et al.* (2005) *An Evaluation of Extended Formulary Independent Nurse Prescribing: Final Report.* London: Department of Health.

2 Bradley E., Nolan P. (2007) Impact of nurse prescribing: a qualitative study. *Journal of Advanced Nursing*, **59**(2): 120–8.

3 Ryan-Woolley B., McHugh G., Luker K, (2007) Prescribing by specialist nurses in cancer and palliative care: results of a national survey. *Palliative Medicine*, **21**: 273–7.

Further reading

Books

BNF (2008) Infections. In *British National Formulary*. London: BMJ Publishing Group Ltd and RPS Publishing.

Clinical Resource Efficiency Support Team (2005) *Guidelines on the Management of Cellulitis in Adults Beleast*. CREST Secretariat.

Eastern Health and Social Services Board. (2004–2005) *Hospital Formulary*.

Twycross R., Wilcock A. (2007) *Palliative Care Formulary*. (3rd edn) Nottingham: www.palliativedrugs.com.

Articles

Brabin E. (2008) How effective are parenteral antibiotics in hospice patients. *European Journal of Palliative Care* **15**(3): 115–125.

(2001). BTS guidelines for the management of community acquired pneumonia in adults. *Thorax*, **56**(Suppl 4): IV1–64.

Clark J. (2002) Metronidazole gel in managing malodorous fungating wounds. *British Journal of Nursing*, **11**(6) (Suppl): 54–60.

Clayton J., et al. (2003) Parenteral antibiotics in a palliative care unit: prospective analysis of current practice. *Palliative Medicine*, **17**(1): 44–8.

Lam, P. T. et al. (2005) Retrospective analysis of antibiotic use and survival in advanced cancer patients with infections. *Journal of Pain and Symptom Management*, **30**(6): 536–43.

Macfarlane J. T., Boldy D. (2004). 2004 update of BTS pneumonia guidelines: what's new? *Thorax*, **59**(5): 364–6.

Mirhosseini M., et al. (2006) The role of antibiotics in the management of infection-related symptoms in advanced cancer patients. *Journal of Palliative Care*, **22**(2): 69–74.

Moncino M. D. a. J. M. F. (1992) Multiple relapses of *Clostridium difficile*-associated diarrhea in a cancer patient. Successful control with long-term cholestyramine therapy. *American Journal of Pediatric Hematology and Oncology*, **14**(4): 361–4.

Mortimer P. P. S. (2007) *Consensus Document on the Management of Cellulitis in Lymphoedema*: London: British Lymphology Society and the Lymphoedema Support Network.

Nagy-Agren S. a. H. H. (2002) Management of infections in palliative care patients with advanced cancer. *Journal of Pain and Symptom Management*, **24**(1): 64–70.

Oh D. Y., et al. (2006). Antibiotic use during the last days of life in cancer patients. *European Journal of Cancer Care*, **15**(1): 74–9.

Oneschuk D., Fainsinger R., Demoissac D. (2002) Antibiotic use in the last week of life in three different palliative care settings *Journal of Palliative Care*, **18**(1): 25–8.

Palace G. P., Lazari P., et al. (2001) Analysis of the physicochemical interactions between *Clostridium difficile* toxins and cholestyramine using liquid chromatography with post-column derivatization. *Biochimica et Biophysica Acta,*, **1546**(1): 171–84.

Pereira J., Watanabe S., Wolch G. (1998) A retrospective review of the frequency of infections and patterns of antibiotic utilization on a palliative care unit. *Journal of Pain and Symptom Management*, **16**(6): 374–81.

Spruyt O., Kausae A. (1998) Antibiotic use for infective terminal respiratory secretions. *Journal of Pain and Symptom Management*, **15**(5): 263–4.

Stroehlein J. R. (2004) Treatment of *Clostridium difficile* infection. *Current Treatment Options in Gastroenterology*, **7**(3): 235–9.

Venkatesan P., *et al.* (1990) A hospital study of community acquired pneumonia in the elderly. *Thorax*, **45**(4): 254–8.

Vitetta L., Kenner D., Sali A. (2000) Bacterial infections in terminally ill hospice patients. *Journal of Pain and Symptom Management*, **20**(5): 326–34.

White P. H., *et al.* (2003) Antimicrobial use in patients with advanced cancer receiving hospice care. *Journal of Pain and Symptom Management* **25**(5): 438–43.

Chapter 5

Oncology and palliative care

The best sentence in the English language is not 'I love you' but 'It's benign'.

Woody Allen, Deconstructing Harry, 1998

The commonest cancers are of the lung, breast, skin, gastrointestinal tract and the prostate gland

Introduction

Cancer is an important cause of morbidity and mortality, particularly in industrialized countries. Currently in the UK one person in three will be diagnosed with cancer during their lifetime and one in four will die of their disease.

Cancer incidence increases exponentially with age, and with increasing life expectancy cancer will become an even more common problem in the future.

Cancers may develop in all body tissues. The cells that form cancers can be differentiated from cells in normal tissues in a number of ways, including:

- Cell division that has escaped the control of normal homeostasis
- Abnormalities of cell differentiation—in general terms cancer cells tend to be less well differentiated than their non-malignant counterparts
- Resistance to programmed cell death
- The potential for cancerous cells to invade local tissues and metastasize.

The development of cancer is associated with the accumulation of defects or 'mutations' in a number of critical genes within the cell.

Many cancers are associated with mutations leading to overactivity of growth-promoting genes, commonly known as 'oncogenes'. Conversely, cancers may also be associated with mutations leading to underactivity of genes which act to suppress growth.

Although our understanding of the genetic abnormalities underlying cancer has grown exponentially over the last decade, the factors that cause these changes are not clear for most cancers.

There is evidence that exogenous carcinogens may be closely linked to some cancers. Smoking, for example, is a causative factor in lung, cervix and bladder cancer.

In other cancers there is an inherited susceptibility to particular types of malignancy. In the majority of common cancers, however, the cause remains elusive. It is likely that for many of these cancers both environmental and genetic factors are implicated.

Organization of cancer care

Optimal care of the patient with cancer requires input from a number of medical disciplines. Typically a provisional diagnosis of cancer is made by a surgeon or physician and confirmed by a pathologist following biopsy or fine-needle aspiration. After staging the cancer a surgeon or an oncologist may then undertake definitive treatment. Support of the patient through treatment may well involve input from a wide range of surgical, medical, allied medical health professionals and laboratory disciplines.

Several factors facilitate this care:
- Good organization of cancer services
- Site specialization for doctors treating cancer
- Multidisciplinary team working
- Well-established links with laboratory and clinical cancer research

The disease journey

A close working relationship between oncology and palliative care professionals is important. Increasingly, the goals are shared and closer working relationships are being forged, at different points along the patient's disease journey (Fig. 5.1).

At the time of original diagnosis

Oncological services, specialist and generalist palliative care services, including the GP and community health team, need to share information quickly so, at this point, when the patient and their family feel particularly vulnerable, informed support can be maximized.[1]

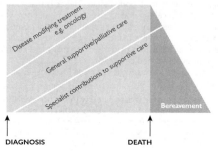

Fig. 5.1 The disease journey.

1 National Council for Hospice and Specialist Palliative Care Services. (2002) *Definitions of Supportive and Palliative Care*. London: NCHSPCS (Briefing Bulletin 11).

Traditionally, palliative care services were only 'offered' to patients when 'there is nothing more that can be done'.

Increasingly, palliative care is involved from the point of diagnosis with increasing input as the oncology needs decrease, maximizing at the time of death and continuing on with bereavement support.

Through the period of staging and/or surgery

This can be a time of great uncertainty for patients, when communicating the often complex prognostic and treatment information is so important. Many find the issues very difficult to grasp, so vast are the associated life implications. An understanding of these issues and of the likely treatments by all those involved in the clinical and supportive care of patient and family can help to consolidate information transfer. It is often only a few days after a crucial oncology outpatient appointment that patients become receptive to important information.

If other healthcare professionals are hesitant or contradictory in their explanations of treatment options patient anxiety will be increased.

'When I was diagnosed with my bowel cancer I was simply devastated. You see, I had watched my father dying from lung cancer and I was sure I would go the same way. I could hardly get out of the hospital quickly enough to get my farm and affairs sorted out. The doctor said something about treatment, but I knew from watching others with cancer that treatment was pointless, so I never went back for the cancer specialist appointment.

It was only after my own doctor came out and we had a good chat that I even thought that they could do anything for me. In the end I decided to go and see what they were offering, still never believing that they could do any good.

I honestly believe if my own doctor hadn't taken the time to come and explain that there really was something they could do to help I would not been alive to enjoy these past six years.'

Through the period of treatment

While the majority of supportive care during this period tends to be linked through the oncology services, specialist and generalist palliative care teams need to be aware of the:

- Goals of treatment
- Side-effects of treatment
- Follow-up plans

The goals of oncology treatment

Before commencing any treatment it is important that both patient and carers are aware of the goals of treatment.

It is possible, particularly if the outlook is not good, that patients will ask different members of the team hoping to find a more optimistic prognosis. Clearly it is not in the patient's interest to hear conflicting opinions about their prognosis and this should be avoided.

Openness regarding realistic treatment outcomes is also important in maintaining staff morale. While the death of a patient is often difficult, particularly for the nurses who are most closely involved in care, this is especially so if unrealistic expectations of treatment are fostered.

Radical oncological treatment

Radical oncological interventions are curative in intent. They may involve surgery, radiotherapy or chemotherapy (or a combination of these modalities).

Because the potential benefits of treatment are great, a relatively high incidence of side-effects is more acceptable.

Providing patients with good symptom control and emotional support through radical treatment is important. They need to be encouraged to complete what is often a very demanding treatment course in order to benefit maximally. Without such encouragement patients may miss the only opportunity they have of cure.

Increasingly, there is an appreciation that such treatments may be associated with long-term toxicities/side-effects (which may be especially relevant for children). Clearly in this potentially curative group care must be taken to minimize the potential for cumulative dose toxicities such as cardiotoxicity caused by anthracyclines.

Adjuvant oncological treatment

Many patients suffer tumour relapse following apparently curative surgery for their primary tumour. This is believed to be due to the presence of micrometastatic disease that is not clinically apparent at the time of the primary treatment.

Anticancer treatment (usually chemotherapy) given at this stage has been shown to improve long-term survival for some tumours. This approach has proven successful even for tumours where chemotherapy is not curative in the metastatic setting, and is presumably related to the increased chemosensitivity associated with microscopic volumes of disease.

The absolute gains in survival from adjuvant chemotherapy are generally small but real. (Adjuvant chemotherapy in premenopausal women with breast cancer, for example, is associated with an approximately 30% relative improvement in 10-year survival). At present there are few predictive factors to identify those patients most likely to benefit from adjuvant therapy. The decision to proceed is often based on the statistical likelihood of relapse, with those at highest risk benefiting most.

The fact remains that the majority of patients will not benefit from adjuvant therapies. Such treatments should therefore have manageable acute toxicities and a low incidence of long-term toxicities.

Palliative oncological treatment

Palliative treatment is indicated when curative treatment is not possible but where treatments may have sufficient anticancer activity to improve cancer-related symptoms. In many cases improvement of symptoms is accompanied by tumour shrinkage detectable clinically or by radiological methods such as CT scan or MRI. It is increasingly recognized that there may be a palliative benefit even in the absence of tumour shrinkage.

As the primary object of therapy is to improve quality of life, such treatments should be well tolerated with a low incidence of acute side-effects. Long-term toxicities are generally not relevant.

In some cases the distinction between radical and palliative treatment may not be absolutely clear-cut. Indeed, the aims of treatment may change as the disease progresses.

Patients presenting with advanced ovarian cancer, for example, have largely incurable disease. However, the tumour is often chemosensitive and lengthy remissions are often seen following primary chemotherapy. In such patients a relatively high incidence of acute toxicity may be acceptable, with efforts being focused on managing chemotherapy-related symptoms. Conversely, a patient presenting with relapsed ovarian cancer following first-line chemotherapy has a low expectation of benefit from further chemotherapy. Consequently only a low incidence of acute toxicity is acceptable with second-line chemotherapy, from which expectation of benefit is very limited.

> For patients and carers who have been through radical or adjuvant therapy the switch to palliative treatment can be difficult to accept.
> In particular, the patient and carers have to be informed that the most important element of assessing palliative treatments is their overall impact on quality of life and that emphasis will shift to a global assessment balance between toxicity and antitumour benefit.

Managing patients receiving oncology treatments

Chemotherapy and radiotherapy are now given largely on an outpatient basis. Surgical patients also spend less time in hospital than in the past. This allows patients to spend more time at home, which inevitably places an increased burden of care on those providing support in the community, particularly where the cancer centre is a long distance from home. Thus a general understanding of the particular side-effects, and the appropriate treatment for such complications, is needed by healthcare professionals in the community and those providing on-call services.

It should not be assumed that a new symptom developing in a patient undergoing treatment for cancer is related to the side-effects of treatment or to the cancer itself, although the high possibility of this must be considered. (*Chemotherapy does not prevent patients developing appendicitis*!) Thus the health professional needs to assess each new symptom independently, and be aware of the side-effects of commonly used oncological treatment regimes. (See the sections on chemotherapy and radiotherapy.)

Supportive teams need to know the significance and *appropriate responses for individual patients* to such side-effects as:
- Clinical anaemia
- Nausea and vomiting
- Pain
- Pyrexia and possible infection
  - *What are the risks of neutropenia for this patient?*
- Increased drowsiness
- Confusion
  - *Could this patient be opioid toxic, hypercalcaemic, or developing renal failure?*
- Hair loss
- Altered sensation, back pain, incontinence
  - *Could this patient be developing spinal cord compression?*

The appropriate response and management will differ according to what the patient and family want, the disease process and where the patient is on their disease journey.

Treatment planning

It is important that treatment plans are communicated adequately to patients, families and professional carers to ensure that appropriate support is given.

A basic management plan should include:
- Details of proposed diagnostic and staging investigations
- Proposed treatment plan for surgery, chemotherapy and radiotherapy where appropriate. The plan should include details regarding the duration of treatment and timing of interval investigations to assess response to therapy. (Patients can be understandably anxious in the days preceding a scan aimed at assessing response to treatment.)
- Changes to treatment dosages or frequency including reasons for change
- Particular side-effects of treatment and specific advice on what to do if these problems develop
- Clear instructions about how long treatments such as antibiotics or steroids should be administered or tailed off
- Treatment goals
- Details of significant conversations with patients and their carers relating to their understanding of their disease and their wishes for further treatment
- Clear details of who to contact in case of treatment complications

No single set of healthcare professionals can manage the many needs that patients have on their disease journey. Holistic, patient-centred, care requires a multiprofessional and multidisciplinary approach that places the patient and family at the centre.

Many centres are now using patient-held records to facilitate improvements in communication. The different professionals record their
findings and management plans, thus improving the continuity of care.
With the increasing demand for transparency in care from patient groups,
and the importance of ongoing care, such systems may well become
commonplace in the UK.

Clinical trials

Clinical research is necessary in order to improve outcomes for patients with cancer. The link between the laboratory and the clinic is developing and increasingly patients are being recruited into trials.

There are three main types of clinical trial:

Phase I

Aim

- To establish the human toxicity of a new drug through delivering carefully selected increasing doses to patients
- To establish the safe dose at which to start further trials with the drug
- To evaluate the body's handling of the drug by pharmacokinetic studies

Eligible patients

- Patients who have progressive disease despite standard oncological therapy or those for whom no standard therapy exists
- Patients must be aware that the primary objective of the studies is to assess toxicity. There is little expectation of benefit to themselves, with a response rate of approximately 5%
- Patients recruited to Phase I trials usually have a good performance status and are highly motivated individuals, since involvement often requires intensive monitoring as an inpatient

Phase II

Aim

- To establish the antitumour activity of the drug for a particular tumour type

Eligible patients

- Patients who have progressive disease despite standard chemotherapy or for whom no standard therapy exists
- Patients usually have a good performance status and are highly motivated
- Patients are closely monitored with toxicity and response assessments, but not as intensively as those in Phase I studies

Phase III

Aim

- To compare the new drug or drug combination with conventional therapy

Eligible patients

- Patients for whom a standard therapy exists. (New drugs may also be compared with 'best supportive care' where no standard therapy exists.)

Important and common endpoints include disease-free survival (in adjuvant studies), and overall survival (in palliative studies). Increasingly, more clinically relevant endpoints such as improvements in pain, performance status and weight gain and quality of life are being used in Phase III trials of palliative agents.

Typically Phase III trials are much larger than Phase I/II trials and patients require less frequent monitoring.

Aims of clinical trials
- Phase I: dose/schedule finding, typically 20–50 patients
- Phase II: disease finding, typically 50–100 patients
- Phase III: comparison of novel treatment/schedule to standard of care, typically 500–1000 patients

Some studies include Phase IV trials. These studies continue after the drug or treatment has been marketed to gather information on the drug's effect in various populations and to identify side-effects associated with long-term use.

Survivorship
Overall survival rates for cancer are increasing but sometimes at a cost. It is estimated that by 2020 there will be over 2 million people living in the UK who have received cancer treatments. This may or may not have resulted in clinical cure, but their health has nevertheless been affected. The majority will be affected in a minor way but some will have significant severe long-term adverse affects. Cancer 'survivors' live with a significantly higher incidence of chronic illness and debility than those without a cancer diagnosis.

Traditionally, oncologists have concentrated on the management of acute rather than more chronic side-effects of cancer treatment. There is no system to record severe outcomes for those who have received radiotherapy or chemotherapy, making it impossible for national trends to be studied or clusters of problems spotted early. This may become an increasing problem as new equipment, surgical techniques and drugs are being introduced at an ever-increasing rate. High profile clinical situations include radiation-induced brachial plexopathy following treatment for cancer of the breast and pelvic morbidity following radical radiotherapy for cancer of the cervix.

The concern is that many professionals will fail to make a connection between a patient's new problem and previous cancer diagnosis/treatment. Even when late effects are recognized the investigation and management of sometimes multiple problems requires the help of a wider multiprofessional team.

There is considerable potential for improvement in the aftercare that our patients should receive and Macmillan Cancer Support has identified a number of priorities:
- A national register of severe late consequences of cancer treatment
- Support to ensure that patients recognize and understand changes in health after cancer treatment and have the information and support to manage these effectively
- Increased understanding of cancer survivorship from a primary care team point of view and provision of information and support
- Innovative ways to bring multidisciplinary specialist expertise to the patients with rare, severe treatment-related chronic illness (estimated as 5–10% of survivors)

Specialists involved in the palliative care needs of patients may be in a position to help in the management of some of those patients with the severest symptoms.

Further reading

Donaldson L. (2007) Reducing harm from radiotherapy. *British Medical Journal*, **334**: 272.

Hewitt M., Rowland J. (2003) Cancer survivors in the United States: age health and disability. *Journal of Gerontological Medical Science*, **58**: 82.

Maher E. J., Makin W. (2007) Life after cancer treatment—a spectrum of chronic survivorship conditions. *Clinical Oncology*, **19**: 743–5.

Tylko K., Blennerhassett M. (2006) How the NHS could better protect the safety of radiotherapy patients. *Health Care Risk Report*, 18–19.

Oncological surgery[2]

Surgery remains the modality of treatment most likely to cure patients diagnosed with solid tumours. It has most potential when the cancer is localized, although results are improving for patients with certain types of metastatic tumours.

Surgery has three main roles in cancer management:
- Diagnosis and staging
- Treatment with curative intent
- Palliative treatment

Diagnosis and staging

In the past, many patients suspected of having cancer required surgery to confirm the diagnosis. The development of cross-sectional radiology and the ability to perform diagnostic biopsies using radiological guidance or endoscopy often allows accurate diagnosis before surgery.

Patient morbidity has significantly reduced since some surgical procedures are avoided. The number of 'open and close' laparotomies for unresectable cancer, for example, has reduced to <5% in recent years, largely due to these advances. The introduction of sentinel node biopsy for patients with breast cancer has been effective in reducing the number of axillary clearances with less morbidity including pain and lymphoedema.

However, surgical staging remains important in a number of common tumours:
- Axillary lymph node dissection for patients with breast cancer, for example, allows assessment of these nodes for tumour involvement. Such information is important in determining prognosis and guiding decisions regarding adjuvant treatments
- Ovarian cancer spreads mainly via the transperitoneal route, leading to tumour deposits in peritoneal surfaces and the omentum—sites poorly visualized on conventional imaging. A laparotomy for patients with ovarian cancer therefore allows a more accurate staging of disease than is currently possible with non-invasive means. Again, such information is vital in determining prognosis and guiding further treatment

Curative surgery

Localized disease

Surgery is most commonly curative in intent for localized cancers and is generally dependent on complete resection of the tumour with a margin of normal tissue.

In some tumours with a propensity to spread to lymph nodes, resection of the draining lymph nodes may improve local control (e.g. vulval tumours). In other tumours the value of lymphadenectomy is uncertain and is the subject of ongoing clinical trials (e.g. endometrial cancer).

Unfortunately surgery still fails to cure many patients. There are a number of reasons for this:
- Development of metastatic disease—this is due to the presence of micro-metastatic disease unidentifiable at the time of surgery.

2 Cassidy J., Bissett D., et al. (2002) *Oxford Handbook of Oncology.* Oxford: Oxford University Press.

This is a common reason for failure of surgery to cure breast and bowel tumours

- Development of local relapse—outcomes from surgery are often closely linked to the margin of normal tissue excised in continuity with the tumour. The amount of tissue that can be resected may be limited by patient-related factors (e.g. only a partial lobectomy may be possible in patients with lung cancer due to the patients' underlying poor respiratory function) or by tumour-related factors (e.g. tumour invasion of a vital structure such as the aorta.)

Metastatic disease

Although much less common, surgery may be curative in a limited number of tumours in the metastatic setting. The role for potentially curative surgery is best established in a small number of instances. These include:

- Pulmonary metastases from osteosarcoma
- Pulmonary metastases from soft tissue sarcoma
- Liver metastases from colorectal cancer
- Isolated brain metastases in special circumstances (📖 see p. 204)

In each of these cases best results are seen with careful patient selection according to well-defined criteria. In general terms, the best long-term results are seen in patients who relapse after a long period from initial tumour diagnosis and who have low volume disease and a good performance status.

Palliative surgery

Surgery may provide very effective palliation in a number of situations. Given the specific problems of oncology patients in the palliative situation (limited life expectancy, poor performance status, rapid tumour progression), the decision to proceed with surgery must involve a careful weighing up of the risk/benefit of such procedures. These decisions are best made with a multidisciplinary approach by surgeons specialized in oncology and experienced in palliative management.

Bowel obstruction

Patients with colonic or ovarian cancer form the majority of patients with bowel obstruction referred for surgery. Surgery to relieve the obstruction is warranted even if disease is incurable (due to liver metastases or locally advanced disease, for example) as such patients may live for many months. Where possible, these patients should have the primary tumour excised and a primary anastomosis performed.

Patients with ovarian cancer commonly present with obstructive bowel symptoms. At initial presentation debulking surgery provides excellent palliation. Patients presenting with relapsed disease and obstructive symptoms often have multiple sites of obstruction due to widespread intraperitoneal dissemination of their disease. In this instance surgery is much less likely to be useful.

Fistulae

Fistulae may arise as a result of pelvic tumours or as a complication of radiotherapy. They are often associated with unpleasant symptoms. Optimum preoperative assessment requires imaging to delineate exactly the site of fistula formation and to guide surgical decisions. Surgery may provide excellent palliation but may not be useful in those with multiple sites of fistulae or rapidly advancing intra-abdominal disease where life expectancy is limited.

Jaundice

Obstructive jaundice due to extrinsic pressure by lymph nodes on the biliary system, or due to intrinsic lesions such as cholangiocarcinoma, is commonly well palliated by radiological and endoscopic placement of stents.

The complications of stents include infection and blockage with consequent need for replacement.

Surgical relief of obstructive jaundice (e.g. by choledochoenter-ostomy) avoids problems associated with stents and may be indicated in a small minority of patients with an excellent performance status and slow-growing disease.

Pain

Surgical debulking of large slow-growing tumours can reduce pain and is justified in patients where the expected morbidity of the procedure is low. Neurosurgical approaches, e.g. cordotomy, are only infrequently considered.

Gastrointestinal bleeding

A wide range of endoscopic techniques have been developed to stop bleeding from benign and malignant causes. This may avoid the need for more major surgery in patients who have a limited life expectancy.

These include:
- Sclerotherapy
- Laser coagulation
- Radiological embolization

Bone metastases

Metastases to bones can cause major palliative problems. Specific problems include pain and pathological fracture. Factors that identify patients most at risk of pathological fracture include:
- Site—lesions in weight-bearing bones
- Extent of destruction—destruction of >50% cent of the cortex
- Symptoms—patients complaining of pain, particularly on weight-bearing
- Type of lesion—lytic lesions > blastic lesions

Such patients may benefit (both in terms of reduced pain and reduced risk of fracture) from prophylactic fixation of a long bone. The type of internal fixation used depends on the site of fracture and the patient's performance status. In all cases internal fixation of the bone should be followed by radiotherapy to control tumour growth and to promote healing.

Techniques such as vertebroplasty are available to manage pain invertebrae.

Chemotherapy

I am dying from the treatment of too many physicians

Alexander the Great

Identification of agents

Chemotherapy generally refers to a group of agents used in the systemic management of cancer. A disparate group, these agents are linked by having demonstrated evidence of anticancer activity and a common range of side-effects.

The anticancer activity of these agents has been identified in a number of ways. For some the discovery of antineoplastic activity was serendipitous. Cisplatin was discovered because of using platinum electrodes in an antibiotic experiment.

For others this activity was identified during screening of a wide range of natural products (e.g. paclitaxel). Some of these agents have been biochemically modified to reduce their toxicity while retaining their antineoplastic activity (e.g. carboplatin).

Mechanism of action

Chemotherapy exerts its anticancer action by a wide variety of mechanisms which are, as yet, incompletely understood (📖 see Table 5.1).

For many, DNA is believed to be the most important cellular target, e.g. irinotecan inhibits the topoisomerase I enzyme thereby causing double-strand breaks in DNA. For other agents, microtubules, particularly those involved in mitotic spindle formation, appear to be the vital target, e.g. paclitaxel promotes tubulin polymerization and so arrests cells in metaphase.

A number of factors determine the likelihood of achieving a useful response to chemotherapy. Some tumours are inherently more sensitive to chemotherapy than others. In general terms, chemotherapy tends to be most effective in tumours with fast cell turnover such as acute leukaemia and high-grade lymphoma. Seminoma, however, a tumour with a long natural history, is also very chemosensitive. Clearly there are other factors, as yet poorly understood, that determine a tumour's chemosensitivity.

Patient-related factors are also important in determining likelihood of response. Patients with poor performance status, for example, respond less well than those with good performance status. The reasons for this are poorly understood but are probably due, at least in part, to a reduced tolerance to the acute toxicity of chemotherapy.

While chemotherapy may induce a partial or even complete response, the tumour may regrow with disease that has become chemoresistant. There is evidence in some cases that the tumour may have become more efficient at actively pumping the drug from the cell. Increasingly it is recognized that the ability of cells either to repair or tolerate the damage inflicted by chemotherapy may lead to chemoresistance. The causes of chemoresistance and the development of agents to overcome such mechanisms are active areas of research at present.

Tumours which divide rapidly with short doubling times respond best to chemotherapy.

Adverse effects of chemotherapy

Although the specific side-effect profile varies between agents, there are a number of side-effects common to most agents.

- **Alopecia** is a common and often distressing side-effect associated with many agents. Patients can be reassured that hair will regrow. On regrowth the hair may develop waves or curls and will revert towards its previous character over many months.
- **Nausea and vomiting** are common with many agents, although the degree to which this is a problem varies both between agents and between patients. The development of 5-HT$_3$ antagonists (e.g. tropisetron, granisetron) has greatly aided the management of this troublesome side-effect. The efficacy of 5-HT$_3$ antagonists can be improved by the addition of steroids
- **Myelosuppression** is a significant cause of morbidity associated with chemotherapy. The white cells (in particular the neutrophils) are most commonly affected between 1 and 2 weeks following chemotherapy. Patients should be warned of the possibility of developing infection during this time and the urgency with which they should seek help, as they will require immediate treatment with broad-spectrum antibiotics. The development of granulocyte colony-stimulating growth factors has reduced this toxicity by shortening the duration of neutropenia. This has allowed higher doses of chemotherapy to be given more safely in certain situations
- **Anxiety** The prospect of chemotherapy is a frightening concept for many patients—not least due to the (often mistaken) view of the difficult side-effects. It is important that the patient and their carers are fully educated about the type of side-effects they are likely to encounter during treatment and how best to deal with them. Most patients are extremely anxious during this difficult time and information may have to be repeated a number of times. It is very useful to have written information to supplement what has been said in consultations. It is also useful if a relative or friend attends with the patient—they will often be able to help the patient review the information at a later date.

Chemotherapy regimens

A wide range of chemotherapy regimens are used in the treatment of patients with cancer. The usual rationale has been to combine drugs that demonstrate activity as single agents but which do not share the same side-effects.

More sophisticated techniques to examine synergy and pharmacokinetic interactions in a pre-clinical setting are now developing, and this will guide a logical approach to the optimal combinations of agents.

Chemotherapy may be given in the following situations:
- Curative
- Adjuvant
- Neoadjuvant
- Palliative

Curative

A small number of solid malignancies are curable by chemotherapy alone; for instance, germ-cell tumours, lymphomas and certain childhood tumours.

Chemotherapy regimens used in the treatment of these diseases tend to be intensive and associated with a high incidence of acute toxicity. It is important that patients receive chemotherapy on schedule as there is evidence that dose reductions and prolonging treatment times may adversely affect outcome. Consequently, treatment can exact a high physical and psychological toll on patients and their relatives.

Given that the long-term aim of treatment is cure, patients and their carers need encouragement to persevere, which will be easier if physical symptoms are optimally managed. The palliative care team can provide expert assistance at this stage of the patient's management.

Increasingly it is becoming clear that patients who are cured following chemotherapy are at risk of long-term toxicity from their treatment. Such problems include secondary leukaemias and solid tumours, fatigue, infertility and cardiomyopathy. These problems have only become appreciated in recent times. Undoubtedly as more people become long-term survivors of cancer, more problems will emerge. For this reason it is important that long-term survivors of cancer remain on long-term follow-up.

Adjuvant

Many patients presenting with apparently localized cancer are known to be at high risk of developing metastatic disease. This is presumed to be due to the presence of micrometastases not apparent by current imaging modalities. Chemotherapy given following successful primary treatment for apparently localized cancer may reduce the risk of developing clinical metastatic disease.

Cancers where adjuvant chemotherapy is commonly used include breast and colorectal cancer where large, multicentre, randomized controlled trials and subsequent meta-analysis have confirmed the survival gain.

At an individual level these gains are small, with absolute improvements in overall survival of 5–15% after five years. At a population level, however, this represents a large number of lives saved in diseases as common as breast and bowel cancer.

Presently, surrogate markers such as tumour size, grade and lymph node involvement are commonly used to assess risk of disease relapse and thereby identify those most likely to benefit from adjuvant therapy. Much current research is directed at developing predictive markers to identify more precisely those most likely to benefit.

Given that the majority of patients treated will not benefit from treatment as their disease will relapse anyway or because primary treatment has been curative, adjuvant regimens must therefore be well tolerated with a low incidence of serious acute side-effects and long-term side-effects.

Again, as with treatment in the curative setting, positive outcomes from treatment are closely linked to dose intensity and to avoiding delays in chemotherapy. Where acute toxicities are a problem, involvement of the palliative care team may improve symptom management and facilitate delivery of treatment on schedule.

Neoadjuvant

Chemotherapy may be used 'up front' in non-metastatic tumours prior to definitive treatment (usually surgery) for the tumour. This may be employed for a large inoperable primary tumour to shrink the tumour and facilitate surgery. Such an approach is standard practice in very large primary breast tumours or those with skin involvement.

Increasingly, neoadjuvant therapy is being utilized for tumours that are operable. Potential advantages of this approach include less extensive surgery in a tumour that has been debulked. From a research point of view, a neoadjuvant approach with biopsies before and after therapy may allow molecular markers that predict chemosensitivity to be identified.

Conversely, there are a number of potential problems with neoadjuvant chemotherapy. First, in a responding tumour there may be a loss of potentially useful prognostic information from the subsequently resected tumour specimen. There is also the risk that such an approach may allow interim tumour progression in a lesion that does not respond to chemotherapy. Finally, performing less radical surgery in a tumour that has responded to chemotherapy may compromise local control.

This approach is being examined with particular interest in a number of tumours including oesophageal, gastric and breast tumours.

> Growth for the sake of growth is the ideology of the cancer cell.
> Edward Abbey 1927–1989

Palliative

The majority of solid cancers are not curable in the metastatic setting. Chemotherapy, however, may have a valuable role to play in the palliative treatment of such patients. Clinical trials now include endpoints such as quality of life and toxicity, which are more clinically relevant in this setting than assessing overall survival as a sole entity.

Given that improvement or maintenance of quality of life is the aim of palliative chemotherapy, acute toxicities must be easily managed and tolerable.

Optimally, a patient is best managed when chemotherapy is administered *in conjunction with* input from the palliative care team. Such input also facilitates the gradual handing over of care to the palliative care team as the patient's disease progresses. Such a team-based approach reduces problems of patients feeling neglected by their oncologist when chemotherapy is no longer useful.

Indications for palliative chemotherapy

'Treatment decisions are based on a consideration of the balance between the benefits expected and the toxicity and risks of chemotherapy which are different for each patient.'[3]

- **Maintaining or improving quality of life**: This is the most important aim of palliative chemotherapy. Chemotherapy may alleviate specific symptoms such as dyspnoea or chest pain in a patient with lung cancer. It may also improve or maintain general well-being with improvements in such factors as appetite and energy. The development of quality-of-life assessment tools, especially those with disease-specific elements, has greatly facilitated the assessment of the effect of chemotherapy on quality of life
- **Improving survival**: While this is a secondary objective in most cases, it is quite clear that chemotherapy given with palliative intent frequently prolongs survival. The extent to which it is expected that survival may be prolonged varies between diseases. Chemotherapy in pancreatic cancer is associated with an improvement in survival of only a few weeks, whereas patients receiving chemotherapy for ovarian cancer may have improved survival of many months or even years
- **In emergency situations**: Potentially life-threatening tumour-related emergencies, such as spinal cord compression or superior vena cava compression, may be treated with chemotherapy where the primary tumour is very chemosensitive. Such tumours include lymphoma and small-cell lung cancer

3 McIllmurray M. (2004) Palliative medicine and the treatment of cancer. In *Oxford Textbook of Palliative Medicine* (ed. D. Doyle, G. et al), p. 213. Oxford: Oxford University Press.

Chemotherapy within the palliative setting is increasingly common because of:

Earlier referral for palliative care services

Chemotherapeutic services and palliative care services can be enhanced by a close working relationship with good lines of communication and early referral. The journey from diagnosis to death is not linear but dynamic, with different interventions governed not by the passage of time but by a patient's particular needs. With an integrated service and earlier referral patterns there will be an ever-increasing number of patients in the palliative care setting who have just had, are having, or are just about to have, chemotherapy. In many cancer centres patients will be introduced to the palliative care team as part of their initial contact with 'the cancer service'.

Increasing indications for chemotherapy

Over the last decade there has been a huge increase in the number of drugs available to treat cancer patients, and clinical trials have identified that these agents may provide palliative benefit in those for whom no treatment would have been available 20 years ago.

Patients undergoing clinical trials

Patients who have relapsed from their initial chemotherapy may well be involved in clinical trials of other agents if their overall fitness and clinical condition permits. As trials often involve treatments where conventional regimens have failed, such patients may have advanced disease, and need increasing palliative care input.

When is chemotherapy offered in the palliative care setting?
The decision to use chemotherapy with palliative intent is often a complex matter, and a number of factors must be taken into consideration:

- **Patient fitness**: Generally patients with an ECOG performance status (see the Box on p. xxxix) >2 tolerate chemotherapy very poorly—chemotherapy is generally contraindicated in such patients. Possible exceptions include those patients with very chemosensitive tumours that may be expected to respond quickly such as small-cell lung cancer and lymphoma
- **Patient symptoms**: Chemotherapy in the palliative setting is usually delayed until the patient develops symptoms. The potential danger with this approach is that the patient may rapidly develop symptoms which render them unfit for chemotherapy. In some cases, therefore, oncologists may choose to monitor disease and institute treatment when there is evidence that disease, although asymptomatic, is progressing
- **Disease sites**: Generally, large volume disease at life-threatening sites, e.g. the liver, requires urgent chemotherapy even when disease-related symptoms are absent as patients are likely to become symptomatic very quickly.
- **Relationships**: Close relationships may build up between doctors and patients over many years. It may be difficult for doctors to withdraw toxic oncological treatment from a patient who continues to demand

it, even if it has now become clearly inappropriate. Thus clear and open discussion with patients and their families about the potential benefits and risks of chemotherapy, the aims of treatment and, in particular, agreed criteria for stopping treatment is important. The palliative care team can support the oncology team in these discussions

How will chemotherapy affect the patient and family?

Each individual patient and family will have their own particular response to chemotherapy in the palliative care setting. Certain themes may be common to many such individuals. The following are some of the scenarios encountered in GP surgeries, oncology services and palliative care units.

- **'We've got to keep on trying.'** Having endured the rigours of their disease and its management, some patients reach the palliative setting protesting their capacity as 'fighters'. (There is now evidence that psychological disposition has no bearing on disease outcome.) They have coped with their disease by trusting in the system and in being 'active' in fighting their cancer. It is very hard to wean such patients off chemotherapy or to stop active treatment, as to do so seems, in their eyes, to admit defeat. Such patients will ask to be put into trials and see their role as patients as being fulfilled only so long as they are participating in active treatment
- **'It was not half as bad as I thought it was going to be.'** Increasingly due to improved symptom control measures and a more holistic approach, patients may be pleasantly surprised by their tolerance of chemotherapy. Most people have had a previous contact with someone going through chemotherapy and their expectations are often adversely affected by this
- **'He has suffered enough.'** Other families come through their disease journey with very ambivalent attitudes towards the system and to chemotherapy. They arrive in the palliative care setting determined that further suffering should be kept to a minimum. They can be reluctant to consider any intervention at all, other than the administration of pain-controlling medications. For such a family the prospect of chemotherapy entering into the palliative setting is anathema, and time may need to be taken to explain the benefits in certain situations, if appropriate
- **'Her hair fell out, then she died.'** Many patients and families come with memories and histories of relatives who have received chemotherapy in the past. Memories seldom show clearly the distinction between problems caused by the illness itself and problems caused by side-effects. The two merge into a mess of suffering leaving the patient and the family convinced that there is only one thing worse than dying with cancer—and that is dying from cancer with the side-effects of chemotherapy. Doctors and nurses are not inured from such emotional responses

- **'Whatever you say Doctor.'** Another group of patients cope with their disease by investing their trust in 'the doctor' looking after them. Such an approach runs contrary to non-patronizing modern trends but is still present particularly among older patients. To present such patients with a meta-analysis of the benefits of one form of chemotherapy or another and to ask the patient which one they want to choose would be inappropriate
- **'What about Mexican dog weed.'** Some patients and relatives may come into the palliative care setting clutching reams of printouts from the Internet about treatments from clinics around the world. They will often be very articulate and questioning of every intervention. Some will have an alternative medicine approach and be very sceptical of western medicine. Honest communication needs to include how health professionals interpret the clinical research literature and what they would be prepared to do in terms of agreeing to provide a treatment that is controversial, unproven and unlicensed. Boundaries need to be set and unrealistic expectations dispelled, alongside not removing hope that a reasonable quality of life can still be achieved
- **'I've had a good life.'** A section of patients come into the palliative setting without illness at the centre of their lives. Instead they are focused on their living and their dying, with its important stages and goodbyes. Such patients have accepted the inevitability of their death and have moved on to preparing for it. They have things that they want to do. When it comes to the possibility of chemotherapy for such people their main concern is, *'Will it interfere with what I still have to do?'* They are strangely neutral about chemotherapy and it is almost as if they are humouring the professionals by agreeing to it, while they get on with the real business of living
- **'I just can't face it.'** Some patients have been so worn down by their disease and treatment that the prospect of any more chemotherapy fills them with fear and dread. Sometimes the fears are justified and sometimes they are not. Sometimes their expression of fear about chemotherapy is a way of verbalizing fears about other matters which should be explored. They face the dilemma of risks and fears whether or not they accept chemotherapy and will need a lot of support in reaching a treatment decision

Cytotoxic drugs (📖 see also Tables 5.1–5.4)

Alkylating agents
Damage DNA by addition of an alkyl group, e.g. cyclophosphamide, ifosfamide, melphalan, busulphan.

Platinum agents
Damage DNA by addition of platinum adducts, e.g. cisplatin, carboplatin, oxaliplatin.

Antimetabolites
Inhibit production of pyrimidine and purine metabolites, e.g. fluorouracil, methotrexate, capecitabine, mercaptopurine, gemcitabine.

Antitumour antibiotics
Variable mechanism, e.g. doxorubicin, epirubicin, mitoxantrone, bleomycin.

Vinca alkaloids
Bind to the tubulin-blocking microtubule and therefore interfere with spindle formation at metaphase, e.g. vincristine, vinorelbine, vinblastine.

Taxanes
Promote tubulin polymerization and arrest cells at metaphase, e.g. paclitaxel, docetaxel.

Topoisomerase I inhibitors
Inhibit topoisomerase I leading to DNA damage, e.g. irinotecan, topotecan.

Hormonal agents
Selective oestrogen-receptor modulators (SERMs)
Partial antagonists of the oestrogen receptor, e.g. tamoxifen.

Aromatase inhibitors
Inhibit extragonadal oestrogen production, e.g. anastrozole, letrozole, exemestane.

Gonadorelin analogues
Inhibit gonadal production of oestrogen and testosterone, e.g. leuprorelin, goserelin.

Anti-androgens
- Testosterone-receptor antagonists
- Cyproterone acetate

Immunomodulatory
- e.g. Interferon

Novel agents

Many anticancer agents currently in development have been rationally developed to antagonize elements of the neoplastic process at a cellular level. While most of these agents are still in preclinical or early clinical testing, a number have already entered routine clinical practice. As a rule these agents are much better tolerated, but do have a different side-effect profile than conventional cytotoxic drugs, with less myelosuppression, alopecia and emesis. Preclinical testing suggests that many may act as cytostatics rather than cytotoxics and that there may be synergistic inter-actions with other drugs. The challenge in the future will be the rational design of clinical trials to investigate how these agents are best used.

Monoclonal antibodies

- **Trastuzumab**—a monoclonal antibody to HER-2—a member of the epidermal growth-factor (EGF) receptors overexpressed in approximately 25% of all breast cancers and associated with a poor prognosis. Trastuzumab has demonstrated activity in HER-2 overexpressing breast tumours both alone and in combination with chemotherapy in the adjuvant and palliative settings
- **Rituximab**—a monoclonal antibody to CD-20, a protein expressed in some lymphomas. Again rituximab is active both alone and in combination with chemotherapy
- **Bevacizumab**—inhibits angiogenesis by binding to circulating vascular endothelial growth factor (VEGF). Bevacizumab increases the efficacy of chemotherapy in patients with cancers such as colorectal and breast
- **Cetuximab**—attaches itself to the extracellular portion of the EGF receptor preventing the receptor from being activated. It has been combined with chemotherapy and radiotherapy and is used in the treatment of colorectal and head and neck cancers

Cancer growth inhibitors

- **Gefitinib and erlotinib**—inhibit the tyrosine kinase activity of the epidermal growth factor receptor (EGFR). Activity is demonstrated as second-line agents in non-small-cell lung cancer. Common side-effects include diarrhoea and skin rashes
- **Imatinib**—inhibits the tyrosine kinase activity of the cKIT proteins found in gastrointestinal stromal tumours and also of the Bcr/Abl fusion protein found in chronic myeloid leukaemia
- **Bortezomib**—inhibits the proteosome, which is the mechanism by which cells dispose of intracellular peptides. It causes a delay in tumour growth and is used in the treatment of multiple myeloma
- **Sorafenib**— is a small molecule inhibitor of Raf kinase, PDGF (platelet-derived growth factor), VEGF receptor-2 and -3 kinases and cKit. It is used in the treatment of renal-cell cancer
- **Sunitinib**—a small molecule multi-targeted receptor tyrosine kinase inhibitor which is used in the treatment of renal-cell cancer and imatinib-resistant gastrointestinal stromal tumour (GIST)
- **Lapatinib**—EGFR and HER-2 dual tyrosine kinase inhibitor which is used in the treatment of HER-2 positive metastatic breast cancer in combination with capecitabine

Table 5.1 Classification of anti-cancer agents

Class of agent		Mode of action	Examples in common usage
Cytotoxics	Alkylating agents	Damage DNA by addition of an alkyl group	Cyclophosphamide, ifosfamide, melphalan, busulphan
	Platinum agents	Damage DNA by addition of platinum adducts	Cisplatin, carboplatin, oxaliplatin
	Antimetabolites	Inhibit production of pyrimidine and purine metabolites	fluorouracil, methotrexate, capecitabine, mercaptopurine, gemcitabine
	Antitumour antibiotics	Variable	Doxorubicin, epirubicin, mitoxantrone, bleomycin
	Vinca alkaloids	Bind to tubulin blocking microtubule and therefore spindle formation at metaphase	Vincristine, vinorelbine, vinblastine
	Taxanes	Promote tubulin polymerization and arrest cells at metaphase	Paclitaxel, docetaxel
	Topoisomerase I inhibitors	Inhibit topoisomerase I leading to DNA damage	Irinotecan, topotecan

Hormonal agents	Selective oestrogen receptor modulators (SERMs)	Partial antagonists of the oestrogen receptor	Tamoxifen, fulvestrant
	Aromatase inhibitors	Inhibit extragonadal oestrogen production	Anastrozole, letrozole, exemestane
	Gonadorelin analogues	Inhibit gonadal production of oestrogen and testosterone	Leuprorelin
	Anti-androgens	Testosterone receptor antagonists	Cyproterone acetate
Immunomodulatory	Interferon		
'Novel' agents	Antibodies	Opsonization, interrupt growth stimulatory pathways	Rituximab, trastuzumab
	Signal transduction inhibitors	Interrupt growth stimulatory pathways	Imatinib, erlotinib, gefitinib, bortezomib, sunitinib, sorafenib, lapatinib
	Vascular targeting agents	Target 'new' vessels associated with tumours—not in use outwith a clinical trial	Bevacizumab, sunitinib, sorafenib, thalidomide

Table 5.2 Commonly used anti-cancer drugs (new drugs are regularly being introduced)

Drug	Administration	Excretion	Side-effects	Indications
Bleomycin *Cytotoxic antibiotic*	IV	Renal	'Flu symptoms; Hyperpigmentation; Allergic reactions; Pulmonary fibrosis— common with doses >300mg	Germ cell tumours Lymphoma
Busulphan *Alkylating agent*	p.o.	Renal	Myelosuppression; Hyperpigmentation Pulmonary interstitial fibrosis; Hepato-venous occlusion	Leukaemia
Caelyx see doxorubicin				
Carboplatin	IV	Renal	Myelosuppression especially thrombocytopenia; Emesis	Ovarian cancer
Capecitabine *Antimetabolite*	p.o.	Renal	'Hand foot' syndrome; Diarrhoea; Stomatitis	GI cancer, Breast cancer
Cisplatin	IV	Renal	Emesis; Renal failure; Peripheral neuropathy Ototoxicity; Allergic reactions	Germ cell tumours Lung & ovarian cancer
Cyclophosphamide *Alkylating agent*	p.o.	Hepatic and renal	Myelosuppression; Alopecia; Emesis Haemorrhagic cystitis (reduced by mesna)	Breast cancer Lymphoma
Cytarabine *Antimetabolite*	IV, IT, SC	Hepatic and renal	Myelosuppression; (Diarrhoea; Stomatitis	Leukaemia
Dactinomycin *Cytotoxic antibiotic*	IV	Hepatic and renal	Myelosuppression; Mucositis; Diarrhoea Alopecia	Choriocarcinoma Ewing's sarcoma
Docetaxel *Taxane*	IV	Hepatic	Myelosuppression; Fluid retention; Alopecia; Peripheral neuropathy	Breast, Prostate and Lung cancer

Doxorubicin (Adriamycin) *Cytotoxic antibiotic*	IV and intravesical	Hepatic	Emesis; Myelosuppression; Mucositis Alopecia; Cardiomyopathy—risk related to total cumulative dose.	Breast cancer Sarcoma
Doxorubicin Liposomal (Caelyx) *Cytotoxic antibiotic*	IV	Hepatic	Palmar-plantar erythrodysaesthesia; Stomatitis	Ovarian cancer Breast cancer Kaposi's sarcoma
Etoposide	IV	Renal	Myelosuppression; Emesis; Alopecia Secondary leukaemia	Lung cancer Germ cell tumour
Epirubicin *Cytotoxic antibiotic*	IV	Hepatic	Similar to Doxorubicin but less cardiotoxic	Breast cancer
Fluorouracil *Antimetabolite*	IV, topical cream	Hepatic and renal	Mucositis; Diarrhoea; Hand-foot syndrome; Myelosuppression; Gastrointestinal upsets; Cerebellar ataxia (rare); Gritty eyes and blurred vision	Colorectal cancer Breast cancer
Gemcitabine *Antimetabolite*	IV	Renal	Myelosuppression; 'Flu like symptoms; Fatigue; Pneumonitis	Pancreatic cancer Bladder cancer Lung cancer
Ifosfamide *Alkylating agent*	IV	Hepatic and renal	Alopecia; Emesis; Haemorrhagic cystitis; Encephalopathy	Sarcoma, germ cell tumours
Irinotecan *Topoisomerase inhibitor*	IV	Hepatic and renal	Cholinergic syndrome—associated with infusion; Delayed diarrhoea; Nausea and vomiting; Myelosuppression; Alopecia	Colorectal cancer
Mercaptopurine *Antimetabolite*	p.o.	Peripheral tissues	Myelosuppression; Hepatic dysfunction; Stomatitis	Leukaemia

(Continued)

Table 5.2 Commonly used anti-cancer drugs (new drugs are regularly being introduced) (Continued)

Drug	Administration	Excretion	Side-effects	Indications
Methotrexate (+ folinic acid) *Antimetabolite*	p.o., IV, IM, IT	Renal	Myelosuppression; Mucositis; Skin pigmentation; Nephrotoxicity	Osteosarcoma Breast cancer Leukaemia and lymphoma
Mitomycin *Cytotoxic antibiotics*	IV or intravesical	Hepatic metabolism	Myelosuppression; Lung fibrosis; Nephrotoxicity; Stomatitis; Diarrhoea; Haemolytic uraemic syndrome	Anal Bladder
Mitoxantrone *Cytotoxic antibiotic*	IV	Excretion: Bile > urine	Myelosuppression; Emesis; Alopecia; Mucositis; Cardiotoxicity	Lymphoma Leukaemia
Oxaliplatin	IV	Renal	Peripheral neuropathy; Myelosuppression; Nausea and vomiting; Laryngeal spasm	Colorectal cancer
Paclitaxel *Taxane*	IV	Hepatic	Myelosuppression; Alopecia; Hypersensitivity reactions; Peripheral neuropathy	Ovarian cancer Lung cancer Breast cancer
Pemetrexed (Alimpta)	IV	Renal	Myelosuppression; Rash; Stomatitis, Drowsiness	Mesothelioma
Temozolomide *Alkylating agent*	p.o.	Renal	Emesis; Myelosuppression	Astrocytomas Melanoma
Tioguanine *Antimetabolite*	p.o. (40mg)	Renal	Myelosuppression; Mucositis; Diarrhoea; Hepatic dysfunction	Leukaemia

Thiotepa *Alkylating agent*	IV	Excreted more in urine than bile	Myelosuppression	Leukaemia
Topotecan *Topoisomerase inhibitor*		Liver metabolism Urine excretion	Myelosuppression; Emesis; Alopecia; Diarrhoea	Ovarian cancer
Vinblastine *Mitotic spindle inhibitor*	IV	Hepatic	Myelosuppression; constipation and stomatitis Rare: hair loss or peripheral neurotoxicity	Lymphoma Germ cell tumours
Vincristine *Mitotic spindle inhibitor*	IV	Hepatic	Peripheral neuropathy; Autonomic neuropathy	Lymphomas Leukaemia
Vindesine *Mitotic spindle inhibitor*	IV	Hepatic	Myelosuppression; Mild neurotoxicity; Autonomic neuropathy	Leukaemia
Vinorelbine *Mitotic spindle inhibitor*	IV	Hepatic	Myelosuppression; Phlebitis; Peripheral neuropathy	Breast cancer Non-small cell lung cancer

Table 5.3 Hormone and antihormone drugs

Drug	Administration	Side-effects	Comments
SERMs			
Tamoxifen	p.o.	Menopausal symptoms Thromboembolic event Endometrial hyperplasia and cancer	Used first line in adjuvant treatment of ER/PR +ve breast cancer
Fulvestrant	IM	Menopausal symptoms	Post menopausal ER/PR + ve breast cancer
Anti-androgens			
Bicalutamide	p.o.	Hepatotoxicity Gynaecomastia	Used in prostatic cancer sometimes in combination with gonadorelin analogues
Aromatase inhibitors			
Anastrozole	p.o.	Menopausal symptoms Increased fractures	Used in post-menopausal breast cancer
Letrozole			
Exemestane			
GNRH analogues*			
Buserelin	SC and intranasal	Gynaecomastia; impotence; nausea; fluid retention	Prostate cancer
Goserelin	Implant		Breast cancer
Leuprorelin	IM	Menopausal symptoms	

* GNRH, gonadotrophin-releasing hormone; Beware initial flare of symptoms when start use in men with prostate cancer. This should be 'covered' with the concomitant use of anti-androgens for the first few weeks of therapy.

Table 5.4 Emetic risk of common chemotherapy drugs

Cytotoxic agents	Risk
Cisplatin*	High
Cyclophosphamide >1000mg/m^2*	
Ifosfamide*	
Melphalan*	
Actinomycin	Moderate
Amsacrine	
Busulphan	
Carboplatin*	
Chlorambucil	
Cladribine	
Cyclophosphamide <1000mg/m^2	
Cytarabine >150mg/m^2	
Dacarbazine	
Daunorubicin	
Daunorubicin liposomal	
Doxorubicin	
Epirubicin	
Lomustine	
Methotrexate >1g/m^2	
Mitoxantrone	
Procarbazine	
Bleomycin	Low
Cyclophosphamide <300mg/m^2	
Cytarabine <150mg/m^2	
Etoposide	
Fludarabine	
Mercaptopurine	
Methotrexate <lg/m^2	
Tioguanine	
Thiotepa	
Vinblastine	
Vincristine	

*Delayed emesis risk.

Radiotherapy

> Radiotherapy is the most important type of non-surgical treatment for patients with common cancers. The proportion of these treated by radiotherapy at some time during their illness has risen steadily and is now well over 50%.
>
> Tobias, UCH London

Introduction

Radiotherapy as a therapeutic modality developed shortly after the discovery of X-rays at the end of the nineteenth century. Clinical and technological advances subsequently have made it one of the most successful modalities in the treatment of patients with cancer, both in the curative and palliative settings.

Mechanism of action

Radiotherapy is the therapeutic use of ionizing radiation to destroy cancerous cells. The critical cellular target is, in common with chemotherapy, nuclear DNA. Double-stranded breaks in the DNA molecule appear to be the lesion responsible for cell death. Cell death takes place during subsequent mitotic cell division, hence the term 'mitotic cell death'. Much less commonly, there are certain tissue types, such as lymphocytes and parotid acinar cells, that undergo cell death without attempting mitosis, a process known as 'interphase cell death'. Not all double-stranded DNA breaks, however, result in cell death, indeed most are repaired by the cell's DNA repair enzyme apparatus (Fig. 5.2). The success or otherwise of the repair process determines the fate of the cell.

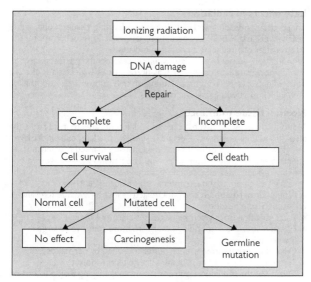

Fig. 5.2 The cell repair process after radiotherapy.

Response of normal tissues to radiation

Different types of normal tissue respond differently to radiation. Homeostatic mechanisms control cell populations by balancing cell death with new cell growth through the proliferation of stem cells. If a proportion of these stem cells are destroyed by radiation, the rate of renewal of normal cells will be reduced. The time of appearance of this tissue damage is determined by the lifespan of the mature cells within that tissue. For certain tissues such as skin and mucosa, this lifespan is short as cells are quickly lost by desquamation, and hence tissue damage is manifest during the radiation course. For other tissues, cell turnover is much slower and radiation damage will only become apparent many months or years after radiation exposure. This gives rise to the distinction between the acute and late effects of irradiation.

Acute effects of radiation

This refers to the normal tissue reactions during a course of radiotherapy. The mucosa and haemopoietic system, i.e. tissues with a fast normal cellular turnover, display the effects of irradiation the earliest. For example, patients receiving radiotherapy to the head and neck area may develop severe oral mucositis, while those receiving radiotherapy to significant volumes of bone marrow may develop bone marrow suppression.

Acute reactions are usually observed during the course of conventionally fractionated radiotherapy (1.8–2Gy per fraction five times a week).

Late effects of radiation

These occur predominantly in slowly proliferating tissues (lung, kidney, heart, liver and CNS). By definition, late reactions occur more than 90 days after commencing a course of radiation.

In addition, some of the tissues which develop their effects early can also demonstrate late effects such as fibrosis or telangiectasia in the skin. This reflects the differing populations of cells (fibroblasts, endothelium, etc.) which exist within a single organ.

Normal tissue tolerance

Not only do different tissues respond at different rates to irradiation, they also vary in their sensitivity. Certain tissues, e.g. the lens, exhibit damage at very low doses while other tissues demonstrate marked resistance to the effects of radiation, e.g. uterine cervix. The situation is analogous among cancers. Lymphomas and seminomas show sensitivity to radiation while renal-cell carcinomas and melanomas are radioresistant.

A number of treatment and patient factors influence tissue tolerance to radiation. These include:

- Total radiation dose given: higher doses are more toxic
- Fraction size: late responding tissues are more sensitive to large fractions
- Overall longer treatment time: better tolerated by normal tissues
- Treatment volume: larger volumes are generally more toxic
- Quality of the radiation: neutrons are more damaging than photons or electrons
- Concomitant therapy: concurrent chemotherapy reduces tolerance

Patient factors adversely influencing tissue tolerance:

- Older age
- Haemoglobin level
- Smoking
- Diabetes mellitus
- Connective tissue disorders
- Genetic syndromes (e.g. ataxia telangiectasia)

Tolerance doses for specific tissues

The following tissues suffer a 5% incidence of toxicity at five years when conventional radiotherapy is given in dose sizes of 1.8–2Gy per fraction at the doses stated for each tissue type (Tables 5.5, 5.6).

Table 5.5 Normal tissue tolerance

Tissue	Injury	Tolerance
Brain	Necrosis	60Gy
Spinal cord	Myelopathy	45Gy (<1% incidence)
Lens*	Cataract	10Gy
Small intestine	Ulceration/perforation	45–50Gy
Kidney*	Clinical nephritis	23Gy
Lung*	Pneumonitis	18–20Gy
Heart*	Pericarditis	40Gy
Ovary	Sterilization	2Gy
Testis	Sterilization	1Gy

* Whole organ.

Re-treatment

Traditional teaching precluded re-treating areas that had already received a maximal radiation dose. Recent studies have shown some tissues and organs have a greater capacity to recover from subclinical radiation injury than was previously thought. For example, the large capacity of long-term regeneration of the CNS allows new possibilities for re-treating recurrent neurological tumours with irradiation.

Table 5.6 Radiation effects within specific tissues (following standard radical doses)

Skin	Acute reaction—erythema begins week 3-4 Dry or moist desquamation later	Reaction settles within 2-4 weeks of completion of therapy
	Late reaction—fibrosis, atrophy, telangiectasia	
Oral mucosa	Acute reaction—erythema/oedema from wk 2-4 Patchy followed by confluent mucositis later	Reaction settles within 2-4 weeks of completion of therapy
Gastrointestinal tract	Acute reaction—mucositis causes nausea, anorexia, cramps, and diarrhoea	Reaction settles within 2-4 weeks of completion of therapy Treat symptomatically
	Late reaction—ulceration and fibrosis leading to strictures, fistulae, and malabsorption	Usually >6 months post RT
Brain	Acute reaction—lethargy common Occasionally cerebral oedema	
	Late reaction—somnolence syndrome at 1-3 months post RT Brain necrosis at 6 months to 3 years	Resolves spontaneously with/without help of steroids Indistinguishable clinically from recurrent tumour
Spinal cord	Late reaction—Lhermitte's syndrome 2-18 months after RT Radiation myelopathy at 6-12 months	Resolves spontaneously. Does not progress to myelopathy. Irreversible
Lung	Early/intermediate reaction—pneumonitis at 1-3 months Results in pulmonary fibrosis	Classical straight-edged appearance on chest x-ray
Kidney	Late reaction—proteinuria, hypertension, renal failure	May take up to 10 years to develop
Heart	Late reaction—pericarditis/effusion Most within 6 months of RT Cardiomyopathy Coronary artery disease	Most resolve spontaneously; may develop into a constrictive process 10-20 years post RT 10-15 years post RT

NB Patients undergoing radiotherapy usually experience lethargy as a general side-effect.

Types of radiation therapy

There are three main types of radiation therapy:

- **External beam radiotherapy**—delivered by radiotherapy machines
- **Brachytherapy**—solid radiation sources delivered directly into tumours
- **Unsealed source or radioisotope therapy**—given by mouth, intravenously or into tissue spaces

External beam radiotherapy

External beam radiation consists of different energies, as shown in Table 5.7.

Table 5.7 External beam radiation

Type of radiation	Energy	Use
Superficial X-rays	80–150kV	Skin tumours
Orthovoltage X-rays (DXT)	200–400kV	Thick skin tumours Superficial tumours, e.g. ribs
Megavoltage radiation		
γ-rays—cobalt 60	1.25MV (mean)	Deep tumours
X-rays—linear accelerator	4–25MV	Deep tumours
Electrons	4–20MeV	Skin tumours Superficial tumours

Superficial X-rays use relatively low-energy X-ray photons in the range 80–400kV. These X-rays are relatively non-penetrating, depositing the majority of their energy in the most superficial few millimetres of skin. They, therefore, deliver a high dose to the skin with rapid fall-off with increasing depth and are thus appropriate for the treatment of superficial skin lesions such as basal-cell cancers.

Orthovoltage energy X-rays are slightly more penetrating and deliver sufficient dose at depth to treat adequately thicker skin or subcutaneous lesions such as rib metastases. (Both superficial and orthovoltage X-rays suffer the disadvantage of delivering a higher absorbed dose to bone compared to soft tissue, thus increasing the risk of osteoradio-necrosis if a lesion is positioned too close to underlying bony tissue.)

Megavoltage X-ray photons possess energies 50–200 times those of superficial X-rays. (1–20MV) In contrast to superficial/orthovoltage X-rays, megavoltage photons are produced by the acceleration of electrons along a linear tube (wave guide) before striking a target. This is done within a machine called a 'linear accelerator'. The interaction of these high-energy electrons with the target material generates high-energy X-rays.

High-energy X-rays are very penetrating and give a much higher dose at a given depth within a tissue than superficial X-rays.

Megavoltage X-rays possess the advantage of relative sparing of the superficial skin tissues as the maximum absorbed dose occurs up to several centimetres below the skin surface. There is also no increased absorption of dose in tissues containing elements of high atomic mass such as bone.

Electron therapy

Electrons may be generated using a linear accelerator. In this situation the accelerated electron beam exits the linear accelerator without striking the target. Electron therapy is used to treat superficial tumours, most often of the skin. It is their characteristic deposition of dose with depth which makes electrons ideal for this purpose: >90% of the dose is deposited in the first few centimetres of tissue with very rapid dose fall-off thereafter, thus sparing underlying structures.

Treatment planning

This is the essential prerequisite step before treatment delivery. During the process of treatment planning questions such as 'where to treat?', 'what to treat?', 'what not to treat?', 'how to treat and how much to treat?' are addressed. It is essentially an iterative process with changes being made at various stages to facilitate the design of an optimal treatment schedule. There are several rungs in the planning ladder (Fig. 5.3).

The complexity of treatment planning depends upon the tumour and the intent of therapy. Radical plans are generally more complicated and time-consuming than those with palliative intent.

Immobilization is relatively more important for tumours positioned close to sensitive normal tissue structures and for radical, high-dose, treatments.

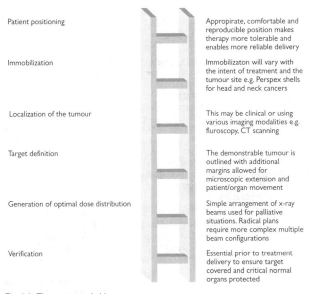

Patient positioning	Appropriate, comfortable and reproducible position makes therapy more tolerable and enables more reliable delivery
Immobilization	Immobilizaton will vary with the intent of treatment and the tumour site e.g. Perspex shells for head and neck cancers
Localization of the tumour	This may be clinical or using various imaging modalities e.g. fluroscopy, CT scanning
Target definition	The demonstrable tumour is outlined with additional margins allowed for microscopic extension and patient/organ movement
Generation of optimal dose distribution	Simple arrangement of x-ray beams used for palliative situations. Radical plans require more complex multiple beam configurations
Verification	Essential prior to treatment delivery to ensure target covered and critical normal organs protected

Fig. 5.3 The treatment ladder.

The tumour is **localized** either by clinical examination, e.g. skin tumours, or by imaging, most commonly fluoroscopy or CT scanning. Newer technology permits the fusing of various imaging modalities, e.g. CT/MRI images, PET/CT images.

Once the tumour is localized the **target volume is defined**. This encompasses the tumour with a safety margin. This margin is added to allow for microscopic tumour extension, the so-called 'clinical target volume'. Additionally, the margin will also accommodate movements in the organ containing the tumour, and uncertainties inherent in the treatment delivery system.

After the target has been delineated differing beam arrangements are generated. The arrangement is chosen which best covers the target volume and most successfully spares the normal tissue structures.

The final step in treatment planning is **verification**. This is an essential step to ensure that a plan generated on a planning computer actually fits the patient, i.e. the tumour is accurately targeted and critical structures such as the spinal cord are adequately spared. The verification process continues through treatment with dose measurements confirming appropriate dose delivery.

Radiotherapy dose prescription

Once the final treatment plan is decided upon, the radiation dose must be prescribed. There are several constituents that together make up the prescription:
- Total dose
- Number of fractions (fraction size)
- Overall treatment time

Total dose/number of fractions

Rather than deliver the entire dose of radiation in a single treatment, the dose is divided up into smaller quanta. This is the process of fractionation, each treatment dose being known as a 'fraction'. Fractionation is performed to permit repair of normal tissue radiation damage. Fractionation will also permit repair to occur within tumour tissue, although this is relatively less efficient. In consequence, when a treatment course is fractionated, the total dose of radiation must be increased. Early studies showed that changing from a single dose to a six-week fractionated course of therapy required an increase in the total dose by a factor of three in order to achieve the same biological effect.
- The relationship between total dose and number of fractions is, however, complex and mathematical models are used to help predict the biological effects

Small numbers of fractions are convenient for the patient as travelling is kept to a minimum. However, the fraction size is in consequence larger; this increases the biological effectiveness of each fraction resulting in more severe damage to late-responding tissues. The total dose in such hypofractionated courses must be reduced to maintain an acceptable level of late tissue damage.

Hypofractionated treatment courses are often employed in the palliative setting because of their convenience for patients and the relative unimportance of adverse long-term radiation effects in patients with limited life expectancy.

Overall treatment time

Standard radical fractionation schedules involve treating once per day, Monday to Friday, for four to seven weeks. As treatment generally extends beyond four weeks, tumour cell repopulation does become a problem.

As the number of tumour stem cells and mature functional tumour cells are depleted as a result of radiotherapy, the remaining stem cells sense this loss and begin to replicate actively to counteract this deficit. This is known as 'tumour repopulation'. It appears that there is a lag period of approximately 3–4 weeks before this phenomenon occurs. Each fraction of radiotherapy delivered after the onset of repopulation is therefore relatively less effective, since part of the fraction must counteract this increase in the number of *tumour cells* resulting from repopulation.

A means of circumventing this effect of tumour repopulation is to *accelerate* the radiotherapy course so that the dose is delivered over a shorter period, preferably less than the 3–4 weeks required for the onset of repopulation. A large, randomized controlled clinical trial[4] of accelerated radiotherapy in non-small-cell lung cancer has demonstrated that such an approach can be effective, with an increased rate of local tumour control and overall survival.

Brachytherapy

Here the radiation source is closely applied to the tumour. (Literally: therapy at a short distance, from the Greek $\beta\rho\alpha\chi\upsilon\varsigma$, brachys, short).

The underlying principle is the inverse square law, which states that the intensity of radiation, R, at a given distance, D, from a radioactive source, and therefore the absorbed dose, is inversely proportional to the square of that distance. Put simply, doubling the distance between the radiation source and the tissue reduces the dose absorbed by the tissue by a factor of four (rather than a factor of two as might be expected if the relationship was linear):

$$R \propto \frac{1}{D^2}$$

The beauty of brachytherapy lies in the ability to administer high doses of radiation to the tumour with relative sparing of neighbouring normal tissue because of rapid fall-off of absorbed dose with distance.

Brachytherapy is also known as '**sealed source therapy**' because the radioactive substance (often a metal), e.g. iridium-192, is usually encased or sealed within a metal casing such that the radioactive substance does not actually physically touch the tissue even when inserted directly into the tumour (see below).

4 Saunders M., *et al.* (1999) Continuous, hyperfractionated, accelerated radiotherapy (CHART) versus conventional radiotherapy in non-small cell lung cancer: mature data from the randomised multicentre trial. *Radiotherapy and Oncology*, **52**: 137–48.

Brachytherapy takes three main forms:

- **Interstitial**: The radiation source is inserted directly into the tumour tissue
- **Intracavitary**: The radioactive source is inserted into a body cavity such as the uterus or the vagina when treating endometrial or cervical cancer
- **Intraluminal**: The radioactive source is positioned in the lumen of a hollow viscus, e.g. bronchus, oesophagus

Brachytherapy, because it involves the placing of radioactive sources in close proximity to the patient, must of necessity make staff vulnerable to the risk of radiation exposure.

Decreasing the time during which exposure might occur, maximizing the shielding between the source and staff, and most importantly increasing the distance from source to personnel all help to diminish risk.

In practice, the brachytherapist places hollow tubes into the tumour, cavity or lumen, through which the source may subsequently be driven mechanically. Thus the radioactive source is brought into very close proximity to the tumour but staff experience no significant exposure.

Unsealed source therapy

This involves administering radioactive substances directly into the patient, either in the form of liquids for ingestion or solutions for intravenous administration.

Unsealed source therapy is most often used as a palliative manoeuvre, although radioactive iodine-131 is employed as an adjuvant to curative surgery for well-differentiated thyroid cancer and indeed is often used to treat thyrotoxicosis, a non-malignant condition.

Radiation protection issues are to the fore as patients emit radiation for a variable period after administration of the radioisotope depending on the half-life of the isotope. They are carefully instructed regarding the precautions necessary to prevent excess exposure to others, most notably family members. Such precautions include double flushing of the toilet after micturition, refraining from close contact with children and avoiding places of entertainment or work for a specified period post-treatment.

A number of radioisotopes are commonly used:

- **Strontium-89 (^{89}Sr)**: Often used for the relief of bone pain due to metastatic bone disease. A disadvantage is the relatively long half-life which poses radiation protection problems, especially if the patient dies within a short period after treatment. Some patients experience a flare up in their bone pain within a few days of treatment. This usually settles with appropriate analgesia. As strontium is absorbed into bone tissue, bone marrow toxicity may occasionally occur, and regular blood count monitoring after treatment is advised
- **Samarium-153 (^{153}Sm)**: Used less commonly than ^{89}Sr but indicated likewise for the relief of pain from bony metastatic disease. It has the advantages of a shorter half-life and the production of photons as part of its decay pathway. These photons permit scintigraphy and thus bone scan images may be obtained. The propensity to pain flare and marrow toxicity pertain as for strontium-89

- **Iodine-131 (^{131}I):** Both normal thyroid and well-differentiated thyroid cancer (papillary and follicular variants) selectively take up and concentrate iodine. This can be exploited therapeutically using ^{131}I. Due to this concentrating effect within thyroid tissue, high doses can be selectively delivered to the normal or malignant thyroid tissue leading to its destruction. In the case of normal thyroid tissue, hyperthyroid patients may be rendered euthyroid with a relatively low dose of ^{131}I; in the case of malignancy, ^{131}I is used as an adjuvant treatment following surgery to ablate the remaining normal thyroid tissue and any potential microscopic residual tumour
- **Phosphorus-32 (^{32}P):** This has proved useful in the treatment of polycythaemia rubra vera, although, because it may increase the risk of subsequent development of leukaemia, it is generally reserved for patients over 70 years of age

Radiation therapy

Radiotherapy is used for about half of the 200,000 patients who develop cancer in the UK each year. It has a curative [or adjuvant] role in two-thirds, and a palliative role in the remainder.

Horwich, Royal Marsden

Radiotherapy may be administered in differing clinical situations and with varying intents.

Treatment can be:
• **Radical**—curative intent
• **Adjuvant**—postoperative
• **Palliative**—symptom control

Radical radiotherapy

Radiotherapy may be administered with the intent of cure either as the preferred primary therapy (e.g. early-stage Hodgkin's disease), or as an alternative to surgery.

In the latter situation it has the advantage of preserving normal anatomy, e.g. anal canal cancer, bladder cancer. Additionally, acute morbidity is often less severe. However, because no surgical specimen is obtained, there can be no pathological data to permit accurate staging. Stage must therefore be assessed by clinical or radiological methods. Late effects of radiation, such as fibrosis, may also make subsequent assessment of the tumour site for local recurrence difficult.

Radical radiation is reserved for tumours which can be encompassed within a reasonable radiation treatment volume, i.e. localized, as opposed to widely metastatic disease; this presupposes accurate staging investigations.

Treatment is often complex, with effort given to rigid immobilization and the use of complicated beam arrangements to obtain a uniform dose distribution confined to the tumour with preservation of normal surrounding structures. A high dose of radiation is necessary for all but the most radio-sensitive of tumours, and treatment is delivered in conventional (small) fraction sizes in order to reduce the late adverse effects of radiation.

Examples of radical radiotherapy include:
• **Head and neck tumours:** Many squamous-cell tumours of the head and neck region can be cured by radical radiotherapy (often combined with synchronous chemotherapy), e.g. early-stage cancers of the larynx are frequently cured with preservation of good-quality voice
• **Anal canal cancer:** A radical approach using concurrent chemo-radiotherapy has been shown to be effective management for epidermoid anal-canal cancer. Additionally, 60–70% of patients retain a functioning anal sphincter after treatment. A common alternative to such an approach is primary abdominoperineal excision of the rectum and anal canal, which results in a permanent colostomy
• **Lung cancer:** Radical radiotherapy can be employed as a second-best option in the management of lung cancer. Although the patients selected for such treatment may not be sufficiently fit to undergo radical surgery, they may be fit for radiation treatment with a cure rate of 15–20%

Adjuvant radiotherapy

Adjuvant radiotherapy is administered as an adjunct to potentially curative surgery. The principle underpinning such treatment is the possibility of microscopic loco-regional residual disease, either within the tumour bed, lymphatic channels or regional lymph node drainage. The aim of adjuvant radiotherapy is the eradication of this microscopic disease and thereby to reduce the rate of local relapse and improve overall survival.

Examples of adjuvant radiotherapy:

- **Breast cancer:** This is perhaps the best example and is certainly the most common exemplifier of adjuvant radiation. Up to 50% of the workload of many UK radiotherapy centres is devoted to adjuvant breast irradiation. Local relapse rates following partial mastectomy may reach 30%. Postoperative breast irradiation can reduce this figure by three- to fourfold. Local control rates then conform to those achieved after mastectomy but with a superior cosmetic outcome
- **Head and neck cancer:** Surgery for squamous tumours of the head and neck is complex. Due to the close proximity of tumours to important structures, surgical margins may often be inadequate because compromise must be made to retain acceptable functional and cosmetic outcomes. Adjuvant irradiation is employed if margins are unsatisfactory or following radical neck surgery that demonstrates multiple involved lymph nodes. Classically, adjuvant radiotherapy is administered after surgery has been performed

However, in some situations, although surgery remains the mainstay of treatment, radiotherapy may be delivered as a prelude to a surgical procedure.

True **neoadjuvant radiation** is administered in order to shrink or downstage the tumour, thus facilitating subsequent surgery. In this case, time must elapse between irradiation and surgery to allow tumour reduction. An illustration of this technique is preoperative rectal radiotherapy for tethered or fixed rectal adenocarcinoma. Treatment is delivered over 4–5 weeks after which there is a gap of about 6 weeks during which tumour shrinkage occurs. This facilitates radical surgery in patients who were initially regarded as technically inoperable.

Short-course preoperative rectal radiotherapy, by contrast, is delivered over the week immediately prior to surgery. No time is permitted for tumour shrinkage. Trials have, however, confirmed a significant improvement in local control and overall survival with this approach.

Adjuvant radiation treatment courses typically extend over 4–6 weeks. The general principles applied to radical radiotherapy also hold for the adjuvant setting as treatment intent is curative, i.e. immobilization, careful avoidance of critical organs at risk, and low dose per fraction. Total doses tend to be slightly lower since the target is microscopic residual disease. It must, however, be remembered that following surgery the vascular supply to tissues is disrupted resulting in areas of tissue hypoxia. **Radiation is relatively less effective in an environment that is poorly oxygenated**.

Palliative radiotherapy

When radiotherapy is administered in the palliative setting, the aim is the control of distressing symptoms. The disease is, by definition, incurable. These factors impact upon treatment in a variety of ways:

• Symptomatic sites of disease are targeted
• Sites at high risk of producing symptoms may receive prophylactic treatment
• Fractionation regimens are kept short
• Moderate doses of radiation are employed
• Palliative benefit must outweigh treatment-related toxicity

Palliative radiotherapy may produce prolongation of survival but this is not its primary aim, rather it is the quality of that survival which is the goal. Palliative radiotherapy often produces significant symptomatic gain.

There are several clinical scenarios in which palliative radiotherapy commonly proves useful.

Pain

Bone metastases, pain due to nerve compression or soft tissue infiltration will usually respond to radiation treatment and will respond to a single fraction of radiotherapy as effectively as more prolonged treatment schedules.

The former are more patient-friendly and may be repeated if necessary. If pain is diffuse, affecting many disparate sites within the skeleton, wide field—hemibody—irradiation often produces relief. An alternative is radioisotope therapy with ^{89}Sr or ^{153}Sm.

Osteolytic tumour deposits in weight-bearing bones are at risk of fracture and are best fixed prophylactically by orthopaedic intervention. This is often followed by postoperative irradiation, although good evidence of benefit is lacking. Rarely, radiation is given without prophylactic surgical intervention.

Haemorrhage

Haemoptysis, haematuria, haematemesis and rectal bleeding all respond to radiation. A hypofractionated treatment course often produces prompt sustained benefit (at least 70% in carcinoma of the bronchus).

Obstruction

Any hollow viscus may undergo obstruction caused by a malignant process. Several organs may commonly be obstructed by cancer:

• Superior vena cava (SVC)
• Upper airways, i.e. trachea, bronchus
• Oesophagus

Prompt, if not immediate, relief is frequently afforded by insertion of a stent under the care of the interventional radiologists for SVC or oesophageal obstruction. There is a role for palliative radiotherapy in some patients who are unsuitable for such procedures, or in the case of stent overgrowth by tumour.

Radiotherapy is most often used for bronchial obstruction due to lung cancer; laser resection or stent insertion are less commonly employed alternatives.

Chemotherapy is also used for SVC obstruction caused by chemosensitive tumours, for example, small-cell lung cancer.

Neurological symptoms
- Spinal cord compression
- Brain metastases
- Cranial or peripheral nerve compression
- Malignant meningitis
- Choroidal or orbital metastases

Radiotherapy is used in treating spinal cord compression. There are a number of important indications for surgical as opposed to radiotherapeutic intervention (e.g. uncertain pathology, unstable spine).

Radiotherapy often improves pain associated with the compression, but neurological recovery is less predictable and mainly depends on the degree of weakness prior to therapy and the particular histological tumour type.

Brain metastases are increasing in incidence as oncological management improves and patients survive long enough to develop relapse within the brain. Steroids can produce significant benefit if the effects are due to oedema or compression rather than tissue destruction. However, their beneficial effects tend to be short-lived. Prolongation of symptom control and a small gain in survival (1–2 months) can additionally be obtained with cranial irradiation, usually at the cost of alopecia and lethargy. Those with good pretreatment neurological function and sensitive tumours stand to gain most.

Cranial or peripheral nerve compression most often occurs with breast or prostate neoplasms. Pain is often improved but nerve palsies seldom show significant recovery.

Fungating tumours
Locally advanced breast tumours, skin tumours, metastatic skin or lymph node deposits, can all lead to fungation. If surgical intervention is not possible or felt to be inappropriate, radiotherapy can reduce the tumour mass, serous ooze or haemorrhage, and promote healing.

Managing side-effects of radiotherapy

Skin
General advice
- Skin reactions tend to be worse in the skin folds, i.e. inframammary fold, axilla, groin and perineum
- Deodorants should be avoided within the treatment area
- Aftershave lotions or astringent cosmetics should be avoided
- Mild soaps are permitted, and washing should be gentle (no vigorous rubbing) and the area patted dry
- Care must be taken not to remove skin markings delineating the treatment fields

Mild reactions
- Skin pink or slightly red
- Apply aqueous cream frequently

Moderate reactions
- Skin red, dry and scaly; some pruritus/tingling
- Apply aqueous cream frequently
- If itch is problematic, 1% hydrocortisone cream q.d.s. is useful

Severe reactions
- Skin is inflamed with patchy areas of moist desquamation
- Epidermis may blister and slough exposing the dermis leading to pain and serous ooze with an increased risk of infection
- Hydrogel or alginate dressing can be applied to moist areas; Diprobase® cream to intact epidermis
- Swab if there is evidence of infection

Mouth and throat care
This is particularly important for patients receiving radiotherapy for head and neck lesions.

General advice
- The patient needs a dental assessment and any dental treatment should be carried out before radiotherapy begins
- A good fluid and nutritional intake is very important and nutritional support by NG feeding is indicated if >10% weight loss occurs
- Cessation of smoking should be strongly encouraged
- Alcohol and spicy foods should be avoided
- The voice should be rested as the radiotherapy reaction becomes established

Treatment of mucositis
- Normal saline or bicarbonate mouth washes often help
- Antiseptic mouth washes, e.g. chlorhexidine, keep the mouth clean but can cause pain due to their alcohol content
- Oropharyngeal candida infection should be actively sought and treated

- Local analgesics include:
  - aspirin (which may be gargled)
  - paracetamol (which may be gargled)
  - benzydamine (Difflam®)
  - local anaesthetics (Xylocaine®)
  - topical steroids (Adcortyl in orobase®, Corlan pellets®)
  - coating agents (Sucralfate®, Gelclair®)

Dysphagia

Thoracic radiotherapy can lead to oesophagitis which needs explanation and symptomatic treatment. Smoking should be strongly discouraged; spirits and spicy food should be avoided.

An antacid, e.g. Gaviscon®, soluble paracetamol or aspirin may all help. An NSAID, either orally or by suppository, may be used. The oesophagus can be coated with some effect by Sucralfate®.

Nausea and vomiting

Radiotherapy to the abdomen often causes nausea due to serotonin release. All patients should thus be considered for prophylactic anti-emetic therapy, e.g. 5-HT$_3$ antagonist.

Diarrhoea

This side-effect frequently accompanies radiotherapy to the abdomen or pelvis. Dietary modification, i.e. reduction in dietary roughage, may sometimes relieve the diarrhoea. Antidiarrhoeal drugs (e.g. loperamide) should be provided to all patients with clear instructions of when and how they should be taken. Proctitis often accompanies rectal or prostatic irradiation and should be treated with rectal steroids either by suppository or enema.

Pneumonitis

Acute radiotherapy-induced pneumonitis can develop one to three months after treatment and is associated with a fever, dry cough and breathlessness. The main differential diagnosis is pneumonia and this should be excluded where possible. The diagnosis can be confirmed by a CXR, which shows lung infiltration confined within the treatment volume. Treatment is with a reducing course of steroids, i.e. a starting dose of prednisolone 40mg.

Cerebral oedema

This can occur during or after cranial irradiation, particularly if no surgical decompression of the brain tumour or metastasis has been undertaken. Oedema usually responds to an increase in the dose of oral steroids.

Somnolence syndrome

This occurs within a few weeks of the completion of brain irradiation and may manifest itself with nausea, vomiting, anorexia, dysarthria, ataxia and profound lethargy. Recovery occurs spontaneously but can be accelerated with steroids.

New developments

Radiotherapy has advanced markedly since the early days of the nine-teenth century. Progress is still being made to improve the quality and effectiveness of treatment for patients.

There are a number of areas of development.

Defining tumour volume

Improvements in imaging have enabled tumours to be targeted more accurately. This reduces the risk of missing the tumour, and also allows the treatment volume to encompass the tumour more closely. The dose of radiation can therefore be higher (giving improved tumour control) without risking additional toxicity to normal tissues.

Imaging

Refinements in CT scanning technology have led to the advent of the multi-slice CT scanner that provides multiple high-quality images rapidly, from which tumour volumes may be defined not only in two but also in three dimensions.

Images can now be fused from different imaging modalities, e.g. MRI/CT image fusion. The new development of co-registered CT/PET scanning. combines functional data (through PET scanning) and high-quality spatial information (through CT scanning) providing opportunity for optimal target volume definition.

Conformal therapy

Imaging improvements provide the ability to identify the tumour target more accurately. This reduces the risk of missing the tumour, but it also provides the opportunity for conforming the treatment more closely to the tumour volume and thereby lessening damage to surrounding normal tissues. Taken further, conformal therapy may permit dose escalation with resulting improved tumour control rates, but without increased toxicity. Multileaf collimators within the treatment unit can automatically shape the treatment field, conforming it to the desired target shape.

Intensity modulated radiotherapy (IMRT) takes this a step further. With IMRT the intensity of the treatment beams are modified in such a way that almost any three-dimensional volume may be generated. Even concave volumes may be created, and so targets which envelop the spinal cord, e.g. thyroid, can be treated much more satisfactorily than with conventional techniques.

Fractionation/combined modality treatment

Advances in the understanding of the principles of fractionation have led to improved treatment outcomes for patients, e.g. CHART in non-small-cell lung cancer. Further research with hypo/hyperfractionation and accel-eration is ongoing in other tumour types.

Integration of chemotherapy with radiation treatment has provided benefit in a number of tumour sites, e.g. cervical cancer. Research seeks to refine this further and also to incorporate the newer molecular agents into radiation therapy.

Individualization of therapy

Two patients with ostensibly similar tumours receiving identical treatments may respond differently, one being cured and the other dying from cancer in a short time. There are clearly factors inherent within tumours which predict for response to radiotherapy. If such variables were identified before treatment the chance of response could be defined. This would help clinicians in deciding whether radiotherapy would be a good treatment option. Furthermore, it might be possible, knowing the particular tumour characteristics, to adapt the treatment course, perhaps by modifying the dose prescribed or the fractionation schedule, to enhance the prospect of cure. Predictive assays are being developed to realize this possibility. New microchip technology may help elucidate the genes behind the differing responses to therapy, and offer patients the possibility of treatment tailored to their individual needs.

Common cancers

Incidence

Huge variations in cancer incidences exist across the globe, reflecting the impact of environmental and genetic factors on the causes of cancer (Tables 5.8 and 5.9).[5]

Table 5.8 The eight commonest cancer types affecting men and women worldwide

Cancer type	Ratio, high:low rate	High incidence	Low incidence
Oesophagus	200:1	Kazakhastan	Holland
Skin	200:1	Australia	India
Liver	100:1	Mozambique	UK
Nasopharynx	100:1	China	Uganda
Lung	40:1	UK	Nigeria
Stomach	30:1	Japan	UK
Cervix	20:1	Hawaii	Israel
Rectum	20:1	Denmark	Nigeria

Table 5.9 The eight commonest cancer types affecting men and women in the UK[5]

Men	Women
Lung	Breast
Colorectal	Lung
Skin	Colorectal
Prostate	Skin
Stomach	Stomach
Pancreas	Ovary
Oesophagus	Cervix
Leukaemia	Pancreas

5 Souhami R. L., Tobias J. D. (2003) *Cancer and its Management* (4th edn). Oxford: Blackwell Science.

In this Handbook it is not possible to outline oncological management of all cancer types. The following cancers are the commonest, and those for which the palliative care team has a particular role to play (Table 5.10).

Table 5.10 Common cancers

Cancer type	Page	Cancer type	Page
Lung	172	Upper GI	194
Colorectal	178	Bladder and ureter	200
Breast	182	Brain	202
Prostate	186	Haematological	208
Gynaecological	190	Unknown primary	210

Patients with lung cancer

Background
- Most common cancer in men and women in the UK and the US
- 90% due to smoking
- 80% are non-small-cell subtype (squamous, adenocarcinoma or large cell)
- 20% are small-cell subtype

Symptoms at presentation
- Cough
- Haemoptysis
- Chest pain
- Recurrent chest infection
- Hoarseness

Diagnosis and staging

Diagnosis
- CXR
- Sputum cytology
- Bronchoscopy with biopsy
- Bronchial brushings and washings
- CT-guided biopsy

Staging
- Bronchoscopy
- CT scan of chest, liver and adrenals
- PET scanning (if available)
- Mediastinoscopy
- Pleural aspiration, pleural biopsy
- Bone and brain scan if symptomatic

Small-cell lung carcinoma (SCLC)

This is generally believed to be a systemic disease at diagnosis; thus surgery generally plays no part in the management of this disease.

Staging
- Limited stage disease—disease confined to one hemithorax
- Extensive stage disease—disease present beyond one hemithorax

Management
- Because of chemoresponsiveness and frequent dissemination at diagnosis combined chemotherapy is the treatment of choice
- Many chemotherapeutic agents have demonstrated activity in this disease. Commonly used regimes include cisplatin/etoposide and cyclophosphamide/doxorubicin/vincristine
- For patients with limited stage disease, thoracic irradiation in addition to chemotherapy improves local disease control and prolongs survival when compared with chemotherapy alone. Prophylactic cranial irradiation reduces the incidence of brain metastases and improves survival in patients who have responded to chemotherapy
- Further radiotherapy may be a useful palliative treatment for patients relapsing after or resistant to chemotherapy

Prognosis

Approximately 80% of patients respond to chemotherapy, but the majority relapse and only approximately 10% of patients are alive two years following diagnosis.

Non-small-cell lung carcinoma (NSCLC)

Non-small-cell lung cancer metastasizes later in its course than small-cell lung cancer and consequently surgery offers the best chance of cure. All patients being considered for surgical treatment must be carefully staged (Tables 5.11 and 5.12) to determine tumour operability. The patient must also be carefully assessed preoperatively to assess their fitness for surgery.

Perioperative mortality rate should be less than 5%.

Table 5.11 TNM staging of lung cancer

T_1	Tumour <3cm diameter; distal to main bronchus
T_2	Tumour >3cm diameter; or involves main bronchus 2cm distal to carina; or invading visceral pleura; or atelectasis extending to hilum
T_3	Tumour invading chest wall, diaphragm, mediastinal pleura or pericardium; or tumour in main bronchus <2cm distal to carina or atelectasis of whole lung
T_4	Tumour invading mediastinum, heart, major vessels, trachea, oesophagus, vertebra or carina; or malignant pleural effusion
N_0	No regional node metastases
N_1	Ipsilateral peribronchial or peribronchial or hilar nodes
N_2	Ipsilateral mediastinal or subcarinal nodes
N_3	Contralateral mediastinal nodes; scalene or supraclavicular nodes

Table 5.12 Stage grouping

I	$T_{1-2} N_0$
II	$T_{1-2} N_1$ or $T_3 N_0$
IIIA	$T_{1-2} N_2$ or $T_3 N_{1-2}$
IIIB	T_4 any N M_0; or any $N_3 M_0$
IV	Any M_1

Management

Surgery

Surgical resection offers the best chance of cure in this disease. The aim of surgery is to resect the primary tumour with clear lateral and bronchial margins with draining peribronchial and hilar lymph nodes. Lobectomy is the most commonly performed operation; however, a bilobectomy or pneumonectomy may be performed for more extensive tumours.

Conversely, in less fit patients with limited respiratory reserve only a partial lobectomy may be tolerated, although the results from this surgery in terms of the risk of tumour recurrence may be inferior.

NSCLC radiation therapy

Radical radiotherapy

Selected patients with stage I–III disease and who are technically unsuitable or medically unfit for surgery may be suitable for radical radiotherapy. Five-year survivals of 15–20% have been reported in this highly selected patient group.

The benefit of adjuvant radiotherapy following surgery for high-risk disease is uncertain but may reduce the risk of local disease relapse.

Palliative radiotherapy

Radiotherapy is a key component of symptomatic treatment for:
• Haemoptysis
• Chest pain
• Dyspnoea due to bronchial occlusion
• Pain from bone metastasis
• Symptoms from brain metastasis

NSCLC chemotherapy

NSCLC is much less chemosensitive than SCLC. Adjuvant platinum-based chemotherapy following surgery confers just a modest survival benefit. Chemotherapy may also be used in the neoadjuvant setting to downstage a tumour prior to consideration of surgery. Cisplatin-based therapy has recently been demonstrated to improve quality of life and survival in patients with good performance status (ECOG performance scale 0–1) in the palliative setting. Commonly used regimens include cisplatin/paclitaxel, cisplatin/vinorelbine and cisplatin/gemcitabine.

Drugs targeting the EGFR tyrosine kinase, such as erlotinib, have shown modest activity in NSCLC. Although response rates are low, a higher proportion of patients gain symptomatic benefit.

Table 5.13 Prognosis

Stage	Five-year survival (%)
I	60–80
II	25–40
IIIA	10–15
IIIB and IV	<5

General issues

Lung cancer, because of its link with smoking, both active and passive, may be associated with emotional distress in the patient and their carers. Lung cancers often occur on top of a background of pre-existing lung disease which may alter the patient's perception of breathlessness and cough.

Specific pain issues
- **Pleuritic pain** may be associated with the tumour itself, metastases in ribs or local inflammation. This type of pain responds well to NSAIDs. It may also be helped by local nerve blockade.
- **Pancoast tumour** at the lung apex can produce severe neuropathic pain by invasion of the brachial plexus which may only be partially opioid-responsive and will need adjuvant analgesics. Early referral for specialist help should be considered
- **Bone metastases** may occur, putting the patient at risk of pathological fractures and spinal cord compression. Management of subsequent pain may be difficult and specialist advice should be sought

Other complications
- **Breathlessness** is common and can be very distressing for carers (see Respiratory section). Treat reversible causes such as anaemia and pleural effusion, where appropriate. Give clear explanations of what is happening. Ensure that practical measures such as sitting upright, opening windows and using fans have been discussed with the family. Regular doses of short-acting oral morphine every 2–4h may decrease the sensation of breathlessness. Other more specialist interventions such as palliative radiotherapy, endobronchial laser therapy and stenting may help some patients. Panic and anxiety are frequently associated with breathlessness and may be helped by simple relaxation techniques. A low dose of an anxiolytic such as diazepam may be helpful
- **Haemoptysis** is a frightening symptom. Palliative radiotherapy may be effective if the patient is fit enough. Oral antifibrinolytics such as tranexamic acid may help. Occasionally frequent small episodes herald a catastrophic haemoptysis. This is rare, but is a difficult situation to manage and early involvement of specialists should be considered. The risks of frightening a family with information about a possible risk of catastrophic haemoptysis need to be balanced against the potential distress that could be caused by leaving a patient and family unprepared
- **Cough** can exacerbate breathlessness and pain, and affect sleep and a patient's ability to eat. Its management will depend on the cause, but it is often appropriate to try and suppress the cough pharmacologically using codeine linctus or morphine. If not responding to simple measures refer for specialist assessment
- **Hypercalcaemia** may occur. It should be considered in any patient with persistent nausea, thirst, altered mood or confusion (even if intermittent), worsening pain and/or constipation. It should be treated with IV hydration and bisphosphonates unless the patient is clearly dying, in which case treatment is not appropriate

- **Cerebral metastases** are common. Decisions about investigation and management may be complex and need to be made on an individual basis. Altered behaviour and personality, as well as problems of comprehension and communication, can be very distressing for relatives. Persistent headache, worse in the mornings and unexplained vomiting may be early signs of this diagnosis. There is a risk of seizures and prophylactic anticonvulsant medication may be appropriate
- **Hyponatraemia** and other biochemical imbalances are particularly common in small-cell lung cancer. Management can be complex and needs specialist input
- **Altered taste and anorexia** are common. Good oral hygiene and effective treatment of oral candidiasis may help. Carers may find it helpful to talk through different ways of encouraging the patient to eat, such as freezing supplement drinks and making frequent small meals, etc.
- **Superior vena cava obstruction (SVCO)** can occur, particularly in patients with right upper lobe lung cancers. Management includes consideration of vascular stenting, radiotherapy and high-dose oral steroids

Mesothelioma

General comments

This usually affects the pleura but can affect other mesothelial linings, most commonly the peritoneum. It is associated with exposure to asbestos, although, unlike patients with asbestosis, the history may be difficult to elicit, as the risk of mesothelioma appears unrelated to the length of exposure to asbestos and may occur many years after such exposure. It is a relentlessly progressive tumour.

It is important that the patient is aware that they may be entitled to *compensation* and should consult a specialist lawyer about this.

All deaths due to mesothelioma should be discussed with the coroner who will most probably order a post-mortem, unless the disease was clearly not related to industry. The patient and family should be made aware that the coroner will be contacted (regardless of any compensation claims or litigation), to minimize distress at the time of death.

Diagnosis

- CXR
- CT scan of chest
- Pleural biopsy
- Thoracoscopic biopsy

There is a high incidence of false-negative biopsies—in some cases these may need to be repeated a number of times to make a diagnosis.

Treatment

Surgery

Radical surgery is of uncertain value, with a high mortality and few long-term survivors reported. Palliative surgery with parietal pleur-ectomy and decortication of the lung may offer excellent palliation with minimal morbidity.

Radiotherapy

The tumour may grow along the track of a biopsy or drainage needle to produce a cutaneous lesion. These areas can become painful, ulcerated and can be difficult to manage. Hence, palliative radiotherapy is given prophylactically following the biopsy. It may also be used locally for established cutaneous spread.

Chemotherapy

The value of chemotherapy in this disease is uncertain. Recent reports, however, suggest that selected patients may respond to combination treatment with platinum and pemetrexed with some palliative benefit.

Specific problems in the management of mesothelioma

- **Pleural effusions** are common, frequently blood-stained and become increasingly difficult to aspirate as the disease progresses. Surgical intervention to prevent re-accumulation of fluid may be helpful if carried out early enough
- **Breathlessness** can be severe due to pleural disease limiting the capacity and expansion of the lung as well as the occurrence of pleural effusions. Give clear explanations of what is happening. Ensure that practical measures such as sitting the patient up, opening windows and using fans have been discussed with the family. Regular doses of short-acting oral morphine every 2–4 hours may decrease the sensation of breathlessness. Panic and anxiety are frequently associated with breathlessness and may be helped by simple relaxation techniques. A low dose of an *anxiolytic* such as diazepam may be helpful. Other treatment options are limited
- **Ascites** occurs with peritoneal mesothelioma. The ascitic fluid is often blood-stained and becomes increasingly difficult to aspirate as the disease progresses.

Specific pain complexes

Mesotheliomas can produce severe neuropathic pain which may only be partially opioid-responsive and may need adjuvant analgesics. Early referral for specialist help should be considered. Local nerve blockades can help in some cases.

Colorectal cancer

Background
- Fourth commonest cancer worldwide
- Approximately 50% of tumours occur in the rectum or sigmoid colon
- Dietary factors are thought to be important
- Tumour often secretes carcinoembryonic antigen (CEA)
- 6–8% of cases are familial
- Associated syndromes include Familial adenomatous polyposis coli and Hereditary non-polyposis coli

Common presentations
- Iron deficiency anaemia
- Abdominal pain
- Altered bowel habit
- PR bleeding

Staging and diagnosis (Table 5.14)
- Sigmoidoscopy
- Colonoscopy—all patients must have full evaluation of the colon prior to surgery
- Barium enema (less useful than colonoscopy)
- CT scan of chest, abdomen and pelvis
- MRI/endorectal ultrasound may be useful to assess local extent of tumour in the rectum

Table 5.14 TNM staging for colorectal cancer

T_1 Invades submucosa	Stage I—T_1/T_2, N_0 M_0
T_2 Invades muscularis propria	Stage II—$T_{3/4}$, N_0 M_0
T_3 Invades subserosa	Stage III—T_{1-4}, N_1/N_2 M_0
T_4 Invades through serosa	Stage IV—T_{1-4} N_{1-2} M_1
N_0 No lymph node involvement	
N_1 1–3 nodes involved	
N_2 4 or more nodes involved	
N_3 Central nodes involved	
M_0 No distant metastases	
M_1 Distant metastases	

Management
Surgery of primary disease
Surgery is the mainstay of therapy for colorectal cancer.

For colonic tumours a segment of colon with its blood supply and draining nodes is excised. Depending on the site of the tumour this may involve a right or left hemicolectomy or a sigmoid colectomy.

Traditionally, surgery for rectal tumours has involved an abdomino-perineal approach. In the absence of radiotherapy local relapse rates of 25–30% have been reported. Previously, radiotherapy has been used post-operatively but increasingly a short course of radiotherapy is being used to 'sterilize' the area prior to surgery. Surgery now typically involves the more meticulous procedure of total mesorectal excision and an anterior resection preserving the anus and reducing local relapse rates to less than 10%.

Surgery for hepatic metastases
The majority of patients develop liver metastases as the first site of disease progression following definitive first-line treatment.

A proportion of these patients may be suitable for metastatectomy. Up to 40% five-year survival has been reported for carefully selected patients.

Chemotherapy
Adjuvant chemotherapy of colorectal cancer
Several large, randomized controlled trials have demonstrated a clear survival advantage to fluorouracil-based or capecitabine therapy for patients with Dukes' C disease. The addition of oxaliplatin to 5-FU (5-fluorouracil) increases the benefit.

The value of adjuvant chemotherapy for patients with Dukes' B disease is less clear, but chemotherapy may be offered to patients with tumours that exhibit adverse prognostic features, such as lympho-vascular invasion.

Advanced colorectal cancer
Fluorouracil-based chemotherapy has also been demonstrated to confer a palliative benefit in patients with metastatic disease. There appears to be a survival advantage with chemotherapy of at least six months. Combination regimes with the addition of oxaliplatin or irinotecan to fluorouracil further prolong survival to approximately 18 months.

Capecitabine is an orally available pro-drug of 5-FU which is equally effective but more convenient and has a different side-effect profile.

Biological therapy

These emerging therapies have considerable potential but their uptake is limited by their expense. Bevacizumab (a VEGF-targeted monoclonal antibody) prolongs survival when added to chemotherapy. Likewise, cetuximab (an EGFR-targeted monoclonal antibody) enhances the activity of irinotecan.

Radiotherapy
Adjuvant treatment
Pelvic radiotherapy with concurrent chemotherapy reduces the risk of pelvic relapse for patients with Stage II and III rectal cancer.

Pelvic chemoradiotherapy may also be useful for patients with large, fixed rectal tumours to reduce tumour volume prior to consideration of surgical resection.

Prognosis (Table 5.15)

Table 5.15 Prognosis

Stage	Five-year survival (%)
Dukes' A (T1)	>90
Dukes' B1 (T2)	>80
Dukes' B2 (T3)	>50
Dukes' C	30–40

General comments

- **Liver metastases** often occur and may cause capsular pain. This usually responds well to NSAIDs or steroids. Liver metastases may also lead to hepatomegaly, causing squashed stomach syndrome with delayed gastric emptying and a feeling of fullness. This may respond to a prokinetic agent such as metoclopramide
- **Perineal and pelvic pain** may be caused by advancing disease or be iatrogenic. There is nearly always a neuropathic element to the pain which will only be partially opioid-sensitive. Tenesmus is a unique type of neuropathic pain which requires specialist assessment
- **Bowel obstruction,** unless it can be palliated surgically, should be managed medically using a syringe driver containing a mixture of analgesics, antiemetics and antispasmodics. Bowel obstruction at multiple levels, which is common in relapsed disease, may make surgery inappropriate. Differentiating between a high blockage (where vomiting is a feature) and blockage lower in the bowel can be useful in targeting treatment strategies. Imaging techniques may also be helpful to delineate the level of obstruction
- **Fistulae** between the bowel and the skin or bladder may occur. These can be very difficult to manage and require a multidisciplinary approach with specialist input
- **Rectal discharge and bleeding** are unpleasant and difficult symptoms to manage. Referral to a clinical oncologist is appropriate as radiotherapy may be of benefit
- **Hypoproteinaemia** is common due to poor oral intake and poor absorption from the bowel and may lead to lower limb oedema
- **Poor appetite** is not uncommon and can be helped with the use of steroids

Breast cancer

Background

- Accounts for 20% of all cancers in Western Europe and the USA
- Lifetime risk for females is 1 in 9
- Factors which increase the risk of breast cancer include increasing age, a family history of breast cancer, nulliparity and the use of HRT or the contraceptive pill
- Incidence of breast cancer is increasing, although overall mortality has decreased by 20% in the UK since 1985
- Five year survival is 80%
- Male breast cancer is rare—accounting for <1% of all breast cancers

Genetics of breast cancer

Some 5–10% of breast cancers are believed to be hereditary. Many of these cancers are due to germline mutations in the tumour-suppresser genes *BRCA1* or *BRCA2*. Prophylactic bilateral mastectomy will reduce the incidence of breast cancer by 90% in patients with proven mutations in the *BRCA1* or *BRCA2* gene.

At present, treatment for a breast tumour arising in a mutation carrier is the same as for non-mutation carriers.

Presentation

- Breast lump (most common)
- Mammographically detected lesion—increasingly common mode of presentation
- Nipple inversion or discharge
- Occasionally rash at nipple (Paget's disease)

Diagnosis

- Mammogram
- Ultrasound (used in younger females or when mammogram unclear)
- Fine-needle aspiration cytology
- Core biopsy

Pathology (Table 5.16)

Table 5.16 Pathology

Preinvasive lesions

Lobular carcinoma *in situ* (LCIS)—significance uncertain
Ductal carcinoma *in situ* (DCIS)—usually detected mammographically, may progress to invasive disease

Invasive lesions

Ductal carcinoma—not otherwise specified—accounts for approximately 80% of all tumours

Lobular carcinoma
Tubular carcinoma
Medullary carcinoma

Presentation and staging

Breast cancer is diagnosed by a 'triple assessment':
- Clinical examination
- Imaging: bilateral mammography (or ultrasound/MRI)
- Biopsy: fine needle aspiration cytology or core biopsy

This approach has >90% sensitivity and specificity.

All patients with proven invasive disease should have the axilla assessed as part of staging. Traditionally, this includes axillary clearance, but increasingly sentinel biopsy is performed instead. Staging investigations in patients without systemic symptoms rarely detects metastases and are recommended only in patients with (4 or more) lymph nodes involved by tumour.

Prognostic factors

Include:
- Axillary node involvement—most important prognostic criterion
- Tumour grade
- Oestrogen receptor (ER)/progesterone receptor (PR) status. More favourable prognosis if ER/PR positive
- HER2 status—*HER2* overexpression is associated with poor prognosis
- Patient age—<35years is an independent adverse prognostic factor

Common problems

- **Bone pain** due to bone metastases which may respond to radiotherapy, bisphosphonates or systemic therapy. Prophylactic surgery may be indicated where there is a risk of fracture
- **Pathological fractures** may occur without obvious trauma
- **Spinal cord compression** requires prompt diagnosis, high-dose oral steroids and urgent referral to the orthopaedic or neurosurgeon or oncologist. The steroids should be continued at a high dose until a definitive plan has been made
- **Neuropathic pain** can be a particular problem especially if there has been spread into the brachial plexus
- **Liver metastases** are common and may require steroids or NSAIDs to reduce the pain of liver capsule distension
- **Hypercalcaemia** may occur. In many cases treatment should be considered with IV hydration and IV bisphosphonates
- **Lymphoedema** can develop, at any point in the course of the disease, affecting the arm following surgery and/or radiotherapy. Early referral to a lymphoedema specialist provides the best chance of minimizing the morbidity and distress caused. Preventive measures include good skin care and avoiding additional trauma to the affected arm (including taking of blood tests and BP measurement). Treatment involves bandaging, lymphatic massage and fitting a compression sleeve
- **Lung and pleural spread** are common causes of breathlessness and cough. These symptoms need to be investigated thoroughly. Drainage of a pleural effusion may be a useful symptomatic procedure and

pleurodesis should be considered. Systemic therapy (chemotherapy or hormone therapy) is indicated in patients of good performance status
• **Psychosocial problems**, some of these patients will be mothers with young children for whom the trauma of disease is worsened by fears for their children. A multidisciplinary supportive approach at a pace dictated by the patient can help to reduce some of the distress for the patient and her family

Management (Table 5.17)

Table 5.17 Management

Non-invasive breast cancer DCIS	Simple mastectomy OR Partial mastectomy and postoperative radiotherapy. Axillary dissection not indicated.
Early breast cancer T_{1-3}, N_{0-1}	**Surgery:** either simple mastectomy or partial mastectomy (lumpectomy) and axillary node dissection.
	Loco-regional radiotherapy: indicated for all patients with partial mastectomy and for mastectomy patients at high risk of local relapse (e.g. patients with T_3 or T_4 tumours or > 4 involved nodes).
	Adjuvant endocrine therapy: Tamoxifen indicated for all ER- or PR-positive tumours and achieves approximately 30% relative reduction in mortality. Aromatase inhibitors are replacing tamoxifen in postmenopausal women because of improved outcomes and tolerability but the optimal role of these drugs is unclear.
	Adjuvant chemotherapy: Combination chemotherapy reduces recurrence and improves overall survival. Anthracycline based regimens are more effective than non-anthracycline based regimens; incorporation of a taxane further improves efficacy. Absolute 10 year survival benefit: 7–11% <50 years; 2–3% >50 years.
	Commonly used regimens include Fluorouracil/epirubicin/cyclophosphamide(FEC), Docetaxel/doxorubicin/cyclophosphamide (TAC), Doxorubicin/cyclophosphamide (AC), cyclophosphamide/methotrexate/fluorouracil (CMF). The benefit risk ratio for chemotherapy must be assessed on an individual patient basis.
	Adjuvant trastuzumab: early results of large clinical trials have shown significant improvements in relapse free and overall survival with the addition of adjuvant trastuzumab in patients with tumours that overexpress HER-2.
	Neoadjuvant therapy: May have some advantage in allowing more patients to have breast conserving surgery. Trials to assess the value of a neoadjuvant approach are ongoing.

Table 5.17 Management (*Continued*)

Locally advanced breast cancer (*Presence of infiltration of the skin, chest wall or fixed axillary nodes*)	The presence of infiltration of the skin, chest wall or fixed axillary nodes requires a *neoadjuvant* approach. Younger patients and those with ER/PR negative disease may need chemotherapy. Elderly patients with ER or PR positive disease may be treated with hormonal therapy alone (aromatase inhibitors are superior to tamoxifen in this setting).
Metastatic breast cancer *The aim is palliation. Usual sites of metastases: lung, liver, bone, brain Bone metastases often respond to hormone manipulation; such patients may survive for many years*	**Endocrine therapy:** indicated in those patients with ER- or PR-positive disease and slowly progressive disease. Responses tend to be slower in onset (3–6 months) than with chemotherapy but also tend to be more durable. Expected response rates of 40–60% to first line hormonal therapy in those with ER- and/or PR-positive tumours. Disease that responds to endocrine therapy and then progresses has a 25% response with second line treatment. Response to a third hormonal agent is 10–15%.
	Chemotherapy: indicated in situations where a high response rate and rapid time to response are required. Anthracycline based regimens are used in patients not exposed to them in the adjuvant setting. First line response rates are of the order of 40–60%. Taxanes are used in patients who have had prior exposure to anthracyclines with similar response rates. In patients with HER-2 over expression, addition of trastuzumab increases response rate and prolongs survival. In patients unfit for chemotherapy trastuzumab may be used as a single agent. Other agents with activity include capecitabine, vinorelbine and liposomal doxorubicin.
	Radiotherapy: useful for palliation of painful bone metastases, brain metastases or of soft tissue metastases causing pressure effects.
	Bisphosphonates: used in the treatment of malignancy related hypercalcaemia. In patients with bone metastases bisphosphonates have been demonstrated to reduce bone pain, skeletal events related to malignancy, and the incidence of hypercalcaemia.

Prostate cancer

Background
- Accounts for approximately 25% of all cancers in men in the UK
- Second to lung cancer as a cause of cancer deaths in men
- Increasing age is major risk factor—70% of men >80 years of age have some evidence of prostatic cancer
- Associated with a 78% 5-year survival
- Appears to be linked to androgen exposure—rare in men castrated before 40 years of age
- Incidence of prostate cancer is rising—due, in part, to increased detection of early disease by PSA screening
- Many PSA-detected cancers are clinically unimportant—more research is needed to distinguish patients with raised PSA levels who are at risk of developing metastatic disease

Presentation
- Urinary outflow symptoms
- Haematuria
- Symptoms of metastatic disease, e.g. back pain
- Asymptomatic elevation of PSA

Diagnosis and staging (Table 5.18)
- PSA assessment: PSA >4ng/mL: clinical suspicion, requires transurethral ultrasound and needle biopsy
- PSA >50ng/mL: often distant metastases
- Transurethral ultrasound and biopsy
- CT/MRI—may help to assess lymph node involvement
- Isotope bone scan

Table 5.18 TNM staging of prostate cancer

T_1—Clinically inapparent
T_2—Palpable tumour confined to prostate
T_3—Tumour extends through capsule
T_4—Tumour is fixed or invades structures other than seminal vesicles
N_0—No regional nodes
N_1—Regional lymph node metastases
M_0—No metastases
M_1—Metastases present

Management
Many prostate tumours are clinically insignificant and will not cause symptoms in the patient's lifetime. It is important, however, to recognize those patients whose tumours are likely to become clinically apparent.

Prognostic factors in patients with cancer confined to the prostate:
- Tumour grade—assessed by Gleason Score
- Tumour stage—assessed clinically and radiologically

- Patient age—younger patients are more likely to develop problems than older patients

Cancer confined to prostate gland

If aged <70 and fit, consider radical local therapy:
- Prostatectomy
- Radiotherapy-external beam or brachytherapy

There are currently no trials directly comparing these approaches. In general terms fitter patients tend to be treated with surgery rather than radiotherapy.

Complications:
- Prostatectomy: 50% impotence; 8–15% long-term incontinence
- Radiotherapy: 40% impotence; rectal stricture/bladder irritation but no incontinence

If over 70 years
- 'Active surveillance policy—active process of examining patient regularly and treating if evidence of disease progression

Locally extensive disease (T_3/T_4) or Node N_1 disease

- Neoadjuvant anti-androgen therapy followed by radical radiotherapy

Metastatic disease

The natural history is very variable, with a number of patients with metastatic bone disease living for >5years following diagnosis.

The majority of tumours are sensitive to androgens. Hormonal manipulation aimed at reducing the effect of androgens (mainly testosterone) at a cellular level will produce responses in around 70% of men with bone metastases with a median response duration of 12–18 months.

Commonly used hormonal treatments include:
- **Medical castration** with luteinizing hormone-releasing hormone (LHRH) agonists. (These can induce a flare of hormone-induced activity on initiating therapy which needs to be suppressed with anti-androgens for the initial two weeks.)
- **Anti-androgens** (cyproterone acetate, flutamide, bicalutamide). These may be used alone or in combination with LHRH agonists. The value of the combination is, however, uncertain.
- **Oestrogens**, such as diethylstilbestrol (stilboestrol) may be used after other hormones have failed. This is used at lower doses than previously to minimize thromboembolic side-effects.
- **Bilateral orchidectomy** is less popular due to the availability of medical methods of castration

The side-effects of these hormone treatments include:
- Loss of libido and potency
- Hot flushes
- Change in fat deposition
- Osteoporosis
- Poor concentration
- Decreased energy and drive
- Metabolic syndrome

Local radiotherapy may be useful as an additional palliative measure particularly for bone pain. Strontium-89 and samarium-153, bone-seeking radioisotopes, have proved effective, though expensive, treatments for reducing bone pain.

Hormone refractory prostate cancer

The prognosis for patients whose disease has progressed through anti-androgen therapy is poor.

Therapeutic options at this stage include:
- **Anti-androgen withdrawal**—this results in a response in a small number of patients
- **Glucocorticoids**—low-dose glucocorticoids, such as, dexamethasone 1mg produce clinical benefit in some patients
- **Chemotherapy**—prostate cancer is relatively chemoresistant. Docetaxel and prednisolone improves symptoms with a modest survival improvement but is appropriate only for fitter patients.

Common palliation issues

- **Pathological fracture** may occur without obvious trauma. It may need orthopaedic intervention (pinning or joint replacement) and radiotherapy. Prophylactic orthopaedic intervention may also be required for bone lesions at high risk of fracture
- **Spinal cord compression** requires prompt diagnosis and treatment with high-dose steroids and radiotherapy. A minority of cases may be suitable for surgical intervention. Such patients include those with a single site of disease and those in whom there is uncertainty regarding the diagnosis. These patients should be discussed with a neurosurgeon
- **Neuropathic pain may be caused by** local recurrence of tumour, pelvic spread or a collapsed vertebra. Such pain is partially opioid-sensitive but adjuvant analgesics are usually required to supplement the effect of the opioid
- **Bone pain,** specialist advice should be sought about the appropriate use of radiotherapy and radioactive isotopes as well as nerve blockade. Bisphosphonates such as pamidronate and zoledronic acid help to reduce bone pain and also reduce the number of cancer-associated skeletal events and incidence of hypercalcaemia
- **Bone marrow failure** may occur in patients with advanced disease. Typically, the patient has symptomatic anaemia and thrombocytopenia. Support with palliative blood transfusions may be appropriate initially, but their appropriateness should be discussed with the patient and their family when there is no longer symptomatic benefit gained from transfusion
- **Retention of urine,** problems with micturition including haematuria may lead to retention of urine. This may be acute and painful or chronic and painless. If the patient is unfit for transurethral resection of the prostate (TURP) then consider a permanent indwelling urinary catheter. Chronic urinary retention can lead to renal failure

- **Lymphoedema** of the lower limbs and occasionally the genital area is usually due to advanced pelvic disease. It needs to be actively managed if complications are to be avoided
- **Altered body image and sexual dysfunction** can result from the disease or any of the treatment modalities. This may be exacerbated by apathy and clinical depression. Specialist mental and psychological health strategies may be required

Gynaecological cancer

Ovarian carcinoma

Background

- Fifth commonest cancer in women
- Median age at diagnosis 66 years
- Approximately 5% are familial
- 95% of tumours are epithelial in origin
- Risk is reduced by factors that reduce the number of ovulatory cycles, e.g. pregnancy, use of oral contraceptive pill

Presentation

Ovarian cancer spreads intraperitoneally and may remain silent until late: 80% of patients present with disease which has spread beyond the pelvis.

Common presenting symptoms include:

- Abdominal distension
- Abdominal pain
- Altered bowel habit
- Weight loss

Diagnosis and staging (Table 5.19)

Table 5.19 Diagnosis and staging

Stage	Description	Five-year survival (%)
Stage I	Confined to ovaries but without pelvic extension	75
Stage II	Tumour with pelvic extension	45
Stage III	Tumour with peritoneal spread outside the pelvis, or involves small bowel; retroperitoneal or inguinal nodes	20
Stage IV	Distant metastases	<5

Preoperatively, a diagnosis of ovarian cancer may be suspected if the marker CA-125 is raised (elevated in approximately 85% of patients with Stage III/IV disease) and the presence of a pelvic mass or ascites on CT scan.

Confirmation of the diagnosis requires histology. Adequate staging and initial disease management requires total abdominal hysterectomy, bilateral salpingo-oophorectomy, omentectomy, lymph node sampling, and multiple peritoneal biopsies.

Management

Radical surgery has an important role in treatment, and retrospective studies demonstrate significantly improved survival rates in patients whose disease has been optimally debulked (i.e. no tumour remaining measuring >1cm in diameter). Where optimal debulking is not possible initially, there may be a benefit to survival from performing debulking surgery after three cycles of chemotherapy—the so-called 'interval debulking'.

First-line chemotherapy

A platinum/taxane combination is considered by most oncologists to be the optimum treatment for ovarian cancer, the most commonly used combination being carboplatin and paclitaxel. Response rates are about 70–80%, and median survival is 2–3 years with such treatment.

Although the introduction of paclitaxel has improved the median survival in this disease, the majority of patients develop progressive disease and 5-year survival is still less than 25%.

Treatment at relapse

The vast majority of patients who relapse after first-line therapy are incurable. Secondary surgical debulking may be useful in selected patients, but its value is uncertain. The choice of further chemotherapy depends on the interval between completion of previous chemotherapy and relapse.

Patients relapsing more than six months after the completion of platinum-based therapy may respond to further chemotherapy and should generally be rechallenged with a platinum agent. If re-challenge takes place more than 2 years from previous chemotherapy the response rate is 60%, whereas re-challenge within 6 months rarely results in tumour response.

Patients relapsing less than six months after completion of platinum-based chemotherapy are unlikely to respond to further platinum-based therapy. Fit patients should be considered for liposomal doxorubicin.

Eventually all patients who relapse following primary chemotherapy will develop chemotherapy-resistant disease. The majority of these patients will have symptoms related to intra-abdominal disease, including abdominal pain and bowel obstruction. Management of these symptoms can be very challenging and requires a multidisciplinary approach with involvement of palliative physicians, surgeons and oncologists.

Carcinoma of the cervix

Background

- Strongly associated with human papillomavirus (HPV)-16 (and also, but less strongly, with HPV-18 and -31)
- 30–40% of patients with untreated cervical intraepithelial neoplasia progress to invasive squamous-cell carcinoma with a latent period of 10–20 years
- Commonest female cancer in South-East Asia, Africa and South America
- In the UK incidence and mortality have fallen by approximately 40% since the 1970s

Presentation

- Unless detected at screening, it is often asymptomatic until the disease is advanced
- Postcoital bleeding
- Intermenstrual bleeding

Staging (Table 5.20)

Table 5.20 Staging

	FIGO staging system
Ia	Micro-invasive disease (max. depth 5mm, max. width 7mm)
Ib	Clinical disease confined to the cervix
IIa	Disease involves upper 2/3 of vagina but not parametrium
IIb	Disease involves parametrium but not pelvic wall
IIIa	Disease involves lower 1/3 of vagina
IIIb	Disease extends to pelvic side wall
IVa	Spread of tumour to adjacent pelvic organs
IV	Spread of tumour to distant organs

MRI plays an increasingly important role in the preoperative staging of these tumours.

Management
Management depends largely on disease stage. Patients with Stage Ia may be treated with simple hysterectomy or a conization procedure in those patients wishing to preserve their fertility.

For Stage Ib or IIa disease, radical hysterectomy appears equivalent to radical pelvic radiotherapy. For those patients with Stage IIb to IVa disease, recent evidence suggests that a combination of radical pelvic radiotherapy with platinum-based chemotherapy gives the best results. Chemoradiotherapy may also be indicated for patients with Stage Ib and IIa disease with adverse prognostic factors, such as those with bulky tumours.

For patients with Stage IVb disease pelvic radiotherapy may be useful in palliating troublesome pelvic symptoms. Cervical cancer is only moderately chemosensitive, with responses to single agents of around 20–30%. Agents with some activity in this disease include cisplatin, ifosfamide and paclitaxel.

Palliative issues in gynaecological cancers
- **Primary treatment** often affects sexual function, fertility and body image, which may impact on coping strategies and need specialist counselling. Ovarian and vulval cancers often present late and specialist palliative care input from the point of diagnosis may be appropriate. Genetic counselling should be considered for close female relatives of patients with ovarian cancer, particularly if there is also a strong family history of breast cancer
- **Perineal and pelvic pain** is common in all three of the common gynaecological malignancies—cervical, ovarian and vulval carcinomas. There is usually a neuropathic element to the pain which may be only partially opioid-sensitive

- **Lymphoedema affecting one or both limbs** develops with uncontrolled pelvic disease. It can develop at any time in a patient's cancer journey and frequently affects both lower limbs. This needs to be actively managed if complications are to be avoided. Management includes good skin care, avoiding additional trauma to the affected leg(s), and appropriately fitting compression garments
- **Ascites** is particularly common with ovarian cancer and can be difficult to manage. Oral diuretics, particularly spironolactone in combination with a loop diuretic such as furosemide, may provide a little help. Repeated paracentesis may be needed. Consideration of a peritoneovenous shunt may be appropriate in some cases where prognosis is thought to be longer than three months
- **Acute or subacute bowel obstruction** is often not amenable to surgical intervention and should be managed medically using SC medication via a syringe driver. Nasogastric tubes are rarely needed, and hydration can often be maintained orally if the nausea/vomiting are adequately controlled
- **Renal impairment** can develop in any patient with advanced pelvic disease. It may be a pre-terminal event. Ureteric stenting may be appropriate depending on the patient's perceived prognosis, the patient's wishes and future treatment options. Renal impairment increases the risk of a patient developing opioid toxicity as renal excretion of opioid metabolites may be reduced
- **Vaginal or vulval bleeding** may respond to antifibrinolytic agents such as tranexamic acid, radiotherapy and/or surgery
- **Offensive vaginal or vulval discharge** can cause considerable distress to both patient and carers. Topical or systemic metronidazole may help as can barrier creams. Deodorizing machines may also help if the patient is confined to one room
- **Vesicocolic and rectovaginal fistulae** need surgical assessment. These can be very difficult to manage and require a multidisciplinary approach with specialist input

Upper gastrointestinal tract cancer

Stomach cancer

Background

- Sixth most common cancer in the UK
- Second most common cancer worldwide—very high incidence in Japan, Korea, central and south America and Eastern Europe
- UK incidence of cancer of the distal stomach is falling but incidence of tumours of the cardia or gastro-oesophageal junction is rising
- More common in males than females (2:1) and in those over 60 years of age
- 90–95% of gastric tumours are adenocarcinomas

Presentation

- Insidious onset
- Anaemia
- Early satiety and anorexia
- Weight loss
- Dyspepsia

Diagnosis and staging

- Full staging is essential if inappropriate surgery is to be avoided
- Endoscopy and biopsy
- Endoluminal ultrasound to assess depth of invasion and lymph node involvement
- CT scan to assess lymph node involvement and distant metastases
- Laparoscopy—may be indicated to assess peritoneal disease if surgery is being considered

Treatment

Resectable disease

Surgery remains the only potentially curative modality of treatment. Partial or total gastrectomy (depending on tumour site and mode of spread) and regional lymphadenectomy is the most commonly performed operation. Factors determining outcome include:

- Tumour location—patients with distal tumours do better than those with more proximally located tumours
- Tumour extent—patients with tumours beyond the gastric wall have a worse prognosis
- Extent of lymph node involvement

Following surgery many patients remain at high risk of local and distant disease relapse. Trials have suggested that such patients may benefit from adjuvant chemotherapy or chemoradiation.

Combined pre- and postoperative chemotherapy has been shown to increase resectability and to reduce relapse rates in patients with operable gastric cancer.

Locally advanced/metastatic disease

Palliative operations can be performed to control pain or bleeding or to relieve obstruction for patients with advanced disease. The type of operation performed depends on the status of the patient and on the anticipated disease course.

Chemotherapy, with cisplatin and 5-fluorouracil with, or without, epirubicin, has a palliative benefit for patients with locally advanced or metastatic gastric cancer, and may also improve survival by some months. Trials exploring the role of drugs such as oxaliplatin, irinotecan, taxanes and capecitabine in this setting are showing encouraging results.

Endoscopic procedures such as stenting or laser coagulation may also provide useful palliative benefits.

Radiotherapy may provide useful palliation for bleeding from locally advanced tumours. It may also be useful in palliating pain caused by metastatic disease, e.g. bone metastases.

Treatment of the rare gastrointestinal stromal tumours (GISTs) has been revolutionized by the biological therapy imatinib which has had dramatic impact in some patients.

Oesophageal carcinoma

Background
- Eighth most commonly occurring cancer in the UK
- More common in males than females (2:1)
- Tumours in the upper two-thirds of the oesophagus are usually squamous-cell cancers
- Tumours in the lower third are usually adenocarcinomas—incidence of adenocarcinoma has been steadily increasing
- Adenocarcinoma often arises in a Barrett's oesophagus—endoscopic screening may reduce the incidence
- Overall survival in the UK is <10% at 5 years

Symptoms
- Dysphagia
- Chest pain
- Dyspepsia

Diagnosis and staging
- Endoscopy and biopsy
- Barium swallow—demonstrate tumour length
- Endoluminal ultrasound—demonstrates extent of local invasion and lymph node involvement
- CT scan—assesses nodal involvement and distant metastases
- Laparoscopy
- Bronchoscopy should be performed if tracheal involvement suspected
- PET scanning is used increasingly to detect nodes and distant metastases, with the result that fewer oesophageal resections are being performed

Treatment

Resectable disease

Surgery remains the key potentially curative modality for tumours in the lower two-thirds of the oesophagus. Unfortunately, however, due to the tumour's tendency to spread longitudinally via the submucosa, circumferentially to other mediastinal structures and to lymph nodes early in its course, the results are poor with a 5-year survival of 20%. Neoadjuvant chemotherapy with cisplatin and 5-FU improves the resectability and reduces the likelihood of local and distant relapse. Studies have not yet established that the increased morbidity is justified in terms of response and survival benefits.

Tumours in the upper third of the oesophagus are inoperable but may be suitable for radical radiotherapy treatment.

Chemoradiotherapy may also be used with radical intent in tumours in the lower two-thirds of the oesophagus in patients who are unfit for surgery.

Unresectable disease

Endoscopic placement of stents or radiotherapy may provide excellent palliation, particularly of dysphagia. Platinum-based chemotherapy may also be useful in palliating symptoms in patients who are fit.

Pancreatic carcinoma

Background

- Seventh most common cause of cancer death in the UK
- 75% arise from the head of pancreas, 15% from the body, 10% from the tail
- Risk factors include:
  - smoking
  - chronic pancreatitis
  - alcohol
- 90% are adenocarcinomas

Presentation

- Insidious onset of symptoms
- Jaundice
- Weight loss
- Pain—the local invasion of tail or body tumours may cause severe neuropathic abdominal pain radiating to the back

Investigations

- LFTs may show obstructive pattern
- CA19–9—elevated in majority of cancers but low specificity
- ERCP with brushings or biopsy
- Endoluminal ultrasound
- Ultrasound scan or CT with FNA or biopsy of pancreatic mass
- CT chest, abdomen and pelvis
- MRI can delineate tumours, ducts and vessels with less morbidity than ERCP
- Laparoscopy—may be required to assess peritoneal involvement prior to surgery

Management

Surgery is the only potentially curative modality of treatment. Unfortunately less than 15% of patients present with surgically resectable disease. A pancreaticoduodenectomy is the operation of choice. But even in those patients who are suitable candidates for this surgery, 5-year survival is less than 10%.

The majority of patients will present with advanced unresectable disease, although surgical bypass procedures may be possible. Primary treatment is aimed at relief of jaundice, which is generally achieved by endoscopic or percutaneous transhepatic placement of a stent.

Pancreatic enzyme supplements may help with malabsorption.

Chemotherapy with gemcitabine can provide a small survival benefit and should be considered in patients with unresectable disease and an ECOG performance status of <3.

Palliative issues for patients with upper gastrointestinal tract cancer

Mild and non-specific symptoms often precede the onset of dysphagia for many months in oesophageal carcinoma. Stomach cancer often presents late and is frequently metastatic at presentation.

- **Liver capsular pain** due to liver metastases is common. This is only partially opioid-responsive but responds well to NSAIDs or oral steroids
- **Oesophageal spasm** may occur and can be difficult to manage. Specialist advice from the palliative care team should be sought. It may be aggravated by oesophageal candidiasis, which needs systemic treatment with oral systemic antifungals
- **Involvement of the coeliac plexus** causes a difficult pain syndrome with non-specific abdominal pain and mid back pain. Blockade of the plexus using anaesthetic techniques can be useful
- **Dysphagia** can occur in both oesophageal and stomach cancer. It may be helped by stenting. Oncological treatment of the tumour may provide temporary relief. Advice about appropriate diet and food consistency may also help. Feeding gastrostomy is sometimes used to improve functional status prior to aggressive treatment. Gastrostomy can also improve nutrition and quality of life in the palliative setting, but should only be inserted after careful multidisciplinary discussion involving the patient and their family.
  Ethical dilemmas can arise towards the end of life when issues of avoiding the prolongation of an uncomfortable dying period (by reducing or stopping artificial feeding) may need to be discussed. There is no evidence that the insertion of feeding tubes in the dying either extends life or improves symptoms
- **Anorexia** is frequent and often profound. There may be a fear of eating because of pain. This may bring the patient and their carer into conflict about food and the 'need to eat'. However, open and honest explanation can help to relieve anxiety and provide practical approaches to dealing with the situation
- **Weight loss and altered body image** can be profound with these cancers and can cause distressing problems for the patient and their family

- **Nausea and vomiting** can be persistent and difficult to control. Specialist advice is often needed and drugs may need to be given by routes other than oral. Small but frequent meals may improve the frequency of vomiting
- **Haematemesis** may be one of the presenting symptoms but can also occur as the tumour progresses. Where possible local treatment may help and brachytherapy and laser therapy, where available, can reduce the incidence. There is risk of a major bleed. This is a difficult situation to manage and early involvement of specialists should be considered.

Cancer of the bladder and ureter

Background
- Account for 1% of all cancers
- 90% are transitional-cell carcinomas (TCC)
- Risk factors for TCC include:
  - smoking
  - occupational exposure to aromatic amines and azo dyes
  - cyclophosphamide therapy
  - phenacetin-containing analgesics
- Squamous-cell carcinoma of the bladder is less common and associated with schistosomiasis, bladder calculi and chronic irritation

Presentation
- Painless haematuria in 90% of cases
- Frequency
- Urgency

Diagnosis and staging
- Cystoscopy and biopsy
- CT/MRI

Treatment
- 70–80% of all bladder cancers are 'superficial'—that is, they do not invade the muscularis mucosa

'Superficial' tumours
- Treated with transurethral resection of the tumour
- Many will recur and follow-up with regular cytoscopy is required
- Factors that identify patients likely to develop invasive disease include:
  - high-grade tumours
  - tumours that have breached the basement membrane
  - multiple tumours

Such patients may benefit from intravesical chemotherapy or immunotherapy.

'Invasive' tumours
Disease which invades the muscularis mucosa of the bladder may be treated with radical cystectomy or radiotherapy. These modalities have not been directly compared and decisions regarding the choice of therapy tend to be based on performance status, with surgery reserved for the younger and fitter patients.

Bladder cancer is moderately chemosensitive. Neoadjuvant chemotherapy confers a 5% benefit in 5-year survival. Patients with locally advanced or metastatic disease may benefit from palliative chemotherapy. The most commonly used regimen is cisplatin/gemcitabine.

Common problems

- **Bladder spasm** can be frequent and troublesome, leading to urinary frequency as well as pain
- **Pelvic pain** is common in advanced disease due to progression of the tumour. This pain can be extremely difficult to control as it is often complex and includes neuropathic elements. Anaesthetic interventions, including intrathecal and epidural procedures, may be needed to gain pain control
- **Recurrent haematuria** is common and may be sufficient to cause anaemia, and urinary retention due to clot retention. Catheter blockage may be a problem
- **Urinary incontinence** may occur
- **Urinary tract infections** due to long-term indwelling catheters are common but are treated only if symptomatic
- **Lymphoedema** of the lower limbs and genital area may occur and requires specialist management to prevent complications
- **Fistulae** may occur which are often suitable for surgery. If surgery is not possible the risks of skin breakdown are high
- **Renal failure** may occur. Stenting the renal tract may be possible but may not be appropriate and needs full discussion
- **Altered body image** and problems with sexual function are understandably common
- **Depression** is common because of the long course of the disease, sleep disturbance and damage to self-esteem

Tumours of the central nervous system

> To expect a personality to survive the disintegration of the brain is like expecting a cricket club to survive when all of its members are dead.
> Bertrand Russell

Background
- Most brain tumours are metastatic from I° sites outside the CNS
- Primary brain tumours account for approximately 2% of all cancers
- Primary brain tumours tend to remain localized to the CNS
- Primary brain tumours include:
  - gliomas (50% of all CNS tumours) comprise:
    - astrocytomas—account for 80% of gliomas, i.e. the most commonly occurring primary brain tumour; grade is important in determining prognosis
    - oligodendrogliomas—account for 10–15% of gliomas and commonly occur in the frontal lobes; longer prognosis
    - ependymomas—account for 5% of gliomas and tend to occur in children and young adults; may metastasize within the CNS
  - pituitary adenomas—account for 20% of CNS tumours; treated medically for endocrine symptoms; treated with surgery or radiotherapy if there are pressure symptoms or visual field problems
  - medulloblastomas—account for 25% of all childhood tumours
  - cerebral lymphomas—1–2 per million per year; are increasing in incidence partly due to HIV-associated malignancy

Symptoms
- Headache (especially in the morning) and vomiting if intracranial pressure is raised
- Seizures
- Neurological symptoms

Investigations
- Contrast-enhanced CT scan
- Gadolinium-enhanced MRI scan
- Isotope scanning (PET, SPECT (single photon emission computed tomography))
- If CSF spread is anticipated (e.g. for high-grade ependymoma) a neuroaxis MRI ± CSF cytology is required
- Biopsy is usually required to confirm diagnosis

Primary brain tumours

Surgery
Where possible surgical resection for some low-grade tumours may be curative. If complete resection of a low-grade glioma is not possible then the timing of surgery is a matter for discussion between both the neurosurgeon and patient. For higher grade lesions decompression of the tumour may provide palliation and facilitate postoperative radiotherapy.

Radiotherapy
For high-grade gliomas postoperative radiotherapy adds to the effectiveness of surgery and increases median survival from 5 to 11 months. For tumours with a propensity for leptomeningeal spread, e.g. high-grade ependymoma or medulloblastoma, then craniospinal irradiation improves prognosis.

Chemotherapy
Chemotherapy has a limited role to play in the treatment of most brain tumours and its use remains to be clearly defined. A survival benefit has been demonstrated for patients treated with a combination of radiotherapy and temozolamide compared to radiotherapy alone in glioblastoma multiforme. Chemotherapy is the principal treatment of CNS lymphoma and is important as adjuvant therapy for medulloblastoma. Some response to temozolamide or the PCV combination— procarbazine, CCNU (lomustine) and vincristine—in recurrent disease can be expected.

Prognosis
As a general rule in patients with brain tumours poorer prognosis is related to:
- High tumour grade
- Neurological deficit at presentation
- Older age at presentation

Secondary brain tumours

Brain metastases
Autopsy reveals that metastases are commoner than revealed clinically: 60% in small-cell lung carcinoma and 75% in melanoma. Carcinoma of the prostate, bladder and ovary rarely metastasize to the brain.

The prognosis for brain metastases is dependent on the extent of systemic disease, the performance status of the patient and the response to treatment.

Assessment—clinical history
Neurological examination of higher cortical function, cranial nerves, musculoskeletal system, sensation, cerebellar function and gait.

Clinical features
Symptoms and signs can evolve over days to weeks. Multiple deposits are present in over two-thirds of patients and clinical signs depend on the anatomical site:
- Focal neurological disturbance consists of motor weakness including hemiparesis (30%), dysphasia and cranial nerve palsies
- Seizures (15–20%)

- Raised intracranial pressure, e.g. headache (50%), nausea, vomiting and lethargy
- Change in mood, cognitive function or behaviour

Investigations

CT scan or MRI scan (better for tumours situated in the posterior fossa or brainstem) show the location of metastases, surrounding oedema and mass effect.

Management

Surgery may be suitable for a very small percentage of patients who are young, fit, with no disease elsewhere, a long treatment-free interval, with a solitary metastasis and depending on the anatomical site of the tumour. If anatomical location is the only contraindication to surgery then highdose localized radiotherapy may be considered.

Patients who might benefit from radical treatment should be identified, including those with chemosensitive tumours such as the haematological malignancies and testicular cancer.

Palliative radiotherapy with corticosteroids is the most usually appropriate treatment and may improve neurological symptoms and function in over 70% of patients (with a median survival 5–6 months), enabling a gentle reduction and sometimes withdrawal of steroids 4–6 weeks following treatment. However, benefit may not be gained in those patients with poor prognostic factors which include poor performance status, over 60 years of age, non-breast primary site, multiple lobe involvement, short disease-free interval and overt uncontrolled metastases elsewhere. As ever, decisions regarding treatment should be tailored to the problems of the individual patient.

Cranial irradiation may cause some degree of scalp and upper pinna erythema and irritation. Temporary alopecia is universal in a population whose prognosis is unlikely to allow regrowth of hair within the remaining lifespan. The start of treatment may induce an increase in cerebral oedema which may require steroid dose readjustment. Other effects include transient somnolence, occurring within a few weeks, and longer term impairment of memory and cognition. These are significant problems in very few people and most patients do not survive long enough for late radiation changes in the CNS to develop.

Corticosteroids

High-dose corticosteroids (dexamethasone 16mg/day initially) reduce cerebral oedema, and associated symptoms of headache and vomiting may be helped rapidly. In certain situations, particularly if metastases are in the posterior fossa, hydrocephalus may be present, in which case a ventricular shunt may be required for symptom control.

The short prognosis for most patients means that the issue of long-term side-effects of steroids may not be a problem. It is best practice, however, to gradually reduce the dose to the lowest possible over a few weeks to minimize potential side-effects since difficulties may build up insidiously.

A stage may be reached when the dose necessary to control the cerebral oedema causes significant side-effects. Disabling problems such as obesity (and associated problems with immobility management), body image problems, proximal myopathy, mood swings, fragile skin and diabetes may then develop. There should be open dialogue (particularly while the patient is *compos mentis* and can join in discussions) about the ongoing use of steroids in the event that quality of life becomes adversely affected. Patients and families may view steroids as agents to control the disease and resist attempts to reduce the dose, fearing the return of symptoms of raised intracranial pressure.

On the other hand, patients may have recognized that their quality of life is deteriorating despite continuing steroids and may then be happy for (or request that) steroids should be withdrawn. This should generally be done slowly while controlling the symptoms of raised intracranial pressure by other means.

When patients become moribund and can no longer swallow, the steroids can generally be stopped but this may depend on the particular clinical circumstances and may need negotiation with the patient and/or their family. There should be adequate medication provision (subcutaneous) including analgesics, antiemetics, anticonvulsants and sedatives as necessary.

Multiple complex physical and psychological problems including poor mobility, heavy care needs, swings in mood and confusion can completely exhaust even the most caring family who need the expert support of an experienced multidisciplinary team.

Prognosis

Although some patients, particularly with metastases from breast cancer, may survive relatively longer, most patients with brain metastases from solid tumours have a survival in the order of a few weeks or months at best.

Metastatic disease of the leptomeninges (meningeal carcinomatosis)

Some 5% of patients with tumours may develop clinical signs and symptoms of leptomeningeal disease, although the autopsy rate is higher (10%). It is most commonly seen in lymphoma and leukaemia, although it may occur in breast cancer, small-cell lung cancer and melanoma.

Clinical features

The presenting features may be varied and fluctuating and the diagnosis should be considered in any unexplained neurological disturbance in a patient with cancer. The most frequently encountered are cranial nerve problems (75%), headache (50%), radicular or back pain (40–45%) and weakness in one or more limbs (40%). Other presentations include meningism, altered consciousness, confusion, sphincter disturbance and seizures. Abnormal physical signs are more prominent than symptoms, with lower motor neurone lesions predominating.

Investigations

- Lumbar puncture if there is no evidence of raised intracranial pressure (90% will have positive cytology and increased protein on CNS analysis)
- Gadolinium MRI scan of the brain and whole spine

Management

This may include intrathecal chemotherapy, depending on the tumour type and radiotherapy. The aim is to halt the progression of disease and relieve symptoms, but is essentially palliative except for a curable subgroup of leukaemia or lymphoma. Steroids and NSAIDs may help symptoms.

Prognosis

Without treatment patients may survive for several months, depending on the tumour type, but with relentless progression of neurological symptoms. Even with treatment, prognosis is usually less than six months and is worst in small-cell lung cancer, widespread disease, poor performance status and where there are widespread neurological signs.

Chronic leukaemia and myeloma

Background

- Balancing opportunities for cure with impact of treatment on quality of life are crucial in assessing the appropriate interventions which are often extremely aggressive and taxing for patients
- Chemotherapy has led to marked improvements in survival over the past 40 years

General comments

The clinical course tends to be very variable, but is characterized by a *protracted cycle of relapses and remissions*. This can cause considerable distress as the patients and their carers have to live with uncertainty about the future. Both patient and the professionals involved with their care may find it hard to accept that the patient is entering the terminal phase.

Infection is a frequent and unpredictable complication of both the disease process and its treatment. It can be fatal and this makes the prognosis even more uncertain.

Chemotherapy may continue in advanced illness because of the possibility of a further remission and/or useful palliation.

Specific pain complexes

- **Bone pain** is very common. The pain is often worse on movement or weight-bearing, which makes titration of analgesics very difficult. The pain often *responds well to radiotherapy and/or oral steroids*. NSAIDs may help but must be used with caution because they may interfere with platelet and renal function
- **Pathological fractures** are particularly common in myeloma due to the lytic bone lesions. These often require orthopaedic intervention and subsequent *radiotherapy*. Prophylactic pinning of long bones and/or radiotherapy should be considered to prevent fracture and to reduce the likelihood of complex pain syndromes developing
- **Spinal cord compression** requires prompt diagnosis, high-dose oral steroids and urgent discussion with an oncologist. The steroids should be continued at a high dose until a definitive plan has been made. They may then be titrated down in accordance with the patient's condition and symptoms
- **Wedge and crush fractures of the spinal column** can lead to severe back pain which is often associated with nerve compression and neuropathic pain. Such pain is partially opioid-sensitive but adjuvant analgesics in the form of antidepressants and/or anticonvulsant medication are usually required to supplement the effect of the opioid. Specialist advice is frequently needed to maintain symptom control

Other complications

- **Bone marrow failure** is usual. Recurrent infections and bleeding episodes can leave the patients and carers exhausted. Patients often feel dependent on the administration of blood and platelet transfusions, unable to consider reducing the frequency of life-sustaining treatment. Difficult decisions about reducing regular transfusions or stopping them if they are providing no further benefit may need to be faced with patients and families.

- **Night sweats and fever** are common, imposing a heavy demand on carers, particularly as several changes of night and bedclothes may be needed. Specialist advice may help in relieving the symptoms, as there are a number of drugs that appear to be effective (📖 see Chapter 6d, p. 361–3).
- **Hypercalcaemia** may occur, especially in myeloma. It should be considered in any patient with persistent nausea, altered mood or confusion (even if this is intermittent), worsening pain and/or constipation. Treatment with IV hydration and IV bisphosphonates should be considered. Resistant hypercalcaemia may be a pre-terminal event when aggressive management would be inappropriate

Palliative care of patients with carcinomatosis of unknown primary

Background

Approximately 3% of patients present with metastases from an unknown primary site. As a group the prognosis for these patient is poor, with a median survival of 3–4 months.

Investigations

- Serological tumour markers including CA19–9, CEA, CA125, αFP, βhCG, PSA, and paraproteins
- Biopsy—thorough pathological assessment with immunohistochemistry may provide clues to the primary site
- CT scan of chest, abdomen and pelvis

In some instances the site of metastatic disease may suggest a probable primary site, e.g. adenocarcinoma in axillary nodes suggests a breast primary.

Particularly in young patients it is important to rule out the possibility of a potentially curable germ-cell tumour. This may be suggested by elevated αFP or β hCG.

In a substantial number of patients a primary site is not identified. In this instance exhaustive investigations may not be appropriate, particularly if the patient is of poor performance status.

Treatment

In some patients where the clinical presentation suggests a primary, even if a tumour cannot be detected in that organ, it may be appropriate to treat the patient in the usual manner. For example, a patient presenting with ER-positive adenocarcinoma in an axillary node could reasonably be treated as if breast cancer was the primary.

For patients in whom there is little evidence of a primary site (e.g. those presenting with liver metastases) the choice is much more difficult. As the primary is unknown it is impossible to give patients an idea of the likelihood of a treatment response or of how durable such a response is likely to be. Any potential benefit of treatment must be carefully balanced against possible toxicity and a decision to proceed with chemotherapy should only be undertaken following a very full discussion with the patient and carers, outlining the uncertainties and limitations of treatment and overall limited prognosis.

Anxiety is common in this group of patients. Not knowing the site of the primary tumour causes considerable distress. Extensive investigations may raise false expectations and may exhaust the patient. Equally, patients and carers may feel cheated of the chance to have effective treatment if the primary is not looked for.

Carers may find coming to terms with the patient's death due to an 'unknown primary' difficult, and are perhaps at greater risk of an adverse bereavement reaction.

Key points
- Anxiety and anger
- Risk of over-investigation
- Adverse bereavement reaction

Investigations (Tables 5.21 and 5.22)

Table 5.21 Tumour markers and associated conditions

Tumour marker	Associated conditions	
	Malignant conditions	*Non-malignant conditions*
CEA	GI tract cancers (particularly colorectal cancer)	Cirrhosis
		Pancreatitis
		Smoking
CA 19-9	Colorectal cancer	Cholestasis
	Pancreatic cancer	
CA-125	Ovarian cancer	Cirrhosis
	Breast cancer	Pregnancy
	Hepatocellular cancer	Peritonitis
αFP	Hepatocellular cancer	Cirrhosis
	Germ-cell cancers (not pure seminoma)	Pregnancy
		Hepatitis
		Open neural tube defects
βhCG	Germ-cell cancers	Pregnancy
	Choriocarcinoma and hydatidiform mole	
PSA	Prostate cancer	Benign prostatic hypertrophy
		Prostatitis
		Prostate instrumentation
		(incl. rectal examination)
		Acute urinary retention
		Physical exercise
		Old age

Table 5.22 Advantages of imaging techniques

Imaging technique	Preferred when evaluating
CT	Lungs, abdominal cavity
Spiral CT	Makes 3-D images of areas inside the body. Detects small abnormal areas better than conventional CT
MRI	Mediastinum, liver, pelvis brain, spinal cord
PET	By using 5-FDG which is avidly taken up by actively dividing cells, helps to:
	Determine functional and metabolic status of tumours
	Distinguish benign from malignant lesions
	Distinguish whether a residual mass after treatment represents fibrosis or residual tumour.

Patient tip

Further information about treatment decisions:
Cancer Research UK 0808 800 4040 ☐ www.cancerhelp.org.uk
Cancerbackup 0808 800 1234 ☐ www.cancerbackup.org.uk
DIPEx Patient experience database ☐ www.dipex.org

Further reading

Books

Cassidy J. et al. (2002) Oxford Handbook of Oncology. Oxford: Oxford University Press.

Souhami R. L., Tobias J. D. (2003) Cancer and its Management (4th edn). Oxford: Blackwell Science.

Thomas K. (2003) Caring for the Dying at Home: Companions on the Journey. Oxford: Radcliffe Press.

Articles

Agarwal J., et al. (2006) The role of external beam radiotherapy in the management of bone metastases. Clinical Oncology. 18(10): 747–760.

Kirkham S. (1988) The palliation of cerebral tumours with high dose dexamethasone: a review. Palliative Medicine, 2: 27–33.

Kvale P. A. (2007) Palliative Care in Lung Cancer. Accp Evidence-Based Clinical Practice Guidelines (2nd edn). Chest, 132: 3685–4035.

Wilkinson A. (2008) Managing skeletal related events resulting from bone metastases. British Medical Journal, 337: 1101–5.

The management of pain

I think the simplest and probably the best definition of pain is what the patient says hurts. I think that they may be expressing a very multi-faceted thing. They may have physical, psychological, family, social and spiritual things all wound up in this one whole experience. But I think we should believe people and once you believe somebody you can begin to understand, and perhaps tease out the various elements that are making up the pain.

Cicely Saunders

The **Specificity Theory** of pain, which was proposed by René Descartes in the sixteenth century, is one of the original pain theories. It states that pain intensity relates directly to the amount of associated tissue injury. Its unidimensional approach to pain implies that 100% of pain is treatable by analgesics.

Dr Henry Beecher recognized the limitations of this theory in the Second World War when he observed that only one out of three soldiers carried into a combat hospital complained of enough pain to require morphine.[1] He noted that a mismatch between pain intensity and injury severity occurs in certain situations.

Melzack and Wall proposed the **Gate Control Theory** of pain in 1965, and suggested that a spinal cord mechanism existed that regulated the transmission of pain sensations between the periphery and the brain.[2] The theory shifted attention away from the peripheral source of injury towards the spinal cord and brain. It provided the first physiological mechanism for psychological interventions to minimize pain (e.g. distraction or relaxation).

Following on from their work an increasingly multidimensional approach to pain was adopted, and clinicians now recognize that pain perception is governed by a multitude of factors (the **Neuromatrix Theory** of pain).[3]

Pain is an unpleasant sensory and emotional experience associated with actual or potential tissue damage, or described in terms of such damage.

International Association for the Study of Pain

1 Beecher H. K. (1959) *Measurement of Subjective Responses.* New York: Oxford University Press.

2 Melzack R., Wall P. D. (1965) Pain mechanisms: a new theory. *Science,* **150**: 971–9.

3 Melzack R. (2005) Evolution of the neuromatrix theory of pain. *Pain Practice,* **5**: 85–94.

Dame Cicely Saunders also recognized that other important factors can influence the pain experience. In parallel with the work of others, she developed the concept of **'total pain'** from her understanding that the origins of pain may be:

• Physical
• Social
• Psychological
• Spiritual

The concept of total pain has become a central tenet of palliative care practice. It recognizes that cancer pain is often a complex, chronic pain with multiple, coexisting causes. Effective management of cancer pain requires a multidisciplinary approach that addresses the patient's concerns and fears, as well as treating the physical aspects of pain. As a result, the provision of analgesics should be combined with the provision of emotional, social and spiritual supports.

One patient in particular, a lady whose name should be recorded, a Mrs. Hinson, there were days that I remember saying to her, 'Tell me about your pain,' and without any more prompting from me, she went on to say, 'Well doctor, it began in my back, but now it seems that all of me is wrong.' And she gave a description about her symptoms. And then she went on to say, 'I could have cried for the pills and the injections, but I knew that I mustn't, the world seemed to be against me, nobody seemed to understand how I felt. My husband and son were marvellous, but they were having to stay off work and lose their money, but it's so wonderful to begin to feel safe again.' So really, she's talked about physical pain, she's talked about emotional pain of feeling shut away and all the emotional burden that she couldn't share. She was talking about social pain, financial in that case, but the impact on her family. And then the spiritual need, I think it is spiritual, of the security, the safety, to look at herself and who she was and just be herself. And then the concept of what I called total pain, and really started to lecture about, really comes from there.

Cicely Saunders

This chapter will focus on the management of physical pain caused by cancer, but the principles of therapy are generally applicable to the management of pain caused by other progressive, non-malignant conditions.

Physical pain in patients with cancer

Pain is a common and feared symptom of cancer (Table 6a.1). Many patients with non-malignant, life-threatening disease also suffer pain. Despite the availability of effective methods of controlling pain, significant numbers continue to receive inadequate pain relief.

Cancer pain may be **acute** or **chronic**, and chronic pain may be further subdivided:

- **Background pain** is a persistent baseline pain. Background pain is managed by the regular administration of analgesics
- **Breakthrough pain** occurs when pain 'breaks through' a regular pain-medicine schedule. The quality of breakthrough pain may feel very much like the background pain, except that it is more severe. Although it generally has the same aetiology as background pain, this is not always the case. Breakthrough pain is relieved with rescue or short-acting medications that are taken only at the time of a breakthrough pain episode (section) p. 232

Table 6a.1 Causes of cancer pain

The cancer itself	Bony/visceral/soft tissue involvement, nerve compression or infiltration, muscle spasm, ulceration, raised intracranial pressure, etc.
Complications of the cancer	Pressure sores, constipation, post-herpetic neuralgia, candidiasis, lymphoedema, etc.
Treatment of the cancer	Neuropathy caused by chemotherapy, mucositis caused by radiotherapy, post-operative pain, etc.
Co-morbidities	Angina, diabetic neuropathy, arthritis, etc.

Incidence of cancer pain

- One-quarter of patients *do not experience pain*
- One-third of those with pain have a single pain
- One-third have two pains
- One-third have three or more pains

The experience of pain can:

- Induce depression
- Exacerbate anxiety
- Interfere with social performance and impair the quality of relationships
- Negatively impact on physical capability
- Prevent work and reduce income
- Challenge existential beliefs
- Constantly impact on the patient's experience of pain

Assessment of pain

What we were aiming at as we started to work together in St Joseph's, was a patient who was alert and themselves and free of pain. For the great majority of patients that isn't that difficult with drugs that are available to anybody in a method that is simple. But it does include the very important careful analysis and assessment at the beginning. One long interview and careful examination can carry an awful lot of shorter ones.

Cicely Saunders

Failure to assess pain is a critical barrier to good pain management.

- Pain is a subjective experience, and so **patient self-report** is the gold standard of pain assessment
- Evaluation and treatment of pain are best achieved by a **team approach**, and the patient should be encouraged to take an active role in his/her own pain management
- Many patients will have more than one type of pain, and **each pain should be assessed separately**
- Patients should be **re-assessed at regular intervals** following initiation of treatment, and also at each report of new or altered pain

Principles of pain assessment

- Seek to establish a relationship with the patient, and encourage the patient to do most of the talking
- Begin with wide-angle open questions before clarifying and focussing on more specific ones
- Watch the patient for clues regarding pain
- Avoid jumping to conclusions

Key components of a pain assessment

- Description of the onset and duration of the pain
- Description of the pain, e.g. location, quality, pattern, character
- Rating of pain intensity (including a current pain rating, and ratings when pain is worst and least)
- Description of aggravating and relieving factors
- Description of associated symptoms and signs
- Description of the effects of pain on functioning and quality of life
- Description of current pain management regimen and assessment of effectiveness
- Summary of the past history of pain management
- Identification of the patient's goals of treatment
- Physical examination
- Diagnostic testing, where appropriate

Pain assessment tools

> I think there's a pain somewhere in the room, but I could not positively say that I have got it.
>
> Mrs Gradgrind (*Hard Times*, Charles Dickens)

Failure to assess pain is the most common cause of poor pain control. Pain scales can be useful tools in the systematic assessment of symptoms. Not only can they can encourage patient communication and facilitate the professional's understanding of the patient's experience, they can also be used to chart the trend of the patient's response to therapy. However, tools should never be seen as substitutes for a complete pain assessment. Moreover, they may need to be tailored to the needs of specific populations, for example generic tools are often unsuitable for use with those people who are cognitively impaired.

The ideal qualities of a pain assessment tool are that:
- It is easy to administer
- It is valid and reliable
- It shows sensitivity to treatment effect
- It has multilingual validity

Pain assessment tools may be **unidimensional** or **multidimensional**:
- Unidimensional tools provide information about the intensity of the pain experienced by the patient, and take the form of visual analogue scales, verbal rating scales and numeric rating scales
- Multidimensional pain measuring tools provide information about additional aspects of the pain such as history, location, affective component and quality of the pain. Examples include the McGill Pain Questionnaire and the Brief Pain Inventory (Fig. 6a.1).

Visual analogue scales (VAS)
The VAS is a line with extremes marked as 'no pain' and 'worst pain'. Patients are asked to mark the point in the line that best describes their pain.

No pain_____Worst pain

Categorical verbal rating scales (VRS)
These involve a sequence of words describing different levels of pain intensity e.g.:
None   Mild   Moderate   Severe

Categorical numerical rating scales (NRS)
These use numbers or gradations that indicate the severity of the pain experience:

0____1____2____3____4____5____6____7____8____9____10
No pain   Worst pain

Brief Pain Inventory

Date: ___/___/___

Name: _____   _____   _____
          Last   First   Middle Initial

Phone: (__) _____   Sex: ☐ Female   ☐ Male

Date of Birth: ___/___/___

1) Marital Status (at present)
     1. ☐ Single   3. ☐ Widowed
     2. ☐ Married   4. ☐ Separated/Divorced

2) Education (Circle only the highest grade or degree completed)
   Grade   0   1   2   3   4   5   6   7   8   9
                 10   11   12   13   14   15   16   M.A./M.S.
                                    Professional degree (please specify) _____

3) Current occupation _____
   (specify titles; if you are not working, tell us your previous occupation)

4) Spouse's Occupation _____

5) Which of the following best describes your current job status?
     ☐ 1. Employed outside the home, full-time
     ☐ 2. Employed outside the home, part-time
     ☐ 3. Homemaker
     ☐ 4. Retired
     ☐ 5. Unemployed
     ☐ 6. Other

6) How long has it been since you first learned your diagnosis? _____ months

7) Have you ever had pain due to your present disease?
     1. ☐ Yes   2. ☐ No   3. ☐ Uncertain

8) When you first received your diagnosis, was pain one of your symptoms?
     1. ☐ Yes   2. ☐ No   3. ☐ Uncertain

9) Have you had surgery in the past month? 1. ☐ Yes   2. ☐ No

10) Throughout our lives, most of us have had pain from time to time (such as minor
    headaches, sprains, and toothaches). Have you had pain other than these everyday
    kinds of pain during the **last week**? 1. ☐ Yes   2. ☐ No

IF YOU ANSWERED YES TO THE LAST QUESTION, PLEASE GO ON TO QUESTION 11
AND FINISH THIS QUESTIONNAIRE. IF NO, YOU ARE FINISHED WITH THE
QUESTIONNAIRE. THANK YOU.

11) On the diagram, shade in the areas where you feel pain. Put an X on the area that hurts
    the most.

                        Front   Back

        Right ☺ Left   Left ☺ Right

12) Please rate your pain by circling the one number that best describes your pain at its
    worst in the last week.
      0   1   2   3   4   5   6   7   8   9   10
     No   Pain as bad as
     Pain   you can imagine

13) Please rate your pain by circling the one number that best describes your pain at its
    least in the last week.
      0   1   2   3   4   5   6   7   8   9   10
     No   Pain as bad as
     Pain   you can imagine

14) Please rate your pain by circling the one number that best describes your pain on the
    average.
      0   1   2   3   4   5   6   7   8   9   10
     No   Pain as bad as
     Pain   you can imagine

Fig. 6a.1 Brief pain inventory. Reproduced with permission from Doyle *et al.*
(eds) (2004) *The Oxford Textbook of Palliative Medicine* (3rd edn). Oxford: Oxford
University Press.

15) Please rate your pain by circling the one number that tells how much pain you have right now.

```
0   1   2   3   4   5   6   7   8   9   10
No                                      Pain as bad as
Pain                                    you can imagine
```

16) What kinds of things make your pain feel better (for example, head, medicine, rest)?
_____
_____

17) What kinds of things make your pain worse (for example, walking, standing, lifting)?
_____

18) What treatments or medications are you receiving for your pain?
_____

19) In the last week, how much relief have pain treatments or medications provided? Please circle the one percentage that most shows how much relief you have received.

```
0%  10%  20%  30%  40%  50%  60%  70%  80%  90%  100%
No                                                 Complete
Relief                                             Relief
```

20) If you take pain medication, how many hours does it take before the pain returns?
☐ 1. Pain medication doesn't help at all   ☐ 5. Four hours
☐ 2. One hour   ☐ 6. Five to twelve hours
☐ 3. Two hours   ☐ 7. More than twelve hours
☐ 4. Three hours   ☐ 8. I do not take pain medication

21) Circle the appropriate answer for each item.
I believe my pain is due to:
☐ Yes ☐ No   1. The effects of treatment (for example, medication, surgery, radiation, prosthetic device).
☐ Yes ☐ No   2. My primary disease (meaning the disease currently being treated and evaluated).
☐ Yes ☐ No   3. A medical condition unrelated to primary disease (for example, arthritis).

22) For each of the following words, check yes or no if that adjective applies to your pain.

Aching	☐ Yes	☐ No	Exhausting	☐ Yes	☐ No
Throbbing	☐ Yes	☐ No	Tiring	☐ Yes	☐ No
Shooting	☐ Yes	☐ No	Penetrating	☐ Yes	☐ No
Stabbing	☐ Yes	☐ No	Nagging	☐ Yes	☐ No
Gnawing	☐ Yes	☐ No	Numb	☐ Yes	☐ No
Sharp	☐ Yes	☐ No	Miserable	☐ Yes	☐ No
Tender	☐ Yes	☐ No	Unbearable	☐ Yes	☐ No
Burning	☐ Yes	☐ No			

23) Circle the one number that describes how, during the past week, pain has interfered with your:

A. General Activity
```
0   1   2   3   4   5   6   7   8   9   10
Does not                                  Completely
Interfere                                 interferes
```

B. Mood
```
0   1   2   3   4   5   6   7   8   9   10
Does not                                  Completely
Interfere                                 interferes
```

C. Walking ability
```
0   1   2   3   4   5   6   7   8   9   10
Does not                                  Completely
Interfere                                 interferes
```

D. Normal work (includes both work outside the home and housework)
```
0   1   2   3   4   5   6   7   8   9   10
Does not                                  Completely
Interfere                                 interferes
```

E. Relations with other people
```
0   1   2   3   4   5   6   7   8   9   10
Does not                                  Completely
Interfere                                 interferes
```

F. Sleep
```
0   1   2   3   4   5   6   7   8   9   10
Does not                                  Completely
Interfere                                 interferes
```

G. Enjoyment of life
```
0   1   2   3   4   5   6   7   8   9   10
Does not                                  Completely
Interfere                                 interferes
```

Pain Research Group, Department of Neurology, University of Wisconsin-Madison

Fig. 6a.1 (Cont)

Assessing pain in people with dementia at the end of life

Pain is under-reported and under-treated in cognitively impaired older people. A comprehensive review of the literature reveals that people dying with dementia represent the 'disadvantaged dying'.[4]

As dementia progresses, and cognitive function and the ability to communicate verbally declines, it becomes increasingly more difficult to ascertain accurately wishes and needs and, consequently, people with dementia often have painful conditions that go unnoticed. This loss of language communication presents a major challenge in assessing pain in this group as self-reporting is required for most pain assessment tools.

In the absence of verbal self-report, nurses and carers are forced to rely increasingly on non-verbal and behavioural cues of physical and emotional pain. They need to use a combination of indicators to determine levels of pain, e.g. crying, facial grimacing, etc. Using observation skills rather than relying on verbal responses is essential, as is consideration that any sign of agitated behaviour may be emotional and not a result of pain.

Behaviour commonly associated with pain may be absent or difficult to interpret; e.g. extrapyramidal signs in people with dementia syndromes may mislead the healthcare professional, who may interpret the movements as an indication of pain.[5] There is no agreed physiological or biological chemical marker of pain and in people who are unable to communicate there is no benchmark that can be used to allow a definitive diagnosis of pain.[5]

A number of pain assessment tools have been developed for use in people with dementia.[6,7] However, it remains a complex area of clinical assessment practice. It is important to select a scale that matches the person's abilities; even their pre-dementia educational level and pre-existing abilities influence their ability to use pain scales.[5,6]

Enlisting the assistance of a carer or family member who is familiar with the usual behaviours and responses of the person with dementia is also essential in identifying behaviour changes that may indicate pain or discomfort.

4 Robinson L., et al. (2006) End-of-life care and dementia. *Reviews in Clinical Gerontology*, **15**(2): 135–48.

5 Scherder E., et al. (2005) Recent developments in pain in dementia. *British Medical Journal*, **330**: 461–4.

6 DeWaters T., Popovich J., Faut-Callahan M. (2003) An evaluation of clinical tools to measure pain in older people with cognitive impairment. *British Journal of Community Nursing*, **8**(5): 226–34.

7 Zwakhalen S. M. G., et al. (2005) Pain in elderly people with severe dementia: A systematic review of behavioural pain assessment tool. *BMC Geriatrics* **6**(3): www.biomedcentral.com/bmc geriatr/

The Abbey Pain Scale is an assessment tool that is presented in a form suitable for clinical use and is both easy and quick to administer. It was developed with care-home residents with end- or late-stage dementia using a combination of quantitative and qualitative data collection and analysis processes.[8]

The Abbey Pain Scale has been shown to be most useful as an aid to intervention where the scale is used to assess changes prior to, and following the administration of analgesia (Fig. 6a.2).

Many of the principles of assessing and managing pain in people with dementia also apply to people with learning disabilities when providing end-of-life care. The Disability Distress Assessment Tool (DisDAT),[9,10] developed to aid in the assessment of distress in people with learning disabilities, may also be of use in guiding practitioners in assessing distress in the dementia group.

8 Abbey J., Piller N., De Bellis A., Esterman A., Parker D., Giles L., Lowcay B. (2004) The Abbey pain scale: a 1-minute numerical indicator for people with end-stage dementia. *International Journal of Palliative Nursing*, **10**(1): 6–13.

9 Regnard C., Mathews D., Gibson L., Clarke C., Watson B. (2003) Difficulties in identifying distress and its causes in people with severe communication problems. *International Journal of Palliative Nursing* **9**(3): 173–6.

10 Regnard C., Reynolds J., Watson B., Mathews D., Gibson L., Clarke C. (2006) Understanding distress in people with severe communication difficulties: developing and assessing the Disability Distress Assessment Tool (DisDAT). *Journal of Intellectual Disability Research*, **51**: 277–92.

Use of the Abbey Pain Scale:

The pain scale is best used as part of an overall pain management plan.

Objective

The pain scale is an instrument designed to assist in the assessment of pain in residents who are unable to clearly articulate their needs.

Ongoing assessment

The scale does not differentiate between distress and pain, therefore measuring the effectiveness of pain relieving interventions is essential.

Recent work by the Australian Pain Society [1] recommends that the Abbey pain scale be used as a movement based assessment.

The staff recording the scale should, therefore, observe and record on the scale while the resident is being moved eg, during pressure area care, while showering etc.

Record results in the resident's notes. Include the time of completion of the scale, the score, staff member's signature and action taken in response to results of the assessment.

A second evaluation should be conducted 1 hour after the intervention taken in response to the first assessment, to determine the effectiveness of any pain relieving intervention.

If, at this assessment, the score on the pain scale is the same, or worse, undertake a comprehensive assessment of all facets of resident's care, monitor closely over a 24 hour period, including any further interventions undertaken, and, if there is no improvement, notify the medical practitioner

---

[1] Gibson, S., Scherer ,S and Goucke , R (2004) Final Report Australian Pain Society and the Australian Pain Relief Association Pain Management Guidelines for Residential Care: Stage 1 Preliminary field-testing and preparations for implementation. November

Australian Pain Society(2005)   Residential Aged Care Pain Management Guidelines, August. http://www.apsoc.org.au

Further details re original validation can be found   : Jennifer Abbey, Neil Piller, AnitaDe Bellis, Adrian Esterman, Deborah Parker, Lynne; Giles and Belinda Lowcay (2004) The Abbey pain scale: a 1-minute numerical indicator for people with end-stage dementia, *International Journal of Palliative Nursing*, Vol 10, No 1pp 6-13.

Fig. 6a.2

Abbey Pain Scale
For measurement of pain in people with dementia who cannot verbalise

How to use scale : While observing the resident, score questions 1 to 6.

Name of resident : ....

Name and designation of person completing the scale : ....

Date : .... Time : ....

Latest pain relief given was...at.........hrs.

Q1. Vocalisation
eg whimpering, groaning, crying
Absent 0   Mild 1   Moderate 2   Severe 3

Q1 ☐

Q2. Facial expression
eg looking tense, frowning, grimacing, looking frightened
Absent 0   Mild 1   Moderate 2   Severe 3

Q2 ☐

Q3. Change in body language
eg fidgeting, rocking, guarding part of body, withdrawn
Absent 0   Mild 1   Moderate 2   Severe 3

Q3 ☐

Q4. Behavioural Change
eg increased confusion, refusing to eat, alteration in usual patterns
Absent 0   Mild 1   Moderate 2   Severe 3

Q4 ☐

Q5. Physiological change
eg temperature, pulse or blood pressure outside normal limits,
perspiring, flushing or pallor
Absent 0   Mild 1   Moderate 2   Severe 3

Q5 ☐

Q6. Physical changes
eg skin tears, pressure areas, arthritis, contractures,
previous injuries
Absent 0   Mild 1   Moderate 2   Severe 3

Q6 ☐

Add scores for 1 - 6 and record here ⟹ Total Pain Score ☐

Now tick the box that matches the
Total Pain Score ⟹

0 - 2 No pain	3 - 7 Mild	8 - 13 Moderate	14 + Severe

Finally, tick the box which matches
the type of pain ⟹

Chronic	Acute	Acute on Chronic

Abbey, J., DeBellis, A., Piller, N., Esterman, A., Giles, L., Parker, D and Lowcay, B.
Funded by the JH&JD Gunn Medical Research Foundation 1998-2002
This document may be reproduced with thisacknowledgement retained

Pain classification

Two main types of pain may be identified on the basis of the mechanism by which pain is produced: **nociceptive** and **neuropathic**. Different types of pain respond with varying degrees of effectiveness to different types of analgesics, and so it is important that clinicians determine what type of pain a patient is experiencing in order to prescribe the most appropriate drug. Many patients with cancer have mixed pain syndromes, i.e. a combination of nociceptive and neuropathic pain, and may need combination therapy.

Nociceptive pain may result from injury to somatic structures (somatic pain) or injury to visceral structures (visceral pain) (Fig. 6a.3.):

- **Somatic pain** results from the stimulation of skin, muscle or bone receptors. The neural pathways involved are normal and intact and the pain is typically well localized, and may be felt in the superficial cutaneous areas (e.g. cellulitis) or deeper musculoskeletal areas (e.g. bone pain). It may be described as aching, stabbing, throbbing or pressure.
- **Visceral pain** results from infiltration, compression or the distension of thoracic or abdominal viscera. It is often poorly localized and may be described as gnawing, cramping, aching or sharp. It may be referred to cutaneous sites (e.g. shoulder-tip pain from diaphragmatic irritation due to liver capsule distension), and the cutaneous site may be tender. Mechanism of action of referred pain is poorly understood.

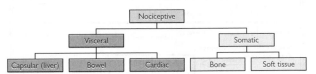

Fig. 6a.3 Somatic pain.

Neuropathic pain is caused by injury to the peripheral and/or CNS (Fig. 6a.4). The underlying mechanisms of neuropathic pain are poorly understood, but broadly speaking, pain occurs because the injured nerves either react abnormally to stimuli or discharge spontaneously.

- Typically, pain that arises from damage to the peripheral nervous system is termed 'deafferentation' pain, while pain that arises from injury to the spinal cord or brain is termed 'central' pain
- Neuropathic pain is typically described as being different in character to nociceptive pain. Patients may describe having a dull ache with a 'vice like' quality, or burning, tingling, shooting or electric shock-like sensations. It may be associated with hyperalgesia and allodynia.

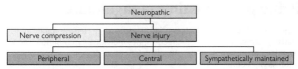

Fig. 6a.4 Neuropathic pain.

Table 6a.2 Definition of pain terms[11]

Allodynia	Pain caused by a stimulus which does not normally provoke pain
Analgesia	Absence of pain in response to stimulation which would normally be painful
Causalgia	A syndrome of sustained burning pain, allodynia and hyperpathia after a traumatic nerve lesion, often combined with vasomotor dysfunction and later trophic changes
Central pain	Pain associated with a lesion in the central nervous system (brain and spinal cord)
Dysaesthesia	An unpleasant abnormal sensation which can be either spontaneous or provoked
Hyperaesthesia	An increased sensitivity to stimulation
Hyperalgesia	An increased response to a stimulus that is normally painful
Hyperpathia	A painful syndrome characterized by an increased reaction to a stimulus, especially a repetitive stimulus, and an increased threshold
Neuralgia	Pain in the distribution of a nerve
Neuropathy	A disturbance of function or pathological change in a nerve
Neuropathic pain	Pain which is transmitted by a damaged nervous system, and which is usually only partially opioid-sensitive
Nociceptor	A receptor preferentially sensitive to a noxious stimulus or to a stimulus which would become noxious if prolonged
Nociceptive pain	Pain which is transmitted by an undamaged nervous system and is usually opioid-responsive
Pain	An unpleasant sensory and emotional experience associated with actual or potential tissue damage or described in terms of such damage
Pain threshold	The least experience of pain which a subject can recognize
Pain tolerance level	The greatest level of pain which a subject is prepared to tolerate

11 Mersky H., Bogduk N. (1994) *Classification of Chronic Pain* (2nd edn). Seattle: ASP Press.

Principles of pain management

The right dose of an analgesic is the dose that relieves pain without causing unmanageable side-effects. Some individuals may simply require regular paracetamol, while others may need doses of oral morphine in excess of 1000mg/day.

More than twenty years ago, the World Health Organization (WHO) published *Cancer Pain Relief*,[12] a book which set out the principles of cancer pain management including the use of the three-step analgesic ladder. The WHO method can be summarized in five phrases:

• By the mouth
• By the clock
• By the ladder
• For the individual
• Attention to detail

The WHO ladder indicates that a structured, yet flexible, approach to the management of cancer pain is important. The steps of the ladder illustrate that the process of selecting analgesics should be dependent on an assessment of the intensity of pain experienced by the patient, rather than aetiology of the pain.

The oral route is the preferred route for analgesics, including morphine. For persistent pain, analgesics should be taken at regular time intervals and not 'as needed'. Adjuvant drugs should be prescribed when required.

Each patient should be regularly re-assessed in order to determine response to treatment, and to ensure that he/she experiences maximum benefit with as few adverse effects as possible. Pain relief can be achieved for about 80% of patients by adopting the basic principles of 'by the mouth, by the ladder and by the clock'.[13]

12 World Health Organization (1986) *Cancer Pain Relief*. Geneva: WHO.

13 Zech D. F. J., et al. (1995) Validation of the World Health Organization Guidelines for cancer pain relief: a 10-year prospective study. *Pain*, **65**(1): 65–76.

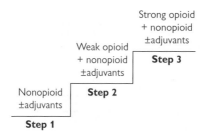

Fig. 6a.5 The analgesic ladder.[14]

Classification of analgesics

The three classes of analgesics referred to in the WHO analgesic ladder are: non-opioids, opioids and adjuvants (co-analgesics) (Fig. 6a.5).

Non-opioids

Non-opioids are analgesic drugs that mediate their effect through receptors other than opioid receptors. Examples of non-opioids are aspirin, paracetamol and NSAIDs.

Opioids

Opioids are drugs that are agonists at opioid receptor sites. There are at least three types of opioid receptor (mu, kappa and delta), which are found in several areas of the brain and throughout the spinal cord. Stimulation of opioid receptors results in a variety of responses, including analgesia, respiratory depression, myosis, reduced gastrointestinal motility and euphoria. Differences between opioids relate, in part, to differences in receptor affinity.

Opioids for mild to moderate pain are so-called because they are conventionally used to treat pain of this intensity. They are sometimes called referred to as 'weak' opioids.

Opioids for moderate to severe pain are used to treat moderate to severe pain and are sometimes called 'strong opioids'. They are available as immediate release and modified release preparations. Immediate–release (i/r) opioids typically reach peak plasma concentrations within one hour of ingestion and have a duration of action of 1–4h, depending on formulation. Modified-release (m/r) opioids typically reach their peak plasma concentrations 2–6h after ingestion, and the plasma levels are sustained over a period of 12–24h, depending on formulation.

14 World Health Organization (1996) Cancer pain relief: with guide to opioid availability (2nd edn). Geneva: WHO.

Adjuvant analgesics

These are drugs which do not function primarily as analgesics but can act to relieve pain in specific circumstances. The choice of adjuvant drug is generally guided by the nature of the underlying pain (i.e. nociceptive or neuropathic). Examples of adjuvant analgesics are listed in Table 6a.3.

Table 6a.3 Adjuvant analgesics

Adjuvant analgesic	Use
Antidepressant	Neuropathic pain
Anticonvulsant	Neuropathic pain
Antispasmodic	Pain due to colic
Bisphosphonate	Pain due to bone metastases
Corticosteroid	Pain due to oedema or nerve compression
Muscle relaxant	Pain due to muscle spasm or cramp
NMDA-receptor blocker	Neuropathic pain

Breakthrough pain

Breakthrough pain is a transient increase in pain intensity over background pain. Usually, breakthrough pain is related to background pain; typically, it is of rapid onset, severe in intensity and self-limiting, with an average duration of 30 minutes.[15]

Three types of breakthrough pain are described:
- **Incident pain:** pain is related to movement (either voluntary or involuntary)
- **Idiopathic/spontaneous pain:** no identifiable cause; lasts longer than incident pain
- **End of dose failure:** prior to scheduled dose of analgesia; gradual onset. Often not regarded as true breakthrough pain[16]

Breakthrough pain affects over 50% of patients with cancer, and also occurs in patients with non-malignant disease. It is a poor prognostic indicator[17] and may lead to decreased functioning, anxiety and depression and longer stays in hospital.[18,19] Every patient on an opioid should have access to breakthrough analgesia in order to ensure optimal pain control.

Management[20]

1 **Non-pharmacological management:** if possible, treat the underlying cause (e.g. surgery, chemotherapy, radiotherapy); avoid precipitating factors (if possible); physical therapy; education about limitations and exacerbating factors; and patient counselling to reduce anxiety
2 **Optimize around-the-clock medication**
3 **Specific pharmacological interventions:**
   - It is generally appropriate to use a short-acting opioid at a dose of one-sixth of the total 24-hour dose of opioid. However, it is recognized that the relationship between the 24-hour dose of opioid and the breakthrough dose is not fixed, and some patients may require individual titration of the breakthrough dose to control their incident pain.
   - Newer analgesics are available that offer more rapid onset and offset of analgesia than traditional short-acting opioids. These agents may offer certain advantages over traditional short-acting opioids because they have a more suitable pharmacokinetic profile. Examples include fentanyl as (a) oral transmucosal lozenges (OTFC/Actiq); (b) sublingual tablet (Abstral); (c) effervescent buccal tablet (Effentora); (d) intranasal spray (Instanyl).

15 Zeppetella G., Ribeiro M. D. Opioids for the management of breakthrough (episodic) pain in cancer patients. *Cochrane Database of Systematic Reviews*, 2006, Issue 1.

16 Payne R. (2007) Recognition and diagnosis of breakthrough pain. *Pain Medicine*, **8**: S2–7.

17 Bruera E., *et al.* (1995) A prospective multi-center assessment of the Edmonton staging system for cancer pain. *Journal of Pain and Symptom Management*, **10**: 348–55.

18 Portenoy R. K., Payne D., Jacobsen P. (1999) Breakthrough pain: characteristics and impact in patients with cancer. *Pain*, **81**: 129–34.

19 Fortner B. V., Okon T. A., Portenoy R. K. (2002) A survey of pain-related hospitalisations, emergency department visits, and physicians office visits reported by cancer patients with and without history of breakthrough pain. *Journal of Pain*, **3**: 38-44.

20 Portenoy R. K. (1997) Treatment of temporal variations in chronic cancer pain. *Seminars in Oncology*, **24**(5) suppl 16 (S7-S12).

Pharmacological management should be tailored to the type of breakthrough pain:

1 **Incident pain:** pre-emptive use of a short-acting opioid at an appropriate interval before activity (if predictable)
2 **Idiopathic/spontaneous:** use of a short-acting opioid when pain occurs
3 **End of dose failure:** alter the around-the-clock medication to increase the dose or shorten the dosing interval

Step 1: Non-opioid ± adjuvants

Patients with mild pain should be treated with a non-opioid analgesic, and if a specific indication exists, the use of the non-opioid analgesic may be combined with that of an adjuvant analgesic.

For example, a patient with mild neuropathic pain may be prescribed paracetamol 500mg–1g q6–8h regularly (max. daily dose 4g) in combination with amitriptyline 25–75mg o.d.

Step 2: Opioid for mild–moderate pain + non-opioid ± adjuvants

Patients who fail to achieve adequate relief after a trial of a non-opioid analgesic, or who present with moderate pain, should be treated with an opioid conventionally used for the treatment of mild to moderate pain. The opioid may be combined with a non-opioid in order to achieve an additive analgesic effect. Adjuvant drugs may also be used as required.

For example, a patient with moderate neuropathic pain may be prescribed codeine 30–60mg q6h in combination with paracetamol 1g q6h and amitriptyline 25–75mg o.d.

Some authors have questioned the usefulness of step 2 of the ladder because, in a systematic review, opioids for mild to moderate pain (either alone or in combination with non-opioids) were shown to be no better than full doses of NSAIDs alone.[21] In practice, however, clinicians have found the range of choices afforded by the ladder to be helpful.

Combination preparations of opioids and non-opioids are available for use at step 2, and are some of the most widely used medicines in the community. e.g. co-codamol

Step 3: Strong opioid + non-opioid ± adjuvants

Patients who fail to achieve adequate relief despite appropriate prescription of step 2 drugs, or who present with severe pain should be treated with an opioid conventionally used for severe pain. Adjuvant drugs may be used as required.

Oral morphine, in either immediate-release (i/r) or modified-release (m/r) form, is the opioid of choice for treating moderate or severe cancer pain for reasons of its familiarity, availability and cost.

21 Eisenberger E. *et al.* (1994) Efficacy and safety of nonsteroidal anti-inflammatory drugs for cancer pain: a meta-analysis. *Journal of Clinical Oncology*, **12**(12): 2756–65.

Step 1 analgesics

Aspirin, paracetamol and NSAIDs are all possible step 1 analgesics, although in practice aspirin is difficult to tolerate at analgesic doses due to its side-effects. The choice between paracetamol and the NSAIDs should be based on a risk/benefit analysis for each patient.

Paracetamol's analgesic and antipyretic activities are similar to that of aspirin, but it lacks an anti-inflammatory effect. Its mode of action for its analgesic effect remains unclear, although serotonin modulation has been suggested. It has minimal toxicity in adults at recommended doses, but at higher doses can cause fatal hepatotoxicity and renal damage.

NSAIDs are a heterogenous group of drugs that are of use in the treatment of pain mediated by prostaglandins, which serve to sensitize nociceptors. They have conventionally been thought to have particular use in the management of bone pain, but their analgesic effect in this area has probably been somewhat over-estimated.

NSAIDs produce their analgesic effect through inhibition of one or both of the isoenzymes of cyclo-oxygenase: **COX-1 or COX-2**.

Non-specific COX inhibitors, such as aspirin, ibuprofen and diclofenac, inhibit both isoenzymes. But their use is associated with a number of adverse effects (notably GI and renal toxicity).

Newer NSAIDs inhibit COX-2 only, and are associated with reduced GI effects. However, they may still adversely affect renal function and they have recently been associated with an increased risk of adverse vascular events. Several epidemiological studies have implied that the increased risk of vascular events is a class effect, and is associated with the use of conventional NSAIDs also; this area is being closely studied

- A dose–response relationship exists in terms of desired effects and both renal and gastrointestinal effects. Therefore, it is good practice initially to use the lowest effective dose of any NSAID, and to increase it only according to need
- Patients appear to vary in their analgesic response to NSAIDs and it may be appropriate to try a drug from a different class if the first-choice drug is ineffective or not tolerated

Tables 6a.4 and 6a.5 provide guides to NSAID selection and dosages, respectively, in palliative care practice.

Table 6a.4 NSAID selection

	No or low NSAID GI risk factors*	**NSAID GI risk factors***
No CVD	Non-selective NSAID ± PPI	COX-2 inhibitor ± PPI, or non-selective NSAID + PPI
CVD	Consider alternative analgesia first (e.g. paracetamol ± tramadol) then a non-selective NSAID ± PPI (cautiously)	Consider alternative analgesia first (e.g. paracetamol ± tramadol) then a non-selective NSAID ± PPI (cautiously)

*Gastrointestinal (GI) risk factors include age >65yrs, a previous history of peptic ulcer disease, concurrent medication, e.g. aspirin, warfarin, selective serotonin-reuptake inhibitors (SSRIs).
Abbreviations: NSAID, non-steroidal anti-inflammatory drug; CVD, cardiovascular disease; PPI, proton pump inhibitor; COX-2, cyclo-oxygenase inhibitor-2.

Table 6a.5 NSAID dosages

Ibuprofen	200–400mg t.d.s. p.o.
Diclofenac	50mg t.d.s. (can be used p.o., SC, or supps.)
Celecoxib	up to 200mg b.d. p.o.
Naproxen	250–500mg b.d. (p.o. or per rectum)
Ketorolac	10–30mg SC every 4–6h p.r.n.; max. 90mg daily (max. 60mg for elderly); max. duration 2 days
Parecoxib	40mg, then 20–40mg every 6–12 h p.r.n.; max. 80mg daily (max. 40mg for elderly)

Step 2 analgesics

Codeine phosphate

Codeine is metabolized by the hepatic cytochrome enzyme **CYP2D6** to morphine. Codeine is a much weaker agonist at mu receptors than morphine, and the analgesic effect is highly dependent on the production of its active metabolite, morphine, by the CYP2D6 system.

Some 7% of Caucasians and 1–3% of Asian people are CYP2D6 poor metabolizers, and do not experience effective analgesia with codeine. CYP2D6 activity may also be inhibited by antipsychotic agents (haloperidol, levomepromazine and thioridazine) and antidepressants (amitriptyline, fluoxetine and paroxetine).

Codeine is available in tablet and syrup formulations. Doses of 30–60mg p.o. q4h are generally prescribed, to a maximum dose of 240mg in 24 hours. It is also available in compound preparations, where it is combined with a non-opioid. The compound preparations may contain either low-dose (8mg) or high-dose (30mg) codeine, and so it is important to stipulate the dose of codeine required in the preparation, e.g. 'paracetamol 500mg/codeine 30mg'. Studies have shown that there is no additional analgesic benefit from preparations that contain only 8mg of codeine combined with paracetamol compared with paracetamol alone.

Tramadol

Tramadol displays weak opioid activity and it is also a noradrenaline and selective serotonin-reuptake inhibitor (SSRI). It is metabolized by both **CYP2D6** to the active metabolite, and additionally by **CYP3A4**. Like codeine, CYP2D6 inhibitors can reduce its analgesic effect. CYP3A4 inducers (e.g. carbamazepine) can also reduce analgesia.

There is some disagreement as to which step of the ladder tramadol should be prescribed. But, traditionally, it has proved suitable as a step 2 analgesic because, at therapeutic doses, its analgesic effect is similar to that of an opioid for mild to moderate pain in combination with a non-opioid.

It is not classed as a 'controlled drug' and this has some practical prescribing advantages. One of the limitations of tramadol in cancer pain is the extent to which the dose can be titrated. It is recommended that, except in special clinical circumstances, doses of 400mg a day should not be exceeded. At doses above this, the risk of convulsions may be increased.

Adverse effects

- Adverse effects include nausea, vomiting, dizziness and drowsiness. Hallucinations and confusion, as well as rare cases of drug dependence and withdrawal, have also been reported. Seizures may occur with use, and appear to be most likely in people taking drugs that lower the seizure threshold, or who have a history of seizures
- Adverse effects may be ameliorated by slow titration
- Tramadol has the potential for serious drug interactions, and may cause serotonin syndrome (particularly when combined with other serotonergic drugs, such as most antidepressants)

Tramadol preparations

- Caps: 50mg; sol. tabs 50mg; sachets effervescent powder 50mg
- Tabs: m/r (12h) 75mg, 100mg, 150mg, 200mg
- Caps: m/r (12h) 50mg, 100mg, 150mg, 200mg
- Tabs: m/r (24h) 150mg, 200mg, 300mg, 400mg
- Inj.: 100mg/2mL

Starting dose: 50mg q.d.s. p.o. or 100mg b.d. p.o. (12h m/r)

Step 3 analgesics

Opioids are safe, effective and appropriate drugs for the management of cancer pain, provided that:

- Appropriate starting doses and titration are observed
- The properties and relative potencies of different opioids are understood
- Opioid-related adverse effects are monitored and managed
- Prescribers are aware that some types of pain are poorly responsive to opioids and require other types of analgesics (adjuvant analgesics)

Morphine is the strong analgesic of choice unless there is a clinical reason to use an alternative opioid (p.245).

- Morphine appears to have no clinically relevant ceiling effect to analgesia. Doses of oral morphine may vary significantly between individuals to achieve the same end-point of pain relief
- The liver is the principal site of morphine metabolism
- Morphine undergoes a significant first-pass metabolism, which results in the production of two main metabolites: morphine-3-glucuronide (M3G) and morphine-6-glucuronide (M6G)
- M6G is believed to be a more potent analgesic than morphine itself, while the pharmacology of M3G remains unclear
- Morphine is well tolerated in patients with mild-to-moderate hepatic failure. In those with more severe hepatic failure it may be necessary to begin with a reduced dose of morphine and titrate to effect
- The products of morphine metabolism are eliminated by the kidney; as a result, patients with renal impairment are at an increased risk of accumulating metabolites and developing adverse effects (p.707)
- Morphine can be administered via oral, rectal, SC, IV, topical, epidural and intrathecal routes. Oral is the preferred route
- If patients are unable to take morphine orally, the preferred alternative route is SC. There is generally no indication for IM morphine for chronic cancer pain because SC administration is simpler and less painful
- The relative potency of morphine varies according to route of administration (p. 244)
- Oral Morphine is available in two formulations: immediate-release (i/r; also known as 'normal release') and modified-release (m/r). Peak plasma concentrations of i/r preparations usually occur within the first hour after oral administration, and the analgesic effect lasts for about 4h. In contrast, m/r preparations produce a delayed peak plasma concentration after 2–6h, and analgesia lasts for 12 or 24h.

Morphine metabolism can be induced or inhibited by a variety of medications:

- Carbamazepine, phenobarbital, phenytoin and rifampicin all accelerate the clearance of morphine
- Phenothiazines, tricyclic antidepressants and cimetidine all interfere with morphine metabolism and increase the effect of morphine
- Lorazepam and other benzodiazepines that undergo glucuronidation competitively inhibit morphine metabolism

Morphine preparations

Morphine i/r (4h)

Oramorph	10mg/5mL; 20mg/1mL
Sevredol	10, 20, 50mg scored tabs
Morphine suppositories	10mg, 15mg, 20mg, 30mg (Equianalgesic dose by oral and rectal routes)

Morphine m/r (12h)

MST and Zomorph can be used interchangeably.

MST Continus	5, 10, 15, 30, 60, 100, 200mg tabs
Morphgesic SR	20, 30, 60, 100, 200mg susp. 10, 30, 60, 100mg tabs
Zomorph	10, 30, 60, 100, 200mg caps (can be opened and administered via an NG/PEG tube, or sprinkled on food)

Morphine m/r (24h)

MXL	30, 60, 90, 120, 150, 200mg caps

Starting morphine (Fig. 6a.6)

The starting dose of morphine depends on whether or not the patient has used opioids before and his/her previous dose.

An i/r morphine regime gives greatest flexibility for initial dose titration, but it may be appropriate to start some patients directly on m/r morphine, e.g.:

- Patients who are already taking step 2 opioids
- Patients with less severe pain
- Patients who have difficulties with compliance
- Outpatients

Immediate-release morphine

- Adult, not pain-controlled on full-dose step 2 analgesics: i/r preparation 5–10mg 4h
- Elderly, cachectic or not taking step 2 analgesics: i/r preparation 5mg 4h
- Very elderly and frail: Oramorph 2.5mg 4h

Modified-release morphine

- Adult, not pain-controlled on full-dose step 2 opioids: 15–30mg morphine m/r 12h
- Elderly, cachectic or not taking step 2 analgesics: m/r 10-15mg morphine 12h
- Very elderly and frail: 5-10mg 12h morphine m/r

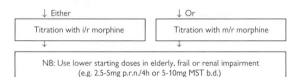

If pain is uncontrolled on WHO step 2 analgesic at full dose
(e.g. codeine 60mg q.d.s., tramadol 100mg q.d.s.)

↓ Either

Titration with i/r morphine

↓ Or

Titration with m/r morphine

↓

NB: Use lower starting doses in elderly, frail or renal impairment
(e.g. 2.5-5mg p.r.n./4h or 5-10mg MST b.d.)

↓

Stop WHO step 2 drug
Start morphine (Oramorph liquid or Sevredol tablets) 10mg 4h (Aim for 5 doses/24hrs; omit dose in night). Also prescribe same dose 'p.r.n.' for breakthrough pain; p.r.n. dose may be given as often as required (up to hourly).

↓

Stop WHO step 2 drug
Start MST 20mg b.d.
Also prescribe Oramorph liquid or Sevredol tablets 5-10mg 'p.r.n.' for breakthrough pain; prn dose may be given as often as required (up to hourly).

↓

Review after 24hrs
If sedated/toxic, reduce dose. If pain controlled, continue same doses & review in further 24hrs.

If pain uncontrolled, adjust regular dose according to number of prn doses taken (dose escalation usually 30-50% of total of p.r.n. morphine taken in 24-hr period). Adjust new p.r.n. dose appropriately.

Review after 24hrs
If sedated/toxic, reduce dose. If pain controlled, continue same doses & review in further 24hrs.

If pain uncontrolled, adjust regular dose according to number of p.r.n. doses taken (dose escalation usually 30-50% of total of p.r.n. morphine taken in 24-hr period). Adjust new p.r.n. dose appropriately.

Review after 24hrs as above
When pain is controlled convert to m/r formulation Add up total morphine use in 24hrs, divide by 2 & prescribe nearest sensible dose as MST. Prescribe appropriate p.r.n. dose. Arrange ongoing review appropriately.

Review after 24hrs as above
When pain controlled, continue same doses. Arrange ongoing review appropriately.

Fig. 6a.6 Flowchart adapted from Cancer Care Alliance of Teeside, Durham and North Yorkshire Network Supportive and Palliative Care Guidelines 2006.

Opioid titration

- Titration is a systematic process of incremental dose adjustment based on the patient's needs and responses
- The goal of titration is to use the smallest dose that provides satisfactory pain relief with the fewest side-effects
- The need for dose adjustment is based on reported severity of pain and frequency of need for breakthrough doses: 'titrating to effect'.
- Titration may be upward (a.k.a. 'dose escalation') or downward (tapering), depending on the patient's needs and responses.

- Dose adjustments are calculated based on a percentage of the total dose of breakthrough analgesia required in previous 24-hour period (most commonly an increase or decrease of 30 – 50%)
- The increment percentage tends to decrease a little as the dose increases, e.g. 5–10–15–20–30–40–60–80–100–130–160–200mg

Opioid adverse effects and toxicity

Adverse effects

The management of opioid-related adverse effects is a fundamental aspect of opioid therapy, and clinicians should adopt a proactive approach, wherever possible. The use of opioid analgesia should not be affected by unfounded fears about pharmacological tolerance, dependence or respiratory depression. **In the palliative care setting, pharmacological tolerance and psychological dependence rarely occur**. There is often significant inter-individual variation in sensitivity to opioid-related adverse effects, and this may be explained, in part, by genetic variability. Other factors influencing the development of adverse effects are:

- The presence of renal and hepatic impairment
- The use of polypharmacy
- The patient's age
- The patient's cognitive function
- The extent of the patient's disease
- The dose and type of opioid
- The route of administration of opioid

Many of the side-effects caused by opioids are non-specific, so it is important as a first step to determine whether the symptoms are related to opioid use or to underlying disease.

Common management strategies for various opioid-related side-effects are listed in Table 6a.6, and are mainly based on a dose reduction of systemic opioid ± use of a specific therapy to treat the adverse effect.

Additional strategies for the management of opioid-related side-effects include:

- Opioid switching (section p. 248)
- Use of adjuvant analgesics that act in a synergistic manner to reduce opioid requirements (📖 p. 269)
- Use of nerve blocks or alternative routes of administration, such as epidural (📖 p. 282)
- Use of anticancer therapies to reduce tumour burden p. 279.

Table 6a.6 Common management strategies for various opioid-related side-effects

Opioid-related nausea and vomiting	Although these symptoms are commonly present during initiation of opioid therapy, they are frequently self-limiting and usually require only a short course of anti-emetic therapy.
	If symptoms persist, metoclopramide 10-20mg p.o. t.d.s. is generally used as first-line anti-emetic. Haloperidol 1.5–3mg o.n. initially is also useful.
Opioid-related constipation	**Prescription of regular, prophylactic laxatives is recommended.**
	Studies comparing laxatives, especially in palliative care patients, are lacking. Various laxatives have been investigated, but findings remain inconclusive and choice of laxative is often dependent on local practice. A combination of a stimulant laxative (senna) and a stool softener (docusate) may be used.
	Methylnaltrexone has been developed specifically for opioid-induced constipation, see p. 319
	If problem persists, laxatives should be titrated upwards, and enemas may be used. The addition of metoclopramide for its pro-kinetic effects may be beneficial.
	If problem is severe, consider prescription of alternative opioid. Fentanyl and buprenorphine may be less constipating.
	Consider non-pharmacological approaches, such as fluid intake, dietary fibre and mobilization. However, in the palliative care population these options may not be appropriate.
Opioid-related drowsiness	This symptom is commonly present in the first days of opioid therapy, and is usually self-limiting. Patients should be advised to expect some sedation during the first days of treatment, and not to drive.
	If persistent, consider treatment of contributing factors: • Sleep hygiene • Review of other centrally acting drugs e.g. benzodiazepines • Correction of metabolic disturbances (e.g. hypercalcaemia) If pain-free, consider a reduction of opioid dose. If pain present, consider addition of a psychostimulant, e.g. methylphenidate
Opioid-related delirium	Opioid-related delirium is often associated with the combined effect of the opioid with other contributing factors, e.g. infection, electrolyte disturbance, CNS metastases or organ failure. Treat contributory causes where appropriate and possible.
	If pain-free, consider a reduction of opioid dose. If pain is present, consider opioid switch or use of adjuvants.
	Discontinue other centrally acting agents.
	Use neuroleptics, such as haloperidol.
Opioid-related xerostomia	Meticulous mouth care.
	Consider stopping anticholinergic drugs where possible.
	Pilocarpine 2% eye drops by mouth or 5mg by mouth 3 times daily may be of use.

Table 6a.6 Common management strategies for various opioid-related side-effects (*Continued*)

Opioid-related pruritus	More common with spinal than with systemic opioids • Use Alternative opioid • If unsuccessful, treat opioid-induced pruritus with 5-HT$_3$ antagonists such as ondansetron
Opioid-related sweating	Exclude other causes of sweating
	Consider alternative opioid
	Consider use of antimuscarinic drugs
Rarely:	Hyperalgesia and allodynia have been reported with high-dose opioids. The symptoms may be associated with signs of toxicity. Characteristically, the patient reports that an increase in the opioid dose leads to worsening pain. Substitution of an alternative opioid often resolves the symptoms. Alternatively, reduction of dose and the addition of an alternative co-analgesic may be useful.

Opioid toxicity
Opioid toxicity may be precipitated by:
• Excessive increase in opioid dose or inappropriate use of opioids for the management of an opioid-insensitive pain
• Dehydration or renal impairment
• Infection
• Other change in disease status, e.g. hepatic function, weight loss
• Reduction in analgesic requirements because pain is relieved by other methods
• Drug interactions, e.g. the co-administration of amitriptyline increases the bioavailability of morphine

Symptoms and signs of opioid toxicity

• Drowsiness
• Hallucinations (most commonly visual)
• Confusion
• Vomiting
• Myoclonus
• Pinpoint pupils
• Respiratory depression (if severe)

Management
• Treat the underlying cause where appropriate (e.g. correct dehydration)
• Reduce opioid dose
• Prescribe haloperidol for management of delirium
• Prescribe benzodiazepine (e.g. clonazepam, midazolam) for symptomatic management of myoclonus
• Consider switch to alternative opioid if dose reduction fails to resolve toxicity or results in uncontrolled pain

Respiratory depression

Pain acts as a physiological antagonist to the central depressant effect of opioids, and strong opioids, when used appropriately, do not cause respiratory depression in patients with pain. Clinicians should take care to distinguish between true respiratory depression attributable to opioids and the slow and irregular breathing that may accompany the terminal phase.

If respiratory depression does occur, reduction of the opioid dose is usually all that is required immediately. Subcutaneous infusions of opioids should be temporarily stopped to allow plasma levels to decrease, before restarting at a lower dose.

Naloxone is rarely used in palliative care practice and is only indicated if significant respiratory depression is present that is attributable to opioids; acute opioid withdrawal symptoms and pain can be severe in patients who have been on long-term opioids.

Indications for use of naloxone
- Respiratory rate <8 breaths/min, **or**
- <10–12 breaths/min, difficult to rouse and clinically cyanosed, **or**
- <10–12 breaths/min, difficult to rouse and SaO_2 <90% on pulse oximeter

Management
- Stop opioid
- Secure IV access
- Dilute 0.4mg naloxone in 10mL sodium chloride 0.9%
- Give 0.5mL (=20mcg naloxone) every 2min IV until satisfactory respiratory status
- Review renal function, pain and analgesic requirements

NB. Naloxone has a half-life of 5–20min. As the half-life of most opioids is longer than this, it is important to continue to assess the patient and give naloxone at further intervals if necessary

Changing route of administration of opioids

In the palliative care setting the IM route is normally avoided because of issues of painful injections, cachexia and reduced muscle mass. The SC route is often used, and is appropriate for those patients who are unwilling or unable to take oral medications for such reasons as:
- Reduced level of consciousness
- Dysphagia
- Nausea/vomiting
- Tablet burden
- Malabsorption

SC administration is not an alternative to ineffective oral treatment. In such cases, the clinician should reassess the patient, determine the reason for their poor response to therapy, and develop a targeted plan to deal with the problem.

Opioids have different analgesic potencies when administered by different routes. Doses of opioids need to be adjusted, therefore, when their route of administration is altered in order to avoid under- or over-dosing. For example, intrathecal and epidural morphine are approximately 100 and 10 times, respectively, more potent than oral morphine.

The average relative potency ratio of oral morphine to subcutaneous morphine is between 1:2 and 1:3 (i.e. 20–30mg of morphine by mouth is equianalgesic to 10mg by sc injection).[22]

Alternative opioids for moderate to severe pain

A number of alternative strong opioid analgesics are available which have their place in palliative care practice (Table 6a.7):

Table 6a.7 Strong opioids

Morphine and similar drugs	Morphine
	Diamorphine
	Hydromorphone
	Oxycodone
Fentanyl and similar drugs	Fentanyl
	Alfentanil
	Sufentanil
Methadone	Methadone
Mixed agonist–antagonist	Buprenorphine
Not recommended	Pethidine

Indications for prescribing an initial opioid other than morphine

- Patient choice
- Past history of unacceptable adverse effects associated with prior use of morphine
- Patient unwilling or unable to take oral morphine regularly, and wishes to take a less invasive form of opioid than morphine administered via a syringe driver—a transdermal opioid such as fentanyl may be appropriate
- Subacute/partial intestinal obstruction—a less constipating opioid such as fentanyl may be appropriate
- Renal failure

Indications for changing to alternative opioids (opioid switching, rotation or substitution)

- Patients who experience poor analgesia or significant side-effects may benefit from a change in their opioids, called 'opioid switching'. Opioid switching involves discontinuation of the previously used opioid and initiation of the new one at the equianalgesic dose

22 Hanks G.W., et al. (2001) Morphine and alternative opioids in cancer pain: the EAPC recommendations. British Journal of Cancer, **84**: 587–93.

- This approach of opioid switching is based on observations that inter-individual response may vary from opioid to opioid, and that switching to another opioid may lead to better opioid responsiveness with fewer side-effects.[23] Switching between opioids complicates pain management and this is a disadvantage for non-specialists (for whom it is not recommended without expert advice).

Choice of alternative opioid

The decision to use alternative opioids in place of morphine is best made by a palliative care specialist. Rigorous evidence favouring the use of one opioid over another is often lacking, but it is generally accepted that individual opioids have characteristics that may result in clinicians preferentially using a particular opioid in certain clinical situations (Table 6a.8).

A number of factors influence choice of an appropriate opioid:

- Individual patient factors (e.g. preference, compliance, renal and other organ function, co-morbidities, out-patient vs in-patient setting, stable vs uncontrolled pain)
- Drug profile
- Possible/desirable routes of administration
- Comparative analgesic effects
- Comparative adverse effect profile
- Other potential therapeutic effects
- Availability

23 Indelicato R. A., Portenoy R. K. (2002) Opioid rotation in the management of refractory cancer pain. *Journal of Clinical Oncology*, **20**: 348–52.

Table 6a.8 Alternative opioids

Diamorphine	More soluble than morphine, and often used as the opioid in a syringe driver for SC infusion
Fentanyl	Of use in those patients experiencing inadequate pain relief or unacceptable toxicity with another opioid
	Of use in those patients with renal impairment
	Associated with less constipation than other opioids, and so may be used in patients for whom constipation is a refractory problem
	OTFC preparations of use in treatment of incident pain
	Transdermal preparation of use for patients who are unwilling or unable to take oral opioids
Buprenorphine	Of use in those patients experiencing inadequate pain relief or unacceptable toxicity with another opioid
	Transdermal preparation of use for patients who are unwilling or unable to take oral opioids
	Of use in renal impairment
Methadone	Of use in patients with refractory pain that has a neuropathic component
	Of use in renal impairment
	Of use where cost is an economic consideration
Oxycodone	Of use in those patients experiencing inadequate pain relief or unacceptable toxicity with another opioid
Hydromorphone	Of use in those patients experiencing inadequate pain relief or unacceptable toxicity with another opioid
	May be of use in renal impairment

Mechanism of opioid switching

The equianalgesic doses of different opioids drugs are only approximations.
A number of factors can affect their accuracy:

- Individual patient variation (differences in absorption, metabolism, excretion)
- The sequence of opioid switching
- Equianalgesic doses can vary according to the dose of opioid (e.g. at higher doses more conservative estimates of opioid conversion are recommended)
- Some estimations are derived from studies of single doses rather than continued therapy, and may therefore require adjustment in clinical practice

Although guidelines and conversion tables should be consulted, each drug must be titrated against pain and side-effects for each individual patient

Suggested regime for opioid switching

- Calculate the equianalgesic dose of the new drug according to guidelines or tables p. 261–266
- Reduce the calculated dose of the new opioid by about 30% to account for incomplete cross-tolerance and inter-individual variability in potency
- Further adjust the dose, if necessary, according to prior pain control (e.g. smaller reductions may be indicated in patients with uncontrolled pain)
- Reassess and titrate new opioid against pain and side-effects

Other opioids

Diamorphine

Diamorphine is more soluble in water than morphine, and is used as an injectable strong opioid in a syringe driver for subcutaneous infusion.

NB It is unusual to give diamorphine IV in a hospice setting. Subcutaneous administration is most commonly used (onset of action is 10–20 minutes) unless the pain is very severe and immediate relief is needed.

Conversion ratio of oral morphine : parenteral diamorphine is 3mg : 1mg

To convert from oral morphine to SC diamorphine, divide the total dose of oral morphine by **three**, e.g. :

10mg 4h morphine
$\cong$ 60mg oral morphine in 24h
$\cong$ 20mg diamorphine by CSCI over 24h

Diamorphine preparations

Inj.: 5mg, 10mg, 30mg, 100mg, 500mg

Oxycodone

Oxycodone is a strong opioid analgesic similar to morphine.

- May be given by p.o., p.r., SC, IM and IV routes
- It is available in 4-h i/r, and 12-h m/r oral preparations, and is used in a similar way to morphine (**remember** to prescribe a laxative
- It is a useful, alternative opioid in selected patients who develop side-effects with morphine
- Although a recent meta-analysis failed to find any clinically significant difference in adverse effect profile between morphine and oxycodone,[24] inter-individual variation means that some individuals who are intolerant of morphine may benefit from an opioid switch to oxycodone
- Oxycodone is metabolized to noroxycodone, oxymorphone and their glucuronides. However, the analgesic activity and profile of the metabolites is not yet known, and caution is advised when using oxycodone in patients with renal impairment
- Oxycodone is metabolized by CYP2D6, but the extent to which its analgesic effect is dependent upon this system is unclear. There have been reports of reduced analgesic effect when used in combination with CYP2D6 inhibitors

Using oxycodone

The conversion ratio of morphine to oxycodone is approximately 2:1.

If a patient is already on morphine, then the total 24-hour dose of morphine should be divided by **two** for the equivalent 24-hour dose of oxycodone; e.g.: morphine 60mg/24h = morphine m/r 30mg b.d. = oxycodone 30mg/24h = oxycodone m/r 15mg b.d.

Oxycodone preparations

- Caps: i/r 5mg, 10mg, 20mg (OxyNorm)
- Tabs: m/r (12h) 5mg, 10mg, 20mg, 40mg, 80mg (OxyContin)
- Liquid: 5mg/5mL, 10mg/1mL
- Injection: 10mg/1mL, 1mL and 2mL amps

24 Reid C. M., et al. (2006) Oxycodone for cancer-related pain meta-analysis of randomized controlled trials. *Archives of Internal Medicine*, **166**: 837–43.

Hydromorphone

Hydromorphone is a strong opioid analgesic very similar to morphine.

- Hydromorphone can be given by p.o., SC, IM, IV and spinal routes
- It is used in a similar way to morphine (**remember** to prescribe a laxative)
- Similarly to morphine, when administered orally it undergoes an extensive first-pass metabolism, resulting in the production of three major metabolites: hydromorphone-3-glucuronide (H-3-G), dihydromorphine and dihydroisomorphine.
- Hydromorphone and its metabolites are eliminated renally
- It is used widely in North America as an alternative to diamorphine, which is not available. It is available in 4h i/r and 12h m/r preparations, but the injection is not routinely available in the UK

Hydromorphone and morphine generally have the same adverse effects, although there may also be individual variation in adverse effect profile between patients.

Conversion ratios with other opioids

- When converting from oral morphine to oral hydromorphone, the manufacturers recommend a ratio of 7.5:1 (i.e. morphine 10mg hydromorphone 1.3mg)

Hydromorphone preparations

- Caps: 1.3mg, 2.6mg (Palladone)
- Caps: m/r (12h) 2mg, 4mg, 8mg, 16mg, 24mg (Palladone SR)
- Caps may be opened and sprinkled on food
- Inj.: 10mg/1mL, 20mg/1mL, 50mg/1mL
  Injections available in UK as a special order from Martindale. See *BNF* for contact details.

Fentanyl

Fentanyl is a semi-synthetic opioid with a high degree of lipid solubility. It is 75–100 times as potent as morphine

- It can be given by IV, IM, SC, transdermal and spinal routes
- It is metabolized in the liver to mainly inactive metabolites, so it is of use in patients with renal failure
- Although both fentanyl and morphine act at the mu receptor, patients switched from long-term morphine to fentanyl may experience withdrawal symptoms despite good pain relief because fentanyl is a highly selective mu agonist.[25] Symptoms may be treated using rescue doses of immediate release morphine until they resolve after a few days

---

25 Marquardt K. A., Tharratt R. S., Musallam N. A. (1995) Fentanyl remaining in a transdermal system following three days of continuous use. *Annals of Pharmacotherapy*, **29**: 969–71.

- Fentanyl shares the side-effect profile of morphine and other opioids, but may cause less constipation, nausea and vomiting. Nevertheless, laxatives are generally still required.[26] In one large trial, although constipation occurred less frequently with fentanyl than with morphine, it was still the most frequent adverse effect reported with each drug (52% and 65% of adverse events reported, respectively).[28] Local skin erythema or pruritus has been reported with use of transdermal fentanyl (<5%)

Transdermal fentanyl

- The transdermal route is of obvious benefit to patients with dysphagia, vomiting or malabsorption. There are two types of transdermal preparations: gel-reservoir and matrix
- Analgesia is delayed for at least 12 hours after application of the first patch, and steady state may not be achieved for 48h . Transdermal fentanyl has a prolonged duration of action; each patch lasts about 72 hours and plasma concentrations are halved about 17 hours after removal
- As a result, transdermal fentanyl should only be used in those patients with stable opioid requirements
- Up to 25% of patients need a patch change every 48h due to pharmacokinetic variability
- Oral i/r morphine is commonly used as the breakthrough analgesic, though oral transmucosal fentanyl citrate may also be used 📖 p. 253
- Used fentanyl patches should be disposed of safely, as a substantial amount of fentanyl can remain in patches (even after 3 days in situ). In a group of patients studied, 28–84% of fentanyl remained in used patches.[27] Patches should be folded with the sticky sides together, wrapped and disposed of either by returning to the pharmacist, or placing in the rubbish well out of reach of children and others
- Clinicians should be aware that increased body heat (e.g. fever, humid climate) and direct heat (e.g. from an electric blanket or heat pad) may increase the rate of absorption of fentanyl
- Sweating may decrease drug absorption because it prevents the patch from sticking to the skin

> **Transdermal fentanyl should be used only in patients with stable pain. It should not be used for titration in patients with uncontrolled pain.**

26 Clark A. J. et al. (2004) Efficacy and safety of transdermal fentanyl and sustained-release oral morphine in patients with cancer and chronic non-cancer pain. *Current Medical Research and Opinion*, **20**: 1419–28.

27 Ahmedzai S., Brooks D. (1997) Transdermal fentanyl versus sustained-release oral morphine in cancer pain: preference, efficacy, and quality of life. The TTS-Fentanyl Comparative Trial Group. *Journal of Pain and Symptom Management*, **13**: 254–61.

Starting a patch

The starting dose of transdermal fentanyl is calculated on the basis of the oral morphine equivalent dose and individual patient factors. Consult tables and adjust appropriately p. 261.

From i/r opioid: apply patch when convenient and use oral i/r opioid only as required

From twice-daily m/r opioid: apply patch at the same time as the last dose of m/r oral opioid

(From once-daily m/r opioid: apply the patch 12h after the last dose of m/r opioid)

Breakthrough/rescue doses of i/r opioids may be needed whilst transdermal absorption is established.

Dose titration

It takes up to 72 hours for a steady state of fentanyl to be achieved. Titration, in 25mcg/hour steps, if required, should take place no more frequently than every 3 days.

Switching from patch to oral m/r opioid

The dose of oral m/r opioid is calculated by consulting dose conversion tables. The dose should be adjusted appropriately for individual factors. Remove patch and give the first dose of oral m/r opioid approx. 8h later.

Use of transdermal fentanyl in the terminal phase

If a patient appears well pain-controlled the fentanyl patch should be continued as normal, and breakthrough doses given as required.

If the patient has uncontrolled pain and death appears to be imminent, it is often not appropriate to stop the fentanyl patch and switch to an alternative opioid administered via syringe driver (because of the adverse effects associated with the inaccurate estimations of dose equivalencies in the terminal phase). In these circumstances, the fentanyl patch may be continued and supplementary regular analgesia may be given by a second opioid infusion via syringe driver.

Note: Care must be taken to use the **total 24-h dose of opioid** as the basis for calculations of breakthrough doses, i.e. fentanyl + SC opioid

Oral transmucosal fentanyl citrate (OTFC)

Fentanyl is rapidly absorbed through the buccal and nasal mucosa, leading to rapid onset of pain relief. These are available in a number of formulations such as those found on Page 232 (Actiq, Abstral, Effentora and Instanyl). The maximum effect is reached within 20–40 minutes with a duration of action of 1–3h. Bioavailability may be as low as 50%.

Indication

Incident pain

Use

The optimal dose of OTFC cannot be predicted from, and is not directly related to, the daily dose of regular opioid being taken for background pain. Therefore, the effective dose has to be found by titration. There is no conversion ratio between fentanyl lozenges and other opioid formulations (including fentanyl patches).

- The lozenge should be placed in the mouth and sucked, constantly moving it from one cheek to the other
- It should not be chewed
- Water can be used to moisten the mouth beforehand
- The lozenge should be consumed within 15min
- Partially consumed lozenges should be dissolved under hot running water, and the handle disposed out of reach of children

Dose titration

- Initial dose is 200mcg, regardless of the dose of the regular opioid. This dose is probably approx. equivalent to morphine 2mg IV
- A second lozenge of the same strength can be used if pain is not relieved after 15 minutes
- No more than two lozenges should be used to treat any individual pain episode
- Continue with this dose for a further 2 or 3 episodes of breakthrough pain, allowing the second lozenge when necessary
- If pain is still not controlled, increase to the next higher dose lozenge
- Continue to titrate in this manner until a dose is found that provides adequate analgesia with minimum adverse effects
- No more than four doses per day should be used (consider increasing regular strong opioid dose for background pain)

Subcutaneous fentanyl

- Administration of fentanyl by subcutaneous infusion will allow therapeutic blood levels to be achieved more rapidly, and also allows for the use of fentanyl in patients with uncontrolled pain
- Calculate dose as equivalent to transdermal patch, e.g. 25mcg/h = 600mcg/24h; for convenience (and considering the widely variable absorption from a patch) use 500mcg/24h CSCI as equivalent to a 25mcg/h patch
- Large volumes are needed for high doses: consider substituting alfentanil (see Alfentanil)
- Compatible with most commonly used drugs in palliative care

Topical use of fentanyl

Fentanyl has been used topically to manage painful skin ulcers.

Fentanyl preparations

- Patches: 12, 25, 50, 75, 100mcg/h (Durogesic DTrans); starting dose: (25mcg/h) patch every 3 days
- Inj.: 50mcg/1mL, 100mcg/2mL, 500mcg/10mL; starting dose: 500mcg/24h CSCI
- Lozenge with applicator: 200, 400, 600, 800, 1200, 1600mcg (Actiq); starting dose: 200mcg lozenge regardless of regular opioid dose
- Sublingual tablet: 100, 200, 300, 400, 600, 800mcg (Abstral)
- Effervescent buccal tablet: 100, 200, 400, 600, 800mcg (Effentora)
- Nasal spray: 50, 100, 200mcg/dose (Instanyl)

Alfentanil

Alfentanil is a selective mu-receptor opioid agonist, similar to fentanyl. However, it has a more rapid onset of action and a shorter duration of action. It is mainly metabolized in the liver to inactive compounds.

Its short-lasting effect means it has been used for incident pain e.g. dressing changes, but it is generally not used for other types of breakthrough pain.

Alfentanil has been given by CSCI in a syringe driver, appears to mix with most other commonly used drugs in palliative care and should be diluted with water. Compared to fentanyl, an equianalgesic dose can be used in a much smaller volume, making CSCI of large doses possible.

Alfentanil preparations

- Injection: 1mg/2mL, 5mg/10mL, 5mg/1mL
Starting dose: 500mcg/24h CSCI (equivalent to diamorphine 5mg CSCI)

Sufentanil

Sufentanil is a synthetic opioid very similar to fentanyl, but with a more rapid onset and shorter half life. It can be used as an alternative to alfentanil if the fentanyl dose necessitates too large a volume for the portable syringe driver in use. It has also been used sublingually. The clinically derived sufentanil to fentanyl relative potency is approximately 20:1.

Buprenorphine[28]

Buprenorphine is a potent semi-synthetic opioid with mixed agonist/antagonist properties. No ceiling dose has been shown for the analgesic effect of buprenorphine in clinical studies, and so it can be used clinically as though it were an agonist at the mu-opioid receptor. The highest reported dose of transdermal buprenorphine in the literature is 140mcg/h.[29]

28 Johnson R. E., Fudala P. J., Payne R. (2005) Buprenorphine: Considerations for pain management. *Journal of Pain and Symptom Management*, **29**(3): 297–326.

29 Mercadante S., Ferrera P., Villari P. (2007) Is there a ceiling effect of transdermal buprenorphine? Preliminary data in cancer patients. *Supportive Care Cancer*, **15**: 441–4.

- It may be given by the epidural, IM, IV, SC and SL routes, but the transdermal route is most commonly used in palliative care practice
- It is available in two forms of transdermal delivery systems. Both delivery systems contain the active drug incorporated into a polymer matrix, which is also the adhesive layer
- The time to reach steady-state plasma concentrations is approximately 24–48 hours, but additional analgesia may be required for the first 24–48 hours of use
- Buprenorphine concentrations decrease to about one-half in 12 hours following patch removal. It has an apparent half-life of about 26 hours
- Buprenorphine is metabolized in the liver, principally to an inactive metabolite, norbuprenorphine
- It may be used in mild-to-moderate liver failure, and in renal failure (📖 p. 707)
- The adverse effect profile of buprenorphine is similar to that of other strong opioids

Transdermal buprenorphine should be used only in those patients with stable pain. It should not be used for titration in patients with uncontrolled pain.

- The use of buprenorphine in association with other opioids, as for example during opioid switching or for the management of breakthrough pain, has been of concern because of a possible partial agonist effect, which might reduce analgesia or induce withdrawal symptoms. However, recent data suggest that no interference between buprenorphine and other opioid mu-agonists exists within the usual clinical dose ranges[30]
- A study evaluated the safety and effectiveness of IV morphine in patients with advanced cancer who were receiving transdermal buprenorphine (mean transdermal buprenorphine dose of 44.5 mg/hour, mean IV-morphine dose of 6.1 mg). It found that morphine provided a strong and rapid analgesic effect, and interference between the two opioids was not noted[31]

30 Kogel B. *et al.* (2005) Interaction of mu-opioid receptor agonists and antagonists with the analgesic effect of buprenorphine in mice. *European Journal of Pain*, **9**: 599–611.

31 Mercadante S., *et al.* (2006) Safety and effectiveness of intravenous morphine for episodic breakthrough pain in patients receiving transdermal buprenorphine. *Journal of Pain and Symptom Management*, **32** (2): 175–9.

- Buprenorphine may have a wider safety profile with regards to respiratory depression compared to other opioids—because of its partial agonist activity it has a demonstrated ceiling effect on respiratory depression
- However, in the event of respiratory depression occurring, higher doses of naloxone may be required compared with other opioids. The effects of naloxone may be delayed, and it may need to be given in repeated doses because of the long duration of activity of buprenorphine
- It has been suggested that buprenorphine's potential for abuse is limited compared to other opioids—because of the fact that the subjective and physiological effects experienced by patients show a ceiling effect. This is due to its partial agonist activity

Buprenorphine preparations

- Transtec: 35mcg/h, 52.5mcg/h and 70mcg/h patches, which release the drug over a 3-4 day period
- BuTrans: 5mcg/h, 10mcg/h and 20mcg/h patches, which release the drug over a 7-day period
- Tabs (sublingual): 200mcg

Sublingual buprenorphine

- The absorption of buprenorphine from the sublingual mucosa is rapid, occurring within 5 minutes. However, the oral bioavailability of buprenorphine is very low (approximately 10%), and additional swallowing of buprenorphine contributes little to overall absorption
- Sublingual buprenorphine is often not tolerated by patients due to its adverse effects profile, which includes dizziness, nausea, vomiting, drowsiness and lightheadedness
- As a result, alternative oral opioids, such as i/r morphine, are generally used to provide breakthrough pain relief for patients using transdermal buprenorphine

Methadone

Methadone is a synthetic opioid agonist at the mu- and delta-opioid receptors, and is also an NMDA-receptor antagonist. Its NMDA-receptor antagonism has led to the clinical impression that methadone has a particular place in the management of neuropathic pain.

- It may be given by the p.o., p.r., IV and SC routes
- Oral administration is followed by rapid gastrointestinal absorption with measurable plasma levels at 30 minutes.

- It is a basic and lipophilic drug that is subject to considerable tissue distribution and sequestration, and it has a characteristically long half-life in plasma of around 24 hours (range 13–100 hours)[32,33,34,35]
- Tissue accumulation of methadone with chronic administration results in the potential for toxicity. Also, there is considerable inter-individual variation in methadone pharmacokinetics, which means that dose conversion and titration is difficult to predict accurately
- Methadone is extensively metabolized in the liver by the cytochrome P450 CYP3A3/4 isoenzyme to inactive metabolites. It is then excreted mainly by the faecal route, and so does not accumulate in renal failure
- Methadone should only be used in the palliative care setting by specialists experienced in its use. Even among experienced physicians, occasional serious toxicity can occur during the administration of methadone.[37] Contrary to what would be expected, toxicity appears to occur more frequently in patients previously exposed to high doses of opioids than in patients receiving low doses

Side-effects

All the typical opioid side-effects can be expected. Methadone also has an antidiuretic effect.

Drug interactions

Methadone has the potential for numerous and complex drug interactions.[32] Its metabolism is increased by a number of other drugs, and their use in combination with methadone may then precipitate pain flare and opioid withdrawal symptoms. Other interactions that inhibit metabolism can lead to overdose and toxicity (Table 6a.9).

Table 6a.9 Interactions which interfere with methadone metabolism

Decrease methadone levels	Increase methadone levels
Phenytoin	Fluconazole
Phenobarbital	SSRIs
Carbamazepine (not sodium valproate or gabapentin)	
Rifampicin	

32 Davis M.P., Walsh D. (2001) Methadone for relief of cancer pain: a review of pharmacokinetics, pharmacodynamics, drug interactions and protocols of administration. *Supportive care in Cancer*, **9**(2): 73–83.

33 Fainsinger R., Schoeller T., Bruera E. (1993) Methadone in the management of cancer pain: a review. *Pain*, **51**: 137–47.

34 Morley J. S., Makin M. K. (1998) The use of methadone in cancer pain poorly responsive to other opioids. *Pain Reviews*, **5**: 51–8.

35 Ripamonti C., Zecca E., Bruera E. (1997) An update on the clinical use of methadone for cancer pain. *Pain*, **70**: 109–15.

36 Hunt G., Bruera E. (1995) Respiratory depression in a patient receiving oral methadone for cancer pain. *Journal of Pain and Symptom Management*, **10**: 401–4.

Use of methadone

Methadone is rarely used as a first-line analgesic in the UK since it has a long half life and is difficult to titrate safely. Equianalgesic ratios of morphine (and other opioids) to methadone are dose-dependent. In single dose studies these ratios may vary from 1:1 at low doses of an oral opioid to as high as 20:1 for those patients receiving oral morphine in excess of 300mg per day. Opioid rotation to methadone is difficult because of the wide variability of equianalgesic ratios, but there have been several guidelines published.[37] (The appropriate conversion ratios should be used when switching from other strong opioids.)

Switching oral morphine to oral methadone

The switch to methadone is successful (i.e. improved pain relief and/or reduced toxicity) in about 75% of patients.

Method Adapted from Palliative Care Formulary[37]

Stop morphine

If switching from immediate release morphine (e.g. oramorph):
• give the first dose of methadone (after stopping morphine) ≥2h
  (if pain present) or 4h (if pain free) after the last dose of morphine.

If switching from modified release morphine:
• give the first dose of methadone (after stopping morphine) ≥6hours (if pain present) or 12h (if pain free) after the last dose of a 12h preparation (e.g. MST), or ≥12h (if pain present) or 24h (if pain free) after the last dose of a 24h preparation (e.g. MXL).
• give a single loading dose of oral methadone 1/10 of the previous total 24h oral morphine dose, up to a maximum of 30mg.
• give oral methadone (1/3 of the loading dose i.e. 1/30 of the previous total 24h oral morphine dose) every 3 hours if needed, up to a maximum of 30mg per dose.

Example 1: Morphine 300mg/24h p.o. = loading dose of methadone 30mg p.o., with 10mg 3hourly p.r.n.

Example 2: Morphine 1200mg/24h p.o. = loading dose of methadone 120mg p.o., with 40mg 3hourly p.r.n.; however, **both are limited to the maximum of 30mg**.
• on day 6, the amount of methadone taken over the previous 2 days is noted and divided by 4 to give a regular 12hourly dose, with 1/6–1/10 of the 24h dose given every 3h p.r.n.

Example: Methadone 80mg p.o. in previous 48h=Methadone 20mg every 12h and 5mg p.o. every 3h p.r.n.

If ≥2 doses/day of p.r.n. methadone continue to be needed, the dose of regular methadone should be increased once a week, guided by p.r.n. use.

37 Twycross R., Wilcock A. (2007) *Palliative Care Formulary* (3rd edn). palliativedrugs.com

Converting oral opioid (other than morphine) to oral methadone
- Calculate the morphine equivalent daily dose and then follow the guidelines for morphine

Converting from oral methadone to SC methadone
- give ½–¾ of the 24h oral dose subcutaneously over 24h

For patients in severe pain and who need more analgesia in < 3h:
- Give the previously used opioid every hour p.r.n. (50–100% of the p.r.n. dose used before switching). (If neurotoxicity was apparent with the preswitch dose, use an appropriate dose of an alternative strong opioid)
- If there has been a rapid escalation of the preswitch opioid dose, calculate the dose of methadone using the pre-escalation dose of the opioid. If a patient becomes over-sedated, reduce the dose generally by 33–50% (some centres monitor the level of consciousness and respirations every 4h for 24h). If a patient develops opioid abstinence symptoms, give p.r.n. doses of the previous opioid until symptoms settle.

Subcutaneous methadone
Although SC methadone has been used, there may be problems with skin reactions, partly because methadone in solution is acidic. If it is necessary to use SC methadone, dilute it as much as possible.

Switching other opioids CSCI to methadone CSCI
Direct CSCI switching between other opioids and methadone is not recommended.

Methadone preparations
- Mixtures: 1mg/1mL, 10mg/1mL
- Tabs: 5mg
- Linctus: 2mg/5mL (for cough)
- Injection 25mg/1mL, 50mg/1mL

Pethidine
Pethidine is a synthetic opioid and has similar agonist effects to morphine. However, it has a short duration of action, and, when given regularly, active metabolites accumulate and can cause convulsions. Although accumulation of metabolites is more likely in patients with renal disease, toxicity has been observed in patients with normal renal function and, as a result, its use is contraindicated in the management of chronic cancer pain.

Topical opioids
Although opioid receptors are not evident in normal tissue, they are found in inflamed tissue. As a result, there has been some interest in the efficacy of topical opioids for the management of ulcers and pressure sores. The use of topical opioids is associated with the potential advantage of a reduction or avoidance of the adverse effect profile associated with the use of systemic opioids.

Most studies describing the topical effects of morphine have mixed the opioid in Intrasite gel, although there are anecdotal reports, in which morphine (or diamorphine) has been mixed with flamazine or metronidazole gel.

A randomized, double-blind, placebo-controlled, crossover pilot study reported an analgesic effect when morphine was applied topically to painful ulcers.[38] However, patient numbers were small and, therefore, the data should be interpreted with caution. Treatment was generally well tolerated by patients, and although local reactions were described during the study, these were mild and possibly not related to morphine. No systemic adverse effects were reported.

Equivalent opioid doses
The following tables show the *approximately* equivalent oral, transdermal and subcutaneous opioid doses.

38 Zeppetella G., Paul J., Ribeiro M. (2003) Analgesic efficacy of morphine applied topically to painful ulcers. *Journal of Pain and Symptom Management*, **25**: 555–8.

Opioid Equivalence for Transdermal Patches – Adult Use

Transdermal patches are not suitable for patients who require rapid titration of strong opioid medication for severe pain and should be restricted to those diagnosed with stable pain.

Dose Equivalence for Transdermal Fentanyl (Durogesic®DTrans®) and Oral Morphine

24 hourly Oral Morphine Dose (mg)	Fentanyl Patch Strength (mcg/hr)	4 Hourly Oral Morphine (mg) (also breakthrough medication dose)
<90	25	<15
90–134	37	15–20
135–189	50	25–30
190–224	62	35
225–314	75	40–50
315–404	100	55–65
405–494	125	70–80
495–584	150	85–95
585–674	175	100–110
675–764	200	115–125
765–854	225	130–140
855–944	250	145–155
945–1034	275	160–170
1035–1124	300	175–185

Please note conversion factors may change depending on direction of conversion
NOTE: Transdermal Fentanyl Patch has 72 hour duration of action i.e. changed every 3 days

Transtec Patch® (Buprenorphine) Conversion Guide

Buprenorphine Matrix Patch/Patches micrograms/hr	24 hr Oral Morphine Dose (mg)
35	50–97
52.5	76–145
70	101–193

NOTE: Transtec Patch is replaced every 3–4 days

Table 6a.10 BuTrans Patch® (Buprenorphine) Conversion Guide

	5 micrograms/hr	10 micrograms/hr	20 micrograms/hr
Oral Tramadol	≤ 50mg/day	50-100mg/day	100–150mg/day
Oral Codeine	~30–60mg/day	~60–120mg/day	~120–180mg/day
Oral Dihydrocodeine	~60mg/day	~60–120mg/day	~120–180mg/day

NOTE: Butrans Patch is replaced every 7 days

Approximate Equivalent Doses of Opioid Analgesics for Adults

Caution should be used when converting opioids in opposite directions as potency ratios may be different

Conversion factors for guidance when converting from one opioid to another
Oral Morphine to Subcutaneous (SC) Diamorphine – Divide by 3 Eg 30 mg Oral Morphine = 10 mg SC Diamorphine
Oral Morphine to Oral Oxycodone – Divide by 2 Eg 30 mg Oral Morphine = 15 mg Oral Oxycodone
Oral Morphine to Subcutaneous Morphine – Divide by 2 Eg 30 mg Oral Morphine = 15 mg SC Morphine
Oral Morphine to Oral Hydromorphone – Divide by 7.5 Eg 30 mg Oral Morphine = 4 mg Oral Hydromorphone
Oral Oxycodone to SC Oxycodone – Divide by 2 (Suggested safe practice) Eg 10 mg Oral Oxycodone = 5 mg SC Oxycodone
Oral Hydromorphone to SC Hydromorphone – Divide by 2 Eg 4 mg Oral Hydromorphone = 2 mg SC Hydromorphone
SC Diamorphine to SC Oxycodone – Treat as equivalent up to doses of 60 mg/24 hrs Caution should be used when converting higher doses (Suggested safe practice) Eg 10 mg SC Diamorphine = 10 mg SC Oxycodone
SC Diamorphine to SC Alfentanil – Divide by 10 Eg 10 mg SC Diamorphine = 1 mg SC Alfentanil
SC Diamorphine to SC Morphine – ratio is between 1:1.5 and 1:2 – Multiply by 1.5 Eg 10 mg SC Diamorphine = 15 mg SC Morphine
Oral Tramadol to Oral Morphine– Divide by 10 (Suggested safe practice)* Eg 100 mg Oral Tramadol = 10 mg Oral Morphine
Oral Codeine / Dihydrocodeine to Oral Morphine – Divide by 10 Eg 240 mg Oral Codeine / Dihydrocodeine = 24 mg Oral Morphine

*Limited evidence suggests that, when converting from Oral Tramadol to Oral Morphine, the dose should be divided by 5. However this may result in too high a dose for some patients hence locally agreed suggested safe practice is to divide by 10 and ensure appropriate breakthrough dose is available.

Table 6a.11 Equivalent oral opioid doses for steps two and three of the analgesic ladder

Opioid	Oral medication		
	Step 2: mild-to-moderate pain	Step 3: moderate-to-severe pain	
Codeine	30–60mg q.d.s.	Not applicable	
Morphine i/r	2.5–5mg 4h	10mg 4h	20mg 4h	30mg 4h	40mg 4h	60mg 4h
Morphine m/r	5–15mg 4h	30mg b.d.	60mg b.d.	90mg b.d.	120mg b.d.	180mg b.d.
Oxycodone i/r	1.5–3mg 4–6h	5mg 4h	10mg 4h	15mg 4h	20mg 4h	30mg 4h
Oxycodone m/r	5mg b.d.	10–20mg b.d.	30mg b.d.	40–50mg b.d.	60mg b.d.	90mg b.d.
Hydromorphone i/r	Not applicable	1.3mg 4h	2.6mg 4h	3.9mg 4h	5.2mg 4h	6.5mg 4h
Hydromorphone m/r	Not applicable	4mg b.d.	8mg b.d.	12mg b.d.	16mg b.d.	20mg b.d.
Tramadol i/r	Not applicable	50mg 4h	Not applicable			
Tramadol m/r	50mg b.d.	100–150mg b.d.	Not applicable			
Approximate 24h oral morphine	**10–30mg**	**60mg**	**120mg**	**180mg**	**240mg**	**360mg**

In all opioid conversions there is uncertainty. It is safer to err on the side of underestimating analgesic requirements when converting between opioids but ensure that the patient has ready access to appropriate breakthrough analgesia. If in doubt about a conversion seek specialist advice if you are unfamiliar with the particular opioid.

Table 6a.12 Equivalent subcutaneous opioid doses for steps two and three of the analgesic ladder

Opioid	Subcutaneous medication				
	Step 2: mild-to-moderate pain		Step 3: moderate-to-severe pain		
Alfentanil CSCI (24h)	1mg 24h	2mg 24h	4mg 24h	6mg 24h	8mg 24h	12mg 24h
Diamorphine SC (4h p.r.n.)	2.5mg 4h	2.5–5mg 4h	5–7.5mg 4h	10mg 4h	15mg 4h	20mg 4h
Diamorphine CSCI (24h)	10mg 24h	20mg 24h	40mg 24h	60mg 24h	80mg 24h	120mg 24h
Morphine SC (4h p.r.n.)	2.5–5mg 4h	5mg 4h	10mg 4h	15mg 4h	20mg 4h	30mg 4h
Morphine CSCI (24h)	15mg 24h	30mg 24h	60mg 24h	90mg 24h	120mg 24h	180mg 24h
Oxycodone SC (4h p.r.n.)	2.5mg 4h	2.5mg 4h	5mg 4h	7.5mg 4h	10mg 4h	15mg 4h
*Oxycodone CSCI (24h)	7.5mg 24h	15mg 24h	30mg 24h	50mg 24h	60mg 24h	90mg 24h
Approximate 24 h oral morphine	**30mg**	**60mg**	**120mg**	**180mg**	**240mg**	**360mg**

Nb. In all opioid conversions there is uncertainty. It is safer to err on the side of underestimating analgesic requirement when converting between opioids but ensure that the patient has ready access to appropriate breakthrough analgesia. If in doubt about a conversion always seek specialist advice if you are unfamiliar with the particular opioid.

* The manufacturer of oxycodone states clearly that the conversion factor between oxycodone sc and diamorphine sc is 1:1. While most clinicians are comfortable with this ratio when converting from oxycodone sc to diamorphine sc, when converting from diamorphine sc to oxycodone sc some would advocate a 2:1 ratio with provision for breakthrough medication. As in every dose conversion the clinician must assess each individual patient and clinical situation.

Intravenous use for pain emergencies

Pain is a more terrible lord of mankind than even death itself.
Albert Schweitzer (1875–1965)

Various protocols have been described:
- Monitor respiratory rate and conscious level regularly
- Draw up morphine diluted to 10mL with water
- If opioid naive dilute 5mg of morphine in 10mL of water
- If patient is on regular opioid use equivalent 4h dose based on previous opioid use in last 24h (📖 see 'Breakthrough doses', p. 232) diluted in 10mL water
- Give appropriate morphine dilution IV at 1mL/minute (total over 10 minutes)
- Stop if pain <5/10 or toxicity develops
- Repeat the above after a further 10–20 minutes if required
- Calculate the total dose of morphine administered and multiply by 6
- Start maintenance infusion with CSCI, or give regular oral morphine equivalent dose over 24h

'Opioid-resistant' cancer pain

Pseudo-resistant?
- Underdosing
- Poor alimentary absorption of opioid (rare, except where there is an ileostomy)
- Poor alimentary intake because of vomiting
- Ignoring psychological aspects of patient care

Semi-resistant?
- Bone pain
- Raised intracranial pressure
- Neuropathic pain

Resistant?
- Muscle spasm
- Abdominal cramps
- Spiritual pain (📖 Chapter 9)

Patients who have chronic unremitting pain from a deteriorating condition are particularly at risk of spiritual pain. Referral for psychological/spiritual support is important, and/or that of a complementary therapist.

Using Hay's seven-model assessment,[39] (spiritual pain) is broken down into:
- Spiritual suffering—interpersonal or intra-psychic anguish
- Inner resource deficiency—diminished spiritual capacity
- Belief system problem—lack or loss of personal meaning system
- Religious request—a specifically expressed religious need

39 Hay M.W. (1989) Principles in building spiritual assessment tools. *The American Journal of Hospice Cafe* **6**(5): 25–31.

ALWAYS REVIEW PATIENT REGULARLY AFTER ANY OPIOID SWITCH AS CONVERSION RATIOS ARE APPROXIMATE AND CONSIDERABLE INTER-PATIENT VARIATION MAY OCCUR.

- When changing from one opioid to another because of toxicity, dose reduction of 30-50% may be necessary.
- Use caution in the elderly and in patients with renal or significant hepatic impairment. Consider reduced doses. In severe renal impairment or dialysis patients, alfentanil may be the preferred opioid. Contact the Palliative Care Team for advice.
- Breakthrough doses for each opioid are calculated as approximately $\frac{1}{6}^{th}$ daily dose (ie 4 hourly dose) but lower doses may be used if effective. eg For a patient on Oral Morphine 60 mg over 24 hours, breakthrough dose is 10 mg orally but a lower dose may be effective in some patients.
- When converting opioids at higher doses, caution should be used. Lower doses (30-50% reduction) may be necessary due to incomplete cross tolerance.
- For further advice contact Palliative Care Team

Neuropathic pain

The medical treatment of neuropathic pain is unsatisfactory, and pain can prove difficult to control in a significant number of patients with this condition.

The early trials of analgesics for neuropathic pain considered neuropathic pain as a uniform entity, but more recent trials have assessed various pain syndromes. It has emerged from this data that analgesics may vary in efficacy according to the type of pain syndrome. Most of the trials on neuropathic pain have studied patients who have post-herpetic neuralgia and painful polyneuropathy. Fewer trials have looked at neuropathic pain due to cancer infiltration, and, as a result, much of the data on the efficacy of different drugs is extrapolated from data collected from patients with non-malignant pain.

The NNT (*number* of patients *needed to treat* to obtain one responder to the active drug) is commonly used as an indication of the overall efficacy of individual drugs. It is a relatively crude measure however, as it can be hampered by methodological variability across RCTs and a lack of consideration for other important outcomes (e.g. quality of life).

Table 6a.13 lists the NNT of analgesics on the basis of data listed in the European Federation of Neurological Societies (EFNS) guidelines. The data was taken from class I/II studies on painful polyneuropathy with 95% confidence intervals (CI). Unless otherwise specified, the NNT used was for 50% pain relief.

Table 6a.13 Efficacy of drugs for painful polyneuropathy (NNT)[40]

Drug	NNT
Amitriptyline, clomipramine, imipramine (TCA—balanced monoamine uptake)	2.1 (CI 1.8–2.6)[*]
Desipramine (TCA—mainly noradrenaline reuptake inhibition)	2.5 (CI 1.9–3.6)[*]
Venlafaxine (SNRI)	4.6 (CI 2.9–10.6)
Duloxetine (SNRI)	5.2 (CI 3.7–8.5)
Oxcarbazepine (antiepileptic)[†]	5.9 (CI 3.2–42.2)
Lamotrigine (antiepileptic)[†]	4.0 (CI 2.1–42)
Gabapentin (antiepileptic)[†]	3.9 (CI 3.2–5.1)
Oxycodone (opioid)	2.6 (CI 1.9–4.1)
Tramadol	3.4 (CI 2.3–6.4)

[*]Most of the data stems from relatively small crossover trials, which may overestimate efficacy
[†]Data from patients with painful diabetic polyneuropathy
Abbreviations: NNT, number needed to treat; TCA, tricyclic antidepressant; SNRI, serotonin and noradrenaline reuptake inhibitor; CI, confidence interval

40 Attal N., *et al.* (2006) EFNS guidelines on pharmacological treatment of neuropathic pain. *European Journal of Neurology*, **13**: 1153–69.

Recommendations for first- and second-line treatments for neuropathic pain in patients with cancer

Painful polyneuropathy (except HIV-associated)
First-line: TCAs, gabapentin, pregabalin, opioids and tramadol
(Use of *amitriptyline and nortriptyline is limited by their adverse effect profiles*)

Second-line: duloxetine and venlafaxine
Venlafaxine lacks the sedative and antimuscarinic effects of the TCAs, but should not be used if there is a high risk of cardiac arrhythmias

Post-herpetic neuralgia
First-line: TCAs, gabapentin, pregabalin, opioids and tramadol
(Topical lidocaine may also be considered as a first-line drug in elderly patients with allodynia and small areas of pain)

Second-line: capsaicin, valproate

Trigeminal neuralgia
First-line: oxcarbazepine, carbamazepine

Central pain
First-line (spinal cord injury): gabapentin, pregabalin and opioids
First-line (post-stroke pain): amitriptyline

Second-line: Lamotrigine

Pharmacological management of neuropathic pain

Antidepressant drugs[41,42]

The mechanism of action of antidepressant drugs in the management of neuropathic pain is unclear. Analgesia is often achieved at a lower dosage and faster (usually within a few days) than the onset of any antidepressant effect (which can take up to six weeks). The pain-relieving properties of antidepressants are independent of any effect on mood.

Two main groups of antidepressants are commonly used:
- The older tricyclic antidepressants (TCAs)
- The newer selective serotonin-reuptake inhibitors (SSRIs) and serotonin–noradrenaline reuptake inhibitors (SNRIs)

Tricyclic antidepressants (TCAs)

TCAs are often listed as first-line drugs for the treatment of neuropathic pain. In terms of NNT, they appear to have a similar efficacy regardless of the underlying condition: diabetes mellitus, post-herpetic neuralgia, traumatic nerve injury or stroke.

TCAs may be subdivided into two categories based on their chemical structure—tertiary and secondary amines:
- The **secondary amines** (e.g. **desipramine** and **nortriptyline)** appear to be as effective as the **tertiary agents** (e.g. **imipramine** and **amitriptyline)** as analgesics in the treatment of neuropathic pain, but they produce markedly fewer adverse effects (Table 6a.14)
- Adverse effects from TCAs can be significant, and may lead to up to 20% of patients withdrawing from treatment. TCAs are contraindicated in those patients with glaucoma and taking MAOIs
- Amitriptyline can increase the bioavailability of morphine, thus leading to toxicity

Table 6a.14 Amitriptyline—adverse effects

Anticholinergic effects	Dry mouth, constipation, blurred vision, urinary retention, dizziness, tachycardia, memory impairment, delirium
Alpha-1-adrenergic effects	Orthostatic hypotension/syncope
Cardiac conduction delays/ heart block	Arrhythmias, Q–T prolongation
Other side-effects	Sedation, weight gain, excessive perspiration, sexual dysfunction

41 McQuay H. J., *et al.* (1996) A systematic review of antidepressants in neuropathic pain. *Pain*, **68**: 217–27.

42 Saarto T., Wiffen P. J. *Antidepressants for Neuropathic Pain* Cochrane Database of Systematic Reviews 2007, Issue 4.

Amitriptyline preparations

- Tabs: 10mg, 25mg, 50mg
- Syrup: 25mg/5mL, 50mg/5mL

Suggested treatment schedule

- Start with amitriptyline 10–25mg nocte
- Slowly titrate, as tolerated
- Some patients do not see a benefit until after 4–6 weeks of treatment, and effective dosages are highly variable, but the average dosage is 75mg/day
  - severity of pain and the patient's prognosis will dictate how long to persevere with antidepressants
  - many patients do not tolerate amitriptyline especially in higher doses, therefore consider changing to a secondary amine

Selective serotonin reuptake inhibitors (SSRIs) and serotonin–noradrenaline reuptake inhibitors (SNRIs)
SSRIs and SNRIs are two newer classes of antidepressants that act by selectively inhibiting the presynaptic reuptake of serotonin and noradrenaline.

SNRIs (e.g. duloxetine and venlafaxine) have the advantage that they are generally safer to use than TCAs.

The most common adverse effects associated with SNRIs are nausea, dizziness, drowsiness, constipation, increased sweating and dry mouth.

Duloxetine is contraindicated in patients with glaucoma and those taking MAOIs.

SSRIs (e.g. citalopram and paroxetine) are believed to be less efficacious in the treatment of neuropathic pain. Generally, they are not regarded as first or second-line agents.

Anticonvulsant drugs
As with epilepsy, neuronal hyperexcitability is thought to be of importance in the pathogenesis of neuropathic pain. Anticonvulsants act through a variety of mechanisms to depress synaptic transmission, elevate the threshold for the repetitive firing of nociceptive neurones and reduce discharges from the dorsal root ganglion cells.
Duloxetine does not cause cardiac conduction abnormalities whereas venlafaxine should not be used in established heart disease with a risk of ventricular arrhythmias.

Gabapentin/pregabalin:

- Gabapentin is associated with diarrhoea and pregabalin with constipation
- Gabapentin and pregabalin bind to voltage-gated calcium channels in the dorsal horn, resulting in a decrease in the release of excitatory neurotransmitters such as glutamate and substance P
- Pregabalin is an analogue of gabapentin; it has the same mechanism of action but with a higher affinity for the presynaptic calcium channel
- Both drugs have a similar adverse effects profile, which includes dizziness, drowsiness, peripheral oedema and dry mouth
- Gabapentin should be titrated slowly according to individual tolerance, and is administered t.i.d.
- Pregabalin has a short onset of action, and is administered b.d.
- Doses should be adjusted in patients with renal impairment

Carbamazepine is associated with frequent and severe adverse reactions, including sedation, dizziness, gait abnormalities, hyponatraemia, hepatitis and aplastic anaemia. Oxcarbazepine shows little risk for crossed cutaneous allergy. Slow dose titration is recommended.

Lamotrigine is generally well tolerated and has shown efficacy in the treatment of diabetic peripheral polyneuropathy. Adverse effects include dizziness, nausea, headache and fatigue. It may induce potentially severe allergic skin reactions. Slow dose titration is recommended.

Sodium valproate, has been used for many years as an anticonvulsant. RCTs have only recently been carried out with this drug in the study of peripheral neuropathic pain; results are conflicting and firm conclusions as to the place of valproate in the management of neuropathic pain are lacking.

Gabapentin

- Caps: 100mg, 300mg, 400mg
- Tabs: 600mg, 800mg

Starting dose: Day 1, 300mg nocte; day 2, 300mg b.d.; day 3, 300mg t.d.s. p.o.

Usual maintenance dose: 0.9–1.2g/24h. Maximum recommended dose 1.8g/24h, but doses up to 2.4g/24h (and even higher) have been used

Sodium valproate

- Tabs: 200mg, 500mg
- Syrup: 200mg/5mL
- Suppositories: available as special orders

Starting dose: 200mg t.d.s. p.o. **or** 500mg nocte p.o.; increase 200mg/day at 3-day intervals

Usual maintenance dose: 1–2g/24h. Max. 2.5g/24h in divided doses

Carbamazepine

- Tabs:100mg, 200mg, 400mg
- Liquid: 100mg/5mL
- Supps: 125mg, 250mg

Starting dose: 100mg b.d. p.o.; increase from initial dose by increments of 200mg every week.

Usual maintenance dose: 0.8–1.2g/24h in two divided doses. Max. 1.6 –2g/24h

Equivalent rectal dosage: 125mg $\cong$ 100mg p.o.

Carbamazepine levels are increased (hence risk of toxicity) by dextro-propoxyphene (co-proxamol), clarithromycin, erythromycin, fluoxetine, fluvoxamine

Pregabalin

- Caps: 25mg, 50mg, 75mg, 100mg, 150mg, 200mg, 300mg

Starting dose: 75mg b.d. (but some clinicians recommend lower starting doses); increase after 3 days to 150mg b.d.; increase after seven days to 300mg b.d.

Opioid analgesics

Opioid agonists may relieve neuropathic pain by binding to the mu-opioid receptors in the CNS and thus dampening neuronal excitability. In addition, opioids may be helpful because many patients with cancer who are experiencing neuropathic pain have a nociceptive component to their pain.

If the pain seems to be resistant to first-line opioid (or opioid toxicity is a problem):

• An alternative opioid analgesic may be tried for better effect
• Medication can be given to counteract side-effects (e.g. psychostimulants for drowsiness)
• The pain may be morphine-resistant

Methadone may be considered to be different from the other opioids with respect to neuropathic pain. It can either be tried as an alternative to a first-line opioid, or introduced later, when other options have failed (📖 see Methadone, p. 258).

The combination of morphine and gabapentin has been shown to be of use in the management of post-herpetic neuralgia. The study demonstrated synergistic effects, with better analgesia at lower doses of each drug than either given as a single agent.[43]

Topical Analgesics (lignocaine)

Topical agents work locally, directly at the site of application, with minimal systemic effects. Lidocaine like other local anaesthetics, seems to act through the inhibition of voltage-gated sodium channels.

Lidocaine patches appear to be safe with very low systemic absorption and only local adverse effects (mild skin reactions). Up to four patches a day for a maximum of 12 hours may be used to cover the painful area. Titration is not necessary.

Capsaicin cream

Capsaicin is thought to elevate the pain threshold by reducing the amount of substance P available to act as a neurotransmitter. The application of the cream can itself cause stinging, which can be relieved by the use of Emla cream applied prior to the capsaicin. Capsaicin is a derivative of chilli pepper and must be applied with glove; it is given 3–4 times a day. Although the pain may increase to start with, perseverance may provide relief.

Capsaicin

• Cream: 0.075% 45g (Axsain)

Starting dose: apply topically 3–4 times daily

---

43 Gilron I., *et al.* (2005) Morphine, gabapentin or their combination for neuropathic pain. *New England Journal of Medicine*, **352**: 1324–34.

Other medications used in the management of neuropathic pain

N-methyl-*D*-aspartate (NMDA) receptors

The NMDA receptor is thought to be involved in the development of the 'wind-up' phenomenon of neuropathic pain.

NMDA receptors are widely spread throughout the CNS, particularly in the spinal cord. Stimulation of pain fibres in the periphery cause the release of excitatory amino acids such as glutamate and aspartate, which in turn activate the NMDA receptor complex. A phenomenon known as 'wind-up' then occurs producing a magnified pain response which, clinically, is associated with the features of neuropathic pain such as allodynia (pain produced by a stimulus that is not normally painful, e.g. light touch) and hyperalgesia (an exaggerated and prolonged pain response to a mildly painful stimulus).

Ketamine and methadone are NMDA antagonists, and this may explain their efficacy in the management of neuropathic pain.

Ketamine

Ketamine is a dissociative anaesthetic which has strong analgesic properties. Its analgesic effect may be partly due to NMDA receptor blockade, i.e. receptor antagonism. Clinical reports indicate that, when added to opioids, low subanaesthetic ketamine doses may give improved analgesia with tolerable adverse effects. However, evidence for the effectiveness of this practice is limited, and insufficient data is available to state definitively that ketamine improves the effectiveness of opioid treatment in cancer pain.[44] High-quality RCTs comprising greater numbers of patients and standardized, clinically relevant routes of ketamine administration, are needed.

- The use of ketamine has been restricted by its adverse effects profile, which includes sedation, nausea, disagreeable psychological disturbances and hallucinations
- It has been used by p.o., SC, IV, epidural and intrathecal routes, and in a very wide range of doses
- Drugs that interact with CYP34A have the potential to affect ketamine metabolism (e.g. azole antifungals, macrolide antibacterials, HIV protease inhibitors and ciclosporin)
- Clinicians with limited experience in using ketamine should seek expert consultation to develop an appropriate treatment plan

44 Gilron I., *et al.* (2005) Morphine, gabapentin or their combination for neuropathic pain. *New England Journal of Medicine*, **352**: 1324–34.

Oral versus parenteral doses

There are no studies comparing various titration or dosing schedules, or routes of administration. Ketamine is effective orally, but it is difficult to assess the potency ratio in view of the wide dose ranges used. Ketamine undergoes first-pass hepatic metabolism to an active metabolite, and one study suggests it may be more potent given orally than parenterally. In general, equivalent daily doses should initially be used when changing route.

Ketamine

Oral route

* Start ketamine 10mg t.d.s–q.d.s. p.o. and p.r.n.
* Increase by 10mg increments once or twice daily. Maximum reported dose 200mg q.d.s.[45,46]

Parenteral route

* Ketamine 10mg SC stat. may be given if indicated for severe pain
* Start infusion of ketamine 50–100mg/24h CSCI (1–2.5mg/kg per 24h)
* Increase ketamine dose by 50–100mg increments as indicated to maximum 500mg/24h CSCI

The use of short-term 'burst therapy' has also been reported:[47]

* Starting dose 100mg/24h
* Increase after 24h to 300mg/24h if 100mg/24h ineffective
* Increase after further 24h to 500mg/24h if 300mg/24h ineffective
* Stop 3 days after last dose escalation

Haloperidol or midazolam may be concurrently prescribed(either orally or parenterally) if the patient experiences dysphoria or hallucinations. Some palliative care practitioners recommend that patients at high risk of experiencing these adverse effects be given these medications prophylactically.

45 Clark J. L., Kalan G. E. (1995) Effective treatment of severe cancer pain of the head using low dose ketamine in an opioid-tolerant patient. *Journal of Pain and Symptom Management*, **10**: 310–14.

46 Vielvoye-Kerkmeer A.P., van der Weide M., Mattern C. (2000) Re: Clinical experience with oral ketamine. *Journal of Pain and Symptom Management*, **19**: 3–4.

47 Jackson K., et al. (2001) 'Burst' ketamine for refractory cancer pain: an open-label audit of 30 patients. *Journal of Pain and Symptom Management*, **22**: 834–42.

Corticosteroids

Although corticosteroids are commonly used to treat neuropathic pain, RCTs have not been used to evaluate their effectiveness. They may act by reducing inflammatory sensitization of nerves, or by reducing the pressure effects of oedema.

Dexamethasone has the least mineralocorticoid effect, and can be used once a day because of its long duration of effect.

A high initial dose may be used to achieve rapid results (dexamethasone 8mg/day will work in 1–3 days); the dose should then be rapidly reduced to the minimum that maintains benefit.

Long-term corticosteroids may be best avoided, although they can sometimes buy useful time whilst allowing other methods (e.g. radiotherapy or antidepressants) time to work (Table 6a.15):

- Hydrocortisone has a high mineralocorticoid effect
- Dexamethasone has a relatively high equivalent corticosteroid dose per tablet and less mineralocorticoid effects than either prednisolone or methylprednisolone, with consequently less problems with fluid retention
- Prednisolone causes less proximal myopathy than dexamethasone.[48]
  If steroids are not helpful for pain within five days, consider stopping them

Table 6a.15 Relative anti-inflammatory steroid doses (approximate)

Steroid	Administration	Equivalent dose (mg)
Dexamethasone	oral/SC	2
Prednisolone	oral/rectal	15
Hydrocortisone	oral/IM/IV	60
Methylprednisolone	oral/IM/IV	12

48 Kingdon R.T., Stanley K.J., Kizior R.J. (1998) *Handbook for Pain Management.* London: Saunders.

Non-pharmacological management of neuropathic pain

- Anaesthetic procedures:
  - spinal (epidural and intrathecal)
  - nerve blocks
  - cordotomy
- Disease-modifying therapy e.g. RT CT
- TENS
- Acupuncture

Management of specific problems

Malignant bone pain

Cancer commonly metastasizes to bone. Although some bone metastases are painless, many frequently cause significant and debilitating pain. The management of patients with metastatic bone pain involves a multidisciplinary approach, and includes analgesia, radiotherapy, surgery, chemotherapy, hormone treatment, radioisotopes and bisphosphonates. Analgesia is generally the first option in most patients. Radiotherapy or surgery can be used for localized metastatic disease, and hemibody radiotherapy may be suitable for patients with disease extending to one region of the body. In patients with widespread painful bone involvement, the use of radioisotopes presents another treatment option.

Radiotherapy[49]

- Radiotherapy has been shown to be effective in decreasing metastatic bone pain and in causing tumour shrinkage or growth inhibition
- Up to 60% of patients will have some pain relief and about one-third of them will have complete pain relief following radiotherapy
- A 'pain flare' is described in around 5% of patients, with the pain worsening in the first few days after treatment before it then settles
- There is no difference in the efficacy between single-fraction radiotherapy and multifraction radiotherapy. However, the re-treatment rate and pathological fracture rate are higher after single-dose radiotherapy

Bisphosphonates[50,51]

- Bisphosphonates form part of the standard therapy for hypercalcaemia and for the prevention of skeletal events in some cancers. There is evidence to support the effectiveness of bisphosphonates in providing some pain relief for bone metastases
- There is insufficient evidence to recommend bisphosphonates for immediate effect as first-line therapy, to define the most effective bisphosphonates or their relative effectiveness for different primary neoplasms

49 Sze W. M. *et al.* (2003) Palliation of metastatic bone pain: single fraction versus multifraction radiotherapy—a systematic review of randomised trials. *Clinical Oncology*, **15**: 345–52.

50 Wong R., Wiffen P. J. Bisphosphonates for the relief of pain secondary to bone metastases. *Cochrane Database of Systematic Reviews* 2002, Issue 2

51 Ross J. R., *et al.* (2003) Systematic review of role of bisphosphonates on skeletal morbidity in metastatic cancer. *British Medical Journal*, **327**(7413): 469.

- Bisphosphonates should be considered where analgesics and/or radiotherapy are inadequate for the management of painful bone metastases
- Patients may experience a 'flu-like' reaction post-treatment
- Doses may need to be altered in renal impairment
- Analgesic effect should be expected within 14 days. Disodium pamidronate, sodium clodronate and ibandronic acid need to be given every 3–4 weeks, but zoledronic acid has a longer duration of action (4–6 weeks)
- It is unclear for how long bisphosphonates should be continued
- The role of oral bisphosphonates has yet to be clarified in patients with metastatic bone disease

Bisphosphonate preparations and bone pain

Disodium pamidronate
Inj.: 15mg, 30mg, 90mg (dry powder for reconstitution)
Dose: 90mg IV in 500mL sodium chloride 0.9% over 4h.

Sodium clodronate
Inj.: 300mg/5mL, 300mg/10mL
Dose: 1.5g IV in 500mL sodium chloride 0.9% over 4h
p.o. 800mg or 520mg b.d.

Zoledronic acid
Inj.: 4mg
Dose: 4mg IV in 100mL sodium chloride 0.9% over 30mins

Ibandronic acid
Inj.: 6mg
Dose: 6mg IV in 500mL sodium chloride 0.9% over 1–2h.
p.o. 50mg daily

Doses adjusted according to renal fucntion. Calcium and Vitamin D supplements may be needed.

Radionuclides[52]
- Strontium-89 and samarium-153 are radioisotopes that are approved in the USA and Europe for the palliation of pain from metastatic bone cancer. Radioisotopes are effective in providing pain relief with response rates of between 40% and 95%. Pain relief starts 1–4 weeks after the initiation of treatment, continues for up to 18 months and is also associated with a reduction in analgesic use in many patients
- Thrombocytopenia and neutropenia are the most common toxic effects, but they are generally mild and reversible

52 Finlay I. G., Mason M. D., Shelley M. (2005) Radioisotopes for the palliation of metastatic bone cancer: a systematic review. *Lancet Oncology*, **6**: 392–400

- Repeat doses are effective in providing pain relief in many patients
- The development and clinical assessment of radioisotopes has focused mainly on their use in prostate cancer. Data also exists for their use in lung and breast cancer. Tumours with little or no osteoblastic reaction, for example renal carcinoma and myeloma, tend to show poor response to radioisotopes
- External beam hemi-body irradiation is an alternative for multiple-site bone pain

Surgical techniques

- The pain of bone metastases may respond to local infiltration or intra-lesional injection with depot corticosteroid ± local anaesthetic. Consideration should be given to the prophylactic pinning of osteolytic metastases in long bones. Vertebroplasty, in which injection of acrylic cement is administered percutaneously, into unstable fractures of the vertebrae may be worth considering if the patient is relatively well. Spinal or epidural anaesthetic blocks may also be needed

Treatment of other causes of poorly controlled pain (Table 6a.16)

Table 6a.16

Pain	Possible co-analgesics
Headache due to cerebral oedema	Dexamethasone
Painful wounds	Metronidazole
Intestinal colic	Hyoscine butylbromide or hydrobromide
Gastric mucosa	Lansoprazole
Gastric distension	Asilone + domperidone
Skeletal muscle spasm	Baclofen/diazepam
Cardiac pain	Nitrates/nifedipine
Oesphageal spasm	Nitrates/nifedipine

Patients with a history of substance abuse

Patients with a history of substance abuse should not be denied effective analgesia for genuine pain. But management is more complex in these patients because:

- Previous users of opioids can have high opioid tolerance and may need higher doses for effective pain relief
- Concurrent use of alcohol and other CNS depressants can have additive effects and place the patient at risk
- There may be a greater risk of dependence in such patients

Involve pain management or drug and alcohol specialists when possible.

Anaesthetic procedures in palliative care

Introduction

The majority of patients with cancer can have their pain needs met by following the WHO analgesic ladder. For the minority of those patients who do not obtain satisfactory pain relief with the WHO three-step ladder, a 'fourth step' (that is, interventional pain management) can be useful in helping to control pain, maintain psychomotor performance and improve quality of life.[53,54] Patients are usually considered for interventional techniques when:

- Conventional oral or parenteral therapies are proving unsuccessful, or where side-effects are intolerable
- A specific nerve block is likely to provide good analgesia, with minimal or acceptable side-effects
- Expertise and support is available

As with all interventions, patient selection is vital for success. General selection criteria include:

- Patient competent/consented
- Patient compliant
- Absence of systemic infection
- Absence of specific allergy
- Absence of significant coagulopathy
- Adequate support for post-procedural care and maintenance
- A clear pathway for the management of complications after the patient is discharged from the primary unit

Unlike the general population receiving anaesthetic input, palliative care patients are often debilitated, have limited mobility and have a limited lifespan. Therefore, it is imperative that all that can be done to alleviate their pain is performed with the least inconvenience and with minimal compromise. Although many spinal procedures can easily be carried out at the bedside, the more involved interventions, such as chemical neurolysis, necessitate the use of radiological guidance, usually in a hospital setting. With this in mind, patients should, therefore, be selected for these procedures according to what is considered appropriate and acceptable to their level of disability.

53 Buchheit T., Rauck, R. S. (1999) Subarachnoid techniques for cancer pain therapy: when, why and how? *Current Review of Pain Cancer Pain*, **3**(3): 173–247.

54 Ballantyne J. C., Carwood C. M. Comparative efficacy of epidural, subarachnoid and intracerebroventricular opioids in patients with pain due to cancer. *Cochrane Database of Systematic Reviews* 2005, Issue 2

General principles of practice

Resuscitation equipment

Infrequently, systemic toxicity can occur from the administration of local anaesthetic or neurolytic agents. If significant hypotension occurs due to spinal sympathetic blockade, boluses of ephedrine 3mg (i.e. 30mg/mL ampoule diluted to 10mL with sterile water, giving 3mg/mL) should be administered IV at 3–4 minute intervals according to response.

Aseptic technique

- All equipment should be sterile and preferably disposable
- Cleaning fluids should be disposed of prior to drawing up the local anaesthetic to avoid error
- Both sterile gloves and a mask should be worn during the procedures

Drug preparation

Drugs and drug mixtures for intrathecal use should be preservative-free and prepared under sterile conditions. If combinations of drugs are used, care should be taken to ensure their stability and compatibility.[55]

Intrathecal and epidural (neuraxial) techniques

Direct delivery of opioids to the spinal cord via epidural and intrathecal techniques has become increasingly popular in recent decades,[56,57,58] and has proven an effective and reversible way to provide profound analgesia with reduced systemic side-effects. Intrathecal opioids bind to the mu- and kappa-opioid receptors in the substantia gelatinosa of the spinal cord. This is achieved to a lesser extent with epidural opioids, which exert a simultaneous systemic and intrathecal effect (10% and 90%, respectively). 📖 See Fig. 6a.7.

55 Classen A. M., Wimbish G. H., Kupiec T. C. (2004) Stability of admixture containing morphine sulfate, bupivicaine hydrochloride, and clonidine hydrochloride in an implantable infusion system. *Journal of Pain and Symptom Management*, **28**: 603–6.

56 Miguel R. (2000) Interventional treatment of cancer pain: the fourth step in the World Health Organisation analgesic ladder? *Cancer Control: Journal of the Moffitt Cancer Centre*, **7**(2): 149–56.

57 British Pain Society (in consultation with the Association for Palliative Medicine and the Society for British Neurological Surgeons) (2006) *Intrathecal Drug Delivery for the Management of Pain and Spasticity in Adults; Recommendations for Best Clinical Practice*. London: British Pain Society.

58 Baker L., Lee M., Regnard C. (2004) Evolving spinal analgesia practice in palliative care. *Palliative Medicine*, **18**: 507–15.

Common indications for the use of neuraxial techniques
- Unacceptable side-effects despite successful analgesia with systemic opioids
- Unsuccessful analgesia despite escalating doses and use of sequential opioids
- Intolerable neuropathic pain which may be amenable to spinal adjuvants
- Sympathetically mediated pain amenable to sympathetic blockade
- Incident pain which may benefit from numbness (local anaesthetic)

Possible contraindications to neuraxial techniques (risk–benefit decision):
- Platelet count $<20\times10^9$/L with clinical symptoms of poor clotting
- Full anticoagulation or INR >1.5
- Active infection with concurrent septicaemia
- Concurrent chemotherapy likely to cause neutropenia
- Occlusion of epidural space by tumour at the site of catheter tip placement (epidural catheters only)
- Allergy or unmanageable side-effects from the anticipated treatment
- Psychosocial issues that make technique untenable
- Inadequate professional support in resolving problems
- Inadequately investigated symptoms

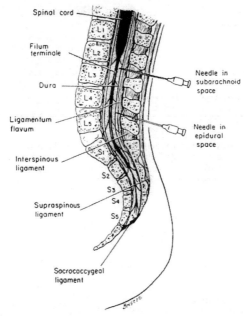

Fig. 6a.7 Schematic diagram of lumbosacral anatomy.

There is a growing body of evidence favouring intrathecal over the epidural administration of opioids.[53,54,58,59] Table 6a.17 compares the two routes of administration.

Table 6a.17 Comparison of intrathecal and epidural opioid administration

Factors	Intrathecal	Epidural
Infection rate	Same as epidural	Same as intrathecal
Pain relief	Better for long-term	Good only for short-term
Dose	Lower (10–20% of epidural dose)	Higher
Pump refills	Less frequent	More frequent (higher volumes)
Side-effects	Fewer	More
Technical difficulty	Easier to place, less likely to become displaced	Potentially more difficult, and catheter may migrate
Long-term complications	Less (approx. 5%)	More (approx. 55%)
Catheter occlusion and fibrosis	Minimal	Higher frequency (leading to loss of analgesia/pain on injection)
Epidural metastases	Less affected	More affected (may compromise drug delivery)
Overall advantage	Effective analgesia with fewer complications	

Catheters may be externalized through the skin at the puncture site or may be tunnelled subcutaneously away from the spine. Alternatively, a totally implantable pump system may be employed if the patient has a life expectancy of several months.[60]

59 Mercadante S. (1999) Neuraxial techniques for cancer pain: an opinion about unresolved therapeutic dilemmas. *Regional Anesthesia & Pain Medicine*, **24**(1): 74–83. [Review]

60 Simpson K. H., Russon L. (2000) The use of intrathecal drug delivery systems in pain management. *CME Bulletin Palliative Medicine*, **2**: 17–20.

Comparison of continuous versus bolus techniques (Table 6a.18)

Table 6a.18 Continuous versus bolus techniques

Factor	Continuous	Intermittent bolus
Dose escalation	Higher	Lower
Analgesic quality	Better	Fair
Local anaesthetic combinations	Minimal motor or haemodynamic complications	Higher risk of motor or haemodynamic complications (**caution** recommended for intraspinal administration)

Ideally, the continuous infusion technique should be used, with a familiar delivery system, e.g. standard Graseby syringe pump delivering the infusion solution over 24 hours. The use of intrathecal bolus administration during pain crises has been described for use in a selected population of patients,[61] but this is not considered routine practice in many institutions.[58]

Technical complications of neuraxial catheters

Mechanical problems (catheter kinking, disconnection, dislodgement or pump failure)

Skin breakdown at insertion site

Infection: local, catheter, epidural abscess, meningitis, systemic infections

CSF leak, causing headache or loss of analgesia

CSF seroma

Haematoma

Catheter displacement, occlusion or migration

Nerve damage (rare but possible): procedure-related, from an inflammatory mass at catheter tip, drug-induced neurotoxicity

61 Mercadante S., *et al.* (2005) Alternative treatments of breakthrough pain in patients receiving spinal analgesics for cancer pain. *Journal of Pain and Symptom Management*, **30**(5): 485–91.

Adverse effects attributable to spinal opioids
Minor sedation: opioid dose excessive
Urinary retention: commonest in males during first 24 hours
Persistent nausea
Pruritis
Respiratory depression: may be severe and insidious if opioid naïve
Hyperalgesia: at higher doses
Myoclonus: at higher doses, indicating toxicity
Constipation

Management of adverse effects

- **Sedation**: reduce dose of opioid
- **Urinary retention**: usually requires once-only catheterization
- **Nausea**: regular anti-emetic
- **Pruritis**:
  - consider adding spinal bupivacaine
  - IV ondansetron 8mg has been shown to be effective[62,63]
  - IV nalbuphine may be effective[64]
- **Respiratory depression** (RR less than 8/min or excessive drowsiness) see p. 244:
  - naloxone 100-400mcg
  - stop intrathecal infusion
  - reduce infusion dose
- **Hyperalgesia**:
  - reduce opioid dose
  - consider addition of adjuvant agent
- **Myoclonus**:
  - reduce opioid dose
  - check renal function
  - encourage rehydration
  - consider low-dose benzodiazepine therapy (myoclonus may not be opioid dose-dependent)
- **Constipation**: regular laxatives from the outset of therapy

62 Twycross R., Zylicz Z. (2004) Systemic therapy: making rational choices in: Zylicz Z et al *Pruritus Advanced Disease.* Oxford: OUP.

63 Borgeat A., Stirnemann H. R. (1999) Ondansetron is effective to treat spinal or epidural morphine-induced pruritis. *Anesthesiology*, **90**: 432–6.

64 Cohen S. E., Ratner E. F., Kreitzman T. R., *et al.* (1992) Nalbuphine is better than naloxone for treatment of side effects after epidural morphine. *Anesthesia and Analgesia*, **75**: 747–52.

Choice of drug: opioids, local anaesthetics, clonidine, ziconotide

Opioids

Morphine is one of the least lipid-soluble opioids available, and when given in the spinal space, it has the slowest rate of uptake into the surrounding vasculature, which gives it a longer and primarily spinal site of action.[57] Intrathecal morphine is regarded as 100 times more potent than a systemically given dose. Data from postoperative pain studies suggest that morphine is twice as potent as diamorphine by the intrathecal route. Intrathecal morphine should be preservative-free.

Diamorphine can be administered intrathecally, with a potency ratio of 1:100 (intrathecal: systemic). Diamorphine should be reconstituted in sodium chloride 0.9%. Alternatives to morphine and diamorphine are used less frequently.

Hydromorphone is an effective and affordable option for the morphine-intolerant patient. The potency of intrathecal hydromorphone is 5 times that of morphine. Of the lipophilic drugs, both **fentanyl** and **sufentanil** are used. Greater lipid solubility may be an advantage to achieve a rapid onset of action, but rapid systemic absorption means a shorter duration of action with a less dose-sparing effect when compared to systemic administration. There is no published data on dose equivalences.

Opioids: typical dosing schedule

- If patient is opioid-naive, start with intrathecal diamorphine 0.5–1mg/24h or epidural diamorphine 2.5–5mg/24h
- If the patient is established on a systemic opioid, the following regimen is recommended for minimizing the withdrawal phenomenon during route conversion:
  - give half of the systemic opioid by the established route
  - convert the remaining half dose numerically to diamorphine, and then divide by 100 to get the intrathecal dose
  - add 2mL of 0.5% bupivacaine to this diamorphine dose
  - add sodium chloride 0.9% up to a total of 10mL
  - infuse this solution over 24h
  - after 24h, reduce the systemic dose by 50% and titrate the intrathecal dose upwards (usually in increments of 10–30%)
  - attempt to discontinue the systemic opioid by day 2 (may not always be possible)

Local anaesthetics

Local anaesthetic agents are sodium channel blockers and are unique in their ability to block nerve impulses conducted proximally (pain relief) and impulses conducted distally (motor blockade). The conduction blockade produced is both painless and reversible. Table 6a.19 shows the most frequently used agents.

Table 6a.19 Comparison of the most frequently used local anaesthetics for spinal use

	Lidocaine	Bupivacaine	Ropivacaine
Onset	Rapid	Slower	Similar to bupivacaine
Duration	Short (hours)	2–3 times longer than lidocaine	Slightly longer than bupivacaine
Typical dosage	2mL 2% over 24h	2mL 0.5% over 24h	2mL 0.75% over 24h
Advantages	Rapid onset and off-set	Synergism with opioids	May preferentially block sensory nerves
	Synergism with opioids		Two-thirds as potent as bupivacaine
			Synergism with opioids

Side-effects of local anaesthetics

- Postural or overt hypotension—sympathetic block
- Numbness—sensory block
- Leg weakness—motor block
- Altered proprioception in low doses, even when motor weakness is not apparent
- Urinary retention
- 'Total spinal'—this potentially catastrophic event can occur if a large dose of local anaesthetic is delivered erroneously to the subarachnoid space. A profound drop in blood pressure is accompanied by motor paralysis of the lower limbs, spreading to the upper limbs and respiratory muscles and ultimately involving the brain. Both cardiovascular and ventilatory support are required until the local anaesthetic effects wear off

Clonidine

Clonidine is an α_2-adrenergic agonist and appears to act at the level of the spinal cord. It acts synergistically with opioids, but is also a powerful analgesic when used alone in the management of neuropathic pain.[55] It is a lipophilic compound and its spinal effect may be more pronounced with intrathecal rather than epidural administration. The dose of clonidine is often limited by the appearance of side-effects, such as sedation, hypotension and bradycardia. Nausea, pruritis and urinary retention have also been reported. Starting doses range from 10 to 20mcg/24h and should be titrated for analgesic effect and minimal side-effects. Doses above 150 mcg/24h should not be necessary.

Ziconotide

Ziconotide is thought to produce its analgesic effects through the blockade of specific N-type calcium channels found at the presynaptic terminals in the dorsal horn.[65] Recognized side-effects of ziconotide include dizziness, gait imbalance, nausea, nystagmus, confusion and urinary retention. These side-effects usually occur after prolonged use, and may be severe. The administration of intrathecal ziconotide has been reported to be useful in the treatment of refractory pain in patients with cancer and AIDS.[55,66] However, clinical experience is limited and longer term data is awaited. The British Pain Society guidelines[57] suggest a starting dose of not more than 0.5mcg/24h, with increases of not more than 0.5mcg/24h no more often than once weekly. Ziconotide is incompatible with morphine.[59]

Other analgesics have been tried as intrathecal agents, including midazolam, ketamine octreotide, calcium channel blockers and neostigmine. As yet, there is no convincing body of evidence to support their use.[57]

Guidelines for percutaneous intrathecal catheter insertion

- Patient consent
- Nurse assistant present
- Adequate space for aseptic trolley
- Patient in sitting or lateral position, with head and knees curled toward the abdomen
- Skin asepsis (e.g. chlorhexidine)
- Local anaesthetic infiltration of skin at chosen level of insertion
- 18G Tuohy needle inserted into spinal space, piercing the dura, until CSF is free-flowing
- Aseptic epidural catheter inserted to 15cm, and free-flow of CSF confirmed
- Catheter secured and dressing applied to insertion site (one which allows daily visual inspection)
- An antibacterial filter should be connected and may remain attached for up to a month
- Connection made to infusion pump or syringe driver

65 Bowersox S., et al. (1996) Selective N-type neuronal voltage sensitive calcium channel blocker, SNX-111, produces spinal antinociception in rat models of acute, persistent and neuropathic pain. *Journal of Pharmacology and Experimental Therapeutics*, **279**: 1234–49.

66 Staats P. S., et al. (2004) Intrathecal ziconotide in the treatment of refractory pain in patients with cancer or AIDS; a randomised controlled trial. *Journal of the American Medical Association*, **291**(1): 63–70.

Follow-up care
- All staff involved in aftercare of the patient should be familiar with the possible side-effects and complications listed, and should be vigilant for signs of infection or problems developing
- The catheter insertion site should be inspected on a daily basis
- A pain chart should be kept initially until the analgesia is considered sufficient
- If the patient is being discharged to the community, there should be liaison with the key members of the primary care team (GP, district nurse and community specialist palliative care nurse) prior to discharge and written guidelines should accompany the patient home
- Patients should not be discharged home until dose escalation has been stabilized

Chemical neurolysis for cancer pain

Neurolysis of nerves by chemical means is indicated for patients with limited life expectancy.[67] The use of neurolytic techniques has diminished over recent years due to advancements in spinal analgesia and increased life expectancies for cancer patients. However, neurolysis should be considered when:

- The pain is severe, intractable and has failed to respond to other measures
- The nociceptive pathway is readily identified and related to a peripheral nerve pathway or sympathetic chain
- A trial block of local anaesthetic has been successful
- The effects of the local anaesthetic block is acceptable to the patient

The goals of neurolysis include reduction in pain and reduction in the need for other pharmacotherapy. Neurolysis rarely is permanent and pain returns as a consequence of regrowth of neural structures or disease progression in the treated area. When used centrally, there is a risk of motor paralysis and sphincter weakness, which are generally unacceptable to most patients. For that reason, patients should be fully consented by the practitioner prior to the procedure.

Neurolytic agents

Alcohol and phenol are the two most commonly used agents.

Alcohol is hypobaric, hence the patient should be able to tolerate a position that allows the alcohol solution to float upwards to the affected nerve root.

Alcohol is usually associated with:

- A burning sensation upon injection along the distribution of the nerve, followed by warm numbness
- An increase in pain relief over a few days, maximal by one week

67 Hill D. A. (2003) Peripheral nerve blocks: practical aspects. In *Clinical Pain Management, Practical Applications and Procedures* (ed. Breivik H., Campbell W., Eccleston C) pp. 197–232. London: Arnold.

Phenol is hyperbaric, so the patient should be able to tolerate a position that allows the phenol to sink down to the nerve roots.
Phenol is characterized as follows:

• Following injection, an initial local anaesthetic effect allows relief of pain which is then maintained by the neurolysis which may take 3–7 days to take full effect.

• The density and duration of block is felt to be less than that of alcohol

Visceral cancer pain is often produced through a combination of visceral afferent stimulation as well as somatic and neuropathic elements. The sympathetic chain carries much nociceptive information, and blockade of the sympathetic chain may improve both visceral- and sympathetic-mediated pain.

• Visceral cancer pain can often be alleviated by a combination of oral pharmacological therapy and neurolytic blockade of the sympathetic axis. Neurolytic techniques have a narrow risk–benefit ratio and, therefore, they should only be performed by experienced pain clinicians in appropriate surroundings[56,68]

• Palliative physicians should be aware of the potential of these blocks and know when it is appropriate to refer patients for neurolytic intervention

Coeliac plexus block

The coeliac plexus is responsible for transmission of nociceptive information from the entire abdominal contents, excluding the descending colon and pelvic structures. It has been successfully used to combat pain from pancreatic cancer and other upper abdominal viscera. It is a relatively safe and simple technique, performed under computed tomography (CT) guidance. Patients referred for this procedure should be able to tolerate lying on an X-ray table, and should have no coagulopathy or local infection (📖 See Figs 6a.8 a and b).
Possible complications include:

• Orthostatic hypotension which may persist for days

• Backache at the site of needle insertion: if backache and hypotension persist, observe serial haematocrit measurements to rule out retroperitoneal haematoma

• Diarrhoea

• Abdominal aortic dissection

• Paraplegia and motor paralysis: rare

Superior hypogastric block

The superior hypogastric sympathetic ganglion transmits nociceptive information from the pelvis, excluding the distal Fallopian tubes and ovaries. Superior hypogastric blocks have been successfully used to manage pain of pelvic origin, other than ovarian pain. Neurological complications have not been reported with this block.

68 de Leon-Casasola O. (2000) Critical evaluation of chemical neurolysis of the sympathetic axis for cancer pain. *Cancer Control: Journal of the Moffitt Cancer Centre,* **7**(2): 142–8.

Ganglion impar block

This ganglion marks the end of the sympathetic chains and is situated at the sacrococcygeal junction. Visceral pain in the perineal area has been successfully treated with neurolytic blockade of this ganglion. These patients often present with a vague, poorly localized perineal pain, accompanied by a burning sensation or urgency, and are often difficult to treat using oral pharmacology alone. No complications have been reported with this block.

Interpleural block

Insertion of an epidural catheter into the pleural space and infusion of local anaesthetic or phenol has been described in the management of visceral pain associated, with oesophageal cancer[69] and rib invasion by bone metastases (Fig. 6a.9). It is a relatively simple technique with few complications, which include:

• Pneumothorax (avoid bilateral blocks)
• Phrenic nerve palsy
• Trauma to local structures caused by the needle, catheter or as a consequence of the phenol injection

Saddle block

This is a modified low spinal technique where phenol is injected into the CSF in the lumbar area, with the intention of causing chemical neurolysis of the low sacral nerve roots that serve the perineum and perianal area. It is useful for patients complaining of pain or excoriation in the 'saddle' area, but carries the potential risk of sphincter compromise (<10%).

69 Lema M. J., *et al.* (1992) Pleural phenol therapy for the treatment of chronic esophageal cancer pain. *Regional Anesthesia*, **17**: 166–70.

(a)

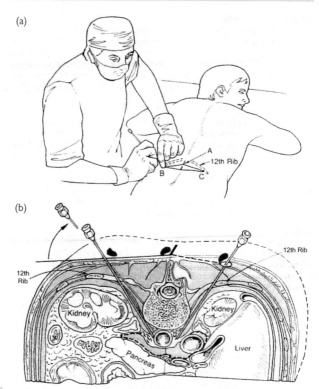

(b)

Fig. 6.8 a & b (a) Positioning for coeliac plexus block; (b) Deep anatomy showing placement of needles for coeliac placement block.

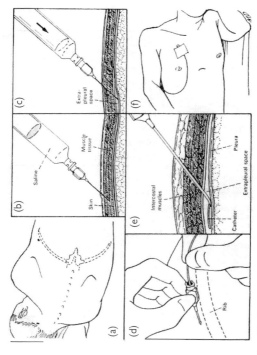

Fig. 6a.9 Technique of intra-pleural block.

Complementary therapies and other non-pharmacological pain interventions

A range of techniques and expertise exists which complement the pharmacological and interventional approaches that have dominated this module thus far (Table 6a.20).

These techniques are not just an adjunct to medication but point to the centrality of holistic patient-centred care. Not all approaches will be appropriate for every patient, but for some traditional medicine has little to offer either.

Table 6a.20 Complementary therapies and other non-pharmacological interventions

Complementary therapies	Other non-pharmacological interventions
Acupuncture	Positioning
Reflexology	Catheterization
Aromatherapy	Reassurance
Art therapy	Good communication
Music therapy	Diversional therapy
Touch therapy	TENS
	Splinting of a fractured limb
	Psychological support

(📖 See also Chapter 11.)

Pain and difficulties in communication

High prevalence of pain in the elderly population is a recognized reality. Almost half of those who die from cancer are over 75 years old. One study showed that 40–80% of elderly people in institutions are in pain. There is evidence that many patients suffering from some form of dementia receive no pain relief at all, despite the presence of a concomitant, potentially painful illness.

The reason for this lies in the difficulty in assessing those with communication difficulties. In addition, the elderly often minimize their pain, making it even more difficult to evaluate. The only indication of pain may be a patient's unusual behaviour that returns to normal with adequate analgesia

Various attempts have been made to evaluate pain in such circumstances. The DOLOPLUS scale,[70] developed in 1993, is based on observations of a patient's behaviour in ten different situations that could be associated with pain. Pain is classified into somatic, psychomotor and psychosocial aspects and scores are allocated. A collective score level confirms the presence of pain.

Examples of unusual behaviours indicating pain[71]

Verbal expression, e.g.:
- Crying when touched
- Shouting
- Becoming very quiet
- Swearing
- Grunting
- Talking without making sense

Facial expression, e.g.:
- Grimacing/wincing
- Closing eyes
- Worried expression

70 Lefebvre-Chapiro S. and the DOLOPLUS group. (2001) The DOLOPLUS 2 scale—evaluating pain in the elderly. *European Journal of Palliative Care*, **8**(5): 191–4.

71 Galloway S., Turner L. (1999) Pain assessment in older adults who are cognitively impaired. *Journal of Gerontological Nursing*, **25**(37): 34–9.

Behavioural expression, e.g.:
• Jumping on touch
• Hand pointing to body area
• Increasing confusion
• Rocking/shaking
• Not eating
• Staying in bed/chair
• Withdrawn/no expression
• Grumpy mood

Physical expression, e.g.:
• Cold
• Pale
• Clammy
• Change in colour
• Change in vital signs if acute pain (e.g. BP, pulse)

Further reading

Book

Scottish Intercollegiate Guidelines Network (2000) *Control of Pain in Patients with Cancer.* Edinburgh: SIGN.

Articles

Back I. N., Finlay I. (1995) Analgesic effect of topical opioids on painful skin ulcers. *Journal of Pain and Symptom Management,* **10**(7): 493.

Cormie P. J. (2008) Control of pain in adults with cancer: summary of SIGN guidelines. *British Medical Journal,* **337**: 1106–9.

Flock P., Gibbs L., Sykes N. (2000) Diamorphine–metronidazole gel effective for treatment of painful infected leg ulcers. *Journal of Pain and Symptom Management,* **20**(6): 396–7.

Gretton S. (2008) Morphine metabolites: a review of their clinical effects. *European Journal of Palliative Care,* **15**: 3: 110–15.

Hoskin P. J. (2008) Opioids in context: relieving the pain of cancer. The role of comprehensive cancer management. *Palliative Medicine,* **22**: 4: 303–10.

Ventafridda V., et al. (1987) Antidepressants increase the bioavailability of morphine in cancer patients. *Lancet* i: 1204. [Letter]

Zeppetella G. (2008) Opioids for cancer break through pain: A Pilot Study Reporting Patient Assessment of Time to Meaningful Pain Relief. *Journal of Pain and Symptom Management,* **35**: 5: 563–7.

Gastrointestinal symptoms

Roast Beef, Medium, is not only a food. It is a philosophy.
Edna Ferber, *Roast Beef, Medium*, 1911

A sizeable proportion of palliative care is concerned with the management of gastrointestinal symptoms. Traditionally, such symptoms have received less attention than pain management, yet the same principles apply.

Patients with pain usually show a response, or a lack of response, to treatment within hours. Patients with gastrointestinal symptoms may take several days to respond to interventions, and the temptation is thus to have a more lax attitude to monitoring gastrointestinal problems. In reality, the doctor and nurse need to be much more attentive to these problems which deceptively cause great patient morbidity, yet may not become obvious until major management difficulties arise.

Example
Every time a patient is prescribed a strong opioid for the first time: Waiting to see if the patient will become nauseated or constipated will lead to major problems. The patient may become so sick that they refuse all morphine again. The patient may become severely constipated with serious and unpleasant consequences.
The patient and family may lose trust in the healthcare professional. Such trust is one of the strongest tools in helping patients and it may be difficult to repair if it is shaken so fundamentally

Therefore
• Every time a strong opioid is prescribed for the first time, or the dose of a strong opioid is markedly increased, always prescribe or increase the dose of a laxative
• Antiemetics should be prescribed for the first 5–10 days of a strong opioid being started or a higher dose being initiated, but after 5 days can and should be stopped as nausea due to the opioid side-effects may wear off. In practice, if patients have tolerated analgesics on step two of the analgesic ladder, they will probably not need anti-emetics when changing to strong opioids

Anticipation of problems before they occur.
Ongoing assessment of treatments and their effectiveness.
Appropriate prescribing of background medication as well as medication for 'breakthrough' symptoms

Oral problems

Oral problems may affect up to 60% of patients with cancer and can impact greatly on quality of life, both physically and psychologically.

Pathology and physiology

A healthy mouth is moist, clean and pain-free with an intact mucosa. Saliva is a major protector of the tissues of the mouth.

About 1500mL of saliva are produced daily by the parotid, submaxillary, sublingual and several minor salivary glands.

Saliva is composed of a serous part (alpha-amylase), which initiates starch digestion, and a mucus component which acts as a lubricant. It also contains calcium, phosphate and bicarbonate which help maintain healthy teeth, and other components such as mucin which protects oral tissue from chemical and mechanical trauma and infections.

The majority of oral problems seen in palliative care are related to a reduction in saliva secretion, although poor oral hygiene is also a major factor. Candidiasis and dry mouth (xerostomia) are two of the most common problems. Other problems include pain, stomatitis, mucositis, ulceration, halitosis, altered taste and hypersalivation (drooling).

During cytotoxic therapy the cells of the oral mucosa are vulnerable due to their high proliferation rate. Other treatment complications may arise due to direct stomatotoxicity or indirectly due to myelosuppressive effects. There are several risk factors for oral problems in patients with advanced cancer:

- Reduced oral intake
- Debility (reduced ability to perform own oral hygiene)
- Dry mouth (often aggravated by medicines, mouth breathing, oxygen therapy)
- Dehydration
- Local irradiation
- Chemotherapy
- Local tumour

General mouth care

The aim of good mouth care is to prevent problems before they arise and to control unpleasant symptoms.

Assessment

- Assess daily for symptoms or signs of problems such as altered taste, oral pain, dry mouth, halitosis, ulcers, oral or pharyngeal candidiasis or dental problems
- Regularly examine lips, tongue, teeth and oral mucosa
- Involve the local dental team if necessary
- Assess the patient's ability to carry out mouth care effectively
- Encourage good oral hygiene for general well being

*An oral assessment tool may be useful. Eilers *et al.*'s oral assessment guide has been found to be appropriate for use in patients with advanced cancer.[1]

---

1 Eilers J., Berger A., Petersen M. (1998) Development, testing and application of the Oral Assessment Guide. *Oncology Nursing Forum*, **15**: 325–30.

Management

Basic oral care—by staff or patient if able.

• Keep mouth moist—encourage regular sips of fluids/oral rinsing
• Brush teeth with toothpaste or clean dentures regularly, especially after meals
• Rinse mouth thoroughly and frequently with sodium chloride 0.9% (helps removal of oral debris and is soothing and non-traumatic[2])
• Gently clean a coated tongue with a soft toothbrush or sponge
• Apply moisturizing cream or white soft paraffin (petroleum jelly) to lips
• Soak dentures overnight in cleansing solution

If the patient is unconscious or too unwell to carry out oral hygiene, instruct and involve family in this important area of care.

Management of oral problems[2,3,4]

Coated tongue/dirty mouth

In addition to basic oral care, if there is no candidiasis:

• Use mouthwashes to remove debris, e.g. cool water or 0.9% sodium chloride
• Gently brush with a soft toothbrush or sponge
• Give pineapple (fresh or tinned) to chew—contains proteolytic enzyme ananase which cleans the mouth. Papaya (papain) acts similarly
• Effervescent vitamin C has been used for a furred tongue. However, it has been blamed for the exacerbation of dental damage through cavitation and the low pH of the tablets.

Dry mouth (xerostomia)

Xerostomia is the subjective feeling of a dry mouth and is often associated with difficulties with speech, chewing or swallowing, the need to keep drinking and loss of taste. This is a common problem in advanced cancer and appropriate management may involve the use of both saliva stimulants and substitutes.

Causes

• Drugs, e.g. antimuscarinics, antidepressants, opioids, diuretics
• Candidiasis
• Dehydration
• Anxiety
• Mouth breathing
• Radiotherapy
• Oxygen therapy (non-humidified)

2 Miller M., Kearney N. (2001) Oral care for patients with cancer: a review of the literature. *Cancer Nursing*, **24**(4): 241–54.

3 Twycross R. (2001) *Symptom Management in Advanced Cancer* (3rd edn). Oxford: Radcliffe Medical Press.

4 Sweeney M. P., et al. (1997) Clinical trial of a mucin-containing oral spray for treatment of xerostomia in hospice patients. *Palliative Medicine*, **11**: 225–32.

Management
- Treat underlying cause if possible, e.g. infection, dehydration
- Review medication
- Provide basic oral care regimen (see the previous page)
- General measures (little scientific rationale[2]):
  - sipping semi-frozen drinks
  - sucking ice-chips in gauze (to prevent mucosal freezing)
  - chewing pineapple pieces
  - sugar-free chewing gum
  - petroleum jelly applied to lips
  - oral sprays may be beneficial[5]

Consider saliva substitutes, especially pre-meals:
- Saliva Orthana (NB pork mucin-based spray—may be no more beneficial than placebo)
- Biotène Oralbalance gel
- Methylcellulose solution, e.g. Glandosane spray
- Saliva stimulation
  - pilocarpine—a parasympathomimetic agent which stimulates salivary gland secretion. (It should be avoided in bowel obstruction, glaucoma, asthma, COPD and cardiac disease) Dose: pilocarpine 5mg tablets p.o. t.d.s; sweating is a common side-effect
  - pilocarpine 4% eye-drop solution has been used in raspberry syrup or peppermint water (2–3 drops taken orally t.d.s.—unlicensed use[6])
  - bethanechol—start with 10mg t.d.s. with meals and increase if necessary (unlicensed use)

Painful mouth and stomatitis
Stomatitis refers to painful, inflammatory and ulcerative conditions affecting the mucous membranes lining the mouth and may be caused by:
- Infection
- Ulceration
- Mucositis post-radiotherapy or chemotherapy
- Iron deficiency (angular stomatitis and glossitis)
- Vitamin C deficiency (gingivitis and bleeding)
- Dry mouth

Other causes of oral pain include:
- Tumour infiltration
- Dental problems

5 Sweeney M. P., *et al.* (1997) Clinical trial of a mucin-containing oral spray for treatment of xerostomia in hospice patients. *Palliative Medicine*, **11**: 225–32.

6 Back I. N. (2001) *Palliative Medicine Handbook* (3rd edn). Cardiff: BPM Books.

Management

Non-drug treatment

- Treat underlying cause if possible, e.g. infection
- Maintain good oral hygiene
- Avoid foods that trigger pain, e.g. acidic foods
- Avoid tobacco and alcohol
- Ensure ENT/oncology review

Drug treatment

Generalized oral pain

- Systemic analgesic
- Analgesic mouthwash, e.g. benzydamine hydrochloride (Difflam) 15mL every 1.5–3h (dilute 1:1 if it stings)
- Chlorhexidine 0.2% (Corsodyl)—rinse mouth with 10mL for 1 minute b.d.
- Sucralfate susp. 10mL as mouthwash 4h (unlicensed use)
- Soluble aspirin 300–600mg q.d.s. (if no contraindications)
- Cocaine mouthwash 2% is used for mucositis in some centres

Some claim there is no evidence that benzydamine, sucralfate or chlorhexidine ease oral pain.[7]

Localized oral pain

- Topical analgesia, e.g.
  - choline salicylate oral gel (Bonjela/Teegel)—apply not more than 3 hourly
  - carmellose paste (Orabase)—protective oral paste—apply p.r.n.
  - lidocaine spray, gel or cream (beware pharyngeal anaesthesia and risk of aspiration)
- Systemic analgesics
  - NSAIDs, e.g. diclofenac (if no contradictions)
  - opioids—consider starting or increasing systemic opioids and monitor response
  - consider ketamine for persistent oral neuropathic pain

7 Regnard C., Hockley J. (2004) *A Guide to Symptom Relief in Palliative Care* (5th edn). Oxford: Radcliffe Medical Press.

Ulceration of oral mucosa

Causes include trauma (chemical or physical), recurrent aphthae, infections, cancer, nutritional deficiencies, haematinic deficiency (iron, folate, vitamin B_{12}) and drug therapy.

Management: Identify and treat cause where possible.

• Consider referral for further investigation if mouth ulcer persists
• Pain relief—as for stomatitis

Aphthous ulcers

• Topical corticosteroids for five days, e.g. Adcortyl in Orabase (triamcinolone 0.1% paste) applied b.d., or Corlan (hydrocortisone) 2.5mg q.d.s. p.o. to ulcerated area
• Tetracycline mouthwash (for resistant ulcers). Caps 250mg—dissolve contents in water and hold in mouth for 2–3 minutes twice daily for three days. Avoid swallowing. May stain developing teeth[7]
• Persistent and severe ulcers may respond to thalidomide (seek specialist advice)

Infection

• Fungal—candidiasis is most common in patients with cancer
• Viral—e.g. herpes simplex
• Bacterial—e.g. coliforms or staphylococci

Predisposing factors

• Reduced salivary flow
• Immunosuppressants
• Chemotherapy
• Antibiotics
• Poor nutritional state
• Diabetes
• Wearing dentures
• Poor oral hygiene

Candidiasis

Present in up to 80% of patients.[8] (Present in normal oral flora of 50% of the general population.) May be asymptomatic.

Presenting features may include:

• Dry mouth
• Loss of taste
• Smooth red tongue
• Adherent white plaques on tongue or mucous membranes
• Soreness
• Dysphagia (remember oropharyngeal/oesophageal candidiasis)
• Angular cheilitis

8 Back I. N. (2001) *Palliative Medicine Handbook* (3rd edn). Cardiff: BPM books.

Investigation
Swabs are not routinely taken in palliative care, although it may be useful since fungal infections may become resistant to standard treatment.

Treatment
- Specific treatments should be accompanied by good oral hygiene
- There is no clear evidence to suggest the superiority of the various antifungal agents in this patient population
- Remember to treat dentures—soak in nystatin or dilute Milton overnight
- Topical:
  - nystatin susp. 100,000U/mL or nystatin pastilles 100^000U
  - Dose: 2–5mL q.d.s. p.o. or 1 pastille q.d.s. p.o. for at least 5 days (reduced activity if nystatin combined with chlorhexidine mouthwash)
  - miconazole oral gel 24mg/mL, apply 5–10mL q.d.s. p.o.
  - amphotericin lozenges 10mg; dose: 1 lozenge q.d.s.
- Systemic:
  - ketoconazole tabs/susp.; dose: 200mg o.d. p.o. (watch liver function)
  - fluconazole tabs/susp.; dose: 50mg o.d. p.o. for 7–14 days

Recurrent candidiasis in patients with AIDS may require prophylactic treatment with fluconazole 50mg daily. Concern is arising that 'azole' (i.e. ketoconazole, fluconazole) resistance may become a clinical problem in palliative care.[9] Note that azoles have important drug interactions, including clinically significant enhancements in the action of warfarin, phenytoin and midazolam.

Herpes simplex infection may require oral aciclovir 200mg 4-h for one week.

Note: Systemic antifungal drugs may interact with several drugs metabolized by the cytochrome P450 enzymes including phenytoin, warfarin, sulphonylureas and midazolam. It is always best to check for possible interactions when co-prescribing.

Bacterial infection
Malignant ulcers or local tumour may be associated with halitosis due to anaerobic bacteria.

Treatment
- Metronidazole 400mg t.d.s. p.o. or 500mg b.d. p.r. × 5 days
- May be used as mouthwash if adverse effects—metronidazole susp. 400mg (10mL) t.d.s. and spit out[8]

9 Davies A., et al. (2002) Resistance amongst yeasts isolated from the oral cavities of patients with advanced cancer. *Palliative Medicine*, **16**: 527–31.

Drooling

May be due to the overproduction of saliva (sialorrhoea) or inability to swallow normal amounts of saliva. Drooling is common in MND (40%) but uncommon in advanced cancer (except head and neck).

Causes

- Neuromuscular:
  - MND
  - CVA
  - cerebral palsy
  - carcinoma of the pharynx
  - Parkinson's disease
  - brain tumours
- Oral factors:
  - ill-fitting dentures
  - deformity post surgery, e.g. oral surgery
  - dysphagia
- Drugs:
  - cholinesterase inhibitors
  - cholinergic agents
  - lithium

Management

Non-drug treatment:
- Head positioning
- Suctioning

Drug treatment (Table 6b.1):
- Antimuscarinic drugs (if patient is able to swallow) will reduce saliva production
- Most patients will not be able to swallow tablets or capsules, or large volumes, and a number will have PEG tube feeding
- Drugs that do not cross the blood–brain barrier minimize the risk of sedation and other central side-effects; however, they may also be poorly and unpredictably absorbed when given orally
- Other drugs with antimuscarinic effects will reduce saliva production, e.g. amitriptyline p.o. 25mg nocte or propantheline 15mg t.d.s., but use is often limited by side-effects
- Choice will depend on local availability and patient's circumstances

Table 6b.1 Drug treatment

Given by injection	
Glycopyrronium 0.1–0.4mg/24h csci	Ideal drug, but requires regular or continuous injection. Most reliable way of establishing effective symptom control rapidly.
Glycopyrronium 25–100mcg b.d. sc increased as needed	
Transdermal patch	
Hyoscine hydrobromide transdermal patch	Central side-effects can occur, especially in the elderly.
Given orally/PEG/sublingual	
Glycopyrronium p.o. 0.6–2mg up to t.d.s.	Solution for injection can be used but may need 3–10mL. Powder for oral solution requires pharmacy to prepare, is not routinely available, and is expensive. Titration to effective dose may take longer.
Atropine eye drops 1% 2 drops p.o./ sublingual q.d.s.	Cheapest; least published experience. Central side-effects may occur, but less than hyoscine hydrobromide.

Further reading

Books

Back I. N. (2001) *Palliative Medicine Handbook* (3rd edn). Cardiff: BPM Books.

Doyle D., et al. (eds) (2004) *Oxford Textbook of Palliative Medicine* (3rd edn). Oxford: Oxford University Press.

Regnard C., Hockley J. (2004) *A Guide to Symptom Relief in Palliative Care* (5th edn). Oxford: Radcliffe Medical Press.

Twycross R. (2001) *Symptom Management in Advanced Cancer* (3rd edn). Oxford: Radcliffe Medical Press.

Twycross R., Wilcock A. (2002) *Palliative Care Formulary* (3rd edn). Oxford: Palliativedrugs.com

Articles

Davies A., et al. (2002) Resistance amongst yeasts isolated from the oral cavities of patients with advanced cancer. *Palliative Medicine*, **16**: 527–31.

Eilers J., Berger A., Petersen M. (1988) Development, testing and application of the Oral Assessment Guide. *Oncology Nursing Forum*, **15**: 325–30.

Miller M., Kearney N. (2001) Oral care for patients with cancer: a review of the literature. *Cancer Nursing*, **24**(4): 241–54.

Regnard C. (1994) Single dose fluconazole versus five-day ketoconazole in oral candidosis. *Palliative Medicine*, **8**: 72–3.

Sweeney M. P., et al. (1997) Clinical trial of a mucin-containing oral spray for treatment of xerostomia in hospice patients. *Palliative Medicine*, **11**: 225–32.

CKS: Topic review: Palliative Cancer Care-Oral problems CKS Website: WWW.CKS.library.nhs.uk

Nausea and vomiting

Last night we went to a Chinese dinner at six and a French dinner at nine, and I can feel the sharks' fins navigating unhappily in the Burgundy. Peter Flemming, Letter from Yunnanfu, 20 March 1938

Nausea is an unpleasant feeling of the need to vomit often accompanied by autonomic symptoms.

Vomiting is the forceful expulsion of gastric contents through the mouth.[10]

Nausea and vomiting are symptoms which can cause patients, and their relatives, deep distress. Of the two, nausea causes most misery; many patients can tolerate one or two episodes of vomiting a day while prolonged nausea is profoundly debilitating. There are many causes of nausea and it is important to try to analyse the likely cause so that appropriate therapy can be initiated.

Evaluation
- Distinguish between vomiting, expectoration and regurgitation
- Separately assess nausea and vomiting
- Enquire if nausea is absent for prolonged periods after vomiting or is persistent
- Review drug regimen
- If there is a likelihood of cerebral secondaries, check the fundi for papilloedema (although its absence does not exclude raised intracranial pressure)
- Examine the abdomen
- Do a rectal examination if faecal impaction is a possibility
- Consider checking plasma concentrations of: creatinine, calcium, albumin and digoxin
- Consider radiological investigations if major doubt remains about the cause
- Note the content of the vomitus, e.g. undigested food, bile, faeculent
- Timing of onset of nausea or vomiting
- Associated symptoms (e.g. the headaches of raised intracranial pressure are coincidental with vomiting)

Causes
Common causes of nausea and vomiting in advanced cancer include:
- Gastrointestinal, e.g. gastric stasis, intestinal obstruction
- Drugs, e.g. opioids, antibiotics, NSAIDs, iron, digoxin
- Metabolic, e.g. hypercalcaemia, renal failure
- Toxic, e.g. radiotherapy, chemotherapy, infection, paraneoplastic
- Brain metastases
- Psychosomatic factors, e.g. anxiety, fear
- Pain

10 Twycross R. (2001) *Sympltom Management in Advanced Cancel* (3rd edn). Oxford: Radcliffe Medical Press.

Treat reversible causes
- Severe pain
- Infection
- Cough
- Hypercalcaemia
- Tense ascites
- Raised intracranial pressure (using corticosteroids)
- Emetogenic drugs—stop or reduce dose
- Anxiety—pharmacological and psychological management

Opioid-induced nausea and vomiting

Opioids can cause nausea and vomiting through a number of different possible mechanisms. These include stimulation of the chemoreceptor trigger zone, increased vestibular sensitivity, gastric stasis or impaired intestinal motility and constipation.

Haloperidol is usually recommended as first-line treatment for opioid-induced nausea and vomiting; however, metoclopramide (for gastric stasis), cyclizine or hyoscine hydrobromide may all be effective in certain patients. $5HT_3$ antagonists have also been shown to be useful but are expensive for long-term use.

Management

Non-pharmacological management of nausea and vomiting
- Control malodour from colostomy, fungating tumour or decubitus ulcer
- Provide a calm, reassuring environment away from the sight and smell of food
- Avoid exposure to foods that precipitate nausea, which may mean transferring the patient to a single room
- Give small snacks, e.g. a few mouthfuls, and not large meals
- Suggest that if the patient is the household cook, someone else may need to take on this role
- Suggest the use of acupressure wrist bands, Sea Bands—these devices are helpful to some patients, particularly those who prefer non-pharmacology treatments

Drug management of nausea and vomiting (Table 6b.2)
There are many neurotransmitter receptors involved in nausea and vomiting. These include those for histamine, acetylcholine, 5-hydroxytryptamine and dopamine located in varying concentrations largely in the vomiting centre and the chemoreceptor trigger zone in the midbrain.

In simple terms, neural impulses from a variety of emetic stimuli are relayed to these sites in the brainstem, triggering the vomiting reflex. A single antiemetic may be adequate to suppress symptoms, but if there are different causes for the vomiting in the same patient, it may be necessary to combine drugs. For instance, if the cause of vomiting is thought to be raised intracranial pressure and uraemia, it may be necessary to combine, for example, cyclizine and haloperidol.

Levomepromazine antagonizes several receptors and may thus be a useful single alternative at a dose of 6.25mg o.d. or b.d. orally, doses higher than this cause sedation.

It may be possible to control nausea with oral medication, but persistent vomiting requires drug delivery by an alternative route such as per rectum or, more reliably, subcutaneously by means of stat doses or continuously via a syringe driver.

Side-effects

All antiemetics have side-effects with which it is necessary to be familiar.

It is very easy to overlook minor extrapyramidal effects of the dopamine antagonists which thus add to a patient's distress. For instance, haloperidol and metoclopramide may cause restlessness and inability to keep still (akathisia). More marked signs include parkinsonian effects such as stiffness and tremor. The effect can be reversed by stopping the drug. If necessary, a small dose of an antimuscarinic drug, such as procyclidine, can be given. Domperidone is an alternative to metoclopramide since extrapyramidal problems are less.

Cyclizine and the phenothiazines (e.g. levomepromazine) are associated with anticholinergic side-effects such as dry mouth, blurring of vision and urinary retention.

$5HT_3$ antagonists cause constipation.

Table 6b.2 Antiemetic drug choice

Cause of vomiting	Choice of antiemetic drug
Drug- or toxin-induced	Haloperidol 1.5mg nocte/b.d.
	Levomepromazine 6.25mg (a quarter tablet)
	6mg tabs now available
Radiotherapy	Ondansetron 8mg stat then 8mg b.d. up to 5 days
	Haloperidol 1.5–3mg nocte/b.d.
Chemotherapy	Ondansetron 8mg stat then 8mg b.d. up to 5 days
	Dexamethasone 4–8mg o.d. (often as part of a chemotherapy regime)
	Metoclopramide 20mg q.d.s.
	Aprepitant 125mg stat, then 80mg o.d. for 2 days, consider adding for resistant nausea and vomiting
Metabolic, e.g. hypercalcaemia	Haloperidol 1.5mg nocte/b.d.
	Levomepromazine 6.25mg nocte
Raised intracranial pressure	Cyclizine 50mg t.d.s./or 150mg/24h SC
	Dexamethasone 4–16mg o.m.
Bowel obstruction[11]	Cyclizine 150mg/24h p.o. or SC
	Hyoscine butylbromide 40–100mg/24h SC
	Octreotide 300–1000mcg/24h SC
	Ondansetron 8–24 mg/24h p.o., IV or SC
Delayed gastric emptying	Metoclopramide 10–20mg q.d.s.
	Domperidone 10–20mg q.d.s.
Gastric irritation	Treat gastritis, e.g. proton pump inhibitor.
	Stop gastric irritants, e.g. NSAIDs
	Cyclizine 50mg t.d.s.
	Ondansetron 8mg b.d.

11 Baines M. J. (2000) Symptom control in advanced gastrointestinal cancer. *European Journal of Gastroenterology & Hepatology*, **12**: 375–9

Management of nausea and vomiting: practical guide

Identify any causes of nausea and vomiting that can best be treated specifically, e.g.:
- Constipation—remember to do a rectal examination
- Gastritis—epigastric discomfort and tenderness
- Raised intracranial pressure—neurological signs
- Oropharyngeal candida
- Hypercalcaemia—dehydration, confusion
- Drug-induced—recent introduction of morphine
- Intestinal obstruction

Choose an antiemetic based on the most likely cause of nausea and vomiting (Fig. 6b.1):
- Drug or metabolic—haloperidol
- Gastric stasis—metoclopramide
- GI tract involvement or cerebral tumour—cyclizine

If first-choice drug is unsuccessful or only partially successful after 24h, increase the dose or use different antiemetic(s):
- Nausea and vomiting in cancer is often multifactorial
- If confident that there is a single cause for the nausea and vomiting, consider increasing the antiemetic dose (especially metoclopramide), or changing to a second-line specific antiemetic (e.g. ondansetron for drug-induced nausea)
- If not confident of cause, empirically try one of the other first-line antiemetics (metoclopramide, haloperidol, cyclizine)
- Combinations of antiemetics with different actions (e.g. at different receptor sites) are often needed and can act additively
- If using more than one antiemetic, one from each class of antiemetics should be considered, 🕮 see Table 6b.3
- Cyclizine and haloperidol are a logical combination
- Levomepromazine acts at several receptor sites, and alone may replace a previously unsuccessful combination
- Levomepromazine may be useful as a non-specific second-line antiemetic for nausea and vomiting of any or unknown aetiology
- Cyclizine may antagonize the prokinetic effects of metoclopramide, and they should not usually be mixed

General points

- Always give antiemetics *regularly*—not p.r.n.
- If vomiting is preventing drug absorption, use an alternative route, e.g. CSCI
- Dexamethasone 4mg daily often contributes an antiemetic effect for nausea and vomiting of unknown mechanism
- Check blood U&E, LFTs and calcium:
  - renal failure—consider lowering the dose of opioids
  - hypercalcaemia—treat with intravenous bisphosphonates
- Monitor carefully if giving prokinetic drugs (e.g. metoclopramide) in intestinal obstruction in case intestinal colic and vomiting increase.

Always reassess the patient regularly as the cause of nausea and vomiting can change with time:
• Levomepromazine tends to cause sedation at doses above 6.25mg b.d.
• Octreotide dries up gastrointestinal secretions tending towards constipation
• Granisetron and ondansetron are also associated with constipation

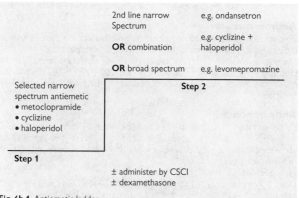

Fig. 6b.1 Antiemetic ladder.

Antiemetic drugs (📖 see Table 6b.3)

Antihistamines

The *vomiting centre* is rich in histamine and acetylcholine receptors. Most antihistamine drugs are also antimuscarinic.

Cyclizine is a commonly used antihistamine antiemetic. Acting at the vomiting centre, it is useful for vomiting of many causes.

Dose: 25–50mg t.d.s. orally or 100–150mg/24h CSCI. *Side-effects*: antimuscarinic effects like dry mouth and drowsiness often abate after a few days.

Antimuscarinics

Hyoscine hydrobromide is a potent antimuscarinic. It is especially useful if there is intestinal obstruction or colic as it reduces peristalsis.

Dose: it is available as buccal tablets (Kwells) and transdermal patches (Scopoderm TTS), and can be used by CSCI: 200–1200 mcg/24h CSCI. *Side-effects*: dry mouth, drowsiness or confusion may be more severe than with cyclizine.

Antipsychotics

Drugs and metabolic disturbances cause vomiting by stimulating the CTZ. Antipsychotics (as potent dopamine antagonists) block this pathway and are very effective against drug- or metabolic-induced nausea and vomiting (e.g. opioids and renal failure).

Haloperidol

Dose: 1.5mg nocte orally (0.5–1.5mg b.d.) or 2.5–5mg/24h CSCI. *Side-effects*: sedation and extrapyramidal effects are rare at these low doses.

Prochlorperazine is relatively more sedative but is available in buccal (Buccastem) and suppository form. Prochlorperazine cannot be given subcutaneously as it is irritant.

Levomepromazine is a sedative, broad-spectrum antiemetic which is effective in low doses. Some patients show a narrow therapeutic window.

Dose: 6.25–25mg nocte or b.d. orally or 6.25–25mg/24h CSCI. Oral bioavailability of levomepromazine is approx. 40%. Use half the daily oral dose by CSCI. *Side-effects*: it also has antimuscarinic, antihistamine and 5HT$_2$ antagonist effects, as well as an anxiolytic effect.

Note: Phenothiazines and haloperidol should be avoided with amiodarone since there is an increased risk of ventricular arrhythmias. The low, antiemetic doses of haloperidol used in palliative care probably carry a low risk.

Prokinetic drugs/drugs altering gastric motility

Metoclopramide acts peripherally on the gut, restoring normal gastric emptying. It also acts at the CTZ and thus helps drug-induced nausea.

Dose: 10–20mg q.d.s. p.o. or 30–80mg/24h CSCI. *Side-effects*: the extrapyramidal effects are rare, but most common in young female patients.

Domperidone is very similar to metoclopramide but is less likely to cause extrapyramidal effects because it does not cross the blood–brain barrier; it is available as suppositories.

5HT₃ antagonists

$5HT_3$ receptors are found in the chemoreceptor trigger zone. Antagonists are very effective against acute-phase chemotherapy and radiotherapy-induced nausea with little to choose between ondansetron and granisetron, but their place in other situations (e.g. intestinal obstruction) is as yet uncertain.

Ondansetron has been shown to be ineffective in the treatment of motion sickness, but effective at treating morphine-induced nausea and vomiting. $5HT_3$ antagonists may work synergistically with haloperidol in some cases.

In the UK, $5HT_3$ antagonists are only licensed for chemotherapy-induced and postoperative emesis.

Other drugs

Corticosteroids often have a non-specific benefit in reducing nausea and vomiting.

Additional drugs

Newer atypical antipsychotics may be expected to show antiemetic effects. Olanzapine has a similar pharmacological profile to levomepromazine and there is weak anecdotal evidence that it may be an effective antiemetic.

Risperidone has potent $5HT_2$ antagonist effects as well as being anti-dopaminergic, but there is no published evidence to date of any antiemetic effect. It should be avoided in patients with cerebrovascular disease.

Aprepitant is the first member of the neurokinin receptor-antagonist class of antiemetics now marketed. To date, its use is specifically for acute and delayed nausea and vomiting associated with platinum-based chemotherapy, in combination with dexamethasone and a $5HT_3$ antagonist.

Table 6b.3 Receptor affinity of antiemetic drugs

Agonist/Antagonist	ACh_M Ant	H₁ Ant	5HT₂ Ant	D₂ Ant	5HT₃ Ant	5HT₄ Ag
Hyoscine hydrobromide	+++					
Cyclizine	++	+++				
Haloperidol				+++(*)		
Ondansetron					+++	
Metoclopramide				++	(+)	++
Domperidone				++		
Levomepromazine	+	+	++	+(*)		

(*) Prokinetic effect of metoclopramide and domperidone is partly attributed to D_2 antagonism—however, there is no evidence that haloperidol or other neuroleptics have prokinetic activity

Avoid dopamine antagonists (particularly haloperidol), in patients with Parkinson's disease.

Constipation

Constipation is characterized by difficult or painful defaecation, and is associated with infrequent bowel evacuations, and hard, small faeces.

Stool frequency varies considerably in the normal population: 45% of patients are constipated on admission to a hospice. Complications of constipation include pain, bowel obstruction, overflow diarrhoea and urinary retention which cause great distress and every effort must therefore be made to avoid them.

Causes
- Disease-related
  - immobility
  - decreased food intake
  - low residue diet
- Fluid depletion
  - poor fluid intake
  - increased fluid loss, i.e. vomiting, polyuria, fever
- Weakness
  - inability to raise intra-abdominal pressure
  - general debility
  - paraplegia
  - inability to reach toilet when urge to defaecate occurs (immobility leads to decreased peristalsis)
- Intestinal obstruction
- Medication
  - opioids (90% of patients taking opioids need laxatives)
  - diuretics
  - antimuscarinics
    - phenothiazines
    - tricyclic antidepressants
    - hyoscine derivatives
  - serotonin inhibitors
    - ondansetron/granisetron/tropisetron
  - somatostatin analogues
    - octreotide/lanreotide
- Biochemical
  - hypercalcaemia
  - hypokalaemia
- Other
  - embarrassment in public setting
  - pain on defaecation, e.g. fissure in ano

Complications of constipation
- Pain—colic or constant abdominal discomfort
- Intestinal obstruction
- Urinary retention or frequency
- Overflow diarrhoea
- Faecal incontinence
- Confusion or restlessness if severe

Management of constipation

- Anticipate this common problem
- Enquire about bowel function regularly
- Start prophylactic laxatives when starting opioid drugs
- Use oral laxatives in preference to rectal measures
- Use a combination of a stimulant laxative with a softener/osmotic laxative if necessary
- Titrate components to achieve optimum stool frequency and consistency

Remember also to:

- Increase fluid intake
- Increase fruit/fibre in the diet
- Encourage mobility
- Get the patient to the toilet, if possible avoiding bed pans
- Provide privacy
- Raise toilet seat for comfort

Laxatives

Choice of laxative

- A number of laxative combinations may be equally effective
- Patient preference may dictate choice
- Mixed preparations of softener/stimulant (e.g. co-danthramer) keep medications to a minimum
- Separate softener and stimulant allows titration of components to give optimum stool frequency and consistency
- Senna has a greater tendency to cause colic than dantron-containing combination laxatives
- One peripheral opioid antagonist capable of relieving opioid-induced constipation is now available. Methylnaltrexone (Relistor®) has shown promise in clinical trials and has at the time of writing been granted approval for use in the UK, and Europe and USA. This agent offers the first prospect of a specific treatment for this condition.

Traditionally, laxatives are divided into:

- Stimulants
- Bulking agents
- Osmotic agents
- Faecal softeners

In reality, these categories are arbitrary as there is much overlap between the agents. For example, an osmotic agent will act as a stimulant by decreasing the GIT transit time by increasing pressure within the bowel. (📖 see Tables 6b. 4 and 5).

Stimulants, e.g. senna, dantron, bisacodyl

Avoid stimulant drugs if there is the possibility of intestinal obstruction. Dantron is useful with a softener such as docusate (co-danthrusate) or poloxamer (co-danthramer) for opioid-induced constipation, but may colour urine red and cause excoriation around the perineum if in contact with skin. (Dantron is only licensed for use in patients with a terminal illness.)

Osmotic agents, e.g. lactulose, magnesium salts, macrogols

In palliative care, the use of such agents is often inappropriate because of the need to drink 2–3 litres per day for the agents to function well. In addition, lactulose may be unpalatable and cause uncomfortable abdominal bloating and flatus.

Macrogol (polyethylene glycol) in the palliative setting, particularly in intractable constipation and faecal impaction, may have a particular role to play.[12]

> Lactulose is usually to be avoided in the palliative care setting because:
> * It can increase abdominal cramps
> * Its sweet taste can be hard for the palliative care patient to tolerate
> * It causes flatulence
> * It should be consumed with large volumes of liquid which palliative care patients are often unable to take

Faecal softeners, e.g. docusate

These are useful in conjunction with a stimulant (e.g. docusate + dantron in co-danthrusate and docusate + poloxamer in co-danthramer). It may be safer to use docusate alone in resolving intestinal obstruction.

Bulk-forming agents, e.g. methylcellulose (Celevac), ispaghula husk (Fybogel)

Patients are rarely started on these preparations in the palliative care setting because they have been implicated in worsening constipation when used with reduced fluid intake. They are also unpalatable and may aggravate anorexia.

Rectal agents (1 bisacodyl suppository + 1 glycerol suppository)

Bisacodyl is a rectal stimulant and should be placed in direct contact with the rectal mucosa. If appropriately placed, it should stimulate an evacuation within one hour.

Glycerol is a faecal lubricant which facilitates defaecation by softening the stool.

For more severe constipation

Arachis oil enema (130mL) overnight to penetrate hard stool, soften and lubricate. Follow with high phosphate enema in the morning to stimulate bowel clearance.

Do *not* attempt *manual evacuation* of impacted stool without some form of sedation or analgesia.

In circumstances of intractable constipation, close consultation with nursing colleagues is vital if a clear strategy for managing the problem is to be achieved.

It is possible that the use of subcutaneous peripheral opioid antagonists such as methylnaltrexone (Relistor ®) will find a place in the routine management of opioid induced constipation. Further studies are required.

---

12 Culbert P., Gillett H., Ferguson A. (1998) Highly effective new oral therapy for faecal impaction. *British Journal of General Practice*, **48**: 1599–600

Faecal impaction

If the patient has faecal impaction, try:

- Bisacodyl suppositories (must be in contact with rectal mucosa)
- Arachis oil retention enema to soften
- Phosphate enema
- An alternative is polyethylene glycol, *Movicol* taken for three days
- Manual removal (with midazolam, morphine, or caudal anaesthesia)
- Once successful it is imperative to start regular oral measures to prevent recurrence of the problem

Table 6b.4 Classification of commonly used laxatives

Category	Examples	Description	Comments
Osmotic laxatives	**Lactulose Polyethylene glycol**	Osmotic laxatives are not absorbed from the gut and so retain water in the lumen by osmotic action (this action may be partial). This increase in volume will encourage peristalsis and consequent expulsion of faeces	Can cause abdominal distension and abdominal cramps. Patients need to drink over a litre a day which may not be practical
Surfactant laxatives	**Docusate Poloxamer**	Act to reduce surface tension and improve water penetration of the stools	
Stimulant laxatives	**Senna Bisacodyl**	Senna and bisacodyl both rely on bacterial transformation in the large bowel to produce active derivatives and so have little small intestinal effect	Can cause abdominal cramps. Should be avoided in patients with intestinal obstruction
	Dantron	Absorbed from the small bowel and undergoes first-pass hepatic metabolism to glucuronide forms. These may be secreted in the bile and converted to the active drug prolonging its action	Dantron is available only combined with a surfactant softener, e.g. co-danthramer with poloxamer, or co-danthrusate with docusate. Dantron-containing preps are subject to licence evidence from animal studies that in high doses it can cause tumours. It is licensed for use in analgesic-induced constipation in terminally ill patients. Dantron may colour urine red. It should be avoided in patients who may be incontinent of urine or faeces, as it can cause severe rashes if it comes in contact with the skin
Peripheral opioid antagonists	**Methylnal-trexone**	Displaces opioids from GI tract. Does not cross blood-brain barrier. Indication for laxative refractory opioid-induced constipation	Given by SC injection 8–12mg depending on weight. Average time to response 30–60 min after dose. Newly introduced. Further preparations in clinical trial

Table 6b.5 Onset of action

• Bisacodyl tablet	10–12h	• Laxoberal	10–14h
• Bisacodyl supps	20–60min	• Methylnaltrexone	30–60min
• Dantron	6–12h	• Microlax enema	20min
• Docusate	24–48h	• Phosphate enema	20min
• Glycerin supps	1–6h	• Senna	8–12h
• Lactulose	48h	• Sodium picosulfate	min

Diarrhoea

Diarrhoea is a less common symptom than constipation amongst patients requiring palliative care and has been defined as the passage of more than three unformed stools within a 24h period.

As with constipation, patients can understand 'diarrhoea' in different ways and clarification of the term is always required.

Up to 10% of patients admitted to a hospice complain of diarrhoea. (In contrast, 27% of HIV-infected patients are reported as having diarrhoea).

Treatment of diarrhoea

A **cause** for the diarrhoea should be looked for prior to giving anti-diarrhoeal agents (Table 6b.6). The presence of fever or blood in the stool should prompt further discussion to ensure the most appropriate treatment.

General measures
- Increase fluid intake, constant sipping
- Reassurance that most diarrhoea is self-limiting

Management
Treat or exclude any speciafic causes

The most common causes of diarrhoea in the palliative care setting

1 **Imbalance of laxative therapy.** (Especially when laxatives have been increased to clear severe constipation.) Diarrhoea should settle within 24h if laxatives are stopped. Laxatives should be reintroduced at a lower dose.

2 **Drugs** such as antibiotics and antacids, NSAIDs or iron preparations.

3 **Faecal impaction** is associated with fluid stool which leaks past a faecal plug or a tumour mass.

4 **Radiotherapy** involving the abdomen or pelvis is likely to cause diarrhoea especially in the second or third week of therapy.

5 **Malabsorption** associated with:
   • *Carcinoma* of the head of the pancreas with insufficient pancreatic secretions thus less fat absorption and resultant steatorrhoea
   • *Gastrectomy* resulting in poor mixing of food with pancreatic secretions and consequent resultant steatorrhoea. Vagotomy can cause increased water secretion into the colon
   • *Ileal resection* reduces the ability of the small intestine to reabsorb bile acids. These acids increase fluid in the colon and contribute to explosive diarrhoea. A resection of over 100cm of terminal ileum will outstretch the liver's capacity to compensate for the bile salt loss, and fat malabsorption will compound the diarrhoea
   • *Colectomy*, immediately following surgery for a total or a near total colectomy, the water in the gut cannot be adequately absorbed. Although this tends to settle over a week, the bowel seldom returns to its pre-surgical function. The small intestine is unable to adequately compensate for the loss of this colonic water-absorbing capacity. This can lead to an ongoing daily loss of an extra 400–1000mL of gut fluid rectally. Such patients often require an ileostomy and need an extra litre of fluid and 7g of extra salt a day with vitamin and iron supplements

6 **Colonic or rectal tumours** can cause diarrhoea through causing partial bowel obstruction or through increased mucus secretion

7 **Rare endocrine tumours** which secrete hormones cause diarrhoea, e.g. carcinoid tumour

8 Concurrent disease such as gastrointestinal infection e.g. *Clostridium difficile*

9 Odd dietary habits

Diagnostic diarrhoea patterns

Defaecation described as 'diarrhoea' happening only two or three times a day without warning suggests anal incontinence

Profuse watery stools are characteristic of colonic diarrhoea

Sudden onset of diarrhoea after a period of constipation raises suspicion of faecal impaction

Alternating diarrhoea and constipation suggests poorly regulated laxative therapy or impending bowel obstruction

Pale, fatty, offensive stools (steatorrhoea) indicate malabsorption due to either pancreatic or ileal disease

Table 6b.6 Cause management

Subacute small bowel obstruction	See intestinal obstruction
Laxatives (including self-administered magnesium-containing antacids)	Discontinue and review
Faecal impaction (with anal leakage or incontinence)	Rectal disimpaction/manual evacuation/macrogol
Antibiotic-associated diarrhoea/pseudomembranous colitis (recent or broad-spectrum antibiotics)	Check stool for *Clostridium difficile* (metronidazole 400mg t.d.s. for 7–14 days) vancomycin 125mg q.d.s
Radiotherapy-induced	Ondansetron, aspirin, colestyramine
NSAID	Try stopping or changing NSAID
Misoprostol	Use a PPI or other alternative
Pre-existing disease, e.g. Crohn's or ulcerative colitis	Corticosteroids or sulfasalazine
Ileal resection (causing bile salt diarrhoea)	Colestyramine
Steatorrhoea/fat malabsorption	Pancreatic enzymes ±PPI (reduces gastric acid destruction of enzymes)
Carcinoid syndrome	$5HT_3$ antagonists, octreotide
Zollinger–Ellison syndrome	H_2 antagonist, e.g. ranitidine
Non-specific profuse secretory diarrhoea	Opioids such as loperamide, codeine and morphine may be necessary (loperamide is not absorbed)

The somatostatin analogue octreotide has a place in the management of severe, profuse, secretory diarrhoea, such as that associated with HIV infection when other agents have failed to work. It is best given by CSCI.

Intestinal obstruction

This most commonly occurs with carcinoma of the ovary or bowel. The obstruction may be intramural, intraluminal or extraluminal due to surrounding peritoneal disease, and is often at multiple sites. In addition, there is often a clinical obstruction in the absence of a mechanical lesion (functional obstruction).

A plain abdominal X-ray may be helpful in excluding constipation.

> If surgical intervention is inappropriate, symptomatic measures using medication are the mainstay of treatment, avoiding the standard 'drip and suck' approach, which may be distressing and is ineffective in 80% of patients.

- In the presence of advanced peritoneal disease, the most likely cause of obstruction is due to malignant tumour. The cause may also be due, however, to benign factors such as adhesions
- If the patient is fit enough, a surgical opinion should be sought and the advantages and disadvantages of laparotomy assessed
- The potential mortality and morbidity associated with surgery should be weighed against quality of life in a patient whose prognosis may only be predicted to be a few weeks or months
- If the obstruction is incomplete or mainly functional, it may resolve. It may therefore be helpful in the first place to try:

Reducing bowel wall oedema
Using: dexamethasone 8–16mg SC before midday
The evidence for such an approach is equivocal, but if a 3-day trial proves beneficial and vomiting subsides it may be useful to consider continuing with reducing doses of oral steroids. Whether improvement is due to steroids or to the passage of time remains the subject of debate.

If dexamethasone is not helpful after three days it should be stopped (unless the patient has been on long-term steroids (more than a week) in which case it should be tailed off slowly).

Stimulating gut motility
Metoclopramide 30–120mg/24h via subcutaneous infusion. Beware of any increase in gut colic and stop if obstruction is not resolving.

For complete obstruction or obstruction not resolving with the above measures in 24–48h, focus on treating the symptoms rather than the underlying cause:
- **Nausea and vomiting:**
  - cyclizine 100–150mg/24h CSCI
  - ± haloperidol 3–5mg/24h CSCI
  - or levomepromazine 6.25–25mg/24h CSCI
  - consider ondansetron 8–24 mg/24h p.o., IV or SC

- **Colic:**
  - hyoscine butylbromide 40–100mg/24h CSCI (morphine may also be needed for background pain)
- **Diarrhoea:**
  - codeine 30–60mg p.o. 4 h, or
  - loperamide 2–4mg p.o. 4 h. *Use with* **caution** *if possibility of reversible obstruction*
- **Constipation:**
  - ensure that reversible constipation is not contributing to the obstruction. Gentle rectal measures or a small dose of a faecal softener such as docusate may be used, particularly if there is no colic and obstruction is thought to be colonic and subacute. More vigorous measures should be avoided for fear of aggravating symptoms

If intestinal obstruction is still not resolving

- Reduce or encourage reabsorption of gut secretions and reduce intestinal motility using:
  - hyoscine butylbromide (Buscopan) 40–100mg/24h CSCI octreotide 300–600 mcg/24h CSCI
- Nasogastric tube
  - *If* vomiting is not subsiding, or *if* very distressing and/or faecal, it may be necessary to use a nasogastric tube after full discussion with patient and carers. Although this is an infrequent practice in a hospice setting, and can be seen as a very undignified approach to patient care, it can bring comfort in exceptional circumstances
- Venting gastrostomy
  - with occasional, clinically stable patients who are distressed by vomiting but who have a prognosis of at least weeks, and who are keen to resume oral intake, it *may* be an option to discuss venting gastrostomy and subcutaneous fluids.[13] In practice, venting gastrostomies are rarely performed

13 Roila F., *et al.*(1996) Comparative studies of various antiemetic regimes. *Supportive Care in Cancer*, **4**: 270–80

Hiccup

Definition: Spasmodic contraction of the diaphragm that causes a sudden breath in, cut off when the vocal cords snap together, creating the characteristic sound

Hiccups result from diaphragmatic spasms caused by diaphragmatic irritation, which is often associated with liver enlargement or gastric distension.

Causes
- Via vagus nerve
  - gastric distension
  - gastritis/gastro-oesophageal reflux
  - hepatic tumours
  - ascites/abdominal distension/intestinal obstruction
- Via phrenic nerve
  - diaphragmatic tumour involvement
  - mediastinal tumour
  - CNS causes including intracranial tumours, especially brainstem lesions and meningeal infiltration by cancer
- Systemic
  - renal failure
  - corticosteroids
  - Addison's disease
  - hyponatraemia

Management of hiccup
Pharyngeal stimulation is effected in a number of ways. The soft palate can be massaged, the patient can try eating dry granulated sugar or holding their breath or rebreathing into a bag, etc. These measures are often effective, at least temporarily. Alternatively:
- Reduce gastric distension:
  - prokinetic drugs, e.g.
    —metoclopramide 10mg q.d.s.
    —domperidone 10mg q.d.s.
  - gastric distension may also improve with a change to small but frequent meals and using a defoaming antiflatulant with an antacid, such as activated dimeticone and aluminium hydroxide (Asilone) 5–10mL q.d.s.
- Relax smooth muscle:
  - nifedipine 5mg p.r.n. or regularly t.d.s., p.o. may be effective
  - baclofen 5mg t.d.s. is an alternative
- **Suppress central hiccup reflex:** If symptoms are severe and not responding to other measures including pharyngeal stimulation it may be necessary to give:
  - chlorpromazine 25mg p.o. Intravenous administration may cause sedation and hypotension and is only used in intractable cases

- **suppress central irritation from intracranial tumour:** This may respond to dexamethasone (starting with high doses, e.g. 16mg daily) or to an anticonvulsant, e.g. phenytoin 200–300mg given at night. **Note**: Corticosteroids can also cause hiccups—consider stopping if recently started.

Anorexia/cachexia/asthenia

Primary anorexia is the absence or loss of appetite for food.

Cachexia (📖 See Chapter 6c) is a condition of profound weight loss and catabolic loss of muscle and adipose tissue. It is often associated with primary anorexia and fatigue.

Asthenia(📖 See Chapter 6c) is characterized by:
- Fatigue or easy tiring and reduced sustainability of performance
- Generalized weakness resulting in a reduced ability to initiate movement
- Mental fatigue characterized by poor concentration, impaired memory and emotional lability[14]

Secondary anorexia is often due to several conditions that may be reversible and should be actively sought:
- Dyspepsia
- Altered taste
- Malodour
- Nausea and vomiting
- Sore mouth
- Pain
- Biochemical:
  - hypercalcaemia; uraemia; hyponatnemia; gastric stasis
- Gastric stasis
- Constipation
- Secondary to treatment:
  - drugs; radiotherapy; chemotherapy
- Anxiety
- Depression

Early satiety (patient hungry but then feels full) occurs with a small stomach, hepatomegaly and gross ascites. Anxiety and depression will contribute to loss of appetite. Patients are 'put off' by too much food and food which is unappetizing.

These symptoms, which are closely interrelated, occur in about 70% of patients with advanced cancer, particularly gastric and pancreatic cancer.

Management
- Assess and treat any reversible causes as outlined above
- Involve the dietician and multidisciplinary team to maximize treatment goals
- Non-drug treatment:
  - explore the patients' and carers' fears of anorexia
  - reassure patients that it is normal to feel satisfied with less food
  - consider if advice on food fortification/supplementation would be appropriate for this patient at this point of their illness
  - suggest smaller helpings to allow patients to eat frequently small amounts of what they enjoy
- Evidence-based drug treatments:
  - **corticosteroids,** e.g. dexamethasone 2–4mg o.d.
    - appetite stimulant, and may help nausea
    - may improve subjective feeling of anorexia and weakness
    - non-specific central euphoric effects

- effects generally short lasting (weeks)
- onset of side-effects rapid
- **progestogens,** e.g. megestrol acetate 160–800mg o.d.
  - improves appetite, nutritional status and calorie intake
  - take 2–3 weeks to produce effect
  - associated with modest weight gain, (though not gain in lean body mass)
  - effects may last for months
  - increased incidence of thrombotic episodes
  - expensive
- **prokinetic drugs,** e.g. metoclopramide 10mg q.d.s.
  - try if early satiety, gastric stasis (many patients with malignancy have associated autonomic dysfunction)

Total parenteral nutrition (☐ See Chapter 10c)

In the case of total parenteral nutrition (TPN) in the palliative care setting, some studies have shown an association with survival shortened with the introduction of TPN.

Universal benefit and efficacy have not been clearly proven with TPN and its routine use is not recommended in view of this, the practical disadvantage and the risk of side-effects and complications.

Aggressive nutritional therapy could perhaps be justified in particular situations such as when patients are recovering from surgery or awaiting chemotherapy.

Hydration (☐ See Chapter 1)

There is often an overwhelming need for relatives and staff to give dying patients food and water, but this must not be allowed to override the patients' need for comfort.

Avoiding overhydration in a dying patient may improve comfort, by minimizing urinary output (and therefore the need for catheterization) and the volume of distressing bronchial secretions. In bowel obstruction gastric secretions will be minimized, thereby reducing the frequency of vomiting and the need for a nasogastric tube. A dry mouth can be treated with local measures.

In contrast, those patients who may survive for many months but who are unable to swallow adequately may find life easier with, for instance, a percutaneous gastrostomy tube. However, when these patients are dying it is necessary to explain to the relatives why it may be helpful to reduce fluid input.[14]

14 Woof R. (1998) Asthenia, cachexia and anorexia. In *Handbook of Palliative Care* (ed. C. Faull, *et al.*). Oxford: Blackwell.

Ascites

The healthy adult has about 50mL transudate in the peritoneal cavity. This has a protein level of about 25% of that found in plasma. Peritoneal fluid turnover is 4–5mL/h in health.

Malignant ascites

- Malignant ascites accounts for about 10% of all cases of ascites and occurs in up to 50% of all patients with cancer
- Malignant ascitic fluid is an exudate with a protein content of about 85% of that found in plasma. This protein-rich fluid is an excellent culture medium for malignant cells and bacteria. It may also have high levels of certain enzymes
- In malignant ascites, the ascitic fluid turnover can be twenty-fold of that found in healthy individuals
- Ascites may be the presenting feature of the malignancy or it may be indicative of a recurrence or metastatic spread. It is often indicative of end-stage disease
- It is caused by malignant peritoneal deposits, blockage of subdiaphragmatic lymphatics and secondary sodium retention

Causes

Malignant ascites

- Ovarian primary (50% of cases)
- Unknown primary (20% of cases)
- Stomach, colon, pancreatic primary (most of the remainder)

Non-malignant ascites

- Cardiac failure, liver failure and renal failure are common causes of non-malignant ascites, accounting for 90% of cases
- The significance of this for patients with palliative care needs is that ascites should not automatically be attributed to underlying malignancy
- Management options, however, are similar for both malignant and non-malignant disease

Management

Treatment of the primary cancer, usually with chemotherapy, may be the most effective measure to reduce ascites. Analgesics and good symptom control may be all that is necessary, particularly for a patient who is bed-bound and has a short prognosis.

Diuretics may alleviate symptoms over several days. Doses must be adequate and include a combination of spironolactone (100mg b.d. and possibly higher) and a loop diuretic, e.g. furosemide (40–80mg o.d.).

Patients with liver metastases are more likely to respond to diuretics; paracentesis will provide more immediate relief (see below).

A peritoneovenous shunt could be considered and inserted under general or local anaesthesia.

Shunts comprise a multi-perforated catheter in the peritoneal cavity which joins to a one-way valve positioned subcutaneously just above the costal margin. From here ascitic fluid is drained into the superior vena cava via a tunnelled catheter which enters the external or internal jugular vein. Fluid flows through the shunt on inspiration.

Patients are encouraged to pump the reservoir to keep fluid flowing through the shunt. The two commonest shunts in use (Denver and LeVeen) have similar performance profiles. Results from the use of such shunts have been mixed as they are prone to blockage.

Paracentesis

General

Paracentesis is a simple procedure, which can be performed as a day case (usually only removing 2–4 litres maximum), or as an inpatient.

- In tense, symptomatic ascites there may be up to 12 litres of ascites present
- Removal of 4–6 litres is usually enough to give symptomatic relief
- Removal of more than 4–6 litres increases the risk of hypovolaemia and adverse effects, but may give symptom relief for longer until the ascites re-accumulates
- For an ill, elderly patient, small-volume paracentesis repeated as needed may be preferable

Indications

- Pain, discomfort or tightness due to stretching of the abdominal wall
- Dyspnoea, usually exacerbated by exertion, due to upward pressure on the diaphragm
- Nausea, vomiting and dyspepsia due to the 'squashed stomach' syndrome
- Patients are usually symptomatic only when the abdominal wall is tensely distended. Patients who are also bothered by ankle (or generalized) oedema, may fare better with diuretic therapy

Complications of paracentesis

- After a large-volume paracentesis, the compensatory large-fluid shifts from circulating volume into extracellular fluid can decompensate the patient's cardiovascular system leading to hypovolaemia, and in severe cases, collapse and renal failure
- A low albumin or sodium level will exacerbate this effect
- The cannula site may continue to leak ascites after removal
- If a limited, partial paracentesis has been performed, this may rarely become a continuing leak over days to weeks (use colostomy bag to collect leakage)
- The patient needs to be warned about possible leaking which may otherwise cause distress
- Bowel perforation is a risk, especially if intestinal obstruction is present
- Infection is a rare complication providing an aseptic technique is used

Investigations prior to paracentesis
- An ultrasound scan will confirm the presence of ascites, and may determine if it is 'pocketed' by tumour adhesions
- A scan should be performed if:
  - ascites is not easily clinically identified
  - there is a chance of bowel obstruction
- A serum albumin and U&E should be taken if:
  - more than 4–6 litres is to be removed and the patient has oedema, *or*
  - the patient is clinically dehydrated *or*
  - the patient has reacted badly to a previous paracentesis
- A platelet count and clotting screen should be measured in at-risk patients

Contraindications to paracentesis
- Local or systemic infection
- Coagulopathy—platelets <40 × 10^9/L or INR >1.4
- Limit paracentesis to 4–6 litres maximum if:
  - hepatic or renal failure (creatinine >250mmol/L)
  - albumin <30g/L or sodium <125mmol/L

Follow-up care to paracentesis
- Ascites will usually re-form after a paracentesis; however, this can vary between one and many weeks
- Diuretics may reduce the rate of re-accumulation, or may prevent it becoming as tense again
- Repeated paracentesis on an as-needed basis is appropriate management for patients with advanced cancer

The procedure of paracentesis
- The patient should be asked to pass urine before the procedure
- Blood pressure should be measured and recorded
- The patient should lie in a semi-recumbent position
- It may be helpful if the patient tilts 30 degrees towards the side of the paracentesis
- Use left iliac fossa unless local disease is present, avoiding scars and inferior epigastric artery (🕮 see Fig. 6b.2)
- Confirm that the site is dull to percussion
- Using an aseptic technique, anaesthetize the skin locally
- **If ascitic fluid cannot be easily located using the anaesthetic infiltrating needle, stop and reconsider**
- A large-bore intravenous cannula or 'Bonanno' catheter can be used
- Avoid clamping the catheter if possible, since malignant ascites can be very proteinaceous and is likely to block it

Large volume paracentesis (>6 litres)
If it is intended to drain to dryness, or >6 litres:
- Stop diuretics (if used solely for ascites) 48h before procedure
- Check blood pressure and pulse every 30 min. during paracentesis, then hourly for 6h
- Some units give plasma substitutes such as intravenous dextran-70 or gelatin infusion (e.g. Gelofusine), 150mL for every litre of ascites drained, during the paracentesis or shortly afterwards in order to reduce hypovolaemia

Note: There is little evidence about paracentesis and hence it is hard to be doctrinaire about it. Our own units' practice is to drain two litres per nursing shift (i.e. up to 6 litres/day) for up to 48 hours (making a possible total drainage volume of 12 litres), the catheter being clamped after each two litres has been obtained. At this rate of removal, routine blood pressure recordings are not found to be necessary. Although catheters certainly can block when clamped, this is not found to be a sufficiently frequent problem to make us use a different procedure. The use of plasma substitutes still occurs occasionally, however it is expensive and without supporting evidence in a palliative context.

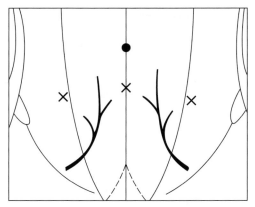

Fig. 6b.2 Usual sites for paracentesis, avoiding the inferior epigastric arteries.

Tenesmus and tenesmoid pain

Tenesmus is the painful sensation of rectal fullness, usually caused by local rectal tumour. There may be an associated spasm of smooth muscle, or neuropathic pain from lumbosacral plexus infiltration causing stabbing or more continuous pain. It may be difficult to distinguish from pudendal neuralgia.

Management

- Prevent and treat constipation
- Opioid analgesia may be helpful but not reliably so
- NSAID, e.g. diclofenac 50mg t.d.s.
- Radiotherapy
- Nifedipine m/r 10–20mg b.d.
- Co-analgesics as for neuropathic pain
- Amitriptyline
- Anticonvulsants
- Corticosteroids
- Lumbar sympathectomy: >80% success rate
- Spinal infusion of local anaesthetic ± opioids

Dyspepsia

Gastro-oesophageal reflux/oesophagitis (GORD)
Assessment
- Exclude or treat oesophageal candida infection
- Consider oesophageal spasm
- Avoid drugs which cause oesophagitis—potassium, NSAIDs
- Consider pain of cardiac origin

Treatment
- Raise head of bed to reduce acid reflux
- Consider paracentesis for tense ascites
- Metoclopramide 10mg t.d.s. if signs of gastric stasis or distension
- Antacid, e.g. Gaviscon Advance 5–10mL q.d.s. for mild symptoms
- PPI, e.g. lansoprazole 30mg daily for moderate or severe symptoms; start with treatment dose then step-down after a few weeks

NSAID and steroid-related dyspepsia
Treatment of drug-related dyspepsia
- Consider stopping or reducing dose of NSAID/steroids
- PPI, e.g. lansoprazole 30mg o.d. for severe symptoms or proven pathology. Start with treatment dose and reduce after four weeks. For milder symptoms start with maintenance dose (15mg) and increase later if needed
- If symptoms persist on treatment dose of PPI, and NSAID needed by the patient to control pain, consider changing to nabumetone, which has a relatively favourable gastrointestinal safety profile in comparison with other NSAIDs and has not been associated with the cardiac adverse effects of selective COX-2 inhibitors[15]

Indications for prophylaxis
- Prescribing NSAID with recent history of dyspepsia
- Prescribing steroids with recent history of dyspepsia
- Co-prescribing NSAID with steroids, anticoagulants, or aspirin
- Prescribing NSAID in elderly patient >70 years (less clear evidence—use judgement)

Drugs for dyspepsia
Proton pump inhibitors (PPIs)
- There is little difference in efficacy between the current PPIs available
- A single daily dose is appropriate for PPIs rather than divided doses
- Lansoprazole and omeprazole can be taken before or after food with equal efficacy

15 Hedner T., *et al.* (2004) Nabumetone: therapeutic use and safety profile in the management of osteoarthritis and rheumatoid arthritis. *Drugs*, **64**(20): 2315–43; discussion 2344–5.

Despite the variations in dose recommendations in the product literature, omeprazole, lansoprazole and pantoprazole display similar dose–
response relationships with similar potency at the same milligram doses.
Daily doses of 15–20mg PPI are appropriate for maintenance therapy,
prophylaxis, or less severe gastro-oesophageal reflux disease. Doses of
30–40mg daily are appropriate for treatment.

Antacids

Aluminium-containing antacids cause constipation whereas magnesium-
containing antacids are laxative. Dimeticone in Asilone is a defoamer,
useful for gastric distension/hiccups.

Prostaglandin analogues

Misoprostol is effective at preventing NSAID-induced ulcers, but is
less well tolerated than PPIs, and diarrhoea is a common side-effect.
Misoprostol is available in combination with diclofenac, which avoids the
problem of non-compliance that can arise when the gastroprotective drug
is given separately from the NSAID.

H_2 antagonists

H_2 antagonists are less effective at acid suppression than PPIs, and are less
effective clinically at healing ulcers. Ranitidine has significantly fewer drug
interactions and adverse effects than cimetidine.

Gastrointestinal bleeding

Gastric bleeding and melaena

Assessment

Consider the commonest causes:
- Tumour bleeding
- Clotting disorders
- Peptic ulcer ±NSAIDs

Management considerations for gastrointestinal bleeding

- Review or stop NSAIDs, aspirin, corticosteroids, warfarin
- Commence PPI in treatment dose, e.g. lansoprazole 30mg o.d. when able to take orally
- Blood tests for clotting screen and platelets and treat if appropriate
- Consider radiotherapy referral if bleeding due to tumour
- Tranexamic acid 1–2g t.d.s. p.o. (or by slow IV until able to take p.o.)
  - stop if no effect after one week
  - continue for one week after bleeding has stopped, then discontinue
  - only continue long term (500mg t.d.s.) if bleeding recurs
  - avoid tranexamic acid with history of thromboembolism/CVA, etc.
- Small bleeds can herald a larger haemorrhage:
  - consider siting an iv cannula to administer emergency drugs
- Intravenous high-dose PPI, e.g. omeprazole 80mg IV stat., then 8mg/h IV infusion
- Arterial embolization
- Oral sucralfate
- Octreotide is an accepted medical management for bleeding from oesophageal or colonic varices. Circumstantial evidence indicates that the actions of octreotide are mainly mediated by a splanchnic vasoconstrictive effect, possibly with gastric acid suppression and enhancement of platelet aggregation. It is uncertain whether it has a role in gastrointestinal bleeding of other aetiology
- Etamsylate

Rectal bleeding

Assessment

Consider the commonest causes:
- Tumour bleeding
- Clotting disorders
- Pelvic infection
- Haemorrhoids

NSAIDs can cause lower gastrointestinal bleeding as well as the better-documented upper GI bleeding.

Treatment

- Review or stop NSAIDs
- Treat any evidence or signs suggestive of pelvic infection
- Consider radiotherapy referral
- Blood tests for clotting screen and platelets and treat as appropriate

- Tranexamic acid 1–2g t.d.s. p.o. (or by slow IV until able to take p.o.)
  - stop if no effect after one week
  - continue for one week after bleeding has stopped, then discontinue
  - only continue long term (500mg t.d.s.). if bleeding recurs
  - avoid tranexamic acid with history of thromboembolism/CVA, etc.
- Small bleeds can herald a larger haemorrhage
- Consider siting an IV cannula to administer emergency drugs
- Arterial embolization
- Etamsylate
- Oral sucralfate for post-radiation proctitis applied topically

Major gastrointestinal or rectal bleeding

If patient's condition is not stable, with history of major haemorrhage or ongoing bleeding:

- Consider if the patient should be transferred to an acute medical/endoscopy unit
- Site an IV cannula to anticipate need for emergency drugs

Treat anxiety or distress as needed:

- Midazolam 2–5mg initially by slow IV titration (diluted 10mg in 10mL with saline)
- If no IV access, midazolam 5–10mg SC (or IM if shocked/vasoconstricted)

The case for PPIs in gastrointestinal bleeding

- Acid suppression in early studies did not help in the management of acute bleeding
- It has more recently been shown that intensive therapy aimed at achieving complete acid suppression does substantially reduce the risk of recurrent bleeding after initial endoscopic treatment
- Pharmacokinetic studies have shown that a bolus of 80mg pantoprazole or omeprazole followed by immediate continuous infusion of 8mg/h will result in an intragastric pH of 7 within 20 minutes. This has been continued for 72h in studies[16]

Support for patient and family

Bleeding is very frightening. Ensure that the patient and family are well supported. Ensure that drugs are readily available for sedation if necessary and that dark bed linen (to disguise the amount of blood loss) is accessible

16 Lau J. Y., et al. (2000). Effect of intravenous omeprazole on recurrent bleeding after endoscopic treatment of bleeding peptic ulcers. New England Journal of Medicine, **343**: 310–16.

Bowel stoma care

A bowel stoma is an artificial opening, created surgically, to allow faeces to leave the patient's body by a new route through a spout or outlet on their abdomen.

The majority of stomas encountered in patients with palliative care needs have been fashioned following surgical resection for cancer, or as a bypass for inoperable or recurrent cancers of the bowel or ovary causing obstruction.

Any patient with a stoma (whether newly created or created many years ago, e.g. in Crohn's disease) and malignant intra-abdominal disease is at risk of a number of different symptoms which need appropriate management. These include abdominal pain (constant or intermittent colic), nausea, vomiting, abdominal distension, constipation, diarrhoea and depression, all of which may impact on the holistic management of the patient.

Bowel stomas are generally created from the colon (colostomy) or ileum (ileostomy). The bowel proximal to the stoma continues to function in the normal way whereas function distal to this is normally lost.

Temporary (de-functioning) stomas

These include loop ileostomies or colostomies, which are usually created to protect an anastomosis or to facilitate decompression or healing in the distal bowel. The bowel loop is usually brought out onto the abdominal wall (right and left iliac fossa respectively for ileostomy and colostomy) and may be supported by a temporary rod or bridge so that it does not retract. The proximal opening allows the passage of stool which is collected in a stoma bag, and the distal opening leads to the redundant section of bowel. Mucus and old faeces may be expelled through the rectum. A temporary transverse colostomy may be created at an emergency operation for bowel obstruction since it is a relatively easy procedure in a sick patient.

Permanent stomas

These are end sections of bowel which are brought to the skin surface. The potential stoma site along the path of the bowel is planned pre-operatively, if possible, to allow optimal positioning of a stoma bag for the individual.

- Panproctocolectomy—a permanent ileostomy is created from the terminal ileum. The rectum and anus are removed
- Total colectomy—an ileostomy is formed and the rectal stump is retained which may be brought out onto the abdominal wall as a mucus fistula
- Abdominoperineal (A–P) excision—here the rectum and anus are removed leaving a colostomy in the left iliac fossa
- Hartmann's procedure—procedure for excision of sigmoid colon or upper rectum. An end colostomy is formed and the rectal stump is closed and left in the pelvis
- Pelvic exenteration—a radical operation removing pelvic organs. A colostomy and urostomy are formed. Men are likely to become impotent. An artificial vagina can be created for a woman

Issues in stoma management

The stool consistency of a sigmoid colostomy is no different from that passed naturally in health through the anus. The stool is less formed the further proximal in the colon the colostomy is. The formation of an ileostomy or colostomy should not in itself interfere with sexual function unless the definitive surgery interfered with the pelvic nerve supply.

Stoma appliances and problems

Stoma appliances are disposable, self-adhesive and skin-friendly. The type of appliance used is determined by several factors which include the shape and position of the stoma itself, including body contours, the type of effluent, skin type and the needs of the individual such as lifestyle and ability to self-care. Adequate adherence, comfort and skin protection are paramount.

Ileostomy appliances are drainable for ease of emptying semi-formed/liquid stool. Modern appliances have integral Velcro-type closures. The bags are emptied several times a day and changed every 1–3 days.

- Colostomy appliances may be in one piece, such that the whole appliance needs removing every time the bag needs changing. Alternatively, a two-piece appliance is used which allows the flange to remain in position for several days, allowing the non-drainable bag to be changed as necessary, thus protecting the skin from the trauma of frequent changes
- The flange size should be cut to fit accurately around the base of the stoma. The peristomal skin must be kept healthy and intact
- A stoma usually shrinks in size during the first few months but should always retain the bright-red colour, indicating a good blood supply
- Checks for colour, odour, consistency and volume should be made routinely

Psychological care

Enjoyment, comfort and satisfaction with life for the patient and his/her family need support from healthcare professionals, giving adequate time for answering questions and responding to needs. Frequently, patients have a short prognosis and the stoma is a visible daily reminder of this. In addition, they may be distressed by a feeling of no longer being in control. They have to learn new skills at a time when it is important to be concentrating on other more important issues, and they may be having to adapt reluctantly to relying on others for care. Relationships with family, friends and particularly spouses may be affected.

Overactive stoma

A cause may need to be identified and treated. Diet may need to be altered until overactivity settles. Foods such as cooked white rice and stewed apple may help. Marshmallows and 'jelly babies' may help in thickening the output from an ileostomy. Extra fluids orally should be encouraged to maintain hydration, especially in hot weather. A drainable bag may be necessary temporarily for a colostomy if the output is liquid. Some medication, particularly longer acting modified-release preparations, e.g. MST, enteric-coated drugs and capsules, may not be absorbed adequately and are not recommended with ileostomies.

Loperamide (taken 45 min before meals) in the form of 'melts' or tablets but not capsules may be helpful in patients with an ileostomy.

If all else fails, systemic opioids and antisecretory agents may be needed. (📖 See the section on diarrhoea, p. 324).

Constipation

A cause should be sought where possible, and may include medication, particularly opioids, partial/complete bowel obstruction and dehydration. It may be necessary to instil warm arachis oil (only 5mL for a short time) through a Foley catheter with the balloon inflated to aid enema retention. The patient will usually be turned on the right side if the stoma is in the left iliac fossa to allow oil to flow across the transverse colon. The oil may cause difficulties with flange adhesion and the possibility of nut allergy should always be considered. Suppositories, phosphate and Microlax micro-enemas may also be useful. As a general rule, bulking aperients such as ispaghula husk (Fybogel) are not used in palliative care.

Odour

This is rarely a problem with modern appliances which contain charcoal filters. Proprietary stoma deodorizing agents are available. A few drops of vanilla essence placed in a bowel stoma bag may help, while topical metronidazole may be helpful for offensive fungating tumours in the region of the stoma.

Bleeding

Stomas may bleed due to clotting deficiencies and fungating tumours. Wafers of Kaltostat soaked in tranexamic acid or adrenaline may help with local pressure. Silver nitrate may be used for oozing granulation tissue. Bleeding from local cancer growth may abate with radiotherapy or cryotherapy.

Skin excoriation

Skin excoriation is a rare occurrence with modern appliances and good skin care. Various preparations are available to aid skin protection, including pastes to make a level surface onto which an appliance can be fitted. This is particularly important in the case of an ileostomy, when damage to the skin from digestive enzymes must be avoided.

Flatulence

Flatulence can usually be minimized by avoiding various foods and medication such as lactulose.

A diet containing fibre such as porridge, root vegetables and brown bread is advised, although the terminally ill may not find these foods palatable. In relatively good health, most people with stomas can eat most foods, although certain food such as vegetables and fruit may cause an increase in stoma activity with embarrassing flatulence and odour. Camomile tea and peppermint tea or capsules may be helpful.

Enterocutaneous fistulae

Enterocutaneous fistulae may occur in 3% of patients with advanced malignant disease. Patients with gastrointestinal tumours and those who have had abdominal radiotherapy are most at risk. A dehisced wound may also need management with a stoma appliance. If the effluent is greater than 100mL per 24h a stoma appliance will probably be needed.

Meticulous preparation of the skin will be needed prior to applying an appliance. Suction may be needed while cleansing and preparing the fistula if there is excessive exudate, or it may need to be spigotted with a balloon catheter for a while. Various pastes, fillers and skin barriers may be needed to protect the skin and ensure a good fit to the edges of the wound. The stoma appliance may need to be adapted with time to take account of the change in size of the tumour and the weight loss of the patient.

Gastrostomy

A gastrostomy is used for the purpose of feeding when the patient is unable to swallow adequately or safely, such as those patients with motor neurone disease, or with head and neck cancers. A venting gastrostomy is occasionally used in a relatively fit patient with intestinal obstruction who wants to be able to eat. In this situation, the patient is able to take nutrients by mouth but food contents are expelled through the gastrostomy.

However, in patients with advanced disease, the decision to insert a gastrostomy has to be judged carefully. It is important to distinguish starvation, which responds to feeding, from cachexia, which does not respond to feeding alone. The latter is more likely in the presence of large tumour masses, certain tumour types or ongoing sepsis.

Types of gastrostomy

Percutaneous endoscopic gastrostomy (PEG)
Inserted under sedation and local anaesthetic using a 'pull' technique. Throughout its lifetime, the PEG tube should be rotated through 360° at least twice a week to prevent adhesion formation.

Radiologically inserted gastrostomy (RIG)
Inserted in the radiology department without sedation by a 'push' technique under fluoroscopic control. The tube is thinner than a PEG tube, and is held in place by its pigtail shape. It should **not** therefore be rotated, or it will dislodge.

Surgical gastrostomy
Carried out under general anaesthetic, usually when it is impossible to insert a PEG or RIG.

Care of the gastrostomy tube
The fixation plate should be maintained at 1–1.5cm from the abdominal exit stoma. A 50mL flush of sterile water should be used before and after every feed or administration of medication and regularly three times a day. Soda water, but not other fizzy drinks (they are too acidic) can be used to unblock stubborn blockages.[17]

Feeding
Patients should be maintained at an angle of 30–45° during feeding and for 2h after to reduce the risk of aspiration. Many centres are less keen for feeding to occur during sleep because of the aspiration risk.

Problems with gastrostomies
- Dislodgement
- Leakage: chemical digestion of surrounding skin
- Overgranulation
- Infection

A major concern with the use of PEG and RIG tubes in the UK involves ensuring that the best possible decision about when to insert a tube is taken.

Often the clinical team that asks for a tube to be inserted is different from the team which carries out the procedure, which in turn is different from the team who manage the tube once it has been inserted.

While tube insertion can play a crucial role for certain patients, especially where clear objectives for the intervention have been discussed and documented with the patient and family, figures show that a large percentage of patients die within weeks of tube insertion, perhaps before they have had time to gain benefit from the procedure and its management.

17 Rabeneck L., Wray P., Petersen N. J. (1996) Long-term outcomes of patients receiving per-cuta-neous endoscopic gastrostomy tubes. *Journal of General Internal Medicine*, **11**(5): 287–93

Further reading

Books

Doyle D., *et al.* (eds) (2004) *Oxford Textbook of Palliative Medicine* (3rd edn). Oxford: Oxford University Press.

Twycross R. (2001) *Symptom Management in Advanced Cancer*. 3rd edn. Oxford: Radcliffe Medical Press.

Watson M., Lucas C., Hoy A. (2006) *Adult Palliative Care Guidance* (2nd edn). London: The South West London and the Surrey, West Sussex and Hampshire Cancer Networks.

Articles

Baines M. J. (2000) Symptom control in advanced gastrointestinal cancer. *European Journal of Gastroenterology & Hepatology*, **12**: 375–9.

Becker *et al.* (2006) Malignant ascites: systematic review and guidelines for treatment. *European Journal of Cancer*, **42**: 589–97.

Coco C., *et al.* (2000) Use of a self-expanding stent in the palliation of rectal cancer recurrences. A report of three cases. *Surgical Endoscopy*, **14**(8): 708–11.

Culbert P., Gillett H., Ferguson A. (1998) Highly effective new oral therapy for faecal impaction. *British Journal of General Practice*, **48**: 1599–600.

Larkin P.J. (2008) The management of constipation in Palliative Care: Clinical practice recommendations. *Palliative Medicine*, **22**: 7: 796–808.

Mertadante S. (1992) Treatment of diarrhoea due to enterocolic fistula with octreotide in a terminal cancer patient. *Palliative Medicine*, **6**: 257–9.

Potter K. (2000) Surgical oncology of the pelvis: ostomy planning and management. *Journal of Surgical Oncology*, **73**(4): 237–42.

Stephenson J. (2002) The development of clinical guidelines on paracenteis for ascites related to malignancy. *Palliative Medicine*, **16**: 213–18.

Sykes N. (2008) Opioid-induced constipation. *European Journal of Palliative Care*. Supplement.

Cachexia, anorexia and fatigue

We must accept finite disappointment, but we must never lose infinite hope.

Martin Luther King, Jr

Background

The symptoms of weight loss and fatigue affect 70% of patients with advanced cancer, particularly gastric and pancreatic cancer. In addition these symptoms are common to many other patients with non-malignant chronic diseases. Apart from marked weight loss and lethargy, there is also an association with physical, emotional and mental symptoms and loss of motivation and social contact.

'Listless, sluggish, faint, despondent, apathetic, tired, slack, indifferent, paralysed', are some of the adjectives used by patients and some even describe the fatigue of advanced disease as 'pain', as it is so profound.

Cachexia and fatigue are multifactorial. They are seldom seen in isolation from other symptoms experienced by patients with advanced disease, thus adding to the disease burden.

Cancer has become more of a chronic rather than an acute illness, because of the improvements in its management. There is an increased awareness of the suffering caused by cachexia and fatigue but they still remain poorly recognized by clinicians. Advances in management have not kept pace with that for other common symptoms in advanced disease.

Definitions

Cancer-related fatigue is defined by the National Comprehensive Cancer Network as 'a persistent, subjective sense of tiredness related to cancer or cancer treatment that interferes with usual functioning.'[1] It has further been described in terms of:

Perceived energy, mental capacity, and psychological status. It rises over a continuum, ranging from tiredness to exhaustion. In contrast with the tiredness sometimes felt by the healthy individual, cancer-related fatigue is perceived as being of greater magnitude, disproportionate to activity or exertion, and not relieved by rest.[2]

---

1 Mock V., *et al.* (2000) NCCN Practice Guidelines for cancer-related fatigue. *Oncology (Huntington)*, **14**: 151–61.

2 Ahlberg K., *et al.* (2003) Assessment and management of cancer-related fatigue in adults. *Lancet*; **362**: 640–50.

Patients may describe fatigue **subjectively** in three dimensions:
Physical sensations—unusual tiredness, and decreased capacity for work
Affective sensations—decreased motivation, mood and energy
Cognitive sensations—decreased concentration and mental agility

Patients may describe fatigue **objectively** as a quantifiable decrease in physical or mental performance. These two experiences of fatigue may not be related, and patients may feel fatigued without any loss of objective performance and vice versa[1]

The Cancer Anorexia Cachexia Syndrome (CACS) is an involuntary loss of weight that is not caused simply by anorexia. The syndrome includes anaemia and immunosuppression along with a number of biochemical changes indicating some systemic effects of malignancy. Cachexia is a term derived from the Greek word *kakos*, meaning bad, and *hexis*, meaning condition.

The Cancer Anorexia Cachexia Syndrome (CACS)

- Weight loss (usually defined as more than 5% of premorbid weight in the previous six months)
- Cancer tumours produce cytokines, e.g. cachectin—TNF (tumour necrosis factor), interleukins I and VI, lipolytic hormones and PIF (proteolysis-inducing factor) which cause metabolic abnormalities such as lipolysis and protein catabolism
- Involves the progressive loss of lean and adipose tissue that is unrelated to anorexia and cannot be reversed by feeding
- It is commonly associated with anorexia (the absence or loss of appetite for food) and asthenia (a syndrome of physical fatigue, generalized weakness and mental fatigue)
- Affects over 80% of patients with advanced cancer and is a major contributor to cancer morbidity and mortality
- Occurs more commonly in solid tumours such as pancreas, lung, stomach, colorectal and oesophagus, but less frequently in carcinoma of the breast and prostate and haematological malignancies
- Creates a major source of distress to patients and families who often seek to reverse it by pressurizing the patient to eat more
- Has a negative psychological impact due to body image changes
- Is a constant reminder to patients of underlying disease
- Decreases social interaction and support
- Decreases ability to tolerate and respond to oncological treatments

Prevalence

Fatigue
- Approaching 100% of patients treated for cancer are affected by fatigue
- Patients report fatigue more commonly when they are undergoing chemotherapy or radiotherapy, or in the presence of advanced malignancy

Cachexia
- More than 80% of patients with advanced cancer are cachexic

Aetiology
Non-malignant causes of cachexia and fatigue all of which can also contribute to symptoms in advanced cancer (📖 see also Fig. 6c.1).

Infection	Metabolic and electrolyte disorders	Pharmacological toxicity
Anaemia		Cachexia due to HIV/ AIDS or progressive illness
Chronic hypoxia	Insomnia	
Neurological disorders	Malnutrition	Chronic pain
Psychogenic causes	Over-exertion	Dehydration

Reversible causes of 'secondary' anorexia should be actively sought and corrected as appropriate. They include:
- Dyspepsia
- Altered taste
- Malodour
- Nausea and vomiting
- Sore mouth
- Pain
- Biochemical
  - hypercalcaemia
  - hyponatraemia
  - uraemia
  - gastric stasis
- Constipation
- Secondary to treatment
  - Drugs
  - Radiotherapy
  - Chemotherapy
- Anxiety
- Depression

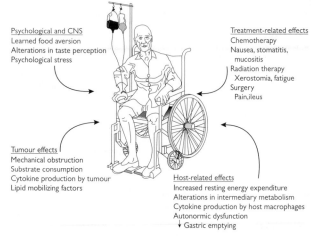

Psychological and CNS
Learned food aversion
Alterations in taste perception
Psychological stress

Treatment-related effects
Chemotherapy
  Nausea, stomatitis,
  mucositis
Radiation therapy
  Xerostomia, fatigue
Surgery
  Pain, ileus

Tumour effects
Mechanical obstruction
Substrate consumption
Cytokine production by tumour
Lipid mobilizing factors

Host-related effects
Increased resting energy expenditure
Alterations in intermediary metabolism
Cytokine production by host macrophages
Autonormic dysfunction
↓ Gastric emptying

Fig. 6c.1 Multifactorial causes of cancer fatigue and cachexia. From Bruera and Higginson (1996) Cachexia–Anorexia in Cancer Patients. Oxford University Press.

Metabolic effects

The metabolic changes seen in cachexia differ from those seen in starvation. In starvation, protein is conserved, energy expenditure reduced and fatty acids and ketones become a major source of energy. This contrasts with cancer cachexia where the resting energy expenditure is *increased* and both protein and fat are inefficiently utilized, in association with increased gluconeogenesis.

The reasons behind these metabolic changes are unknown, but postulated mechanisms may include the following:

• A non-specific response to the tumour or factors released by the tumour. The presence of a tumour may cause chronic stimulation of the body's inflammatory system leading to classic cachexic metabolic changes, including an increase in carbohydrate, fat and protein catabolism.

• Solid tumours metabolize glucose anaerobically and thus inefficiently, increasing the resting energy expenditure of the body

• The neuroendocrine axis appears to be important in the regulation of appetite

• There is evidence of increased insulin resistance in patients with cancer, and reduced glucose tolerance, perhaps caused by an imbalance of cortisol, insulin and glucagons

• An increase in protein turnover, particularly in skeletal muscle, is associated with the striking loss of lean muscle mass occurring in malignancy associated cachexia

• The acute phase response is the systemic response to inflammation or tissue damage occurring in trauma and sepsis, as well as cancer cachexia. This response appears to be mediated by cytokines.

The activity of this response has been shown to correlate with the development of cachexia in patients with malignancy (Fig. 6c.2)

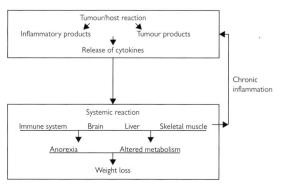

Fig. 6c.2 The systemic inflammatory response and cancer.

Management

Cachexia and fatigue can often be anticipated and various potentially correctable causes **actively** sought. A multidisciplinary approach maximizes the potential to improve symptoms.

National Comprehensive Cancer Network cancer-related fatigue guidelines propose the following:[1]

- Regular screening of patients using an instrument to evaluate degree of fatigue
- For those who describe mild fatigue, the subject is discussed and education provided. For those who describe moderate or severe fatigue a fuller, primary assessment is required, looking in particular for the presence of:
  - pain
  - emotional distress
  - sleep disturbance
  - anaemia
  - hypothyroidism

If such primary factors are detected, they should be treated according to practice guidelines.

If primary factors are not detected a *secondary* comprehensive assessment is advocated, with referral to other healthcare professionals as appropriate, including:

- Review of medications
- Assessment of co-morbidities, e.g.:
  - nutritional/metabolic evaluation
  - assessment of activity level

If specific causes (and therefore treatment) of fatigue and weakness cannot be found, symptomatic interventions should be considered.

Non-drug interventions
- There is a large body of evidence to suggest that a moderate exercise programme can improve functional capacity, reduce fatigue and also improve mood
- Nutritional advice—to eat when hungry, what is enjoyed, in frequent small amounts
- Pacing activity so that important activities can be carried out. Pacing allows gradual adaptation to lower levels of energy
- Promotion of good sleep hygiene
- Helping the family: listen to their concerns and explain cachexia. They may need to find other ways of expressing their love rather than being obsessional about quantities of food that can no longer be eaten and that will not alter prognosis, but may threaten to isolate patients who withdraw from the social interactions of mealtimes due to being put under pressure to eat.

Drug interventions

Corticosteroids (i.e. dexamethasone 4mg o.d.)
- Rapid onset of benefits within 2–3 days
- Role is limited by the rapid onset of side-effects (i.e. proximal myopathy, fluid retention and insulin resistance) and loss of effectiveness after only a few weeks
- They do not increase lean body mass
- They may be useful to improve appetite and well-being, particularly when prognosis is limited and a fast response is needed

Progestogens (i.e. megestrol acetate 160–320mg/day; medroxyprogesterone acetate 200mg t.d.s.)
- Onset of benefit may take up to two weeks
- Clear evidence of appetite improvement but less clear evidence of anything other than minimal weight gain. Fluid retention may be a problem
- Does not increase lean body mass
- Higher doses of progestogens above 800mg/day not noted to be more effective than lower doses
- Comparisons between corticosteroids and progestogens show no survival advantage, but more side-effects are noted with corticosteroids

Metoclopramide
- Useful in situations where there is gastric stasis
- Prokinetic action counteracts autonomic dysfunction—common in malignancy
- Reduces nausea

Erythropoietin

- For patients with anaemia, erythropoietin on a weekly basis has been shown to reduce fatigue
- It is unclear if the beneficial effect is due to the correction of the anaemia or to a direct erythropoietin effect on its receptors, which have been isolated in several different tissues including the brain
- Expensive treatment
- Most efficient dosage schedules still to be determined

Future treatment possibilities

There is growing understanding as to the complex nature of the pathophysiological basis of cachexia. Cytokine activity has been strongly implicated in much of the recent research. The cachexia-promoting cytokines are opposed by weight-promoting cytokines. However, the relationships are not straightforward and research is still exploring potential interventions. It may be that the specific causes of CACS in patients may respond best to specific treatments, but it is very unlikely that one solution will impact on all patients with CACS.

Both procatabolic and anticatabolic cytokine involvement, altered inflammatory responses, neuroendocrine effects and the interactions of both tumour and host will all have to be taken into account.

The causes of cachexia and fatigue are so multifactorial that it is now increasingly realized that the most potentially successful approach to treatment will require a multifactorial approach. Such work has been pioneered in Montreal in the Cancer Nutrition Rehabilitation programme where a small team of a dietician, therapists and palliative physicians have been working to impressive effect among patients with lung cancer, particularly those noted to have a high CRP level suggestive of an acute phase response.

Such a strategy requires an individualized response based on taking a careful clinical history and examination in order to decide which interventions are appropriate. Unfortunately, such a low-tech approach to the problem does not always attract the attention achieved by a drug product.

Considerable research activity is taking place into CACS at various centres across the world, and the future holds much promise that some interventions may become available that may, at the very least, reduce the speed of onset of CACS, thus allowing patients the opportunity for increased quality of life and to consider further disease-modifying treatments as their functional status is maintained (see Table 6c. 1).

Table 6c.1 Possible mechanisms of action of established and emerging pharmacological agents in the management of cachexia

Possible mechanism	Agent
Central nervous system effects	Metoclopramide
	Corticosteroids
	Progestational agents
	Cannabinoids
	Thalidomide
Modulate immune response/reduce inflammation	Corticosteroids
	Progestational agents
	Polyunsaturated fatty acids
	Thalidomide
	Melatonin
	NSAIDs
Anabolic effect	Growth hormone/insulin growth factors
	Anabolic agents
	Beta-2 adrenergic agents
Stimulate gastrointestinal motility/increase gastric emptying	Metoclopramide
Stimulate appetite	Ghrelin

Further reading

Books

Bruera E., Higginson I. (1996) *Cachexia–Anorexia in Cancer Patients*. Oxford: Oxford University Press.

Doyle D., et al (eds) (2004) *Oxford Textbook of Palliative Medicine* (3rd edn). Oxford: Oxford University Press.

Articles

Argiles J. M., et al (2008) Novel approaches to the treatment of cachexia. *Drug discovery Today*, **13**(1–2): 73–8.

Inui A. (2002) Cancer anorexia–cachexia syndrome: current issues in research and management. *CA: A Cancer Journal for Clinicians*, **52**(2): 72–91.

Krzystek-Korpacka M. et al. (2007) Impact of weight loss on circulating IL-1, IL-6, IL-8, TNF-alpha, VEGFA, VEGF-C and midkine in gastroesophageal cancer patients. *Clinical Biochemistry*, **40**(18): 1353–60.

MacDonald N., et al. (2003) Understanding and managing cancer cachexia. *Journal of the American College of Surgery*, **197**(1): 143–61.

McMillan D. C., et al. (2001) Albumin concentrations are primarily determined by the body cell mass and the systemic inflammatory response in cancer patients with weight loss. *Nutrition and Cancer*, **39**(2): 210–13.

McMillan D. C. et al. (1999) A prospective randomized study of megestrol acetate and ibuprofen in gastrointestinal cancer patients with weight loss. *British Journal of Cancer*, **79**(3–4): 495–500.

Monk J. P., et al. (2006) Assessment of tumor necrosis factor alpha blockade as an intervention to improve tolerability of doseintensive chemotherapy in cancer patients. *Journal of Clinical Oncology*, **24**(12): 1852–9.

Nelson K. A., Walsh D. (2002) The cancer anorexia–cachexia syndrome: a survey of the Prognostic Inflammatory and Nutritional Index (PINI) in advanced disease. *Journal of Pain and Symptom Management*, **24**(4): 424–8.

Radbruch L. (2008) Fatigue in palliative care patients-an EAPC approach. *Palliative Medicine* **22**: 13–32.

Stewart G. D., et al (2006) Cancer cachexia and fatigue. *Clinical Medicine*, **6**(2): 140–3.

Stone P., et al. (2000) Cancer-related fatigue: inevitable, unimportant and untreatable? Results of a multi-centre patient survey. Cancer Fatigue Forum. *Annals of Oncology*, **11**(8): 971–5.

Wang H. S., et al (2007) Elevated serum ghrelin exerts an orexigenic effect that may maintain body mass index in patients with metastatic neuroendocrine tumors. *Journal of Molecular Neuroscience*, **33**(3): 225–31.

Sweating and fever

Definition
- Sweating (diaphoresis) is the secretion of fluid onto the skin surface to aid cooling
- Hyperhydrosis is the production of large volumes of sweat
- Sweating is a normal phenomenon in the regulation of body temperature, but in illness can be a troublesome and distressing symptom
- Severity of sweating can change with climate, and perception of the symptom may differ with varying cultural norms

Measurement tools include
- Symptom diary
- Three grade severity scale[1]
- Six-point rating scale[2]

Causes (common)
- Sepsis
- Tumour burden[3]
- Lymphoma (neoplastic fever)
- Disseminated malignancy, especially hepatic and renal metastases (neoplastic fever)
- Sex hormone insufficiency due to cancer treatment, especially breast cancer (tamoxifen, induction of menopause by chemotherapy or by radiotherapy) and prostate cancer (gonadorelin analogues)

Causes (less common)
- Endocrine disturbance, e.g. hypoglycaemia, hyperthyroidism
- Thermoregulation in response to increase in temperature, exertion or nutrition
- Weakness
- Hypoxia
- Severe pain (infarction, fracture)
- Fear and anxiety
- Medication, e.g. opioids (rare), antidepressants, ethanol
- Drug reactions; blood products (transfusion reaction)
- Neuropathy (diabetic, autonomic); autoimmune disease, idiopathic

1 Quigley C. S., Baines M. (1997) Descriptive epidemiology of sweating in a hospice population. *Journal of Palliative Care.* **13**: 22–6

2 Deaner P.B. (2000) The use of thalidomide in the management of severe sweating in patients with advanced malignancy: trial report. *Palliative Medicine.* **14**: 429–31

3 Chang J. C. (1988) Antipyretic effect of naproxen and corticosteroids on neoplastic fever. *Journal of Pain and Symptom Management*, **3**: 141–4.

Management

- Exclude reversible cause(s) and treat if appropriate
- Supportive measures:
  - decreasing ambient temperature
  - lowering humidity
  - increasing airflow around patient (fan)
  - clothing (modern synthetic materials, e.g. Gore-Tex, allow evaporation)

Pharmacological measures

- Sepsis
  - antibiotics if appropriate
  - paracetamol 1g p.o./p.r. q.d.s. (effective in palliating sepsis-induced sweating)
- Neoplastic fever
  - naproxen 250–500mg p.o. b.d. can relieve neoplastic fever for 10–14 days; once stopped, fever recurs in 66% of patients[3]
  - patients may benefit from switching to an alternative NSAID[4]
  - corticosteroid therapy with dexamethasone has been shown to reduce symptoms, independently of NSAIDs. However, there is no agreement on starting dose. Suggestion:
    - start dexamethasone at 1–2mg o.d. and titrate to effect (or to corticosteroid side-effects)
- Sex hormone insufficiency
  - venlafaxine 37.5mg p.o. o.d. is effective, as is clonidine 0.3–0.4mg p.o. nocte
  - higher doses of venlafaxine may be required, though this drug can also *cause* sweating[5]
  - diethylstilboestrol 1–3mg p.o. o.d. improves symptoms in men, but risk of thromboembolic events is increased
  - progestogen therapy is effective in women, but has a high side-effect profile
- Non-specific treatments
  - antimuscarinic therapy can block parasympathetic-mediated sweating, e.g. propantheline p.o. 15mg nocte
  - drugs used for other antimuscarinic effects, such as glycopyrronium, may also help
  - thalidomide 100mg p.o. nocte[2] has been used in the hospice setting with some effect, though controlled studies are still required

4 Tsavaris N., *et al.* (1990) A randomised trial of the effect of three non-steroid anti-inflammatory agents in ameliorating cancer induced fever. *Journal of Internal Medicine*, **228**: 451–5

5 Loprinzi C. L., *et al.* (2001) Management of hot flashes in breast cancer survivors. *Lancet Oncology*, **2**(4): 199–204.

- other drugs of reported benefit include:
  - cimetidine (for opioid induced sweats)
- beta-blockers
- calcium channel blockers (e.g. diltiazem)
- benzodiazepines
- gabapentin[6]
- olanzapine[7]
- thioridazine[8]

Further reading

Books

Back I. (2001) *Palliative Medicine Handbook*. Cardiff: BPM Books.

Doyle D., *et al.* (eds) (2004) *Oxford Textbook of Palliative Medicine* (3rd edn). Oxford: Oxford University Press.

Watson M., Lucas C., Hoy A. (2003) *Adult Palliative Care Guidance*. (2nd edn) London: The South West London and the Surrey, West Sussex and Hampshire Cancer Networks.

Articles

Chang J. C. (1988) Antipyretic effect of naproxen and corticosteroids on neoplastic fever. *Journal of Pain and Symptom Management*, **3**: 141–4.

Chang J. C. (1989) Neoplastic fever: a proposal for diagnosis. *Archives of Internal Medicine*, **149**: 1728–30.

Economos K. (1995) The effect of naproxen on fever in patients with advanced gynaecologic malignancies. *Gynecologic Oncology*, **56**(2): 250–4.

Loprinzi C. L. *et al.* (2001) Management of hot flushes in breast cancer survivors. *Lancet Oncology*, **2**(4): 199–204.

Miller J. I., Ahmann R. D. (1992) Treatment of castration induced menopausal symptoms with low dose diethylstilboestrol in men with advanced prostate cancer. *Urology*, **40**(6): 499–502.

Penel N., *et al.* (2000) Are there criteria for the diagnosis of paraneoplastic fever? *La Revue de Médecine Interne*, **21**(8): 684–92.

Quigley C. S., Baines M. (1997) Descriptive epidemiology of sweating in a hospice population. *Journal of Palliative Care*, **13**(1): 22–6.

Zhukovsky D. S. (2002) Fever and sweats in patients with advanced cancer. *Hematology/Oncology Clinics of North America*, **16**(3): 579–88.

6 Porzio G., *et al.* (2006) Gabapentin in the treatment of severe sweating experienced by advanced cancer patients. *Supportive Care in Cancer*, **14**(4): 389–91.

7 Zylicz Z., *et al.* (2003) Flushing and sweating in an advanced breast cancer patient relieved by olanzapine. *Journal of Pain and Symptom Management*, **25**(6): 494–5.

8 Abbas S-Q. (2004) Use of thioridazine in palliative care patients with troublesome sweating. *Journal of Pain and Symptom Management*, **27**(3): 194–5.

Respiratory symptoms

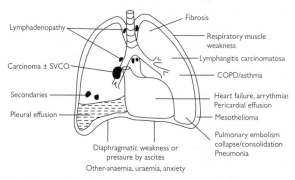

Fig. 6e.1 Causes of breathlessness.

Breathlessness[1,2]

- Breathlessness is 'an uncomfortable awareness of breathing'
- Breathlessness is common in palliative care (40–80% prevalence in some series) and in patients with cancer
- Breathlessness is a complex symptom involving physiological, psychological, environmental and functional factors
- The pathophysiology of breathlessness is complicated and not fully understood
- Normal breathing is maintained by regular rhythmical activity in the respiratory centre in the brainstem. This is stimulated by *mechanical receptors* (stretch receptors in the airways, lung parenchyma, intercostal muscles and diaphragm) and by hypoxia and high levels of CO_2 (detected by *chemoreceptors* in the aortic and carotid bodies and in the medulla)
- In malignant lung disease, breathlessness is usually due to distortion and stimulation of the mechanical receptors, and blood gases may be normal
- Fatigue and respiratory muscle weakness are both significant factors contributing to breathlessness among patients with cancer

1 Bruera E. (2000) The frequency and correlates of dyspnoea in patients with advanced cancer. *Journal of Pain and Symptom Management*, **19**: 357–62.

2 Dudgeon D. J., Lertzman M. (1998) Dyspnea (sic) in the advanced cancer patient. *Journal of Pain and Symptom Management*, **16**: 212–19.

Assessment and investigation

Aim to identify reversible/treatable causes of breathlessness

- A good history and examination are vital
  - assess timing and speed of onset of breathlessness
  - consider exacerbating and relieving factors
  - identify co-morbidities and relevant past medical history
- Targeted investigations as appropriate for the individual patient, e.g.
  - full blood count to identify anaemia
  - chest X-ray to reveal consolidation, pleural effusion, etc.
  - V/Q scan or CTPA if pulmonary emboli suspected

Note: Do not assume that breathlessness is directly caused by cancer.

Principles of management

Consider:

- General measures
- Treatment of reversible causes
- Disease-specific treatments
- Symptomatic management—including pharmacological and non-pharmacological measures

General management

Explanation of the factors contributing to breathlessness is vital, along with discussion of steps to be taken in its management. Remember the importance of reassurance and building patient confidence, that the awareness of breathing can be reduced by the drugs and that he or she can feel more in control.

Patients and carers may find it helpful to discuss fears openly, and to acknowledge the impact of breathlessness on their lives. A calm, positive, logical approach can do much to alleviate the distress of the patient and their family as well as other members of the healthcare team.

Consider the need for adjustments to the patient's lifestyle or expectations.

Treatment of reversible causes and disease-specific measures

Reversible or treatable causes of breathlessness should be identified and managed appropriately (📖 see **Table 6e.1** below).

- Interventions need to be considered in terms of the potential benefits versus risks posed to each individual patient, taking into account disease stage, performance status as well as the patient's wishes
- Breathlessness due to lung cancer per se, can be alleviated in a high proportion of patients with radiotherapy or chemotherapy

Symptomatic treatment

An approach focused on managing the symptom of breathlessness rather than addressing specific causes may be needed in some individuals, depending on their ability to tolerate specific treatments, stage in disease and symptom burden. Symptomatic management includes both pharmacological and non-pharmacological strategies and involves the multidisciplinary team.

Table 6e.1 Management of treatable causes of breathlessness

Cause	Management options
Lung tumour	Radiotherapy (**RT**) or chemotherapy
Bronchospasm	Bronchodilators Corticosteroids
Infection	Antibiotics Add corticosteroids if infective exacerbation of COPD
Pleural effusion	Therapeutic pleural aspiration Drainage and pleurodesis
Pulmonary embolism	Anticoagulation (low molecular weight heparin may be safer in some cases than warfarin)
Heart failure	Diuretics, nitrates, anti-arrhythmics if indicated
Anaemia	Blood transfusion Iron Erythropoietin
Lymphangitis carcinomatosa	Corticosteroids Diuretics?? Bronchodilators
Large airway obstruction	**RT** Stenting if extrinsic compression Laser treatment Brachytherapy Corticosteroids
SVC obstruction	**RT**/chemotherapy Stent Corticosteroids

Pharmacological measures

Bronchodilators

Even in the absence of an obvious 'wheeze', there may be an element of reversible bronchoconstriction—consider a trial of bronchodilators.

- Beta-adrenoceptor agonists
  - salbutamol 2.5–5mg p.r.n/6h via nebulizer or 2 puffs p.r.n. via spacer (**Beware** of increased anxiety, tremor and tachycardia if used regularly)
- Anticholinergic bronchodilators
  - ipratropium bromide 250–500mcg 6h via nebulizer, or 2 puffs q.d.s. via spacer device—can be given in combination with salbutamol

  (Nebulized saline may liquidize tenacious secretions and aid expectoration)
- Sodium chloride 0.9% 5mL via a nebulizer p.r.n.

Corticosteroids

Steroids are thought to reduce tumour-associated oedema and may improve breathlessness due to multiple lung metastases, tracheal obstruction, SVCO or lymphangitis carcinomatosa. Benefit should be apparent within four to seven days.

- dexamethasone 4–8mg p.o. o.d., **stop** if no improvement within 7 days

Theophyllines

Oral theophyllines are bronchodilators, but their use is limited by a high incidence of side-effects. It is important to be alert to significant interactions with other drugs and remember that there are differences in bioavailability between various brands of oral theophyllines. Brand name must be specified when prescribing. See up-to-date edition of the *BNF* for full details.

Try:
- Theophylline m/r e.g. Uniphyllin Continus 200mg b.d.
- Aminophylline m/r e.g. Phyllocontin Continus 225–450mg b.d.

Caution:
- The half-life of theophylline may be **increased** in hepatic impairment, heart failure, elderly patients and by drugs including cimetidine, ciprofloxacin and erythromycin
- The half-life is **decreased** in smokers, heavy drinkers and by phenytoin, carbamazepine and barbiturates

Opioids

Morphine reduces inappropriate and excessive respiratory drive and substantially reduces the ventilatory response to hypoxia and hypercapnia. By slowing respiration, breathing may be made more efficient, reducing both the sensation of breathlessness and associated anxiety.

Morphine does not cause CO_2 retention or clinically significant respiratory depression if used appropriately. There is evidence to support its use among patients with cancer, heart failure, chronic obstructive pulmonary disease and pulmonary fibrosis.

Try:
- Oral morphine 2.5mg p.o. p.r.n. or regularly 4h if dyspnoea is continuous
- Substitute SC morphine or diamorphine if patient cannot swallow

Morphine modified release (MST) seems to be less effective for breathlessness than immediate release morphine preparations given 4h.

A recent article suggests dosing regimes for use of opioids in breathlessness, including use among patients already receiving opioids for pain.[3]

There is currently no evidence to support the use of nebulized morphine, and in some individuals there is a risk of bronchospasm with its use.

There is some interesting work being done on the use of oral transmucosal fentanyl citrate for shortness of breath. Initial findings look promising.[4]

---

3 Brown D. J. F. (2006) Palliation of breathlessness. *Clinical Medicine*, **6**(2): 133–6.

4 Gauna A.A, *et al.* (2008) Oral transmucosal fentanyl citrate for dyspnea in terminally ill patients: an observational cases study. *Journal of Palliative Medicine*, **11**(4) 643–8.

Benzodiazepines

Panic with hyperventilation and the fear of suffocation may worsen breathlessness.

- Longer acting benzodiazepines may be particularly helpful if there is severe anxiety, or at night when breathlessness and associated panic disturb sleep
  - diazepam 2–5mg nocte, b.d. or p.r.n.
- Benzodiazepines with shorter half-lives can be useful in crisis situations, but there is a risk of reactive agitation/anxiety as the effect wears off
  - lorazepam 0.5–2mg p.r.n. (fast onset, short half-life and is well absorbed sublingually—it can be useful for self-administration by patients)
  - midazolam 2.5–5mg SC or buccal stat

Cannabinoids

Nabilone 0.1–0.2mg orally up to four times a day may be given for patients who are continually breathlessness, anxious and who do not tolerate other conventional respiratory sedatives. Sedation and dysphoria may occur with higher doses. Side-effects can be minimized by starting with 0.1mg nocte and gradually titrating the dose. It is unsuitable for patients with heart disease or severe hepatic impairment.

Oxygen[5]

Oxygen may help breathlessness (and/or confusion) in those patients who are hypoxic either at rest or on exertion Fig 6e.2. It may help other breathless patients (with a normal PaO_2) because of the effect of facial or nasal cooling, or as a placebo.

Hypoxic respiratory drive usually only starts with PaO_2 <8kPa (roughly equivalent to an oxygen saturation (SaO_2) of 90%); hypoxic drive is often not significant until PaO_2 <5.3kPa (approx. SaO_2 75%). Most breathless cancer patients are not hypoxic to this degree and will not benefit from oxygen physiologically. It is difficult to predict which patients will derive benefit from supplemental oxygen therapy purely from their oxygen saturation. Hypoxia is not an absolute indication for oxygen use.

The use of supplemental oxygen therapy needs to be considered on an individual patient basis, taking into consideration possible adverse effects, which include:
- psychological dependence
- bulky heavy equipment which restricts mobility and daily activity
- delivery device may become a barrier to communication
- fire hazard and risk of burns to those who smoke
- financial cost of providing oxygen, particularly in the community
- drying effect on the upper airways

Domiciliary oxygen

Intermittent or continuous domiciliary oxygen can be prescribed for palliation of breathlessness in patients with cancer. An oxygen concentrator is generally more cost-effective for patients requiring oxygen more than 8h/day, unless it is only very short term. The 1360L size of cylinder is the one usually dispensed in the community and at 2L/min this gives about 11h of use.

Oxygen concentration

Method	Flow rate (L/min)	O_2 delivered (%)
Nasal cannulae	1	24
	2	28
Ventimask	2	24
	6	35

5 Goody R., (2007) Using oxygen therapy in the palliative care setting. *European Journal of Palliative Care*, **14**(3): 120–3.

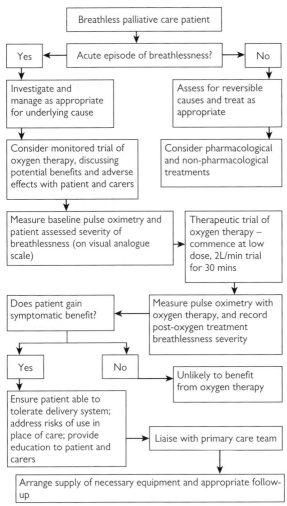

In patients with underlying COPD beware of Type 2 respiratory failure when supplemental oxygen therapy is given. There may be a risk of carbon dioxide retention, with increased drowsiness and reduced respiratory drive. Check local arrangements for prescribing of long term oxygen therapy, including liaison with respiratory physicians where necessary.

Fig. 6e.2 Suggested guidelines for use of oxygen in a hospice inpatient unit.[5]

Pharmacological approaches in the terminal phase
- Occasionally breathlessness is very difficult to control despite general measures and medication, especially in the terminal phase of disease
- Sedation may then be necessary to alleviate patient and family distress
- Medications to manage breathlessness, such as opioids and midazolam, can be delivered using a syringe driver to provide a continuous infusion

Non-pharmacological management of breathlessness

A non-pharmacological approach to breathlessness in lung cancer works well alongside existing medical treatment. This approach may be helpful to patients suffering from breathlessness due to end-stage non-malignant disease. In earlier stages of disease the majority of management strategies employed may be non-pharmacological in nature.

- A draught of air from a fan, or open window may be helpful
- Massaging the patient's back during an episode of respiratory panic can encourage muscular relaxation and may be comforting
- Positioning of the patient in bed is important:
  - upright position uses gravity to assist in lung expansion and to reduce pressure from the abdomen on the diaphragm
  - lying high on one side can be helpful to the patient with copious secretions by preventing aspiration
  - sitting forward and resting the arms on the thighs with the wrists relaxed assists relaxation of the upper chest muscles and encourages freer use of the diaphragm
- Physiotherapy or occupational therapy input for breathing exercises
- Teaching relaxation techniques
- Use of cognitive behavioural therapy to help manage fears and negative thoughts associated with breathlessness
- Complementary therapies, including acupuncture, may be helpful
- Multidisciplinary breathlessness clinics are available in some centres
- Advice on adapting and planning daily activities

Exploring the patient's experience of breathlessness

An essential prerequisite to managing breathlessness involves understanding what it means to be that person in that particular situation.

- Ask the patient to describe his/her breathlessness experience
- Encourage open acknowledgement of the feelings of 'terror' associated with breathlessness
- Gently help the patient to confront their fears of suffocation, choking, not being able to get another breath, or dying during an episode of acute breathlessness. Offer reassurance that these fears are unlikely to be realized
- Ascertain the patient's exercise tolerance and ask him/her to identify things which either trigger or alleviate breathlessness
- Explore the impact of breathlessness on the patient's daily life and assist him/her in coping with and adjusting to the loss of roles and activities. It is important to be aware of the extent to which depression may be a component of breathlessness
- Give time to talk sensitively and at the patient's pace about their disease and associated feelings

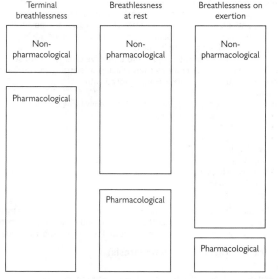

Fig. 6e.3 The relative contributions of pharmacological and non-pharmacological approaches for the management of breathlessness in patients with cancer according to the severity of the breathlessness and the patient's prognosis. From J.Corner *et al* (1997) The palliative management of breathlessness. London: European Congress for Palliative Care.

Teaching skills to assist the patient in managing breathlessness

The patient is offered an educational programme, consisting of a number of skills and strategies, to manage breathlessness. The programme is dependent on a partnership and therapeutic working relationship between the patient and professional, and has three main aims:

1. To enable efficient and effective breathing, where possible.
Breathing re-training is a core part of this approach. This involves teaching the patient to use diaphragmatic breathing exercises as a controlled breathing technique when they feel breathless (as opposed to the tendency to breathe rapidly using the upper respiratory accessory muscles which tire easily leading to inefficient lung aeration).

- Diaphragmatic breathing exercises involve a combination of:
  - pursed lip breathing which promotes control, slows the respiratory rate, increases tidal volume and decreases the possibility of airway collapse
  - controlled breathing with the diaphragm, or lower chest, which helps to improve function and breaks the pattern of upper chest breathing

2. To enable the patient to feel in control by reducing anxiety and panic. The effect of tension and anxiety versus the effect of relaxation on breathlessness, and the concept of the mind–body link are fully discussed with the patient. Relaxation and distraction techniques are taught with the purpose of reducing residual tension, and for use when anxiety and panic are exacerbating breathlessness

3. To enable the patient to adjust and conserve energy for those activities that are important to them. Pacing, prioritizing and problem-solving in relation to activity are all explored with the patient.

- Advice is offered on managing activities of daily living such as:
  - washing/showering/bathing
  - talking on the telephone
  - dressing and undressing
  - making love
  - bending
  - carrying shopping/heavy objects
  - climbing stairs
  - gardening

Goal-setting for learning breathing techniques, in relation to activity, is encouraged. It is important that this is realistic and achievable. The patient is given both verbal and written information focusing on the skills taught.

Pleural aspiration (thoracocentesis)

General

Aspiration of a pleural effusion can give symptomatic relief from dyspnoea. A pleural effusion large enough to cause dyspnoea will be detectable clinically. Aspiration of 300–500mL fluid will usually give some symptomatic improvement, but up to 1.5 litres may be aspirated in some cases.

Complications
- Bleeding or haemothorax—either from damage to the lung/spleen/liver or from vascular pleural tumour
- Pneumothorax—a significant pneumothorax is unlikely after an uncomplicated aspiration if simple precautions are taken
- Infection is a rare complication, providing an aseptic technique is used

If a small IV cannula is used for aspiration rather than a large-bore chest drain, very little air can enter through the cannula if reasonable care is taken. A routine check X-ray after aspiration is not essential in a palliative care setting. Aspiration of a very large effusion that is causing the heart and mediastinum to be displaced may cause cardiovascular embarrassment.

Investigations
A chest X-ray will show a pleural effusion, but it can be difficult to differentiate an effusion from collapse/consolidation or a mixture of the two. An ultrasound scan will confirm the presence of a pleural effusion, and many radiologists will mark a site for aspiration if requested.

Chest X-ray or ultrasound scan should be performed if:
- A clinically diagnosed pleural effusion has not been confirmed radiologically
- The clinical signs are not straightforward

Platelet count and a clotting screen should be checked if the patient has any symptoms of bleeding or unexplained bruising.

Contraindications
- Local skin infection
- Coagulopathy—platelets <40 or INR >1.4
- Presence of local pleural tumour is a relative contraindication, as tumour cells may be 'seeded' in the chest wall

The procedure
- The patient should sit leaning forward, resting their head on folded arms which are leaning on a pillow on a bedside table
- Ensure the patient is in a comfortable position which they can maintain during the procedure
- Use the site marked by ultrasound scan, *or*
- Choose a point in the posterior chest wall, medial to the angle of the scapula, one intercostal space below the upper limit of dullness to percussion (the mid-axillary line can also be used)
- Confirm that the site is dull to percussion
- Avoid the inferior border of the rib above since the neurovascular bundle runs in a groove inferior to the rib
- Clean the skin and use an aseptic technique throughout
- Infiltrate the area with local anaesthetic from skin to the pleura
- It is helpful to advance the needle until pleural fluid is obtained to confirm that the site is suitable for aspiration and to gauge the depth of pleural fluid beneath the skin surface
- Introduce a large-bore IV cannula with syringe attached until fluid is just obtained, then advance a further 0.5–1cm to ensure that the cannula is in the pleural space

- Asking the patient to exhale against pursed lips (to increase intrathoracic pressure), remove the metal trochar or needle and immediately attach a 50mL syringe via a three-way tap
- Tip: A piece of tubing (e.g. cut from a fluid giving set) can be attached to the other port of the three-way tap for ease of disposal of fluid into a suitable container
- Aspirate fluid 50mL at a time, until:
  - 1 litre has drained (1500mL maximum)
  - **or** the patient starts to cough excessively
  - or giddiness, light-headedness or chest discomfort occur
- Remove the cannula, having asked the patient to take a breath, and immediately seal with flexible collodion BP, and cover with a dressing

Non-invasive positive pressure ventilation (NIPPV)

Non-invasive positive pressure ventilation is used to support deteriorating respiratory function. It is most commonly used in palliative care for patients with motor neurone disease (MND).[6, 7]

Indications of deteriorating respiratory function may be: disturbed sleep with morning headaches; daytime fatigue and sleepiness; breathlessness at rest with excess use of the accessory muscles of respiration; increased respiratory rate; and a weak cough.

At present, NIPPV can only be assessed for and provided by specialist centres. Ventilation can be delivered either as intermittent positive pressure or bi-level positive pressure where different pressures are delivered in the inspiratory and expiratory phases.

There are several different systems but all include a ventilator in a portable case and tubing attached to either a nasal or facial mask. It is advisable to have a battery back-up system and some can be adapted to plug into the cigarette lighter in a car.

Following assessment, a period of adjustment may be necessary when the patient uses the NIPPV for periods of 10–15 minutes. Often the patient will only require additional ventilatory support at night but progress to longer periods of use as respiratory function deteriorates.

Common problems associated with NIPPV:
- Mask leak—repositioning the mask and adjusting the straps may help
- Skin irritation—pressure area care is essential and it may be necessary to rotate nasal and facial masks or use dressings to alleviate pressure
- Difficulty eating and drinking—the mask should be removed to allow oral intake and reduce the risk of aspiration
- Psychological impact of use of NIPPV—careful assessment and support
- Body image—awareness of impact on patient and carers
- Ethical issues over stopping ventilation—timeliness of end-of-life discussions is of utmost importance

6 Oliver, D., Borasio, G. D., Walsh, D. (2006) *Palliative Care in Amyotrophic Lateral Sclerosis.* (2nd edn) Oxford: Oxford University Press.

7 MND Association. Information Sheets No.14A, 14B and 14D, available from www.mndassociation.org

Further reading

Books

Ahmedzai S. (1998) Palliation of respiratory symptoms. In *Textbook of Palliative Medicine* (2nd edn) (ed. D. H. Doyle *et al.*), pp. 567–600. Oxford: Oxford University Press.

Booth S., Dudgeon Dm (eds) (2006) *Dyspnoea in Advanced Disease: a Guide to Clinical Management.* Oxford: O.U.P.

Davis C.L., Percy G. (2006) Breathlessness, cough and other respiratory problems. In *ABC of Palliative Care* (eds. M. Fallon, G. Hanks) (2nd edn) pp.13–16.

Edmonds P. (2004) Breathlessness. In *Management of Advanced Disease*, (4th edn) (ed. N. Sykes, P. Edmonds, J. Wiles), pp.70–80. London: Arnold.

Wilcock A. (1997) Dyspnoea. In *Tutorials in Palliative Medicine*, (ed. P. Kaye), pp. 211–33. Northampton: EPL Publications.

Articles

Allen S., et al (2005) Low dose diamorphine reduces breathlessness without causing a fall in oxygen saturation in elderly patients with end-stage idiopathic pulmonary fibrosis. *Palliative Medicine*, **19**(2): 128–30.

Anderson T. (2008) The use of cognitive behavioural therapy techniques for anxiety and depression in hospice patients: a feasibility study. *Palliative Medicine*, **22**: 7: 814–22.

Booth S., et al. (1996) Does oxygen help dyspnoea in patients with cancer? *American Journal of Respiratory and Critical Care Medicine*, **153**(5): 1515–18.

Bredin M., et al. (1999) Multicentre randomised controlled trial of nursing intervention for breathlessness in patients with lung cancer. *British Medical Journal*, **318**: 901–4.

Brown D. J. F. (2006) Palliation of breathlessness. *Clinical Medicine*, **6**(2): 133–6.

Bruera E., et al. (1990) Effects of morphine on the dyspnoea of terminal cancer patients. *Journal of Pain and Symptom Management*, **5**: 341–4.

Connolly M., O'Neill J. (1999) Teaching a research-based approach to the management of breathlessness in patients with lung cancer. *European Journal of Cancer Care*, **8**: 30–6.

Goody R., et al. (2007) Using oxygen therapy in the palliative care setting. *European Journal of Palliative Care*, **14**(3): 120–3.

Philip J., et al. (2006) A randomized, double blind, crossover trial of the effect of oxygen on dyspnea [sic] in patients with advanced cancer. *Journal of Pain and Symptom Management* 32(6): 541–50.

Reuben D. B., Mor V. M. (1986) Dypsnoea in terminally ill cancer patients. *Chest*, **89**(2): 234–6.

Ripamonti C. (1999) Management of dyspnea (sic) in advanced cancer patients. *Supportive Care in Cancer*, **7**(4): 233–43.

Seamark D., et al. (2007) Palliative care in chronic obstructive pulmonary disease: a review for clinicians. Journal of the Royal Society of Medicine 100(5): 225–33.

Van der Molen B. (1995) Dyspnoea: a study of measurement instruments for the assessment of dyspnoea and their application for patients with advanced cancer. *Journal of Advanced Nursing*, **22**(5): 948–56.

Zhao I. (2008) Non-pharmacological interventions for breathlessness management in patients with lung cancer: a systematic review. *Palliative Medicine*, **22**: 6: 693–702.

Cough

Cough is a complex physiological mechanism to protect the lungs and airways. There are numerous causes of pathological cough and may be malignant or non-malignant. Cough may be present in up to 50% of patients with terminal cancer and in up to 80% of patients with lung cancer. It occurs as a result of the mechanical and chemical irritation of receptors in the respiratory tracts.

Prolonged bouts of coughing are exhausting and frightening, especially if associated with dyspnoea and haemoptysis, and can lead to vomiting, pain, disturbed sleep and syncope.

Management
- Where possible, treat any reversible underlying causes
- Consider disease-specific treatments—palliative radiotherapy or chemotherapy relieve cough in a significant number of patients
- Symptomatic treatments—as outlined below

Symptomatic management of cough

It is important to distinguish between a *productive cough* and *non-productive cough* when considering symptom management.

Productive/wet cough

Promotion of an easy, effective cough to clear the mucus should be the aim, unless the patient is dying and too weak to expectorate. Antibiotics may be appropriate, even in very ill patients, as symptomatic treatment for cough.

Occasionally, bronchorrhoea (voluminous amounts of clear frothy sputum, occurring in 6% of cases of alveolar-cell cancer of lung and 9% of other lung cancers) may be very debilitating. Radiotherapy should be considered; however, other suggested symptomatic treatments are largely anecdotal.

For patients still able to cough effectively with help:
- Steam inhalation or nebulized sodium chloride 0.9% 2.5mL q.d.s. and p.r.n. may help to loosen tenacious mucus and aid expectoration
- Carbocisteine (500–750mg t.d.s. p.o.) may reduce sputum viscosity
- Percussion, postural drainage and advice on breathing techniques may help
- Bronchospasm should be treated with nebulized salbutamol

In patients with a chronic persistent infection causing cough, nebulized gentamicin can be considered.

Antitussives should ideally be avoided, but may be helpful at night to aid sleep (📖 see Table 6e.2 for choice of antitussive). *For patients who are dying and too weak to cough:*
- Antimuscarinic drugs (e.g. ipratropium (nebulized) *or* glycopyrronium (SC) *or* hyoscine (SC))
- Cough suppressants (see below—usually diamorphine CSCI if the patient is dying)
- Corticosteroids

Dry cough

A dry cough should be suppressed once reversible causes are treated.

- Nebulized sodium chloride 0.9% 2.5mL q.d.s. may be helpful, by reducing the irritation of dry airways (breathing oxygen or mouth-breathing) and helping to loosen the normal bronchial secretions

Cough suppressants

As an alternative to relieving the cause of the cough or to aiding expectoration, it may be more appropriate to aim to suppress the cough, particularly in a patient who is terminally ill.

- Peripheral suppressants:
  - bupivacaine (5mL of 0.25% t.d.s.)
  - lidocaine (5mL of 0.2% t.d.s.)

Both have been used via **ultrasonic nebulizers** with effect—these agents act by anaesthetizing those sensory nerve endings involved in the cough reflex.

Note: Pharyngeal anaesthesia occurs, so food and drink should be avoided for an hour or so after treatment to avoid aspiration. The first dose should be given as an inpatient in case of reflex bronchospasm.

Cause	Treatment
Pharyngeal irritation	Simple linctus
Bronchial irritation	Nebulized bupivacaine

- Non-opioid cough suppressants:
  - simple linctus 5mL up to q.d.s.
  - inhaled sodium cromoglycate 10mg q.d.s. has been used for cough in lung cancer, it usually acts within 48h
- Opioid cough suppressants:
  - codeine 30mg q.d.s.; increased if needed to 60mg q.d.s.
  - codeine linctus (15mg/5mL) 5–10mL q.d.s.
  - pholcodine 5–10mL q.d.s. is non-analgesic, causes less sedation and constipation than codeine
  - morphine, initially 5mg 4-h p.o.
  - diamorphine 5–10mg/24h CSCI is an alternative, especially towards the end of life

(If a patient is already taking opioids a dose increment or two can be tried, but there is little evidence supporting the use of high doses of opioids for cough.)

  - the efficacy of hydromorphone, oxycodone and fentanyl is not well described
  - methadone linctus can be used under specialist guidance: it may be more effective than morphine but it has a longer duration of action and tends to accumulate

Diazepam may also be needed to relieve anxiety and distress and as a central cough depressant.

Table 6e.2 Opioid and antitussive dose

	Comparable antitussive dose
Pholcodine	10mg
Dextromethorphan	10–15mg
Codeine	15mg
Dihydrocodeine	15mg
Morphine	2.5–5mg
Methadone	2mg
Benzonatate (not UK)	100mg

Haloperidol and antitussives

Studies on experimental models have shown that pre-treatment with haloperidol markedly reduces the antitussive effect of pentazocine and dextromethorphan. Haloperidol is a potent sigma-ligand and it is suggested that the antitussive effect is mediated by sigma-sites. Clinical relevance is unknown, but a trial of an antiemetic other than haloperidol may be worth trying if a patient has intractable cough resistant to antitussives.

Antibiotics

Chest infections commonly occur in the last few days of life. It may be inappropriate to treat those with relatively asymptomatic bronchopneumonia. However, infected chest secretions may be copious and more effectively treated with antibiotics than with symptomatic measures alone. Frequently, patients have had several prior courses of antibiotics, in which case a short course of a broad-spectrum antibiotic may be justified. Offensive sputum, which is suggestive of anaerobic infection, may respond to metronidazole.

Nebulized gentamicin is used quite frequently in patients with cystic fibrosis. Purulent secretions colonized with Gram-negative organisms can be treated with nebulized gentamicin 80mg b.d t.d.s. with a significant reduction in the volume of secretions. Negligible systemic absorption has been shown.

Further reading

Books

Ahmedzai SH, Muers M.F. (2005) *Supportive Care in Respiratory Disease* (3rd edn) Oxford: OUP.

Doyle D. H., et al (eds) (2004) Oxford Textbook of Palliative Medicine (4th edn). Oxford: Oxford University Press.

Articles

Ahmedzai S. H. (2004) Cough in cancer patients. *Pulmonary Pharmacology and Therapeutics,* *17*: 415-23.

Kvale P. A. (2006) Chronic cough due to lung tumors (sic): ACCP evidence-based clinical practice guidelines. *Chest,* **129** (1): 147s-153s.

Zylicz Z., Krajnik M. (2004) The use of antitussive drugs in terminally ill patients. *European Journal of Palliative Care,* **11**: 225–29.

Skin problems in palliative care

A man's illness is his private territory and, no matter how much he loves you and how close you are, you stay an outsider. You are healthy.

Lauren Bacall, *By Myself*, 1978

Wound care in cancer

Skin infiltration with subsequent ulceration or fungating wounds can be distressing. A small metastatic skin nodule is a visual reminder of disease progression and a fungating carcinoma with malodour, discharge and bleeding add to the misery of advanced and uncontrolled metastatic disease.

Loco-regional skin involvement (e.g. breast fungation) should be distinguished from generalized skin metastases which imply very late disease. Local extension of malignant tumour leads to embolization of blood and lymphatic vessels, compromising tissue viability. Infarction of the tumour leads to necrosis with subsequent infection, particularly anaerobic.

The ideal aim is complete healing through either local or systemic treatment, which may involve surgery, radiotherapy, hormonal manipulation or chemotherapy. If such treatment is inappropriate, then care is directed to the minimization of:

- Pain
- Infection
- Bleeding
- Exudate
- Odour
- Psychological trauma

Treatment should be realistic and acceptable to the patient and carers. The primary aim is the promotion of comfort (as opposed to healing) and the enhancement of quality of life, which may hitherto have been severely impaired.

Following assessment of the problems, choose a dressing regime to meet the needs of the patient. Be prepared to change and experiment since there are no rights or wrongs. The aim is to contain problems and improve quality of life.

Continually re-evaluate

There are numerous commercially available products: hydrocolloids, hydrogels, alginates, semi-permeable films, cavity foams, desloughing agents and charcoals. All may have a place in the management of chronic wounds. The health professional must keep abreast of the merits of established and newer products. The simplest products may be the best and the most cost-effective.

The criteria are comfort, acceptability and availability.

Choosing a wound care regime

Consider:

- Pain
- Exudate
- Necrotic tissue
- Bleeding
- Comfort
- Odour
- Infection
- Cosmesis
- Patient's lifestyle
- Psychological effects

Pain

Ensure that pain is caused neither by infection nor the dressing itself. Try to stick to simple regimes, limiting the frequency of dressing changes. Non-stick and sealed dressings may be useful. Prior to applying the dressing, use short-acting analgesia, or relaxation techniques after discussing the options with the patient. Use of a hydrogel sheet dressing may provide topical analgesia and comfort, e.g. Actiform Cool® hydrogel sheet dressing (Young & Hampton, 2005), in addition such dressings aid by removing bacteria and debris from a wound surface via sequestration.

Exudate

Fungating wounds often produce copious amounts of exudate, this poses a danger of maceration to peri-wound skin. If there are bleeding points within the wound it may be necessary to apply a combination dressing; an absorbent dressing with haemostatic properties e.g. Aquacel®, Sorbsan Plus® or Kaltostat®, plus a highly absorbent outer dressing which provide a high fluid handling capability, plus atraumatic removal from both wound bed and surrounding skin are advisable e.g. Versiva XC® gelling foam dressing, Allevyn® foam, Sorbion Sachet®, Mepilex foam®, the latter has a soft silicone wound contact layer to ensure atraumatic removal (White, 2005). Large sizes in these dressings are available and if needed they can be customised by an adept healthcare professional.

While it might seem economical and patient friendly to change only the outer dressing when saturated, this is false economy since, it is not likely to prolong the wear time of the dressings and exposes the patient to potential maceration of their skin.

Protection of the surrounding skin using a durable barrier cream, e.g. Cavilon® or if the skin is broken Cavilon No-sting Barrier Film® is essential If necessary additional support may be gained by using flexible tubular bandaging (Netalast™), sports bra or firm pants.

Necrotic tissue

With surgical debridement there may be significant potential for heavy bleeding. Autolytic debridement may be needed using products such as honey dressings.

Bleeding

Gauze soaked in adrenaline 1:1000 or sucralfate liquid, or alternatively Kaltostat may be used over bleeding points. Gentle removal of the dressing with a normal saline spray, Steripods or irrigation with a syringe containing warm sodium chloride 0.9% or warm water prevents trauma at dressing changes. Kaltostat becomes a jelly-like substance and can be easily lifted off using forceps or gloved fingers. Sorbsan dressings become liquefied and can be washed off with sodium chloride 0.9%. It is preferable to use dressings that can be left in place for a few days to prevent frequent dressing changes—these include the alginates Kaltostat, Sorbsan and Sorbsan Plus.

Odour

Wounds are naturally colonised with bacteria, problems arise when the balance between aerobes and anaerobes is disturbed, this may often result in heavy anaerobic colonisation which leads to malodour. In addition the presence of any necrotic tissue will naturally lead to heavy anaerobic colonisation. Charcoal dressings may be useful as odour absorbers, but only while they remain dry, once wet the charchoal is no longer effective as a filter. Consequently it is advisable to place a charcoal dressing over a primary absorbent dressing prior to appliction of an outer adhesive dressings. Once the dressings are clearly saturated all should be changed to maintain odour control.

Another means of odour control is to use metronidazole intravenous solution topically to the wound area, either positioning the patient and filling the cavity for 5–10 minutes then gently suctioning away the solution or applying gauze soaked in the solution for 5–10 minutes then removing. If applied weekly this can control anaerobic colonisation and keep malodour at bay.

Infection

This is usually chronic and localized. The wound should be cleaned with sodium chloride 0.9% or preferably under running water in the shower or the bath. If the surrounding areas are inflamed, especially if there is spreading inflammation, not just a red rim, antibiotic(s) should be used. The commonest organisms grown in fungating, cancerous wounds and in pressure sore areas include coliforms, anaerobes, *Staphylococcus aureus* and group G beta-haemolytic streptococcus. *Staphylococcus aureus* is probably the commonest pathogen.

Antibiotics such as flucloxacillin or, failing this, trimethoprim or erythromycin should cover most common infections, but anaerobic infections may need to be treated with metronidazole: metronidazole topical gel is particularly useful for eradicating the associated noxious smell.

Methicillin-resistant *Staphylococcus aureus* (MRSA) is difficult to eradicate. It may not necessarily result in morbidity to the patient, but there is clearly a transmission risk to other immunocompromised individuals. Present guidelines for inpatients suggest isolating patients who are MRSA-infected or -colonized and observing of strict 'standard' isolation precautions.

Note: Remember that agents such as cephalosporins, which cover a wider spectrum of bacterial infections, increase the risk of *Clostridium difficile* diarrhoea.

Comfort

By trial and error, a combination of dressings and top packing that is most comfortable for the individual patient will be needed.

Cosmesis

The best cosmetic effect possible should be achieved, in order to boost confidence.

Lifestyle

Patients may need different regimes for different occasions. For social occasions, avoid bulky unsightly dressings. Large sheet hydrocolloids are limited in their exudate handling capacity, a better option may be large sheets of dressings designed to hold euxdate (i.e. Eclipse, New Allevyn, Mesorb).

Daily relaxing baths, perfumes and cosmetics should be encouraged to promote well-being and confidence. Use minimal skin strapping by fixing dressings with vests, cling film, Netelast or incontinence pads (which may be more comfortable).

Psychological effects

Attention to detail and, in particular, ensuring leakproof/odourproof appliances and giving information and an explanation will lessen the sense of isolation and enhance confidence and morale.

Further reading

Books

Grocott P, Dealey C. (2004) Nursing Aspects. In *Textbook of Palliative Medicine* (3rd edn) (ed. D. H. Doyle, *et al.*), pp. 612–24. Oxford: Oxford University Press.

Miller C. (1998) Skin problems in palliative care: nursing aspects. In T*extbook of Palliative Medicine* (2nd edn) (ed DH Doyle eta) p.626–640. Oxford: OUP.

White R. (2005) Evidence for atraumatic soft silicone wound dressing use. *Wounds UK.* 1(3):104–109

Young SR, Hampton. (2005) Pain management in leg ulcers using Actiform Cool™ . *Wounds UK.* 1(3): 94–101.

Pruritus (itch)

Pruritus may be defined as 'an unpleasant sensation that provokes the desire to scratch'. The prevalence is 27% with the common cancers and 80% in the presence of cholestasis.

Pathogenesis of pruritus

This is complex and not fully elucidated, but it is known that both central and peripheral mechanisms are involved. A number of mediators including serotonin, neuropeptides, cytokines, prostaglandins and growth factors are being studied to generate future treatment options.

Complications of pruritus

- Excoriation ± secondary infection
- Lack of sleep, social unacceptability and interference with daily functioning
- Depressive symptoms in up to one-third of patients with generalized pruritus

Medical history assessment of the pruritic patient

- Generalized or localized itch
- Drug history
- Exacerbating factors
- Previous medical history

Causes of pruritus in patients with cancer

These can be divided into general causes of pruritus (which occur in the healthy population as well as those with cancer) and those specifically related to malignancy. In either case pruritus may be localized or generalized.

Senile itch

This is experienced by 50–70% of those over the age of 70 years. The majority have xerosis and skin atrophy, while in others the cause is unknown. It is best treated with general measures (see below) and the application of emollient cream.

Iatrogenic itch

The following drugs are common causes: opioids, aspirin, amphetamines and drugs that can cause cholestasis such as erythromycin, hormonal treatment and phenothiazines.

Iron deficiency

This can cause pruritus with or without anaemia, and responds to iron replacement.

Hormonal itch

Pruritus occurs in up to 11% of thyrotoxic patients, particularly long-term untreated Graves' disease, and less commonly in hypothyroidism. The link between diabetes mellitus and pruritus is controversial.

Management of pruritus

Removal of causative agents (e.g. drugs) as well as the appropriate investigation and treatment of underlying disease are essential first-line measures. Management can be divided into *general* and *cause-specific*.

Evidence for the use of different systemic agents in the treatment of pruritus is limited, but specific drugs may be useful for specific situations as outlined below.

General management

For intact skin

- Ensure that the skin is not dry
- Discontinue using soap
- Use emulsifying ointment or aqueous cream as a soap substitute, or add oilatum to bath water
- Avoid hot baths. Bathe in cool or lukewarm water
- Dry skin gently by patting with soft towel (not rubbing)
- Apply aqueous cream or alternative emollient ('moisturizer') to the skin after a bath or shower each evening
- Avoid overheating (wear light clothes) and sweating day and night (may need an antimuscarinic agent)
- Use sedatives, such as benzodiazepines, to help improve associated anxiety and insomnia
- Discourage scratching; keep nails short; allow gentle rubbing; wear cotton gloves at night
- Avoid exacerbating factors such as heat, dehydration, anxiety and boredom
- Avoid alcohol and spicy foods which may worsen itch
- Consider behavioural treatments and hypnotherapy, which may help ease associated psychological issues and break the cycle of itching and scratching
- Consider TENS and acupuncture
- Use a humidifier, especially in winter

For macerated skin

- Dry the skin and protect from excessive moisture
- Use a hairdryer on a cool setting
- Apply surgical spirit to assist evaporation
- Apply a wet compress t.d.s. and allow it to dry out completely
- If infected, use an antifungal solution, e.g. clotrimazole
- If very inflamed, use 1% hydrocortisone solution for 2–3 days
- Avoid adsorbent powders, e.g. starch, talc, zinc oxide which may form a hard abrasive coating on the skin and be abrasive

Cause-specific management

Itchy skin rashes and insect bites

A 1–2% menthol solution in aqueous cream or oily calamine lotion with 0.5% phenol (which can be increased up to 1%) may be useful. Antihistamine creams should be used when the cause of itch is thought to be histamine-related, e.g. acute drug rash. Prolonged topical use, however, may lead to contact dermatitis, which is best treated with 1% hydrocortisone until it has settled.

Paraneoplastic itch

Cancer per se is an infrequent, but important, cause of generalized pruritus (paraneoplastic itch), the mechanism for which is unknown. Pruritus is particularly associated with haematological malignancies such as Hodgkin's lymphoma and polycythaemia rubra vera.

Treatment of an underlying lymphoma with steroids (dexamethasone 4–8mg o.d. or prednisolone 30–60mg o.d.) may be helpful. There is some evidence that paroxetine 5–20mg o.d. (see below), mirtazepine 7.5–15mg o.n. or cimetidine 800mg o.d. (or other H_2-receptor antagonists) may be effective (see below). Thalidomide may also be useful, but its association with teratogenicity and peripheral nerve damage may be difficult to manage.

Cimetidine, an H_2-receptor antagonist, has been shown to be helpful in itch associated with lymphoma and polycythaemia rubra vera. This is not thought to be a direct antihistaminic effect as it has little effect on itching caused by histamine, but is thought to be related to its inhibitory action on liver enzymes which are involved in the synthesis of endogenous opioids, and possibly other agents, causing pruritus.

Paroxetine, a selective serotonin-reuptake inhibitor (SSRI) antidepressant, has been shown to relieve itch in a case series of patients with advanced cancer with paraneoplastic and opioid-induced itch probably due to down regulation of 5 HT_3 receptors, but side-effects (nausea, vomiting and sedation) may limit its use.

Opioid-induced pruritus

Itch is a well recognized side-effect of opioids and a switch to another opioid (or stopping if possible) may be helpful.

Ondansetron has been shown to be useful in opioid-induced itch at traditional antiemetic doses, although most studies pertain to its success in treating the pruritus associated with opioids given by infusion into the epidural/spinal area. Opioid antagonists are theoretically useful in reducing pruritus but may reverse the essential analgesic effects.

Cholestasis

In palliative care, cholestasis (causing itch) occurs most commonly due to obstruction of the common bile duct from primary or secondary tumours involving the pancreas and biliary tree. (It may also occur as a result of gallstones, drugs or intrahepatic disease.) Stenting of the common bile duct and relief of jaundice should relieve the itch, and dexamethasone may be of some help. Drug treatment may include an opioid antagonist (e.g. naltrexone 12.5–25mg o.d.) which may be helpful if the patient is not taking opioids for pain relief or an androgen (e.g. methyltestosterone 25mg sublingually o.d., or danazol 200mg o.d. t.d.s.). Alternatively, rifampicin 75mg o.d.–150mg b.d. may be used or colestyramine (but this is unpalatable and not effective in complete biliary obstruction) or charcoal which is equally unpalatable.

Renal failure

The pathogenesis of pruritus in renal failure has not been fully defined, but is thought to be multifactorial. Pruritus may be localized (in 70%) or generalized, and is more common in patients receiving dialysis than in those who are not. Ultraviolet light/phototherapy may be helpful. Opioid antagonists such as naltrexone may be effective but cannot be used in patients already receiving opioids because of the risk of reversing analgesia. Ondansetron, mirtazepine and thalidomide have been shown to be effective for generalized itch, whereas topical capsaicin cream can be effective for localized itch.

Further reading

Books

Doyle D. H., et al (eds) (2004) *Oxford Textbook of Palliative Medicine* (3rd edn). Oxford: Oxford University Press.

Zylicz Z., et al. (eds) (2004) *Pruritus in Advanced Disease.* Oxford: Oxford University Press.

Articles

Borgeat A., Stirnemann H. R. (1999) Ondansetron is effective to treat spinal or epidural morphine-induced pruritus. *Anesthesiology,* **90**: 432–6.

Breneman D. L., et al. (1992) Topical capsaicin for treatment of hemodialysis-related pruritus. *Journal of the American Academy of Dermatology,* **26**: 91–4.

Connolly C. S., Kantor G. R., Menduke H. (1995) Hepatobiliary pruritus: what are effective treatments? *Journal of the American Academy of Dermatology,* **33**: 801–5.

Daly B. M., Shuster S. (2000) Antipruritic action of thalidomide. *Acta Dermato-Venereologica,* **80**(1): 24–5.

Ebata T., et al. (1998) Effects of nitrazepam on nocturnal scratching in adults with atopic dermatitis: a double blind placebo-controlled crossover study. *British Journal of Dermatology,* **138**(4): 631–4.

Krajnik M., Zylicz Z. (2001) Understanding pruritus in systemic disease. *Journal of Pain and Symptom Management,* **21**(2): 151–68.

Sheehan-Dare R. A., Henderson M. J., Cotterill J. A. (1990) Anxiety and depression in patients with chronic urticaria and generalized pruritus. *British Journal of Dermatology,* **123**(6): 769–74.

Zylicz Z., Smits C., Krajnik M. (1998) Paroxetine for pruritus in advanced cancer. *Journal of Pain and Symptom Management,* **16**: 121–4.

Lymphoedema

Lymphoedema is a collection of excessive interstitial fluid with a high protein content and is associated with chronic inflammation and fibrosis. It may occur in any part of the body, although generally in a limb. It is progressive and may become a grossly debilitating condition. Acute inflammation and trauma cause a rapid increase in swelling. In patients with cancer, lymphoedema is usually due to the blockage of lymphatic vessels and glands by malignancy or by fibrosis as a result of previous radiotherapy or surgery.

The aim of treatment is to prevent complications developing, and to achieve maximum improvement and long-term control. Success requires full patient cooperation and treatment strategies devised by a lymphoedema therapist (often a nurse or physiotherapist).

Treatment comprises two phases: intensive and maintenance. The intensive phase is indicated for those patients with moderate/severe lymphoedema and is therapist-led. It comprises daily treatment for a period of 2–4 weeks. Treatment includes manual lymphatic drainage, multilayer lymphoedema bandaging, skin care and exercise.

The maintenance phase focuses on self-management and includes simple lymphatic drainage, the use of compression hosiery, skin care and exercise.

Additional management
- Explanation, information and encouragement
- Scrupulous skin care
- Avoidance of trauma, such as sunburn, or venepuncture to minimize infection risks
- *Manual lymphatic drainage* is a very gentle form of massage used to encourage lymph flow from areas of congestion to areas of normal lymphatic drainage
- *Simple lymphatic drainage* is taught to patients and their carers and, paradoxically, involves very gentle, slow massage beginning from areas of healthy lymphatic drainage towards the areas of lymphatic obstruction, 'opening up' the drainage channels
- Compression pumps and intensive low-compression bandaging may also be needed for slowly resolving oedema

Contraindications to compression include local extensive cutaneous metastases, truncal oedema (since fluid from a limb may be diverted to an already congested area), infection or venous thrombosis. Various drugs which influence capillary protein flux and filtration and reduce protein viscosity in interstitial spaces are currently under evaluation but are not in regular use.

Chronic lymphoedema leads to changes in both subcutaneous tissue and skin which make them vulnerable to infection:
- Careful hygiene reduces the risk of infection and moisturizing skin creams should be liberally applied to prevent drying and cracking.
- Any suggestion of impending infection requires prompt treatment with antibiotics

- Diuretics are of limited value in the treatment of lymphoedema, unless the swelling has deteriorated since the prescription of a NSAID or systemic corticosteroid, or there is a cardiac or venous component
- Patients with lymphoedema are vulnerable to infection (acute inflammatory episodes (AIE)). Symptoms can be 'flu-like' symptoms, pain, redness and an increase in swelling. Immediate administration of antibiotics is essential. Patients with repeated infections should be offered prophylactic cover.

Further reading

Books

British Lymphology Society (2007) *Strategy for Lymphoedema Care*. Cheltenham: British Lymphology Society.

Doyle D. H., *et al.* (eds) (2004) *Oxford Textbook of Palliative Medicine* (3rd edn). Oxford: Oxford University Press.

Twycross, R., Jenns K., Todds J. (2000) *Lymphoedema*. Oxford: Radcliffe Medical Press.

Articles

Board J., Harlow W. (2002) Lymphoedema 2: classification signs, symptoms and diagnosis. *British Journal of Nursing*, **11**(6): 389–95.

Fally J., *et al.* (2007) The use of subcutaneous drainage for the management of lower extremity edema in cancer patients. *Journal of Palliative Care*, **23**(3): 185–7.

Genitourinary problems

Anatomy and physiology of the bladder and micturition

Patients with palliative care needs may suffer a variety of symptoms attributable to dysfunction of the urinary system. In order to focus treatment appropriately, it is helpful to understand the basic anatomy and physiology.

Bladder wall

- Made up of detrusor muscle, which is a smooth muscle with an adventitial outer covering together with a supporting inner submucosa for a specialized transitional-cell epithelium
- Detrusor muscle forms a functional syncitium with relatively indistinct muscle layers. The outer and inner layers of muscle bundles tend to be longitudinal in orientation with a middle layer circularly orientated
- Bladder emptying is accompanied by detrusor contraction
- The trigone is a smooth, sensitive triangular area at the base of the bladder with apices formed by the ureteric orifices and the internal urinary meatus or bladder neck

Sphincter active urethra

- The distal sphincter mechanism is situated just beneath the prostate in males and in the distal half of the urethra in females. There is a smooth muscle component and a striated muscle component within the wall of the urethra
- The striated muscle component, the intrinsic rhabdosphincter, is the most important component for maintaining continence
- The striated sphincter contains fatigue-resistant, slow-twitch fibres that are responsible for passive urinary control. Voluntary contraction of the levator ani musculature is responsible for active continence

Nerve supply of the bladder and urethra

- Normal micturition is partly a reflex and partly a voluntary act
- Parasympathetic nerve fibres in the anterior sacral roots of S2 to S4 are the principal motor supply to the detrusor muscle. Parasympathetic (cholinergic) nerve stimulation results in bladder contraction and bladder neck sphincter relaxation, allowing micturition
- Smooth muscle in the region of the bladder neck and prostate is regulated by sympathetic fibres from the hypogastric plexus arising from T11 to L2. Sympathetic stimulation relaxes the detrusor muscle (beta-adrenoceptors) and contracts the bladder neck sphincter, thus preventing micturition. The role of the sympathetic nervous system in the female is less exact
- The functional innervation of urethral smooth muscle is adrenergic
- Somatic innervation comes from S2 to S4 as the pudendal nerve to the striated muscle of the sphincter

- The neurovascular bundles running alongside the prostate carry the autonomic innervation of the sphincter active urethra as well as the cavernous nerves responsible for erections. It is these nerves which may be damaged during radical prostatectomy with resulting erectile dysfunction

Clinical relevance of the nerve supply

Anticholinergic drugs, including hyoscine and tricyclic antidepressants, cause urinary retention by effecting relaxation of the detrusor muscle and contraction of the bladder neck mechanism. Alpha-blockers (including doxazosin and tamsulosin) increase urinary flow in bladder outflow obstruction by relaxing the smooth muscle of the bladder neck and prostate.

Bladder pain

Bladder discomfort or pain presents in the hypogastric (suprapubic) area and may be associated with other symptoms such as dysuria, frequency, nocturia and urgency, as well as urine retention and/or incontinence. If the trigone is affected the pain may radiate to the tip of the penis. Pain may be constant (e.g. urinary tract infection) or intermittent (e.g. bladder spasm). It may vary in intensity from a dull ache (e.g. urinary tract infection) to acute disabling pain (e.g. acute obstructive pathology causing retention of urine).

Commonest causes of bladder pain in palliative care

- Urinary tract infection (UTI)
  - bacterial (☐ see Chapter 4d and p. 396) including tuberculous cystitis
  - fungal (immunocompromised patients)
  - urethritis
  - genital herpes
  - vaginitis
- Anatomical
  - pelvic mass
  - urethral obstruction
  - cystocoele
- Neoplastic
  - bladder cancer
  - urethral cancer
- Foreign body
  - urethral or suprapubic catheter (usually comfortable unless infected or blocked)
  - bladder calculus
- Bladder instability
  - bladder spasm may be idiopathic or more commonly due to contraction around the balloon of an indwelling catheter, blood clots, tumour and infection
- Inflammatory
  - radiotherapy
  - chemotherapy—cyclophosphamide
  - intravesical chemotherapy or immunotherapy for bladder cancer
  - interstitial and eosinophilic cystitis
  - amyloid

Treatment of bladder pain/irritability

Treat reversible causes.

Non-drug management

Regular toileting, good fluid intake (which may be difficult for the terminally ill), avoiding caffeine and alcohol, drinking real cranberry juice (although evidence is limited).

Drug management

- Antimuscarinic drugs may be helpful but should be avoided in significant bladder outflow obstruction or urinary retention
- Antispasmodics
  - oxybutynin 2.5–5mg b.d.–q.d.s. (also has a topical anaesthetic effect on the bladder mucosa and can be given intravesically as 5mg in 30mL o.d.–t.d.s.). Modified preparations are available, including a transdermal patch
  - tolterodine 2mg b.d. (better tolerated than oxybutynin, use lower dose if hepatic impairment). Modified release preparations are available
  - propiverine hydrochloride 15mg o.d.–t.d.s
  - trospium chloride 20mg b.d.—undergoes negligible metabolism by cytochrome P450 (CYP450), and can therefore be useful in patients on drugs such as benzodiazepines which are also metabolized by CYP450
- Tricyclic antidepressants
  - amitriptyline 25–50mg nocte.
  - imipramine 25–50mg nocte
- NSAIDs may be useful
- Corticosteroids may reduce tumour-related inflammation of the bladder and thereby improve bladder comfort
- Local anaesthetic and opioids can be used intravesically. Lidocaine 2% (diluted in sodium chloride 0.9%) can be instilled through an indwelling catheter, which should then be clamped for 20 min to 1h. Bupivacaine 0.5% can be combined with morphine 10–20mg and instilled t.d.s. through an indwelling catheter which should be clamped for 30 minutes[1]

Terminal situation

- Antimuscarinics can be given via a CSCI: hyoscine butylbromide 60–120mg over 24h; glycopyrronium 0.2–0.4mg over 24h

Blood supply of the bladder

The bladder has a considerable blood supply from the vesical arteries and from branches of the anterior division of the internal iliac arteries. This facilitates reconstructive surgery of the bladder but makes the management of haemorrhagic cystitis difficult.

---

1 McCoubrie R., Jeffrey D. (2003) Intravesical diamorphine for bladder spasm. *Journal of Pain and Symptom Management*, **25**: 1–2.

Urinary tract infection (UTI)

UTI is common in palliative care patients and presentation may be non-specific. The clinical picture may vary from asymptomatic to severe symptoms to septicaemia.

Presentation

Dysuria, incontinence, urinary retention, haematuria, suprapubic pain, loin pain, pyrexia of unknown origin, confusion.

Risk factors

Low urinary output (dehydration), bladder dysfunction (outlet obstruction, neuropathic bladder), catheterization, atrophic vaginitis, renal calculi, diabetes mellitus, immune impairment, vesical fistulae

Pathogens

Escherichia coli commonest, also *Streptococcus faecalis* and *Proteus*, *Klebsiella*, *Pseudomonas* spp.

Management

Bedside testing for protein, blood, leucocytes and nitrates (any or all may be positive). UTI unlikely if all bedside tests negative. MSU for culture: clinical diagnosis and positive bedside testing sufficient to start treatment in most patients. Catheter *in situ*—do not treat unless patient symptomatic or undergoing re-catheterization/instrumentation. Encourage increased fluid intake.

- Antibiotic regime:
  - trimethoprim 200mg b.d. for three days is effective in most uncomplicated infections
  - other regimes:
  - ciprofloxacin 250–500mg b.d. p.o./i/v, co-amoxiclav 375mg t.d.s. p.o./IV, cephalexin, 250mg q.d.s. p.o., cefuroxime 125–250mg b.d. p.o./IV
  - recurrent symptomatic UTI (proven on MSU):
  - prophylaxis with trimethoprim 200mg o.d. or nitrofurantoin 50–100mg nocte

Renal pain

Renal pain is characteristically a dull ache in the loin caused by capsule distension, irritation or obstruction.

Causes

- Infection—pyelonephritis, abscess
- Haematoma (trauma)
- Infarct
- Tumour—renal-cell carcinoma, transitional-cell carcinoma, oncocytoma, bleed into angiomyolipoma
- Hydronephrosis

Diagnosis

Urine culture, ultrasound scan, CT scan (MRI may be useful if contrast contraindicated).

Management
Treat the underlying cause if possible, consider dexamethasone 8–16mg for enlarging tumour, analgesics (WHO ladder).

Ureteric colic

Ureteric colic is a severe constant pain, usually located to the loin and may radiate to the ipsilateral groin and testicle. Its onset is typically over 15–20 min building to an intense plateau of pain with fluctuations in intensity but never disappearing, as for example in small bowel colic. It relates to acute ureteric obstruction, and, depending on the cause, may abate with a similar time course to its onset. The patient will become agitated, unable to settle and roll around in agony, unlike the patient with peritonitis who lies still.

Causes
Calculus, tumour, clot, renal papillae, fungal infection

Treatment
NSAIDs will inhibit the renal response to acute urinary obstruction (*avoid with impaired renal function*) and opioid analgesia may also help. Treating tumour-related oedema with dexamethasone 8–16mg may be useful. Anticholinergics (e.g. hyoscine butylbromide) play no role in the management of acute ureteric colic. Tamsulosin (400 mcg o.d.) may be helpful in those with distal ureteric calculi.

Pelvic pain

Can be highly problematic and multifactorial. Assessment needs a logical and thorough approach.
- Consider which structures may be the site of pain:
  - GU tract:
    - males: ureters, bladder, prostate, urethra, penis, testes
    - females: ureters, bladder, urethra, ovaries, uterus and fallopian tubes, vagina
  - perineum
  - GI tract: distal colon, rectum, anus
  - bones: sacrum, pelvis
- Consider pathological process leading to pain:
  - cancer—can be nociceptive (visceral or somatic), musculoskeletal or neuropathic and due to the tumour itself/local invasion/metastases/extrinsic compression of nearby structures
  - concurrent non-cancer disease (e.g. UTI)
  - iatrogenic (caused by cancer treatment or non-cancer treatment, e.g. radiotherapy, surgery, constipation)
- Treat underlying cause—but also consider:
  - medical treatment
  - specific to the cause (e.g. antibiotics for infection)
  - symptomatic: follow WHO ladder, adjuvant analgesia as appropriate to type of pain
  - consider dexamethasone 8–16mg daily for extrinsic compression from tumour as a 3-day trial
  - surgery: e.g. stabilization of fractures such as neck of femur

- oncological treatment: palliative chemotherapy or radiotherapy, hormone therapy (hormone-sensitive tumours)
- anaesthetic analgesic interventions: interruption of the pre-sacral sympathetic nerve supply may help relieve pelvic pain. A caudal or lumbar epidural may be useful. **Note:** neurolytic techniques may result in lower limb paralysis and double incontinence[2]
- non-physical treatments: complementary therapies, psychological support, spiritual input, social support

Urinary retention

Urinary retention is common in palliative care patients and should always be considered in those showing non-specific symptoms such as confusion, restlessness and agitation. Patients presenting with retention often have a previous history of urological difficulties. Risk factors for retention include drugs (such as opioids, anticholinergics), constipation, poor mobility and inadequate toileting facilities and should be avoided as far as possible.

Causes

Local
- Urinary tract infection
- Benign prostatic hypertrophy (BPH)
- Pelvic tumours (any)—primary or secondary
- Constipation
- Urethral stricture—rare, since it usually presents with bad lower urinary tract symptoms first
- Haematuria with clot retention

Drugs
- Tricyclic antidepressants
- Phenothiazines
- Opioids
- Anticholinergics, e.g. oxybutynin, hyoscine, glycopyrronium
- Alpha-agonists (contained in some proprietary cough medicines)

Neurological
- Spinal cord compression
- Pre-sacral plexopathy
- Intrathecal/epidural anaesthesia

Debility
- Immobility/weakness
- Decreased conscious level

Acute obstruction
  Symptoms: hesitancy and poor urinary stream, post micturition dribbling, early morning frequency and nocturia. Subacute symptoms may have been present previously but may be of sudden onset.

Diagnosis:
- Severe lower abdominal pain
- Intense desire to urinate

2 Wilsey N., Ashford N., Dolin S., (2002) Presacral neurolytic block for relief of pain from pelvic cancer. *Palliative Medicine*, **16**: 441–4.

- Anxiety/irritability—may be the only symptom in terminal or unconscious patient
- Distended, tense bladder: tender to palpation, increases desire to urinate, dull to percussion
- >500mL on catheterization in presence of symptoms

Chronic obstruction

Symptoms: classic and cardinal symptom is nocturnal enuresis. The onset is often slow and insidious, and is often missed or misdiagnosed as incontinence

Diagnosis:
- Dribbling incontinence
- Large, non-tender bladder (low pressure chronic retention)
- Dull percussion note in lower abdomen (may extend to above the umbilicus)
- High residual volume (>300mL) post micturition. (May otherwise be symptomless). Acute on chronic volumes may be >800mL on catheterization

Complications
- Urinary infection (📖 see also infection as cause in acute obstruction, p. 400) and bladder stones
- Hydronephrosis and post renal failure (high-pressure chronic retention)
- Constipation refractory to laxatives
- Agitation, confusion
- Post-catheterization diuresis: due to released pressure on the renal cortex and osmotic effects of high urinary urea. A record should be kept of urine output and if excessive (e.g. >200ml/h), intravenous fluid should be used for replacement. To avoid driving the high urine output, 80% of the output, on an hourly basis, can be replaced as a combination of oral ± IV fluids with measurement of serum biochemistry. It is no longer good practice to clamp catheters to allow slow drainage

Treatment

Acute retention
- Immediately catheterize with 10–14Fr gauge urethra catheter
- Leave catheter in place if the patient is in agreement. There are risks of bacteraemia when catheters are both inserted and removed. In the terminally ill, this will prevent the risk of further retention and aid in nursing management
- Measure residual volume
- Perform rectal examination in males and vaginal examination in females as appropriate

If it is not possible to pass a urethral catheter, a suprapubic catheter will be needed. In a hospice setting in the terminally ill, a Bonanno catheter can be used. It should be inserted in the midline away from scars, two finger breadths above the symphysis pubis. This is a short-term measure and the catheter should be changed by a urologist to a more appropriate tube if appropriate for the patient. A suprapubic catheter is contraindicated with clot retention.

Chronic retention
- Catheterize—as above
- Check fluid balance and monitor electrolytes Na^+ and K^+
- Consider IVI if needed to supplement oral intake

Clot retention
- This should ideally be managed by the urologists who will use a stiff 22Fr catheter and may need to use an introducer. In a hospice setting with a terminally ill patient an 18Fr catheter should be tried. It may be necessary to use a 3-way catheter to irrigate the bladder.

Treat underlying cause as appropriate for the patient
- Give laxatives for constipation
- Treat UTI
- Review medication and reduce or stop drugs causing retention (if possible)
- Clot retention—stop anticoagulants and correct bleeding diathesis if possible. **Note:** Tranexamic acid should be used with caution since it might exacerbate the situation
- Consider and treat spinal cord compression. Investigate/treat pelvic tumour (surgery, radiotherapy or chemotherapy according to type)
- Place urethral stent, e.g. in patients too unwell for surgery
- Debilitated patient—ensure regular toileting, use commode rather than bedpan (women), sit/stand at edge of bed (men), privacy—anxiety will inhibit micturition

Further investigations (unnecessary if patient is in terminal decline)
- CSU for culture and sensitivity
- Urea and electrolytes, creatinine—uraemia not improving after catheterization may indicate other cause, e.g. NSAID nephropathy or a high obstruction not corrected by catheterization
- Consider urinary imaging: IVU, USS, cystoscopy if patient is well and corrective treatment is contemplated

Ureteric obstruction
This may be unilateral or bilateral and is caused, in palliative care, largely by pelvic tumours, e.g. carcinoma of the cervix in women and carcinoma of the prostate in men. A reduction in urine volume, abdominal pain and/ or serial blood tests of deteriorating renal function alert the team to the possibility of bilateral obstruction and impending renal failure. Renal ultrasound will confirm the diagnosis of ureteric obstruction due to tumour and rule out other contributing factors.

Obstructing stones are best diagnosed on plain abdominal X-ray. In the presence of ureteric obstruction, cystoscopy and retrograde pyelograms can be carried out which should outline the level/s and cause of obstruction. An indwelling ureteric stent can then be passed under cystoscopic control if there appears to be reasonable potential for regaining function. If this is not possible a percutaneous nephrostomy could be considered under ultrasound guidance. This can sometimes be replaced by the antegrade insertion of ureteric stents. In some circumstances, antegrade ureteric insertion into an ileal conduit may be appropriate. With modern equipment and techniques, long-term nephrostomies are a possible option, but this needs very careful discussion with patients who may already be suffering from pelvic pain, fistulae or other tumour-related problems. They may not want artificial prolongation of life at the expense of relentlessly distressing symptoms.

In palliative care, this discussion with the patient and their family is crucial in guiding the patient to the correct management for them. Clearly, if restoration of renal function with reasonable quality of life and minimal symptoms and disruption to life is a possibility, then interventional management will be in the patient's best interests. On the other hand, if the patient is in the terminal phase of cancer with a known large pelvic mass that is already causing pain and debility, the patient might not wish to undergo procedures that might not be successful and that, if technically successful, might prolong life for a short time but with the added burden of further discomfort. This is the choice of the patient and should be discussed adequately with him/her.

Urinary incontinence

This is a distressing symptom for patients, affecting their lives physically, psychologically, socially and sexually. Patients may become isolated from family and friends as they try to maintain their own personal hygiene, fearing to lose their dignity in public. A good history is essential and may indicate that the cause is simply an inability to mobilize and reach the toilet in time. Pelvic disease in a female patient may result in a vesicovaginal fistula leading to constant urinary drainage through the vagina.

Total urethral incontinence

This type of incontinence is relatively common for those patients with advanced malignant disease. An uncontrollable loss of urine occurs secondary to local incompetence of the urethral sphincter (due to direct tumour invasion or previous surgical intervention) or central loss of sphincter control (due to confusion or dementia).

Treatment includes regular toileting for the central loss of control to allow continence to be regained. Females will need a urethral catheter. A male sheath catheter can be tried first, but these are often problematic since they may be difficult to fit securely and twist easily.

Neurological incontinence

Loss of neurological bladder control may be due to damage to the sacral plexus or spinal cord/cauda equina compression. A hypotonic neuropathic bladder may result in overflow incontinence and a reflex/automatic bladder empties automatically. Patients who are well, willing and dextrous enough may be taught intermittent self-catheterization. Other patients will require long-term catheterization. Anticholinergics may help.

Overflow incontinence

This is associated with obstruction of the bladder outlet or a poorly contractile floppy bladder. Small volumes of 'overflow' urine may be passed without control. A palpable, distended bladder alerts the clinician to overflow incontinence, although a large distended but floppy bladder, particularly in a patient with other abdominal pathology, may be difficult to diagnose. Permanent catheterization will probably be necessary. Definitive treatment may be possible if the patient is well enough and if the obstruction is amenable to surgery or other intervention such as an intraurethral stent.

Urge incontinence

A sudden urge to urinate and subsequent urinary loss may be particularly distressing for patients with poor mobility who are unable to reach the toilet in time. The causes of urge incontinence include all factors that contribute to an irritable bladder. The underlying cause should be treated, and anticholinergic agents may help. Patients may be able to manage timed voiding.

Stress incontinence

The involuntary urethral loss of urine with increased intra-abdominal pressure from coughing, sneezing, laughing, jumping or even walking in severe cases in the absence of bladder contraction may occur. It is more common in multiparous women and is associated with poor urethral support and reduced pelvic floor tone. Support prostheses (e.g. ring pessary) and urethral inserts may be a possibility in the absence of local tumour.

Haematuria

A normal urinary tract does not usually bleed, even if the patient is on warfarin. Haematuria is a frequent presentation of urological disease. It ranges from microscopic haematuria discovered incidentally on urinalysis to frank haematuria with the passage of clots and clot retention of urine. The extent of the bleeding does not always correlate with the severity of the underlying aetiology. The bladder is a very vascular organ and hence will not have a chance to stop bleeding unless it is collapsed. Dantron (a stimulant laxative) may tint the urine pink or orange, which may be confusing.

Causes

- Tumour—renal, ureteric, bladder, prostate (post radiotherapy or locally advanced)
- UTI
- Drug-induced—aspirin or NSAIDs do not usually cause gross haematuria in a normal urinary tract, but any bleeding associated with surgical interventions may be exacerbated. Cyclophosphamide and ifosfamide may cause haemorrhagic cystitis (🕮 see p. 144)
- Systemic coagulation disorder—usually evidence of bruising or bleeding elsewhere. Platelets may be low due to leucoerythroblastic anaemia and marrow infiltration
- Urinary calculus

Investigations

- Urinalysis, microscopy and urine culture
- Intravenous urography
- Ultrasound scan
- Cystourethroscopy (visualizes the bladder and urethra)

Treatment

Treat any reversible causes, i.e. treat UTI and systemic coagulation disorder and stop precipitating drug.

General measures

- Encourage oral fluids to promote a good urine output (to avoid clot retention)
- Transfusion may improve symptoms due to anaemia
- Etamsylate: (reduces bleeding by enhancing platelet adhesion). The use of tranexamic acid (prevents fibrinolysis by inhibiting plasminogen activation) is controversial. It may result in the formation of hard clots which then need to be irrigated cystoscopically; urological surgeons describe bladders lined with clot which can be difficult to manage. But, as ever, the decision must be made on an individual basis. Terminally ill patients may prefer to risk clot retention than to continue with gross haematuria and significant blood loss
- Palliative radiotherapy often reduces haematuria from a bleeding urinary tract cancer
- Instilling 1% alum, formalin, 0.5–1.0% silver nitrate or epsilon aminocaproic acid solutions may be tried. (Discuss with urologists)
- Internal iliac artery embolization may provide effective relief from severe bladder haemorrhage[3]; renal artery embolization may be useful in renal-cell carcinoma
- Bleeding from the prostate may respond to finasteride 5mg o.d. (a specific inhibitor of 5 alpha-reductase which metabolizes testosterone to the more potent androgen, dihydrotestosterone) even if patients are on other drugs
- Cystectomy may be the final option in a patient able to undergo the procedure, which, however, would be most unusual in the palliative care situation

Clot retention

The principle in the management of clot retention is to evacuate the bladder clots. A non-distended bladder bleeds far less than a distended bladder. An 18Fr catheter will be needed. Patients may need referral to a urologist for insertion of a 3-lumen catheter (to permit irrigation with sodium chloride 0.9% and allow removal of clots) which is stiff and may need to be inserted with an introducer. Cystoscopic bladder washouts may be necessary. Percutaneous insertion of a suprapubic catheter is contraindicated in the presence of clot retention since the catheter is of insufficient diameter to allow satisfactory irrigation; there is also the potential for seeding of bladder tumour through the percutaneous tract.

Haemorrhagic cystitis

This may require clot evacuation and irrigation, and instillation of alum. Intravesical prostaglandin E2 may be helpful. In selected fit patients, urinary diversion, cystectomy or selective embolization of the internal iliac artery may be appropriate, but this would be very rare in the palliative care population.

3 Gujral S., et al. (1999) Internal iliac artery embolisation for intractable bladder haemorrhage in the perioperative phase. Postgraduate Medical Journal, 75: 167–9.

Catheterization

Indications

Urinary retention (acute and chronic), incontinence, patients in whom toileting is problematic, e.g. pathological fracture femur.

Indwelling urethral catheterization

The French scale of catheter size is measured in mm. A 10–14Fr silicone catheter is most commonly used in adults since smaller diameters tend to coil in the urethra. A larger size may be needed (e.g. 18Fr) if debris and infection is suspected. A size 18Fr will be needed for clot retention (see below). Long-term catheters should be changed every six weeks to avoid blockage, encrustation and formation of stones in the catheter.

For male urethral catheterization:
- Retract the foreskin to view the urethral meatus
- Clean the glans with sodium chloride 0.9% or aqueous chlorhexidine
- Anaesthetize and lubricate with 10mL lignocaine 2% gel via syringe
- Wait for a few minutes and gently pass the catheter using an aseptic technique. Resistance may be encountered at the level of the distal sphincter complex or bladder neck. Sphincter spasm will diminish in a few minutes. Asking the patient to cough, may facilitate passage of the catheter
- A catheter introducer should only be used by experienced urological surgeons

For female catheterization:
The female meatus may be difficult to identify and is often situated in the vaginal introitus or along the anterior vaginal wall
- Inflate the catheter with the required volume of saline to prevent the catheter dislodging

Urethral catheter problems[4]

- Trauma and false passages—refer to urological team
- Haematuria
- Infection is extremely common with long-term catheterization. The incidence of UTIs is related to the duration of catheterization, bacteriuria developing at a rate of about 5% per day of catheterization. Antibiotic treatment should be given if the patient is symptomatic (fever, urinary symptoms, delirium, etc.)
- Bladder spasm—caused by irritation of trigone of bladder by the balloon. Often this is relieved by removing water from the balloon, although most long-term silicone catheters have only a 10mL balloon and there is the risk that the problem will not be solved and the catheter will fall out. Antispasmodics (e.g. oxybutynin) may help
- Blockage may occur from debris or clots. Flushing the catheter with antiseptic (0.02% chlorhexidine) or sodium chloride 0.9% may relieve

4 Zylicz Z., Krajnik M. (1999) Improvement of transurethral catheterization in male patients. *Palliative Medicine*, **13**: 261–2.

the situation but at the risk of encouraging further infection. This decision will depend on the particular clinical circumstances
- Bypassing is due to a blocked catheter or bladder spasm
- Paraphimosis—failure to reposition foreskin may lead to constriction causing swelling and pain of glans penis. Reduction with gentle squeezing pressure over 30 min using swabs soaked in 50% dextrose may allow foreskin repositioning
- Undeflated balloon—if the balloon will not deflate to allow removal of the catheter, it will need deflating with a wire, usually under US control

Suprapubic catheter

A suprapubic catheter is indicated if passing a urethral catheter has failed. This may be due to a stricture, obstruction due to intrinsic or extrinsic compression or distorted anatomy of the urethral meatus due to tumour or lymphoedema. It may also be used as an alternative to a urethral catheter in a patient with an unstable bladder in whom the balloon is constantly irritating the trigone. A suprapubic catheter is contraindicated in clot retention.

For suprapubic catheterization:
- Palpate the distended bladder is suprapubically
- Place the patient with the foot of bed raised
- Infiltrate the skin with lidocaine 1% about two finger breadths above the pubis in the midline and aspirate urine with a 21G needle
- Insert a suprapubic catheter using an aseptic technique. A pigtail (e.g. Bonanno) catheter may be needed as a short-term measure if the patient is not well enough for transfer for the more appropriate insertion of a 16Fr silicone catheter, which should be sited by a urologist
- **Caution**: midline scar, previous pelvic surgery, unsuccessful urine aspiration with needle. In these situations, the insertion should be under ultrasound control

Intermittent self-catheterization[5] is unusual in patients with palliative care needs. It may be used in patients with a neuropathic bladder, e.g. after spinal cord compression. Clean catheter insertion at least four times daily frees patients from indwelling catheterization, gives them control and prevents renal damage from urinary retention. Patients need to be highly motivated, have manual dexterity and be well enough to perform the task. Refer to incontinence advisor for counselling/instruction.

General management of catheters

Catheters (especially suprapubic) need skin protective agents around the base of the catheter to stop leakage spilling directly onto the skin. Secretions around the catheter site should be removed with soap and water. Over-granulated areas can be removed with silver nitrate. Meatal cleaning around urethral catheters is necessary since secretions are increased due to urothelial irritation. The secretions form crusts which, when removed, form areas of exposed damage that are prone to bacterial colonization and which can then ascend into the bladder.

---

5 Hunt G., Oakeshott P., Whitaker R. (1996) Intermittent catheterisation: simple, safe, and effective but underused. *British Medical Journal*, **312**: 103–7.

Genitourinary fistulae

Fistulae (abnormal communications between two hollow viscera or viscera and body surface) are common in those patients with advanced cancer, causing considerable morbidity and distress. They may be associated with previous RT and are managed, where possible and appropriate for the clinical circumstances, with bypass surgery.

General management

Includes:

- Meticulous skin protection—barrier creams, e.g. zinc and castor oil, Sudocrem or Cavilon (applied as a spray or stick protector and dries to form a protective membrane). Lutrol gel (solidifies when warmed in contact with skin, forming a protective layer) is not commercially manufactured but some hospital pharmacies may be able to prepare it
- Water absorbent pads or tampons
- Treatment of odour: metronidazole 400mg t.d.s. may reduce odour from anaerobic infection. Charcoal dressings and charcoal placed in the room may have some effect. Masking the smell with lavender oil, etc. has been tried but is often ineffective

Vesicoenteric fistulae

A fistula may develop between the bladder and any segment of bowel. The cause in palliative care is usually colonic malignancy, although diverticulitis or small bowel inflammatory disease may also be responsible. Vesicoenteric fistulae rarely occur secondary to bladder pathology. A characteristic symptom is pneumaturia (passage of gas or froth in the urine) and there may also be a foul odour to the urine, persistent urinary tract infections and the presence of faecal matter in the urine (especially with large fistulae). Cystoscopy, contrast cystography or intestinal barium studies will normally demonstrate the fistula. Ideally, the management is surgical removal of the segments of bowel and bladder, together with repair of the bowel and bladder. Otherwise a bypass procedure may be performed, a colostomy or ileostomy may provide complete relief. Some patients may be too unwell for surgery or prefer not to have a stoma.

Vesicovaginal fistulae

These are characterized by a continuous leakage of urine from the bladder into the vagina and need to be distinguished from total urethral incontinence. Intravenous urography will identify a ureterovaginal fistula and a cystogram will identify a vesicovaginal fistula. Cystoscopy and retrograde ureterography may be helpful. Surgical excision provides the most effective solution but is often not feasible. Urinary diversion, e.g. ileal conduit, may be necessary if the patient is well enough, but this a formidable undertaking in patients who have had radiotherapy. Bilateral nephrostomy is a potential but radical alternative. As ever, the advantages and disadvantages of procedures need to be discussed with the patient.

Sexual health in advanced disease

Patients with palliative care needs who are very ill and symptomatic may not be interested in sexual intercourse, although they may want to maintain intimacy with their partner. Discussions of sexuality issues may be very helpful for patients and their partners.

Background
- Individuals with advanced cancer may remain sexually active
- Problems may be physical, psychological or relational and are frequently multifactorial and complex
- Many sexual problems are solvable
- Patients with cancer often fear transmission of cancer (especially genitourinary) to their partner, or partners fear contracting cancer themselves
- Patients often find it difficult to ask for help and are embarrassed, fearing that professionals might see sexual difficulties as frivolous in the context of serious disease. They also assume that nothing can be done
- Healthcare professionals without specialist knowledge find it difficult to address this area since they too may be embarrassed

General issues
- Lack of libido in both sexes can be caused by: change in body image (surgery to/disfigurement of the face, the presence of stoma, etc.), depression, relationship problems, hormone deficiency, drug-related side-effects (📖 see Chapter 4)
- Physical problems such as breathlessness, weakness and pain may lead to difficulties, some of which may be addressed. Catheterization does not preclude sexual intercourse, a male catheter may be folded inside a condom

Issues for males
- Impotence:
  - drug causes (📖 see Chapter 4)
  - disease/treatment effects: spinal cord compression, pelvic malignancy, pelvic surgery/radiotherapy, orchidectomy, brain neoplasm
  - concurrent disease: diabetes, peripheral vascular disease, age-related
  - psychological: fear of failure to acquire or maintain erection for fear of experiencing or causing pain
- Treatment:
  - stop or change medication
  - discuss trial of sildenafil with urologist. Patients with psychogenic ejaculatory dysfunction, spinal cord injury, nerve-sparing prostatectomy and hypertension may get a response of about 80%. Absolute contraindications include the use of nitrates, liver impairment, hypotension and recent stroke or myocardial infarction (MI). Relative contraindications include poor libido, history of priapism (may be associated with myeloma, sickle-cell disease and leukaemia), bleeding disorders and active peptic ulceration
  - intercavernosal drugs (prostaglandin E), vacuum devices and prosthetic implants may very rarely be appropriate for selected patients in palliative care

Issues for females
- Lack of libido:
  - change in body image: disease/surgery of breast, genitals, reproductive organs. Associating gynaecological cancer with 'punishment' for previous lifestyle. Fear of pain on intercourse
- Dyspareunia:
  - vaginal dryness: lack of oestrogen, infection, e.g. candidiasis, vaginal stenosis following radiotherapy or surgery
  - post-pelvic surgery, pelvic tumour, pelvic infection
- Treatment:
  - local oestrogen creams, HRT, treat infections, lubrication using KY jelly, use of vaginal dilators post-surgery/radiotherapy (needs to be started early and used persistently), encourage regular intercourse to maintain vaginal passage

Approach to management
- Pre-treatment counselling, regarding sexual issues, may help to avoid problems
- Exploration of issues with open questions—e.g.: 'Has your disease affected the way you view yourself?', 'Has it affected your relationships?'—while allowing the patient to guide the consultation into more specific areas
- General patient information literature available
- PLISSIT model framework for exploring/managing sexual problems
- Referral for further counselling with specialists who will have the information/skills for addressing this area. Psychosexual counsellors are available for complex situations

Drugs associated with sexual dysfunction
- Antihypertensives
  - thiazide diuretics
  - beta-blockers
- Psychotropic drugs
  - phenothiazines, e.g. levomepromazine
  - butyrophenones
  - anxiolytics and hypnotics
  - antidepressants
- Endocrine drugs
  - antiandrogens
  - oestrogens
  - gonadorelin analogues
- Other
  - recreational drugs
  - digoxin
  - spironolactone
  - ranitidine
  - metoclopramide
  - carbamazepine

Further reading

Books

Back I. N. (2001) *Palliative Medicine Handbook* (3rd edn). Cardiff: BPM Books.

Norman R. W., Bailly G. (2004) Genitourinary problems in palliative medicine. In *Oxford Textbook of Palliative Medicine*, (3rd edn) (ed. D. Doyle, *et al*), pp. 631–42. Oxford: Oxford University Press.

Tomlinson J. (ed.) (1999) *ABC of Sexual Health*. London: BMJ Books.

Twycross R., Wilcock A. (2001) *Symptom Management in Advanced Cancer* (3rd edn). Oxford: Radcliffe Medical Press.

Articles

Dienstmann R. (2008) Palliative percutaneous nephrostomy in recurrent cervical cancer: a retrospective analysis of 50 consecutive cases. *Journal of Pain and Symptom Management* **36**: 2: 185–90.

Gujral S., *et al.* (1999) Internal iliac artery embolisation for intractable bladder haemorrhage in the perioperative phase. *Postgraduate Medical Journal*, **75**: 167–9.

Hunt G., Oakeshott P., Whitaker R. (1996) Intermittent catheterisation: simple, safe, and effective but underused. *British Medical Journal*, **312**: 103–7.

Law C. (2001) Sexual health and the respiratory patient. *Nursing Times*, **97**: 12 NT Plus XI–XII.

McCoubrie R., Jeffrey D. (2003) Intravesical diamorphine for bladder spasm. *Journal of Pain and Symptom Management*, **25**: 1–2.

Penson R., *et al.* (2000) Sexuality and cancer: conversation comfort zone. *Oncologist*, **5**: 336–44.

Wilsey N., Ashford N., Dolin S. (2002) Presacral neurolytic block for the relief of pain from pelvic cancer. *Palliative Medicine*, **16**: 441–4.

Zylicz Z., Krajnik M. (1999) Improvement of transurethral catheterization in male patients. *Palliative Medicine*, **13**: 261–2.

Palliation of head and neck cancer

Basic epidemiology and pathology

Head and neck cancer makes up about 3% of all cancer deaths in the UK. It is commoner in France, Italy, Poland, Thailand and the Indian subcontinent. About 50% of patients overall are cured while 50% die of their disease, though the mortality varies widely according to site, histology, stage at diagnosis and degree of tumour differentiation. Most patients who survive two years without recurrence are likely to be cured. Second primaries are very common, occurring in around one in eight patients. The effects of these on prognosis are often dire[1]. These may be due to:

- **Field change:** Carcinogens produce widespread epithelial changes, which easily develop into malignancy
- **Clonal expansion and migration** of malignant cells
- Common aetiological factors include:
  - smoking
  - alcohol: the effects of these two factors are synergistic, and they are the strongest factor in the causation of head and neck squamous-cell carcinoma (HNSCC).
- Tumours at particular sites also have local risk factors:
- Betel nut chewing: vitamin deficiencies for oral cancer
- Nickel, chromate, hardwood dusts: airway tumours
- Viruses: Epstein–Barr virus in nasopharyngeal carcinoma
- Iron deficiency: Patterson–Brown–Kelly syndrome (iron deficiency, koilonychia, glossitis, upper oesophageal web) are associated with postcricoid carcinoma
- Familial: increased risk of head and neck squamous cell carcinoma if there are two or more first-degree relatives with HNSCC.

Histology
- Most tumours are **squamous cell carcinomas,** these:
- Are often moderately chemosensitive but not curable with chemotherapy
- Tend to develop hypercalcaemia. This is usually due to the secretion of parathyroid hormone-related peptide (PTHrP).

Less common tumours include adenocarcinomas, adenoid cystic carcinomas (salivary glands), anaplastic carcinomas, lymphomas, melanomas of the mucosa and other rare tumours.

1 Dhooge I., De Vos M., Van Cauwenberge P. B. (1998) Multiple primary malignant tumors in patients with head and neck cancer: results of a prospective study and future perspectives *Laryngoscope*, **108**, 250–6.

Staging

Squamous cell carcinoma tends to progress from local disease, along lymph node levels in a stepwise manner to distant disease quite late. This allows radical treatment to be staged (📖 see p. 118–128), with treatment of the important lymph node groups, e.g. radical neck dissection. Treatment has now improved such that the cause of death is changing: as local control has improved, distant metastases are the cause of death in perhaps one-third of patients and are found in many others[2]. This has obvious implications for the likely problems to be encountered and the management of the terminal phase.

2 Taneja C., et al. (2002) Changing patterns of failure of head and neck cancer. *Archives of Otolaryngology—Head & Neck Surgery,* **128**: 324–7.

The patient with head and neck cancer

Many patients with head and neck cancer will have a history of heavy alcohol and tobacco use. Those with a history of heavy alcohol intake may also have inadequate coping strategies, poor family and social networks to fall back upon and sometimes very damaged close relationships. Understandably, the psychological toll can be considerable.[3] All this has to be kept in mind during assessment, rehabilitation and discharge planning as well as the provision of psychosocial support to the patient and their family to help them cope with possible severe disfigurement, communication problems and often frightening potential complications such as severe airway obstruction or bleeding. They need explanation, sensitively given information about the likely future, and special care for isolated relatives, young children and those with severe health or other problems of their own.

Possible psychiatric complications

- Adjustment reactions can occur around the time of surgery or other treatment, as well as when function alters rapidly in advanced disease. They can take the form of anxiety, depressive reactions or mixed states.
- Adjustment reactions are commoner and more severe if severe disfigurement or communication problems are anticipated. They often settle with time, particularly in a supportive environment, but they need active management if severe
- Depression[4] has been found in over half the patients with advanced disease. Counselling and antidepressants may be needed
- Suicidal ideation: the suicide risk is said to be considerably higher than with other cancers. Professional psychiatric assessment (psychiatrist or social worker) should be sought if the risk is judged to be significant.
- Anxiety may be related to fears that one's airway is about to close off, or of an impending serious bleed or other catastrophe. The underlying fears, if any, need to be addressed. Always explain, and also consider counselling, cognitive therapy, relaxation training, anxiolytics
- Alcohol withdrawal can cause confusion and agitation. Detoxification, often under benzodiazepine cover, may be necessary.

3 Moadel A. B., Ostroff J. S., Schanz S. P. (1998) Head and neck cancer. In *Psycho-oncology* (ed. J. C. Holland), pp. 298–307. New York: Oxford University Press.

4 de Leeuw J. R. J., *et al.* (2001) Prediction of depression 6 months to 3 years after treatment of head and neck cancer. *Head and Neck*, **23**(10): 892–8.

Tumour treatment: Implications for the palliative stage

Head and neck tumours can be treated by surgery, radiotherapy or chemotherapy.[5]

Surgical treatment operates on the principle that HNSCC spreads in an orderly manner through successive lymph node groups, so bloc dissection taking out tumour, nodes and intervening lymphatics will control disease. Excision of structures invaded by tumour may be needed. Therefore major reconstruction is frequently required.

Cervical nodal metastases are found in 40% of patients with HNSCC at diagnosis. **Radiotherapy** can sterilize small neck nodes or those from certain tumours (nasopharynx, thyroid) effectively, but surgery is needed in other cases. **Radical neck dissection** removes all the nodes on that side, the sternomastoid, internal jugular vein and spinal accessory nerve, which supplies the trapezius and sternomastoid. This is effective but disabling, and more limited forms of neck dissection are now employed when appropriate,[6] often associated with radiotherapy or chemotherapy. Damage to the axillary nerve can result in the **shoulder syndrome** (□ see 'Pain' p. 421)

Radical radiotherapy often retains function better than surgery, but it has side-effects: mucositis, dry mouth (xerostomia), tissue fibrosis and complications to other organs within the radiotherapy field, e.g. the spinal cord. Radiotherapy can be given by **external beam** or **brachytherapy** (radioactive implants, e.g. needles in the tongue). Various fractionation regimes are used. In addition, radiotherapy can be given preoperatively (neoadjuvant), postoperatively (adjuvant) or as an accompaniment to chemotherapy.

Palliative radiotherapy can address various problems such as bone pain, dysphagia or stridor from paratracheal nodes, or bleeding or infection from fungating tumours.

Chemotherapy is potentially curative in some tumours, for example lymphomas, but never in HNSCC. However, adjuvant or neoadjuvant chemotherapy has a place alongside surgery and/or radiotherapy.

5 Gleich L. L., *et al.* (2003) Therapeutic decision making in Stages III and IV head and neck squamous cell carcinoma. *Archives of Otolaryngology—Head & Neck Surgery*, **129**: 26–35.

6 Myers E. N., Gastman B. R. (2003) Neck dissection: an operation in evolution. *Archives of Otolaryngology—Head & Neck Surgery*, **129**: 14–25.

Some notes on specific tumours, with emphasis on advanced disease

Oral cavity tumours

- Anterior two-thirds of the tongue
- Lips
- Buccal mucosa
- Alveola of the teeth
- Hard palate
- Floor of mouth
- Retromolar trigone

These are the most frequent head and neck cancers. They are usually well-differentiated SCC, but tumours of minor salivary gland origin are also seen. Spread is predominantly local and to nodal groups in a stepwise manner. Larger tumours are more likely to have spread and have a poor prognosis. Midline tumours metastasize quickly to deeper cervical nodes. Anterior tongue carcinomas tend to spread or recur despite adequate primary treatment.

Oral tumours can initially be treated with surgery, with or without radical neck dissection. Radiotherapy causes less functional impairment, but mucositis and xerostomia is invariable. Dental care is essential with radiotherapy: dental sepsis can contribute to osteoradionecrosis. Late disease, or treatment, may cause dysarthria, dysphagia if the tongue is not mobile, and local ulceration and extension. A third of patients with tongue tumours develop multiple primaries.

Carcinomas of the sinuses

Paranasal sinus tumours (maxillary, ethmoid, frontal, sphenoid) are commonly well-differentiated SCC. They present late with local swelling, pain, ocular symptoms if the orbit is involved and nasal or palatal extension with dental symptoms. Treatment is a combination of surgery and radiotherapy.

Salivary gland tumours

Malignancy is likely if a parotid mass is associated with facial palsy, or if a salivary gland mass is rapidly growing, hard and infiltrative.

Adenoid cystic carcinoma is the commonest salivary cancer. It is slow growing and ulcerative. The tumour spreads along perineural sheaths, with the potential for neuropathic pain. It also infiltrates marrow cavities, so X-rays may miss its true extent

Adenocarcinomas often have a relatively good prognosis because of their differentiation

Squamous cell carcinomas are more aggressive, cause pain, and metastasize early. They are more often metastatic than primary.

Undifferentiated carcinomas progress rapidly, and may mimic sarcomas. A small proportion of **pleomorphic adenomas** become malignant.

Management is usually surgical, with radiotherapy for residual or recurrent disease, high grade tumours or lymphomas.

Malignant melanoma

Commonest on the hard palate, also occurs on lower jaw, lips, tongue or buccal mucosa. It is infiltrative and metastasizes early to lymph nodes. It often ulcerates and bleeds.

Carcinoma of the larynx

May present with voice changes, dysphagia or stridor.

Glottic (vocal cord) carcinoma is commonest. Nodal metastases occur late. The main determinant of prognosis is the T stage. Initial treatment consists of radiotherapy, or surgery. Combined radiosurgical or radiochemotherapeutic approaches are often needed in cases of advanced disease

Supraglottic carcinoma presents late, with vague dysphagia, referred ear pain, or cervical lymphadenopathy; hoarseness may signify involvement of the cords or adjacent structures. Progression is by local extension (to the oropharynx, especially posterior third of the tongue, hypopharynx, or glottis) or lymph node spread. Treatment is commonly by radical radiotherapy; surgery has to be radical (total laryngectomy[7]), but has to be used in certain settings, e.g. airway obstruction. Radical neck dissection may be warranted. Restoration of the voice has to be considered after total laryngectomy (📖 see p. 132)

Subglottic carcinomas are rare but highly invasive. Pyriform fossa tumours behave like supraglottic tumours and have a poor prognosis. Postcricoid tumours may be associated with iron deficiency (Patterson–Brown–Kelly syndrome) and invade the hypopharynx circumferentially. Radiotherapy, (sometimes very) radical surgery and chemotherapy have a role in management, depending on the exact site and stage

Carcinomas of the pharynx

Usually these are squamous cell carcinomas, though lymphomas are fairly common, especially for the tonsils and nasopharynx.

Nasopharyngeal carcinomas cause nasal obstruction, epistaxis and otitis media from eustachian tube obstruction. Lower cranial nerve palsies from base of skull extension, or third, fifth and sixth nerve palsies from cavernous sinus invasion, signify advanced disease. Growth into the posterior orbit also takes place. These may spread haematogenously

Tumours are often **anaplastic**. Radiotherapy is the treatment of choice. Unusually for head and neck cancers, irradiation of the neck is as effective as radical neck dissection, though very occasionally may cause damage to the upper spinal cord. Xerostomia is common from salivary gland irradiation. Chemotherapy is sometimes very effective. Late recurrences (over 2 years) can be retreated

Oropharyngeal carcinomas frequently present late. They produce dysarthria, pain and risk of aspiration. Radical radiotherapy is usual but extensive surgery with radical neck dissection followed by RT may be indicated in locally advanced disease

Hypopharyngeal carcinomas are uncommon but have a poor prognosis as they occur in a silent area with late diagnosis. Aggressive treatment has to be used judiciously

7 Ward E. C., et al. (2002) Swallowing outcomes following laryngectomy and pharyngolaryngectomy. *Archives of Otolaryngology—Head & Neck Surgery*, **128**: 181–6.

Pain

Pain is widely prevalent in head and neck cancers[8] (up to 100% has been reported), particularly in those with advanced disease. With the complex anatomy of the head and neck, diverse anatomical structures are compressed or invaded by tumour in a small space. Thus pain is often mixed somatic (bone, muscle, skin) and neuropathic, and treatment may need to combine:

- Opioids[9]
- NSAIDs
- Antidepressants, anticonvulsants, etc. for neuropathic pain
- Other drugs
- Non-pharmacological techniques

Sources of pain in cancer of the head and neck

- Local infiltration with tumour, e.g. ulceration, infection
- Vascular and lymphatic occlusion producing oedema, lymphoedema and sometimes pain
- Bone invasion or extension of soft tissue infection causing osteomyelitis
- Nerve involvement or pressure: adenoid cystic carcinoma, in particular (but to a lesser extent most head and neck tumours) can show perineural invasion and extension
- Referred pain is very common, e.g. earache from most structures in the face, neck and mouth
- Treatment-related, e.g. chemotherapy- or RT-induced mucositis

Approach to pain assessment[10]

1 Take a detailed pain history, with special emphasis on character, exacerbating factors and accompanying dysfunction. Functional disturbances need treatment in their own right: they are distressing and disruptive to the patient
2 Examine the head and neck for masses and deformities
3 Check the movement of involved joints
4 Carry out a cranial nerve assessment
5 Occasionally, radiology or other tests are helpful in elucidating the cause of pain

8 Talmi Y. P., et al. (1997) Pain experienced by patients with terminal head and neck carcinoma. *Cancer*, **80**(6), 1117–23.

9 Mercadante S. (1998) Opioid responsiveness in patients with advanced head and neck cancer. *Supportive Care in Cancer*, **6**, 482–5.

10 Vecht C. J., et al. (1992) Types and causes of pain in cancer of the head and neck. *Cancer*, **70**(1), 178–84.

Table 6h.1 Specific pain syndromes

Syndrome	Location, features	Causes	Notes
Shoulder syndrome	Pain in shoulder, difficulty with certain movements, e.g. putting on jacket	• Radical neck dissection (due to axillary nerve sacrifice/damage)	Patient can only abduct arm to 75° and flex arm to 45°
Trigeminal neuralgia-like syndrome	Lancinating, continuous/paroxysmal. Distribution of Va, Vb and/or Vc, not crossing midline, though very occasionally bilateral	• Middle/posterior fossa tumours • Base of skull metastases • Meningeal metastases	Trigger areas or activities such as chewing, talking, breeze of air. May be accompanied by neurological signs ± diplopia, dysarthria, dysphagia, headache
Glossopharyngeal neuralgia	Severe unilateral paroxysmal pain in throat or beneath the angle of the jaw, may radiate to ear, often precipitated by swallowing	• Meningeal metastases • Disease around jugular foramen • Local disease around the base of the tongue or oropharynx	Occasionally associated with syncope or postural hypotension
Jugular foramen syndrome	Pain occiput to vertex, ipsilateral shoulder or neck	• Base of skull metastases[11] • Meningeal metastases	Horner's syndrome, lower cranial nerve signs ± local tenderness Worse on head movement

[11] Greenberg H. S., Deck M. D. F., Vikram B., Chu F. C., Posner J. B. (1981) Metastasis to the base of the skull: clinical findings in 43 patients. Neurology, **31**(5): 530–7.

(Continued)

Table 6h.1 Specific pain syndromes (*Continued*)

Syndrome	Location, features	Causes	Notes
Clivus syndrome	Vertex headache worse on head flexion. ± VI–XII signs	• Base of skull metastases • Meningeal metastases	
Orbital syndrome	Retro-orbital/frontal headache	• Orbital metastases • Meningeal metastases • Metastases around sella turcica, with sphenoid bone or cavernous sinus invasion	± Diplopia, visual loss, proptosis, extraocular nerve palsies
Sphenoid sinus metastases	Bifrontal headache radiating to both temples, intermittent retro-orbital pain	• Base of skull metastases: sphenoid sinus • Meningeal metastases	± Nasal stuffiness, diplopia, VI palsy
Occipital condyle invasion	Severe occipital pain exacerbated by movement	• Occipital condyle invasion	± XII palsy

Further pain management options

- **Tumour mass reduction** by surgery, radiotherapy or chemotherapy is usually the best way of reducing pain
- Radiotherapy is particularly useful for bone metastases, e.g. base of skull
- Steroids, e.g. dexamethasone 4–8mg p.o. daily, may contribute to analgesia by reducing swelling inside restricted fascial spaces. They are also useful temporizing measures while effective doses of other antineuropathic pain agents are built up. Doses are then usually able to be tailed off gradually
- **Antibiotics** can relieve pain by reducing pressure in tight fascial compartments or by controlling osteomyelitis.
- **Nerve blocks** are often difficult due to the distorted anatomy following disease or treatment

Mouth problems in head and neck cancer

Apart from disease and therapy, other contributory factors include:
• Smoking and alcohol
• Dry mouth: medication, treatment, dehydration
• Poor dental hygiene – e.g. made difficult by intraoral mucosal tenderness or friable tumour
• Infection and bleeding from fungating tumours
• Trismus, restricting mouth opening
• Vitamin deficiencies associated with poor nutrition
• Underlying osteomyelitis

Dry mouth is extremely common due to:
• Radiotherapy involving salivary glands
• Antimuscarinic drugs, opioids
• Blocked nose leading to open-mouth breathing
• Dehydration, including diuretics

Xerostomia can lead to decreased taste perception, poor appetite; food becomes more difficult to swallow, and intraoral infections and dental caries become much more likely.

Management of xerostomia[12]

Includes:
• Dental hygiene: (See Oral problems p. 302.) May occasionally require specialist advice
• Adequate hydration
• General measures, e.g. sucking on fruit drops, pineapple chunks
• Synthetic salivas, e.g. Saliva Orthana: little evidence of effectiveness in these circumstances
• Simple sialogogues, e.g. Salivix tablets
• Pilocarpine tablets[11] or eye drops instilled in the mouth: but can induce sweating or gastrointestinal complaints
• Treat underlying causes when possible

Dribbling

Usually indicates either a problem with swallowing saliva or a mass in the mouth, such as an infected fungating tumour. It is also associated with poor lip closure, as in facial palsy. This is managed by *antimuscarinic drugs* e.g. transdermal or sublingual hyoscine, *tricyclic antidepressants*, and occasionally surgery.

12 Johnson J. T., *et al.* (1993) Oral pilocarpine for post-irradiation xerostomia in patients with head and neck cancer. *New England Journal of Medicine*, **329**(6), 390–5.

Sticky, viscous saliva

Common and underreported. It is a frequent complication of radiotherapy, as serous salivary glands are more sensitive to its effects than the mucous glands. Antimuscarinics, apart from reducing the volume of saliva, also render it more viscous. Beta-blockers can make saliva looser, as can hydration. Antibiotics for intraoral infections as well as frequent, meticulous oral hygiene help.

Mucositis

Usually follows radiotherapy or chemotherapy with certain agents, e.g. fluorouracil, methotrexate or cyclophosphamide. There are reports of a reduction of mucositis by treating intraoral infections.[13] Treatment usually requires a combination of oral analgesics and topically applied local anaesthetic agents or anti-inflammatories. Benzydamine, an anti-inflammatory with local anaesthetic properties, is often used as a mouthwash and has been claimed to reduce the duration of mucositis, as has sucralfate. However, a recent Cochrane review shows that neither of these two drugs is effective; nor is chlorhexidine. On the other hand, allopurinol and vitamin E appear to be.[12] The evidence is, however, weak even for these.

13 Worthington H. V., Clarkson J. E., Eden O. B. (2007) Interventions for preventing oral mucositis for patients with cancer receiving treatment Cochrane Database of systematic Reviews.

Tracheostomy

Tracheostomies:
- Relieve respiratory obstruction
- Reduce anatomical dead space, improving respiratory failure
- Aid removal of respiratory secretions
- Can protect the airway in aspiration
- Allow prolonged artificial ventilation with less trauma to the airways

However, bypassing the nose and upper pharynx also removes:
- Patient's voice (📖 see p. 430, section on speech)
- Warming and humidification of inspired air
- Filtering function of the nose
- First line of the immune response: the tonsils
- The narrower bore of the tracheostomy tube compared to the natural airway increases airways resistance
- Tracheostomies impair swallowing performance

To prevent drying and damage to the tracheal mucosa, or an increase in sputum production, tracheal or lung infection, the nasopharyngeal functions need to be compensated for by good tracheostomy care.

Types of tracheostomy

Most tracheostomies seen in palliative care will be established surgical tracheostomies, and this section concentrates on these. For percutaneous tracheostomy, used mostly in intensive care for airways management, and for the management of new surgical tracheostomies, look in appropriate ENT texts.

A guide to types of tracheostomy tube[14]

It is crucial to know what type of tracheostomy tube you are dealing with:

Metal or plastic: Metal is less irritant, but is rarely used as prolonged intubation with plastic tubes is now possible. Metal tubes interfere with CT and MRI scans and radiotherapy.

Cuffed or uncuffed: An inflatable cuff at the lower end of the tracheostomy tube seals air leaks around the tube. This permits artificial ventilation and protects the airway if there is a risk of aspiration. However, prolonged cuff inflation causes ischaemic damage to the tracheal wall. Prevention requires frequent pressure checks and periods of cuff deflation. Apart from some high aspiration risk patients, all patients seen in general wards, palliative care settings or the home environment are almost certain to have uncuffed tubes.

---

14 *National Library of Guidelines: Best practice Statement: Caring for the patient with a tracheostomy.* (2007) NHS Quality Improvement Scotland. www.nhshealthyquality.org/nhsqis/files/tracheorev_bps_mar07.pdf

Three essential warnings about cuffed tubes

1. For resuscitation, the cuff must be inflated for bag ventilation to be effective. In most palliative care patients, of course, resuscitation may be inappropriate.

2. If the tracheostomy is occluded, e.g. by secretions or a decannulation cap, and the balloon is inflated, the airway will be totally blocked and the patient will suffocate. Open the cap, deflate the balloon or remove the tracheostomy tube immediately.

3. Speaking valves should, in general, not be used with cuffed fenestrated tubes as the extra resistance increases the work of breathing considerably.

With or without inner cannula: An removable inner cannula is nowadays almost always used. This prolongs the life of the tube before it needs changing (30 days instead of 7–14 days with a single lumen tube), and allows cleaning to reduce risks of occlusion and infection. The inner cannula should be removed, inspected for encrustation and cleaned every four hours or if respiratory distress develops.

Fenestrated tubes: Fenestrated tubes have little windows in their wall to allow air flow round the tube as well as through it. **Note**: *Patients at risk of aspiration should not have fenestrated tubes.* If suctioning though a fenestrated tube, ensure there is a non-fenestrated inner cannula in situ, to avoid sucking the tracheal mucosa into the fenestrations.

Humidification: Ventilated patients need heat-moisture exchanger devices. Long-term tracheostomy or laryngectomy patients will usually use a Buchanon bib or foam filter dressing, which needs changing every 24 hours. Regular saline nebulizers with tracheostomy fittings also help keep the mucosa healthy.

Suctioning: This can clear up excessive secretions but carries risks. Suction pressures should be between 13.5 and 20kPa. The suction catheter should not be inserted for more than a third of its length, should not make the patient cough and suctioning should not be used for longer than 15 seconds.

Signs of problems with a tracheostomy
- Stridor, difficulty breathing
- Bleeding
- Increasing thickness and volume of sputum
- Difficulty expectorating

If these develop, you may need specialist advice.

Tracheostomy tube obstruction (📖 See Emergencies, p. 436.)

Swallowing problems[15]

Swallowing requires:
- Good lip closure: prevents food leakage
- Teeth: break food down
- Mobile tongue: crushes bolus and pushes it back into pharynx
- Saliva: lubrication
- An intact palate
- Functioning cheek musculature for food not to collect in gingival sulcus
- Intact oral and pharyngeal musculature and innervation (V, VII, IX, X, XI, XII)

Remember innervation:
- Lingual nerve, from Vc, supplies sensation
- Chorda tympani (VII) supplies taste to anterior two-thirds of tongue
- Glossopharyngeal (IX) supplies sensation and taste to posterior third of tongue
- Hypoglossal (XII) supplies tongue musculature

A tongue lacking sensation produces more long-term swallowing difficulties than a tongue with restricted mobility.

Obstruction by a mass, or functional problems (muscle dysfunction, nerve damage), pain, dry mouth or tooth loss contribute to dysphagia.

Improving swallowing

Perhaps the commonest cause of difficulty swallowing is dry mouth. (For management see p. 302.)

Other helpful manoeuvres

- Chilled food helps re-educate lost sensation, e.g. after surgery
- Encouraging the patient to chew or even just manipulate the bolus in the mouth for a few seconds facilitates initiation of the swallow
- Alternating the temperature, taste and texture of food in a meal keeps awareness of the swallowing process high, important while the process has to be deliberate
- Carbonated drinks increase the sensation of the liquid bolus
- Placement of food boluses in parts of the mouth where sensation is still intact aids patients with diminished sensation
- Viscous boluses, e.g. thickened liquids, purees, permit poorly co-ordinated muscles to mount a much more effective swallow than thin liquids
- Head or body tilting in the appropriate direction can utilize gravity in the swallowing process or protect the airway

15 Kendall K. (1997) Dysphagia in head and neck surgery patients. In *Dysphagia Assessment and Treatment Planning: A Team Approach* (ed. R. Leonard, K. Kendall K.), pp. 19–27. San Diego, Singular Publishing Group.

Is the patient at risk of aspiration?

Hints include:
- Wet or gurgling noises with breathing: fluid in the airways
- Altered voice during eating: food on vocal folds
- Cough associated with swallowing
- Fatigue during a meal: leads to prolonged meal times
- Lower cranial nerve palsies
- Aspiration pneumonia

Seek a speech and language therapy (SALT) assessment if appropriate, considering the patient's clinical state.

Gastrostomies

Many patients come into palliative care with a gastrostomy tube (a feeding tube bypassing the mouth) in place. In patients with advanced disease, inserting a gastrostomy has to be judged carefully[16], considering not only the small risks of the procedure itself but later risks as well, for example diarrhoea, vomiting or a feeling of fullness may occur especially in the first weeks after insertion. It is important to distinguish starvation, which responds to feeding, from cachexia, which does not respond to feeding alone. The latter is more likely in the presence of large tumour masses, metastatic disease, certain types of tumours or ongoing sepsis.

Types of gastrostomy

Nasogastric tubes (NGT): Can be used for feeding temporarily (for up to four weeks).

Percutaneous endoscopic gastrostomy (PEG): Inserted under sedation and local anaesthetic using a 'pull' technique. Throughout its lifetime, the PEG tube should be rotated through 360° at least twice a week to prevent adhesion formation.

Radiologically inserted gastrostomy (RIG): These are inserted in the radiology department without sedation by a 'push' technique under fluoroscopic control. The tube is thinner than a PEG tube, and is held in place by its pigtail shape; it should **not** therefore be rotated, or it will dislodge.

Surgical gastrostomy: Carried out under general anaesthetic, usually when it is impossible to insert a PEG or RIG.

Care of the gastrostomy tube

The fixation plate should be maintained at 1–1.5cm from the abdominal exit stoma. A 50mL flush of sterile water should be used before and after every feed or administration of medication, and regularly three times a day. Soda water, but not other fizzy drinks (too acidic), can be used to unblock stubborn blockages.

Feeding

Patients should be maintained at an angle of 30–45° during feeding and for 2 hours after to reduce the risk of aspiration. Many centres are less keen for feeding to occur during sleep because of the aspiration risk.

Problems with gastrostomies

- Dislodgement
- Leakage: chemical digestion of surrounding skin
- Overgranulation
- Infection
- Blockage: more common with narrower gauge tubes

16 Rabeneck L., Wray P., Petersen N. J. (1996) Long-term outcomes of patients receiving percutaneous endoscopic gastrostomy tubes. *Journal of General Internal Medicine*, **11**(5): 287–93.

Speech problems

Head and neck cancer and its treatment impair communication in various ways:
- Dysarthria, e.g. tongue fixed by tumour
- Laryngectomy
- Recurrent laryngeal nerve palsies
- Loss of facial expression: VII palsy, facial disfigurement
- Kissing: tumour/body image problems
- Reception of communication by others: hearing or visual impairment

Studies show that up to 92% of patients with head and neck cancer have difficulties with speech. This has been found in surveys to be the single most important correlation to quality of life after treatment.

Production and articulation of speech

The vocal cords produce sound which is then modified by the action of tongue, lips and mouth to produce intelligible speech. For example, good lip closure is needed to say 'p' or 'b', while a mobile tongue is necessary to produce 't' and 's'. Thus problems with any part of this apparatus can produce difficulties with intelligible speech.

Laryngectomy

This produces the most profound speech deficit, as the production of sound is removed. Various techniques have been developed to address this:[17]

Oesophageal speech: produced by swallowing air and then expelling it while mouthing the necessary sounds. Various techniques are available for learning this, and it is taught by a speech therapist. Only 25–50% of patients master this technique, and it is useless in noisy environments or from any distance.

Speaking valves, e.g. Blom–Singer valve: here an opening is made between the larynx and oesophagus, and a valve is fitted which allows oesophageal air to be used to produce sound. Fluency rates of 70–90% have been reported. However, the dynamics of sound production may change again if there is major local disease recurrence.

Electrolarynx: this produces clear intelligible words, although in an 'electronic' voice. It occupies one of the patient's hands to keep it against the neck while talking.

17 Blalock D. (1997) Speech rehabilitation after treatment of laryngeal carcinoma. *Otolaryngologic Clinics of North America*, **30**(2): 179–88.

Recurrent laryngeal nerve palsy

This causes hoarseness if it is unilateral, sometimes worse as the day wears on, but reduces the voice to a whisper if bilateral. The recurrent laryngeal nerves are motor to the intrinsic muscles of the larynx; they also supply sensory fibres to the mucosa below the level of the vocal folds. Therefore, in bilateral palsy the sphincter effect of the vocal folds during swallowing is lost and aspiration can result in adductor paralysis. In addition, aspiration will not be detected due to the sensory loss, and the risk of aspiration pneumonia is high. Bilateral abductor paralysis can produce stridor.

There are various techniques for treating vocal fold palsies:

- Behavioural techniques and biofeedback may be taught by speech therapists
- Injection of Teflon, fat or collagen into a paralysed vocal fold
- More invasive techniques (thyroplasty, arytenoid adduction, re-innervation, vocal cord lateralization) are very rarely indicated in patients with advanced disease
- Patients who aspirate from bilateral vocal fold paralysis are temporarily helped by vocal fold injection. More extensive surgery is unlikely to be indicated in this patient group with end-stage illness

Articulation problems

Result from:

- Tongue problems: glossectomy, tumour
- Facial palsy
- Dry mouth
- Poor lip closure
- Poor control of jaw movement: e.g. Vc palsy
- Defect in palate (excision) or teeth
- Other lower cranial nerve palsies: base of skull metastases

How to communicate with patients with articulation problems

- Choose a quiet place where you can hear better
- Sit in a position where you can see the patient talk. Make sure there is enough light to see properly
- Sit close enough to hear
- Take time: you get tuned in
- Encourage the use of gestures which give useful clues to the meaning
- If necessary, remind the patient to keep their sentences short and uncomplicated
- Encourage the patient to articulate each syllable clearly but not to overarticulate
- Learn lip reading
- Encourage the family to participate
- Involve a speech and language therapist
- Be aware of the range of procedures on offer

Remember:

Lack of fluency does not just result in loss of ability to speak. Patients are often embarassed into reducing their communication so that **the _content_ of speech also becomes poorer and deals only with the concrete.** These patients need time to express their deeper thoughts, and utilization of alternative means of communication, e.g. as above and pen and paper. Also think about non-verbal expression, e.g. art therapy, which can often express feelings better than words.

Infection and fistulae

Local infection

This has devastating consequences in advanced tumours:
• Septicaemia
• Wound extension
• Pain, from: inflammation; pressure build-up within fascial spaces; erosion into adjacent tissues; maceration, e.g. of skin by exudates
• Fistula formation
• Vascular erosion: catastrophic bleeds
• Cachexia in unchecked sepsis
• Thick saliva: heavy intraoral exudate makes speech and breathing difficult

Osteomyelitis

Particularly in the jaw, this is common and it produces discharging sinuses, pain and tooth loss; necrosis is particularly extensive in irradiated bone. Two very rare localized infections deserve mention. First, base of skull infections spread via the retropharyngeal space to the anterior mediastinum (the cervical vertebrae are protected by thick fascia). Such infections are, however, commonly tubercular. Second, infections of the submental space (Ludwig's angina) cause pain, high fever, trismus and hypersalivation; floor of the mouth swelling occasionally causes respiratory obstruction.

Treatment

Most infections are caused by anaerobes and Gram-positive cocci which are commensals in the mouth. Gram-negative bacteria are less frequently found. Options include metronidazole and a penicillin, or clindamycin (concentrated in bone, but remember risk of pseudomembranous colitis), or a third-generation cephalosporin. Do not ignore the indispensable role of antibiotics in analgesia and reduction of intraoral exudates: gratifyingly rapid effects are often seen on both, enabling the patient to communicate properly and breathe easily for the first time in months. The conditions which set off the infection in the first place usually persist, so consider continuous prophylactic antibiotics at a lower dose (little trial evidence, but clinical experience suggests it is a very effective ongoing symptomatic measure).

Fistulae

Once formed, fistulae are maintained because:
• There is something in the depths of the wound needing to be discharged, usually infectious exudates: bony sequestrate in chronic osteomyelitis
• The chemical composition of the exudate prevents healing: e.g. saliva, small bowel fistulae

In palliative care there is usually an untreatable deep necrotic tumour, but bear in mind drainable abscesses and osteomyelitis.

Avoid exudates or saliva bathing the great vessels (e.g. presence of fistulas between oropharynx and skin), which greatly increases the risk of catastrophic bleeding, through:

- Dressings
- Drying up saliva (📖 see Mouth care, p. 300)
- Continuous antibiotics
- Making a silicone elastomer plug to fit large fistulae. Unfortunately, malignant fistulae enlarge, so this plug will need to be renewed regularly. Such plugs are only used in single, clean, open cavities: plugging complex cavities impedes drainage, extending deep infection and encouraging new fistulae to form where they can drain freely.

Remember: fistula effluent will find the route of least resistance—this can sometimes be used to divert fistulae away from 'tiger country'.

Emergencies

Catastrophic bleeds (partly based on British Association of Head and Neck Oncology Nurses guidelines[18])
These are among the most feared complications of cancer of the head and neck, although they are rare.

Risk factors
- Previous neck irradiation
- Fungating tumour invading the artery
- Postoperative: flap necrosis
- Infection
- Salivary fistula
- Systemic factors, such as malnutrition, cachexia, increased age

Warning signs
- Minor bleeding from wound, tracheostomy or mouth
- 'Pulsations' from artery or tracheostomy or flapsite—false aneurysm formation
- Sternal or high epigastric pain several hours before rupture if carotid
- The patient may become restless and irritable

Management
1 If the patient is thought to be at risk, discuss a plan within the multidisciplinary team. Can the risk be reduced, e.g. embolization or ligation of the implicated artery?
2 What should the patient and family be told?

To tell or not to tell about potential bleeding?

Consider:
- Bleeds are often feared but rarely occur
- No preparation for a very severe bleed can make it any less frightening
- Can the patient or family do anything to reduce the risk of bleeding, e.g. embolization?
- Are there special circumstances, e.g. children in the house who would be especially traumatized by a catastrophic bleed?
- Is the patient doing anything that might increase the risk, e.g. neglecting an infection in a dangerous area?
- Has the patient had any warning bleeds or are there other severe risk factors which would indicate that a major bleed is more likely

---

18 BAHNON website: www.bahnon.org.uk

Obviously, if the patient or family ask specifically about catastrophic bleeds this should be discussed with them, giving information in small steps and letting them decide how much they want to know. It is also useful to ask in a general way if they have any special fears about how the patient will die, as this may bring out unspoken fears. Otherwise, one needs to be careful not to raise fears of unlikely complications, which are terrifying and about which nothing may be able to be done.

3 Stop anticoagulants, aspirin, NSAIDs (COX-2 inhibitors may be safe)—though this will make no difference to a major bleed. Correct any platelet abnormalities if warning bleeds occur.

Checklist
- Treat infection
- Ensure the family, and staff, know who to contact in an emergency
- Have emergency sedative drugs in the home: morphine, midazolam.
- Ensure all professionals involved know the plan, e.g. district nurses, GP, etc.
- If in a hospice or hospital, nurse the patient in a side room to avoid potential distress of other patients or relatives
- Discreetly have trolley available with blue towels, gloves, apron, emergency drugs
- If there is a bleed, a senior member of staff must stay with the patient. Nothing is as reassuring as a calm human presence, nothing as frightening as panic. Call for help
- Be respectful of the family's wishes about whether they wish to stay with the patient. Support them
- Apply towels to the bleeding site and absorb the bleeding if possible.
- Apply gentle suctioning to the mouth and trachea as necessary
- Give IV/IM midazolam, e.g. 10mg; if necessary, repeat in 10–15 min. Subcutaneous drugs are poorly absorbed in shock
- Occasional families might be taught to administer rectal diazepam or buccal midazolam. Few will be calm enough to do this, and, in most cases, it loads them with an extra responsibility they can do without.
- After the event, debrief the family and staff, and point them in the direction of their normal supportive networks. Extensive counselling just after an event has actually been shown to be more likely to do harm than good
- Offer family and staff (including non-clinical involved staff, such as domestics) a chance for a follow-up meeting later to deal with any questions they might have

Tracheostomy tube obstruction

Causes
- Infection
- Excessive mucus production
- Pressure sores
- Tube displacement
- Granulation tissue

Management
- Call for help
- Reposition the patient in semi-recumbent position
- Ask the patient to cough, use suction
- Manipulate the head to eliminate tube kinks
- Give oxygen
- Remove inner cannula
- Suction
- Resuscitate if appropriate
- If severe problems breathing, sedate as for haemorrhage (📖 see p. 494)

Quality of life

Cancer of the head and neck not only has the usual overtones of any cancer but also has a major impact on appearance, communication and the basic functions of life—feeding and breathing, for example. It is, therefore, to be expected that it will have a massive impact on patients' quality of life. In other cancers it has been shown that patient-rated quality of life is a more accurate prognostic indicator than performance status as rated by clinicians.

There is a plethora of scales which look at quality of life in head and neck cancer. The most widely used are:

- **EORTC (**European Organization for Research and Treatment of Cancer) **QLQ-C30 and QLQ+ H&N35:** The two parts make up a 66-item questionnaire. Some questions in the general module are of little relevance to most terminally ill patients (e.g. difficulty carrying a suitcase)
- **FACT H&N** (Functional Assessment of Chronic Illness Therapy): Again consisting of a general module—FACT G—and a site-specific module, FACT H&N for head and neck cancer. These questionnaires look at physical, social and family, emotional and functional well-being as well as particular concerns for the specific condition. http://www.facit.org/facit_questionnair.htm.
- **University of Washington Quality of Life scale, UWQoL:** This looks at pain, appearance, activity level, recreation, swallowing, chewing, speech, shoulder function, taste and saliva production. Version 4 includes questions about depression and anxiety.[18] http://depts.washington.edu/soar/projects/dxcat/hnca/qol_uw.htm
- **SEIQoL(Schedule for the Evaluation of Individual Quality of Life):** In this scale the patient decides which domains of quality of life are most important for them at this time. The patient sets the agenda.

Most QoL studies have been done on patients at or around the time of primary treatment and the interval after that. There are now some studies that look at QoL in later disease but very few which pursue it longitudinally throughout an illness.

It is impossible to summarize here the key findings of these studies,[19] but let us highlight one aspect. There is a subset population who judge their QoL to be very good despite major disease and deeply disfiguring treatment. It has become clear that what gives life quality can change as an illness progresses—the so-called '**response shift**'. Understanding this, and understanding how disability and disfigurement affect quality of life, will allow us both to adapt our management to promote a better life for patients, and to understand better the process of coping and adaptation to illness, which might in turn lead us to ways of helping people develop coping strategies.

18 Rogers S. N., et al. (2002) The addition of mood and anxiety domains to the University of Washington quality of life scale. Head and Neck, **24**(6): 521–9.

19 Rogers S. N., Fisher S. E., Woolgar J. A. (1999) A review of quality of life assessment in oral cancer. International Journal of Maxillofacial Surgery, **28**: 99–117.

Body image and sexuality

Slade defined **body image** as the picture we have in our minds of the size, shape and form of our bodies, and our feelings concerning these characteristics and our body parts. There is little gender or age difference in the impact of appearance changes on body image. The degree to which people can be rehabilitated after facial disfigurement also does not depend on the degree of disfigurement but correlates with perceived social support and with the degree of dysfunction.

Factors which have been associated with poor body image include:
- Poor self-esteem
- Social anxiety
- Self-consciousness
- Depressive features

Sexuality is a closely related field. One study found how, a year after head and neck surgery, marital and sexual relationships still suffer, and alcohol use (a marker of depression, particularly in men) is higher in a very significant number of patients. Almost half of patients at least a year after treatment in another small study had problems with libido, arousal, sexual activity; a significant minority still never or almost never kissed and held hands with their partner.

Working with body image and sexuality

Questions about body image and sexuality feel difficult and embarrassing to raise, yet must be explored. Sometimes a broad question can be asked which the patient will often interpret as referring to their sexual relationship if it is preoccupying them:
- 'How has this affected your relationship with your wife?'
- 'What things that really matter to you do you miss?'
- 'How did you feel about yourself after the operation?'

Often a more direct approach, which tells the patient that it is all right to talk about issues of sex and intimacy, is needed:
- 'How did your husband/wife cope with the change in your appearance after the operation?'
- 'What impact did it have on your sex life?'
- 'How have you dealt with that as a couple?'

Normalizing embarrassing fears in this manner is one important step in dealing with them.

It is obvious from all the above that body image and sexuality depend more on perceived social support and the existence of supportive relationships than on the degree of disfigurement or disability. This again brings us back to one of the central, though often unsaid, tenets of palliative care: that ultimately what matters most to people is being cared for and respected and loved. There is now good work showing how after cancer treatment, social rehabilitation through a simple behavioural approach is effective. Medical staff play an important role by modelling attitudes and allowing patients to practise new behaviours in a safe environment. For example, patients can be trained to prepare a number of responses for when people inevitably comment to them about their appearance, or when they walk into a pub and everyone stares. Changing Faces, a UK charity, runs courses about this.[20] But the situation in advanced cancer, where appearance rapidly worsens rather than being static as after surgery, where it is accompanied by generalized bodily deterioration and by a shrinking social world, has not been explored properly yet.

20 www.changingfaces.org.uk

General medical problems in patients with head and neck cancer

When one recalls that the main risk factors for head and neck cancer are smoking and alcohol, it is not surprising that concurrent medical problems are common in these patients:

- **Malignancies in other organs** are common,[21] particularly lung, but also other smoking- or alcohol-related tumours: bladder, kidney, pancreas, liver. This may both have physical consequences to the patient, e.g. due to metastatic disease from a distant malignancy, and have a psychological toll on them. It should be kept in mind that many patients are more prone to other head and neck cancers too, so patients with a history of two or three head and neck primaries and a distant primary are encountered as well
- **Ischaemic heart disease**: keep in mind that such patients are less tolerant of anaemia
- **Alcohol-induced cardiomyopathies**: may limit the use of some agents for neuropathic pain
- **Strokes**: if these are present in addition to neurological damage from the tumour, almost total disability can result
- **Chronic obstructive airways disease**: airways problems from head and neck cancer can precipitate decompensation and respiratory failure
- **Thromboembolic disease**: may necessitate difficult decisions about continuing anticoagulation if there is a risk of bleeding. Sometimes conversion to heparin will allow rapid responsiveness if bleeding occurs.
- **Alcoholic liver disease**: may contribute to clotting problems or to altered handling of medication
- **Nutritional deficiencies**: from poor diet, dysphagia, alcohol, cachexia
- **Psychiatric problems**: depression, anxiety
- **Substance abuse**: watch out for alcohol withdrawal in particular.

Syncope

This is common among patients with cancer of the head and neck.[22] It may be carotid sinus syncope from metastatic compression or post-radiotherapy fibrosis. Glossopharyngeal neuralgia can lead to sinus arrest, perhaps as intense glossopharyngeal nucleus stimulation overflows to the vagal nucleus leading to parasympathetic suppression of the cardiac pacemaker.

Do not ignore the fact that many patients will have been on high doses of steroids for prolonged periods. This may mean that if they are in crisis steroids may need to be restarted if an acute and potentially fatal crisis is to be avoided.

21 Crosher R., McIlroy R. (1998) The incidence of other primary tumours in patients with oral cancers in Scotland. *British Journal of Oral and Maxillofacial Surgery*, **36**(1): 58–62.

22 MacDonald D. R., et al. (1983) Syncope from head and neck cancer. *Journal of Neuro-Oncology*, **1**: 257–67.

Further reading

Books

Close L., et al. (1998) Essentials of Head and Neck Oncology. New York: Thieme.

Leonard R., Kendall K. (eds) (1997) Dysphagia Assessment and Treatment Planning: A Team Approach. San Diego: Singular Publishing Group.

Watkinson J. C., Gaze M. N., Wilson J. A. (2000) Stell and Maran's Head and Neck Surgery (4th edn). Oxford: Butterworth Heinemann.

Articles

Chua K. S. G., et al. (1999) Pain and loss of function in head and neck cancer survivors. Journal of Pain and Symptom Management, 18(3): 193–202.

Forbes K. (1997) Palliative care in patients with cancer of the head and neck. Clinical Otolaryngology & Allied Sciences, 22(2): 117–22.

Endocrine and metabolic complications of advanced cancer

Understanding the association between endocrine and metabolic complications in advanced cancer is increasingly complex as knowledge of the processes involved at the genetic and biochemical level grows.

Malignancy produces endocrine effects in two ways:

- Directly interferes with the function of endocrine glands by invasion or obstruction
- Remotely produces effects without direct local spread—paraneoplastic syndromes

Paraneoplastic syndromes are caused by:

- Tumour cells secreting hormones, cytokines and growth factors
- Normal cells secreting products in response to the presence of tumour cells (such as antibodies in the Lambert–Eaton syndrome)

Paraneoplastic syndromes

- Hypercalcaemia
- Cushing's syndrome
- Syndrome of inappropriate antidiuresis
- Hypoglycaemia (non-islet cell)
- Carcinoid syndrome

Non-paraneoplastic

- Diabetes mellitus

Paraneoplastic Syndromes

Hypercalcaemia (📖 see Chapter 16, Emergencies in palliative care)

Hypercalcaemia is the commonest life-threatening metabolic disorder associated with advanced cancer. As it is a condition which is usually amenable to treatment and is both distressing and fatal if untreated hypercalcaemia must always be sought in patients who are deteriorating for no clear cause.

Epidemiology

- Some 10% of patients with cancer develop hypercalcaemia
- Malignancy is responsible for 50% of the patients with hypercalcaemia who are treated in hospital
- Up to 20% of patients develop hypercalcaemia without bone metastases
- Most patients with hypercalcaemia of malignancy have disseminated disease—80% will not survive beyond one year
- The prognosis is poor, with a median survival of 3–4 months

Table 6i.1 Clinical features of hypercalcaemia of malignancy

General	Gastrointestinal	Neurological	Cardiological
Dehydration	Anorexia	Fatigue	Bradycardia
Polydipsia	Weight loss	Lethargy	Atrial arrhythmias
Pruritus	Nausea	Confusion	Ventricular arrhythmias
	Vomiting	Myopathy	Prolonged P–R interval
	Constipation	Seizures	Reduced Q–T interval
	Ileus	Psychosis	Wide T waves

Treatment
Rehydration followed by the administration of calcium-lowering agents is the mainstay of treatment. Drugs promoting hypercalcaemia (thiazide diuretics, vitamins A and D) should be withdrawn.

The corrected serum calcium should be calculated from the formula:

Corrected calcium = measured calcium + [(40 − serum albumin g/L) × 0.02]

In practice, most laboratories now correct for albumin routinely.

Intravenous fluids
Dehydration due to polyuria and vomiting is a prominent feature of acute or symptomatic hypercalcaemia. While large fluid volumes will lower serum calcium, calcium levels will seldom return to normal by rehydration alone and care to avoid fluid overload must be taken.

Rehydrating with 2–3L/day of fluid is now accepted practice, with daily serum electrolyte measurements to prevent hypokalaemia and hyponatraemia developing. There is little evidence that there is any benefit in using diuretics in conjunction with rehydration and they should be avoided.

Corticosteroids
While steroids have been shown to inhibit osteoclastic activity and calcium absorption from the gut *in vitro*, their use *in vivo* is limited. They are most effective in haematological malignancies when oral prednisolone 40–100mg/day is usually effective.

Bisphosphonates
These synthetic pyrophosphate analogues reduce bone resorption by inhibiting osteoclastic activity. They are highly effective at reducing hypercalcaemia, but take 48h to be effective. Infusions of bisphosphonates following rehydration are the mainstay of hypercalcaemia treatment. Many patients receive monthly infusions as outpatients to maintain calcium levels within the normal range.

Oral bisphosphonates have been used for maintenance therapy, but low bioavailability and gastrointestinal side-effects have limited their widespread use. Oral ibandronic acid, 50mg daily, is increasingly used. Tablets should be swallowed whole with plenty of water while sitting/standing, 30 minutes before breakfast or other medication.

Some 20% of patients with hypercalcaemia of malignancy will be resistant to bisphosphonate infusion therapy.

One of the following intravenous bisphosphonates may be used:

- Disodium pamidronate 30–90mg/over 2–4h
- Zoledronic acid 4mg over 15 minutes
- Clodronate 1.5g over 4h
- Ibandronic acid 2–4mg iv 1–2h

The more expensive zoledronic acid (4mg) has been found to achieve a normal corrected calcium in more patients, faster and for longer (4–6 weeks).

Complications of bisphosphonates

There has been an increase in recent reports of osteonecrosis of the jaw with intravenous bisphosphonates. Updated guidance indicates that early diagnosis and management is needed. Patients who need intravenous bisphosphonates should have a dental assessment and complete procedures if possible prior to commencing treatment. Good oral hygiene with regular dental visits should be advised. Exposed bone in the mouth should be reported with urgency to a dental professional.[1]

Calcitonin

Calcitonin inhibits osteoclastic bone resorption and encourages calcium excretion. It is effective in around a third of patients and usually causes a fall in calcium within 4h.

Doses of salmon calcitonin 100 units can be used subcutaneously every 6–8h. It is rarely used in palliative care since it needs frequent administration and correction of hypercalcaemia is short lasting.

Cushing's syndrome

- Ectopic secretion of corticotrophin (ACTH) by non-endocrine tumours is rare
- Associated pro-peptide secretion is more common, producing a more complex mosaic of symptoms
- Up to 20% of cases of Cushing's syndrome is caused by ectopic ACTH, often from an occult tumour
- Some 50% of cases of ectopic ACTH secretion is due to small cell lung carcinoma
- Some 15% of cases of ectopic ACTH secretion is due to carcinoid and neural crest tumours
- Long-term survivors of malignancies with associated ectopic ACTH secretion will often continue to have elevated ACTH levels

1 Weitzman R., et al. (2007) Critical review: updated recommendations for the prevention, diagnosis, and treatment of osteonecrosis of the jaw in cancer patients–May 2006. *Critical Reviews in Oncology/Hematology*, **62**(2): 148–52.

Clinical features	
Hypokalaemic metabolic alkalosis	Mental changes
Weak muscles	Glucose intolerance
Oedema	Weight loss
Raised blood pressure	

The more classical features of Cushing's syndrome, e.g. truncal obesity moon facies and striae, may suggest a benign tumour such as bronchial carcinoid or thymoma.

Investigations
- Increased free urinary cortisol
- Loss of diurnal variation of plasma cortisol
- Failure of cortisol suppression in low-dose (2mg) dexamethasone test
- Failure of cortisol to suppress ACTH levels following high-dose dexamethasone (2mg q.d.s. or 8mg nocte)

When the above investigations are still equivocal, more complex imaging techniques are available at specialist centres.

Treatment
The mainstay of treatment is inhibition of steroid synthesis.

Metyrapone
A dose of 250–750mg q.d.s. inhibits 11βhydroxylase, the final enzymatic step in steroid production, but again side-effects (nausea and vomiting) are common. The use of ketoconazole, bromocriptine and octreotide have also been advocated in case reports.

Treatment efficacy should be monitored by measuring 24h urinary cortisol excretion. As levels return to normal, hormone replacement therapy, as in Addison's disease, may be required (e.g. hydrocortisone 20mg at 0800h and 10mg at 1800h with fludrocortisone 0.05–0.15mg daily).

Syndrome of inappropriate antidiuresis (SIAD)

Hyponatraemia is common in patients with advanced malignancy due to many factors, including cardiac and hepatic failure, hyperglycaemia, diuretics and sick-cell syndrome. However, the presence of concentrated urine in conjunction with hypo-osmolar plasma, suggests abnormal free water excretion and the presence of the syndrome of inappropriate antidiuresis. (The SIAD acronym is more appropriate than SIADH, as there is no vasopressin hormone secretion in approximately 15% of cases.)

The vasopressin gene codes for peptide products, including arginine vasopressin (AVP) and vasopressin-specific neurophysin II (NP II). In malignancy-related SIAD, tumours secrete ectopic AVP.

SIAD is most frequently associated with small cell lung carcinoma or carcinoid tumours, but has also been noted in pancreatic, oesophageal, prostatic and haematological cancers.

Causes of SIAD

- Ectopic AVP
- Infections: lung, cerebral and meningeal
- Drugs: morphine, phenothiazines, tricyclics antidepressants

      NSAIDs

      vincristine

      cyclophosphamide

Clinical features

Significant symptoms of hyponatraemia develop at plasma sodium levels below 125mmol/L, with confusion progressing to stupor, coma and seizures. Nausea, vomiting and focal neurological signs may also develop.

The clinical features depend on both the levels of plasma sodium and the rate of decline. With gradual falls the brain cells can compensate against cerebral oedema by secreting potassium. Asymptomatic hyponatraemia suggests chronic SIAD, whereas symptomatic hyponatraemia suggests acute SIAD.

Diagnosis

Essential criteria

- Plasma hypo-osmolality (plasma osmolality <275 mosmol/kg H_2O and plasma sodium <135 mmol/L)
- Concentrated urine (with plasma osmolality >100 mosmol/kg H_2O)
- Normal plasma/extracellular fluid volume
- High urinary sodium (urine sodium >20mEq/L) on a normal salt and water intake
- Exclude: (i) hypothyroidism, (ii) hypoadrenalism and (iii) diuretics

Supportive criteria

Abnormal water load test (unable to excrete >90% of a 20mL/kg water load in 4h, and/or failure to dilute urine to osmolality <100mosmol/kg H_2O).

Management

Management depends on the rate of onset of symptoms and neurological complications.

Acute symptomatic hyponatraemia has a mortality rate of 5–8% and patients will need prompt correction with intravenous hypertonic saline with meticulous monitoring, as over-rapid correction can lead to central pontine myelinosis with quadriparesis and bulbar palsy.

Chronic asymptomatic hyponatraemia is best treated with fluid restriction. In effect, this means reducing dietary input or urinary output to less than 500mL/day, which may take several days to produce an effect. This may not be appropriate in the terminal care setting, when patients may prefer to eat and drink what they like without strict regimes.

Drug treatments involve the use of distal nephron inhibitors that prevent water reabsorption (e.g. demeclocycline) and oral osmotic diuretics (e.g. urea).

Demeclocycline (desmethylchlortetracycline) inhibits vasopressin and causes nephrogenic diabetes insipidus: 900–1200mg/day will reverse chronic SIAD over 3–4 days and should be followed by a maintenance dose of 600–900mg/day. Side-effects include gastrointestinal disturbances, hypersensitivity reactions and reversible nephrotoxicity.

Urea is effective in controlling SIAD by both intravenous and oral routes. Oral urea, 30g dissolved in orange juice to mask the taste, is the daily dose. (Using urea obviates the need to fluid-restrict the patient.)

Non-islet cell tumour hypoglycaemia

Hypoglycaemia in malignancy is often associated with beta-cell tumours which secrete insulin. More rarely, non-islet cell tumours produce hypoglycaemia by increased tumour usage of glucose, secretion of insulin-like growth factors (IGFs) (formerly somatomedins) and disruption of the balance maintaining normal homeostasis.

Increased use of glucose by tumours has been clearly documented, with daily consumption sometimes reaching levels of 200g/kg per day. Hepatic glucose production may also fall, and suppression of compensatory growth hormone and glucagons also contribute to the hypoglycaemic state.

> In advanced malignancy the commonest cause of hypoglycaemia is oral hypoglycaemic medication.

Epidemiology

Insulin-secreting tumours are usually large (average 2.4kg), and often retroperitoneal or intrathoracic with liver invasion. The tumours may be growing over a relatively longer time course than many other cancers (often several years).

- Approximately 60% are mesenchymal tumours (mesothelioma, neurofibroma, leiomyosarcoma, etc.)
  - 20% are hepatomas
  - 10% are adrenal carcinomas
  - 10% are gastrointestinal tumours

Clinical features

Hypoglycaemic symptoms often do not appear until the terminal stage of the disease. Symptoms are associated with cerebral hypoglycaemia and the associated secondary response of catecholamine secretion. The neurological features include agitation, stupor, coma and seizures, usually following exercise or fasting, and occur most often in the early morning or late afternoon. Other causes of hypoglycaemia should be excluded, such as overtreatment of diabetes.

Treatment

The reversal of symptomatic hypoglycaemia initially requires intravenous glucose infusion. Central lines may be needed for hyperosmolar glucose solutions. Up to 2000g/day of glucose may occasionally be needed. Frequent feeding, including during the night, and steroids may be helpful.

Debulking surgery, arterial embolization of tumours or chemotherapy can all have a place in the palliation of tumor-related hypoglycaemia.

Carcinoid syndrome

Carcinoid tumours are a diverse group of tumours of enterochromaffin-cell origin. The incidence is 1.5 per 100,000. The carcinoid syndrome develops in up to 18% of patients with such tumours and these patients almost invariably have hepatic metastases.

The commonest site of origin is the appendix (25%) and rectum but they have also been reported in the pancreas, lungs, thymus and gonads. Tumours may be benign but 80% that are greater than 2cm in diameter metastasize.

Clinical features

- Flushing and diarrhoea occur in at least 75% of patients
- Cardiac manifestations involving the right side of the heart are late manifestations in a third of patients
- Wheeze/right ventricular heart failure (RVF) (tricuspid valve regurgitation or stenosis and pulmonary valve stenosis) are seen
- Asthma and pellagra are less common

Clinical features are mediated by several active substances secreted by tumours including:

- Numerous vasoactive amines and hormones
- Serotonin (5HT), 5-hydroxytryptophan (5HTP)
- Prostaglandins
- Catecholamines
- Tachykinins (Substance P, neuropeptide K)
- Histamine
- Alcohol or psychological stress may precipitate symptoms.

The features of carcinoid tumours vary by their sites of origin (Table 6i.2).

Table 6i.2 Comparison of carcinoid tumours by site of origin

	Foregut	Midgut	Hindgut
Site	Resp. tract, pancreas, stomach, proximal duodenum	Jejunum, ileum, appendix, Meckel's diverticulum, ascending colon	Transverse and descending colon, rectum
Tumour products	Low 5HTP, multihormones	High 5HTP, multihormones	Rarely 5HTP, multihormones
Blood	5HTP, histamine, multihormones	5HT, rarely ACTH, multihormones	
Urine	5HTP, 5HT, 5HIAA, histamine	5HT, 5HIAA	Rarely 5HT or ACTH
Carcinoid syndrome	Atypical	Frequently with metastases	Rarely occurs
Metastases to bone	Common	Rare	Common

5HIAA, 5-hydroxyindole acetic acid; 5HTP, 5-hydroxytryptophan; 5HT, 5-hydroxytryptamine; ACTH, adrenocorticotrophic hormone

'Multihormones' include tachykinins, neurotensin, enkephalin, insulin, glucagons, glicentin, VIP, somatostatin, pancreatic polypeptide subunit of human chorionic gonadotrophin

Diagnosis

This is usually established by:
- Measuring urinary excretion of 5HIAA (metabolite of 5HT)
- Platelet 5HT levels (unaffected by diet)

Tumour localization may be achieved with somatostatin scintography or PET scanning.

Management (See Table 6i.3.)

Palliative debulking surgery, hepatic artery embolization, somatostatin analogues and chemotherapy may be appropriate palliative treatment for selected patients, while symptomatic treatment of diarrhoea and wheezing, using more traditional agents, also has a place in the management of patients with advanced carcinoid tumours.

Ketanserin has been used in some centres, ameliorating flushing in 50% but only providing 20% relief of diarrhoea. Selective $5HT_3$ receptor inhibitors may reduce diarrhoea.

Table 6i.3 Pharmacological management of carcinoid syndrome symptoms

Drug	Mechanism	Diarrhoea may reduce	Flushing may reduce	Comments
Octreotide	150–1500 mcg/day			CSCI ± alpha interferon
Sandostatin LAR	20mg–30mg every 28 days Somatostatin analogues	yes	yes	First-line therapy. 80% Reduced hormonal output and blocks action. Effects diminish with time. Doses need to be adjusted after three doses Very expensive
Lanreotide	30mg every 7–10 days IM			
Verapamil 40–120mg t.d.s/q.d.s	Calcium channel blocker	Yes	(?)	Limited value
Cyproheptadine 4–10mg t.d.s.	5HT₂ antagonism Antihistamine	yes (60%)	yes (47%)	Mean duration of response 8 months Limited value

Non-paraneoplastic complications

The incidence of hyperglycaemia in patients with cancer is higher than in the general population. Several theories to account for this have been postulated:

- Increased gluconeogenesis
- Increased conversion of lactate to glucose
- Diminished glucose tolerance
- Insulin resistance
- Increased use of medications such as corticosteroids promoting hyperglycaemia

These changes may arise as a result of liver damage, altered glucose metabolism by tumour cells and secretion of insulin antagonists.

Diabetes mellitus

Management of diabetes in palliative care (📖 See Tables 6i.4–6.)

A limited prognosis for a patient makes *close* control of blood glucose (aimed at reducing long-term sequelae) unnecessary, thereby allowing a less invasive/interventional approach.

Changes in the patient's condition (e.g. cachexia), infection or treatment (e.g. corticosteroids) commonly alter the diabetic treatment needed—the management may have to change rapidly at different phases of the illness.

Aims of management

- To prevent symptoms
  - maintaining the blood glucose at <15mmol/L is usually sufficient to prevent symptoms of hyperglycaemia (polyuria, thirst, nausea and vomiting, feeling 'unwell', drowsiness). Hyperglycaemic patients are susceptible to infection
  - a dry mouth is commonly due to drugs (morphine or antimuscarinics) and is not a good indicator of dehydration
- To prevent hypoglycaemia occurring
- To minimize intervention, i.e. frequency of blood sugar measurement and number of injections

Hyperglycaemia in advanced malignancy

In addition to pre-existing diabetes mellitus (including previously undiagnosed cases, which may present in the terminal stages), there are two particular causes of hyperglycaemia that may occur in patients with advanced malignancy:

- Corticosteroid-induced diabetes
- Insulin deficiency/resistance in pancreatic cancer

Hypoglycaemia

Common clinical changes that occur in patients with advanced malignancy, leading to reduced insulin or oral antidiabetic drug requirements in pre-existing diabetics are:

- Cancer cachexia in advanced illness (reduced body mass)
- Reduced food intake due to anorexia, dysphagia, 'squashed stomach' or nausea/vomiting, etc.
- Liver replacement by tumour causing low glycogen stores and limited gluconeogenesis

Corticosteroids

Corticosteroids are commonly used in advanced malignancy. They have a direct metabolic hyperglycaemic effect, but may also increase appetite, sometimes dramatically.

Hyperglycaemia is a dose-related effect in any patient (one in five patients on high doses will develop steroid-induced diabetes), but there is wide variability between patients in their response. The hyperglycaemia is usually asymptomatic and requires no therapy unless polyuria or polydipsia develop, in which case a short-acting sulphonylurea (e.g. gliclazide) may be useful. The dose of steroids should be reduced to the minimum possible.

Treatment options for diabetes

Oral hypoglycaemic drugs
- Gliclazide is a short-acting hypoglycaemic agent. It may be given once or twice daily at a starting dose of 40–80mg mane
- Increase as required to a maximum total dose 160mg b.d.
- Avoid metformin in patients with advanced cancer

Insulin

It is sensible to use only two or three insulins, such as:
- Human insulin glargine (long-acting)
- Human isophane insulin (e.g. human Insulatard or Humulin I) (intermediate acting)
- Human soluble insulin (e.g. human Actrapid or Humulin S) (short acting)

Use either:
- A single dose of human glargine daily (given at bedtime), *or*
- Isophane insulin: two-thirds daily dose mane, one-third dose nocte

If converting from a mixed insulin regime (e.g. isophane + human soluble insulin) to single daily human glargine:
- Calculate the total daily insulin requirement
- Reduce the dose by about 20–30% to account for the conversion
- Adjust the dose as necessary if blood glucose has been high or low
- Give this dose once-daily as human glargine

For a patient who has been uncontrolled on oral hypoglycaemics, start with human glargine 10u daily.

Initiating treatment in new diagnosis hyperglycaemia
- Restrict diet *if overeating*: Do not impose a strict diet on a patient with advanced illness. It is more important to try and achieve a regular caloric input from one day to the next
- Reduce the dose of corticosteroids if appropriate
- Consider infection as a factor causing the hyperglycaemia
- Thin, cachectic patients are less likely to respond to oral hypoglycaemic drugs, and insulin should be considered early if not responding to simple measures, e.g. gliclazide 80mg o.d.
- If the patient is peripherally vasoconstricted, give insulin by IM route, rather than SC

Sliding-scale insulin regimen
Monitor blood glucose and give soluble insulin sc as indicated. Use 8-hourly if patient not eating, or before mealtimes. Adjust sliding-scale doses according to response.

Fasting blood sugar mmol/L	Soluble insulin
10–14	4u
15–18	6u
19–22	8u
>22	10u

Drugs used in hyperglycaemia
Gliclazide
- Tabs 80mg
- Dose: 80mg mane p.o.
- Blood levels increased by fluconazole and miconazole (hypoglycaemia)

Human insulin soluble
- Inj. 100u/mL (human Actrapid or Humulin S)

Human insulin glargine
- Inj. 100u/mL (Lantus)

Human isophane insulin
- Inj. 100u/mL (human Insulatard or Humulin I)

Drugs used in hypoglycaemia
Glucagon may be ineffective in a starved patient, as it depends on an adequate liver glycogen level.

Glucagon
- Inj. 1mg
- Dose: 1mg IM (<12years, 0.5mg)
- Do not give by sc route, as the patient may be peripherally vasoconstricted

Glucose/dextrose
- Oral gel 10g (Hypostop gel). Inj.: 20%, 25mL; 50%, 25mL
- Dose: 25mL of 50% IV or 10g p.o.

Table 6i.4 Management of hyperglycaemia

Blood sugar (mmol/L)	Action
11–17	Dietary advice
	Reduce steroids if possible
	Start gliclazide 40mg daily and increase as necessary every few days
17–27	Start gliclazide 80mg mane if no, or mild, ketonuria
	If moderate or severe ketonuria the patient will need insulin—start human glargine 10u nocte
	If ketonuria and symptomatic, consider reducing blood glucose more rapidly using human soluble insulin 4–8u 4h until glucose <17mmol/L, or IV regimen below
>27	Consider if admission to acute medical unit is appropriate, especially if ketonuria present
	Use IV regimen if intensive treatment appropriate, or human soluble insulin 4–8u every 4h until glucose <17mmol/L

Table 6i.5 Managing diabetes when vomiting or not eating

Diabetes type	Action
Oral hypoglycaemics	Reduce dose by 50% if oral intake reduced, or discontinue if no oral intake.
Insulin-dependent	Insulin is required to prevent ketosis even with no oral intake. Use the iv regimen if intensive control is appropriate, or use sliding scale of human soluble insulin 8-h

Table 6i.6 Managing diabetes in the terminal days

Diabetes type	Action
Oral hypoglycaemics	Discontinue when unable to take oral intake.
Insulin-dependent	Insulin is required to prevent ketosis, even with no oral intake.
	• If patient unconscious/unaware, discontinue insulin and monitoring
	• If the patient is still aware/conscious, several strategies may be appropriate, depending on the patient's/relatives' attitude to burden of treatment (and monitoring) and prognosis:
	• use sliding scale soluble insulin 8h
	• give approximately half of the patient's recent insulin requirement as a single dose of human glargine as a single daily injection, with or without blood sugar monitoring

Further reading

Books

Back I. (2001) *Palliative Medicine Handbook* (3rd edn). Cardiff: BPM Books.

Doyle D., *et al.* (eds). (2004) *Oxford Textbook of Palliative Medicine* (3rd edn). Oxford: Oxford University Press.

Watson M., Lucas C., Hoy A (2006) *Adult Palliative Care Guidance*. (2nd edn). London: The South West London and the Surrey, West Sussex and Hampshire Cancer Networks.

Articles

Alsirafy S.A., *et al.* (2007) Pattern of electrolyte abnormalities among cancer patients referred to palliative care: a review of 750 patients. *Progress in Palliative Care*. **15**(4): 182–185.

Dev R., Dell Fabbro E., Bruera E. (2007) Association between megestrol acetate treatment and symptomatic adrenal insufficiency with hypogonadism in male patients with cancer. *Cancer*, **110**(6): 1173–7.

Ford-Dunn S., *et al.* (2007) Management of diabetes during the last days of life: attitudes of consultant diabetologists and palliative care physicians in the UK. *Palliative Medicine*, **20**(3): 197–203.

McCann M., *et al.* (2006) Practical management of diabetes mellitus. *European Journal of Palliative Care*, **13**(6): 226–9.

Poulson J. (1997) The management of diabetes in patients with advanced cancer. *Journal of Pain and Symptom Management*, **13**(6): 339–46.

Neurological problems in advanced cancer

Local nerve damage

(📖 For spinal cord compression see Chapter 15, 'Emergencies in palliative care'.)

Brachial plexopathy

Cause
Invasion or compression by tumour, or fibrosis secondary to radiotherapy.

Clinical features
Shoulder or arm pain (suggestive of tumour), numbness or allodynia in an arm or hand, muscle weakness, atrophy, Horner's syndrome.

Investigations
CT or MRI scan of the brachial plexus.

Management
Palliative radiotherapy or chemotherapy may reduce the pain if tumour is the cause, but there is rarely an improvement in function. Otherwise, appropriate analgesia, including an agent for neuropathic pain, will be necessary.

Lumbosacral plexopathy

Cause
Invasion or compression by tumour, radiation fibrosis or abscess (rare).

Clinical features
Lumbosacral pain radiating into the legs. Leg weakness is usually unilateral and sensory dysfunction is apparent.

Investigations
CT or MRI scan of the pelvis.

Management
Palliative radiotherapy or chemotherapy, if tumour is the cause, reduces pain and can occasionally improve function.

Paraneoplastic neurological syndromes

- These are neurological disorders which occur in up to 7% of patients with cancer
- The aetiology is unclear, although the production of a specific antibody may be involved

- Syndromes can occur as a presenting feature before the diagnosis of cancer is made
- The commonest implicated cancers include small cell lung cancer (SCLC) (30%), breast and ovarian cancer and lymphoma
- Symptoms are usually subacute and there may be more than one syndrome in the same patient

Syndromes include:
- **Peripheral neuropathy** involving distal sensory and/or motor or autonomic nerves. Removal of tumour (which is usually SCLC, myeloma, Hodgkin's disease, breast and gastrointestinal cancers) does not usually produce an improvement in symptoms, which are generally progressive. Steroids may help, but only for short time.
- **Cerebellar degeneration** may present rapidly, sometimes before the primary tumour becomes apparent. Response to treatment, however, is disappointing
- **Lambert–Eaton myasthenic syndrome** is a disorder of neuromuscular transmission occurring in 3% of patients with small cell lung cancer who account for 60–70% of cases. It is seen occasionally with other cancers including thymoma, breast cancer and lymphoma. There is a presynaptic deficit in neuromuscular transmission caused by a reduction in the amount of acetylcholine released at the motor nerve terminal

   There is some evidence of an autoimmune aetiology, with the presence of autoantibodies to calcium channels at the neuromuscular junction. Common symptoms include proximal muscle weakness, particularly of the legs, and an associated waddling gait. Fatigue, diplopia, ptosis and dysarthria may also be a problem. Unlike classical myasthenia, weakness may be improved by repetitive activity and there is a poor response to edrophonium. It may improve with treatment of the underlying malignancy
- **Encephalomyelopathies** can affect the limbic system, brainstem and spinal cord
- **Other clinical presentations** include dementia, opsoclonus–myoclonus, limbic encephalitis (presenting rapidly with confusion, memory disturbance and agitation) and necrotizing myelopathy

Corticosteroid-induced proximal myopathy

- This can occur within a few weeks of starting dexamethasone, 8–16mg a day
- Patients experience difficulty in rising from a sitting position and in climbing stairs
- Disabling symptoms may not be readily volunteered and direct questioning may be needed. Management includes reducing the dose of steroid to the minimum possible and considering a change to prednisolone, which may not cause as much muscle wasting (but is associated with more fluid retention)
- Weakness should improve in 3–4 weeks of steroid withdrawal

Drug-induced movement disorders

- Certain drugs may induce extrapyramidal symptoms and signs
- These include akathisia (motor restlessness in which the patient may frequently change position or pace up and down if able), dystonia and parkinsonism.
- Implicated drugs are those which block dopamine receptors such as antipsychotics (particularly haloperidol and the phenothiazines) and metoclopramide
- Antidepressants and ondansetron may also cause problems
- **All these drugs should be avoided as far as possible in patients with Parkinson's disease**

Convulsions and seizures

Common causes of seizures in palliative care include:
- Brain tumour (primary or secondary)
- Biochemical disturbance (e.g. severe hyponatraemia)
- Previous cerebrovascular accident
- Long-standing epilepsy

Isolated tonic–clonic seizures sometimes occur but rarely last more than a few minutes: treatment should be initiated since they may herald status epilepticus or grand mal seizures.

A grand mal seizure should be treated promptly since it is very distressing and frightening for families to witness. Efficient management is therefore needed.

If a patient develops a grand mal seizure or status epilepticus, give:
- Midazolam 5–10mg buccal/sc or slow IV (dilute 10mg with water to 10mL) and repeat after 15 and 30 minutes if not settled. Midazolam is not licensed as an anticonvulsant, but is usually readily available in palliative care units. A number of alternative benzodiazepines can be used:
  - lorazepam 4–6mg slow IV or sublingually
  - diazepam solution 10mg p.r. or emulsion 2–10mg slow IV
  - clonazepam 1mg slow IV (into large vein)

If the patient has not responded to a repeated dose of benzodiazepine or seizures recur, consider:
- Phenobarbital 100mg SC or IV after diluting 1 in 10 with water for injection ⌨ on p. 92.
- Repeat phenobarbital if necessary and set up a syringe driver with phenobarbital 200–600mg SC over 24h
- Once seizures have been controlled, review anticonvulsant therapy

General notes

- For patients with intracranial tumours, consider starting, or review dose of, corticosteroids
- Remember to advise the patient about restrictions on driving and to contact the DVLA
- Consider parenteral thiamine if alcohol abuse is suspected
- Consider and treat hypoglycaemia in at-risk patients
- Consider drug interactions that alter anticonvulsant levels (e.g. steroids)

Initiating anticonvulsant therapy

- It is usually appropriate to initiate anticonvulsant therapy after one seizure in patients with terminal illness
- Sodium valproate is an appropriate first-line anticonvulsant for almost all types of convulsions or seizures, including focal and partial seizures, and those caused by intracranial tumours
- Aim to increase the dose to lower end of quoted 'usual maintenance dose' unless side-effects occur, or the patient is frail and elderly (doses given below)
- Carbamazepine and phenytoin may be suitable alternatives

Patients unable to take oral medication

- Patients who are unable to take oral medication due to dysphagia, vomiting or because they are in the terminal stages may need to be given anticonvulsants by another route
- The half-life of most anticonvulsants is quite long (>24h), therefore no parenteral anticonvulsant is usually needed if there is a low risk of seizures, **and** only a **single dose** is missed
- **The risk of seizures is higher if the patient:**
  - has decreased or stopped steroids (intracranial tumours)
  - has increasing headache, vomiting or other signs suggesting rising intracranial pressure (intracranial tumours)
  - exhibits myoclonus or other twitching
  - has a history of poor seizure control or recent seizures
  - has previously needed more than a single anticonvulsant to achieve control
- Because of the long half-life of anticonvulsants, parenteral treatment can be started at any time within 24h after the last oral dose

Choice of non-oral anticonvulsant

Choice may be determined partly by availability (Table 6j.1):

Table 6j.1 Choice of non-oral anticonvulsant

Phenobarbital CSCI or daily SC	Well-proven anticonvulsant for all types of seizures. Experience suggests it is effective in doses of 200mg/24h.
	Phenobarbital is incompatible with most other drugs in a syringe driver, therefore a second syringe driver may be necessary. Stat doses of 100mg SC or IM can sting
Midazolam CSCI	Midazolam is more useful as a sedative than as an anticonvulsant. Anticonvulsant efficacy of 'standard' doses is unknown, but probably requires 20–30mg/24h minimum. Unlicensed use
	If low risk of seizures, and midazolam indicated for, e.g. terminal agitation, then additional anticonvulsant probably unnecessary. If higher risk of seizures, use phenobarbital in addition
Clonazepam CSCI	Main advantage is that clonazepam is compatible with many other drugs used in CSCI. Much less experience supporting its use in this way; doses recommended: 2–4mg/24h (4–8mg/24h if sedation acceptable or desired)
Carbamazepine or valproate suppositories	Occasionally suitable for patients well-controlled on one of these drugs who develop a temporary inability to take oral medication (e.g. vomiting and who would find rectal administration acceptable)

Phenobarbital as the anticonvulsant

- If a patient is dying, and sedation is acceptable, it is better to err on the generous side and give:
  - phenobarbital 200mg SC stat. as a loading dose
  - phenobarbital 200mg/24h by CSCI, *or*
  - if high risk of seizures—phenobarbital 400mg/24h by CSCI
- If needing to minimize sedation, use 100mg SC stat. as a loading dose followed by 100–200mg/24h by CSCI

Phenobarbital is compatible with diamorphine and hyoscine if given by CSCI

Management of seizures at home

Most seizures are self-limiting and require only supportive care. For more prolonged seizures occurring at home, a number of measures can be arranged in anticipation which can avoid inappropriate emergency admission to hospital.

- Diazepam rectal solution 10mg p.r.—administered by district nurse or carer
- Midazolam 5–10mg SC (or preferably IM)—administered by district nurse

- Midazolam buccal 10mg/2mL can be administered by a carer if the rectal route for diazepam is unacceptable: it appears to be as effective and may be quicker-acting than rectal diazepam 10mg. An oral solution is available as a 'special' or the injectable preparation can be used

In an inpatient unit, midazolam 5–10mg SC (or preferably IM) may be given first before treating status epilepticus as above.

Non-convulsive status epilepticus

Non-convulsive status epilepticus (NCSE) is a possible cause of confusion or delirium in terminally ill patients. The clinical presentation varies from altered mental status to comatose patients, without visible convulsions. In comatose patients unilateral tonic head and eye-movement is often observed. Other symptoms include myoclonic contractions of the angle of the mouth, mild clonus of an extremity or rarely epileptic nystagmus. EEG is the most important diagnostic tool to identify epileptiform activity. Treatment should be initiated following a step-wise model (e.g. phenytoin, sodium valproate, levetiracetam together with benzodiazepines), avoiding intubation and transfer to the intensive care unit. Although mortality rates are high, in some patients NCSE can be reversed by treatment.

Anticonvulsants (📖 see Chapter 4, 'Principles of drug use in palliative care')

Carbamazepine and phenytoin levels are decreased (risk of fits) by corticosteroids. Carbamazepine, phenytoin and phenobarbital can reduce the efficacy of corticosteroids.

This two-way interaction is common when managing patients with cerebral tumours. Carbamazepine, phenytoin or phenobarbital plasma levels are also reduced by St John's Wort (risk of fits).

Sodium valproate

- Tabs: 200mg, 500mg; chewable tabs: 100mg; syrup: 200mg/5mL
- Dose: 200mg t.d.s. p.o.
- Increase 200mg/day at three-day intervals. Usual maintenance dose, 1–2g/24h. Max. 2.5g/24h in divided doses. Suppositories are available as special orders

Carbamazepine

- Tabs: 100mg, 200mg, 400mg; liquid: 100mg/5mL; supps: 125mg, 250mg
- Dose: 100mg b.d. p.o.
- Increase from initial dose by increments of 200mg every week. Usual maintenance dose 0.8–1.2g/24h in two divided doses. Max. 1.6–2g/24h. Equivalent rectal dosage: 125mg p.r. ≅ 100mg p.o.
- Carbamazepine levels are increased (risk of toxicity) by clarithromycin, erythromycin, fluoxetine and fluvoxamine

Phenytoin

- 250 mg b.d. increasing step-wise by 250mg b.d. to a maximum dose 1.5mg b.d.
- Caps: 50mg, 100mg, 300mg: chewable tabs: 50mg; susp.: 30mg/5mL, 90mg/5mL
- Dose: 90mg b.d. p.o.
- Start 150–300mg daily. Usual maintenance dose: 300–400mg daily. Max. 600mg/24h. Single or two divided doses
- Phenytoin levels are increased (risk of toxicity) by clarithromycin, metronidazole, trimethoprim, fluconazole, miconazole, omeprazole, fluoxetine, fluvoxamine, aspirin, diltiazem, nifedipine and amiodarone
- Because phenytoin has a very long and variable half-life, it can take several days and even up to 3–4 weeks for changes in dosage to take complete effect: this should be borne in mind in determining the interval after dosage is altered before measuring the plasma phenytoin concentration again

Levetiracetam

- Tabs: 250mg, 500mg, 750mg, 1000mg; susp.: 100mg/mL
- Dose: 500mg b.d. p.o.
- Start 250 mg b.d. increasing step-wise by 250mg b.d. to a maximum dose 1.5mg b.d.
- Levetiracetam is widely used in addition to phenytoin or sodium valproate, but it may also be used alone. No interaction with other antiepileptic drugs or other drugs have been reported

Barbiturates

Phenobarbital (phenobarbitone)

- Inj.: 60mg/1mL, 200mg/1mL; tabs: 15mg, 30mg, 60mg; elixir: 15mg/5mL
- Elixir in various strengths can be made to order, e.g. 10mg/mL
- Phenobarbital is a barbiturate with both sedative and anticonvulsant effects. It is rarely used nowadays as a first-line anticonvulsant, as it is too sedative. It can be given by CSCI, but usually needs to be given in a separate syringe driver. It can be given by daily SC or IM injection, but the preparation is very viscous and stings on injection. *Doses: see above*

Benzodiazepines

Midazolam

- Inj.: 1mg/1mL, 2mg/1mL, 5mg/1mL. **Caution is needed**.
- Dose: 30mg/24h CSCI
- Oral solution available as special order, or use injection for buccal use
- Sedative effect markedly enhanced by itraconazole, ketoconazole and possibly fluconazole

Lorazepam

- Tabs: 1mg, 2.5mg; inj.: 4mg/1mL
- Dilute inj. with an equal volume of water or saline for IM use

Diazepam

- Tabs: 2mg, 5mg, 10mg; oral solution: 2mg/5mL, 5mg/5mL
- Rectal tubes: 5mg/2.5mL, 10mg/2.5mL; supps.: 10mg
- Inj: (emulsion) 10mg/2mL (Diazemuls)—IV use only
- Inj: (solution) 10mg/2mL— IM use

Clonazepam

- Tabs: 500mcg, 2mg; inj.: 1mg/1mL
- Starting dose: 1mg nocte
- Increase gradually to usual maintenance dose of 4–8mg/24h. Oral solutions in various strengths are available from several sources

Further reading

Books

Back I. (2001) *Palliative Medicine Handbook* (3rd edn). Cardiff: BPM Books.

Doyle D., et al. (eds). (2004) *Oxford Textbook of Palliative Medicine*. (3rd edn) Oxford: Oxford University Press.

Watson M., Lucas C., Hoy A. (2006) *Adult Palliative Care Guidance*. (2nd edn) London: The South West London and the Surrey, West Sussex and Hampshire Cancer Networks.

Articles

Cavaliere R., et al. (2006) Clinical implications of status epilepticus in patients with neoplasms. *Archives of Neurology*, **63**: 1746–9.

Heafield M. (2000) Managing status epilepticus. *British Medical Journal*, **320**: 953–4.

Danell R. B., Posner J. B. (2006) Paraneoplastic syndromes affecting the nervous system. *Seminars in Oncology*, **33**: 270–98.

Sleep disorders

Sleep disorders are a frequent complication of both medical illnesses and the medications used in their treatment; and can occur in up to 70% of those with advanced cancer,[1] particularly where pain is a complicating factor. Sleep problems in cancer patients have been found to be associated with changes in mood, decreased pain tolerance and a decreased quality of life. However, sleep disorders have received relatively little attention from healthcare providers despite their prevalence in patients with advanced disease.[2]

Human sleep is an essential, active, dynamic and complex physiological function in which stages are repeated in a cyclical pattern throughout the night. There are two distinct states of sleep: non-rapid eye movement sleep (NREM) and rapid eye movement (REM). NREM sleep accounts for 75% of the night, in a staged process from light to deep sleep, and is a period of relative physiological and cognitive quiescence. REM sleep, on the other hand, is characterized by muscle atonia, dreaming and autonomic variability.

The sleep–wake cycle is a component of the body's overall circadian rhythm, synchronized with other biological rhythms including temperature oscillation and cortisol and growth hormone secretion. The onset and maintenance of normal sleep patterns depends on the appropriate timing of sleep within the 24-hour circadian rhythm. Adequate physical comfort, an acceptable sleeping environment, an intact central nervous system function and the relative absence of psychological distress and psychophysiological arousal are also necessary for sleep.

The restorative functions of sleep are dependent on a well-organized and reasonably uninterrupted sleep structure (sleep architecture). Sleep tends to be lighter with advancing age and in many medical conditions. The percentage of REM sleep, however, remains relatively constant in a healthy elderly population, but is decreased when cognitive impairment or certain other medical conditions are present.

Insomnia

Insomnia is a subjective complaint by the patient of poor sleep, usually associated with daytime consequences. This can encompass complaints of insufficient sleep, difficulties in getting off to sleep (sleep initiation) and remaining asleep (sleep maintenance), poor sleep quality, non-restorative sleep or episodes of sleep occurring at the wrong time in the day–night cycle. Physical, psychological and environmental factors contribute to poor sleep in medical conditions.

1 Solano J. P., Gomes B., Higginson I. J. (2006) A comparison of symptom prevalence in far advanced cancer, AIDS, heart disease, chronic obstructive pulmonary disease and renal disease. *Journal of Pain and Symptom Management*, **31**(1): 58–69.

2 Berger A. M, *et al.* (2005) Sleep wake disturbances in people with cancer and their caregivers: state of the science. *Oncology Nursing Forum*, **32**(6): E98–126.

Sleep deprivation may result in progressive fatigue, sleepiness, impairment of concentration, irritability and depression. Deep stages of NREM sleep may be critical in tissue restoration and in maintaining a healthy immune system.

Disorders of the sleep–wake cycle

A normal sleeping pattern depends on a well-established schedule of sleep and wakefulness. Patients who are terminally ill are prone to disturbances in the sleep–wake cycle because of frequent disruptions to night-time sleep, an absence of their usual daytime schedule and relative inactivity during normal waking hours. A lack of sleep at night leads to late awakening, daytime napping and late settling to sleep the following night (delayed sleep phase syndrome) or early morning waking and early bedtime (advanced sleep phase syndrome). This can create a vicious cycle of disturbed sleep. For some, a rhythm disappears altogether and is replaced by a pattern of multiple shorter sleep periods interspersed with wakefulness throughout the 24h cycle. Hospitalization can also lead to fragmented sleep due to factors such as noise, nocturnal disturbance and patient anxiety.

Excessive daytime sleepiness

It is common for patients receiving palliative care to complain of general tiredness and fatigue. But this should be distinguished from excessive daytime sleepiness, which is defined as an inability to stay awake and alert during major waking episodes of the day leading to unintended lapses into drowsiness and sleep. A degree of daytime sedation can be desirable in some cases; however, excessive sleepiness can be disabling, leading to inactivity and poor motivation. Patients may become less capable of participating in treatment and may find it difficult to retain information and to interact socially. They may also become unnecessarily depressed, irritable and withdrawn during the important last weeks or months of life.

Causes of disturbed sleep in the terminally ill which should be actively sought and treated where appropriate

Symptoms

- Uncontrolled pain—contributes to a lack of sleep in up to 60% of patients. Sleep deprivation lowers pain thresholds
- Nausea and vomiting
- Respiratory disturbances, e.g. dyspnoea, cough, respiratory distress, obstructive sleep apnoea
- Restless legs syndrome—may be associated with potentially manageable causes such as sedative hypnotic withdrawal, anaemia, uraemia, peripheral neuropathy, iron deficiency, diabetes mellitus
- Bladder or bowel discomfort and incontinence
- Depression—at least 90% of depressed patients have abnormal sleep patterns. Depression is common and it is a significant cause of sleep pathology in the terminally ill
- Anxiety and fears—anxiety may be directly related to the illness or treatment and is often associated with pain. Early delirium, withdrawal from drugs and breathlessness can frequently cause anxiety. During the daytime, fears are masked by distractions

- Cognitive impairment disorder—delirium is not uncommon in the terminally ill and reversible causes should be actively sought. Sleep disturbance itself may lead to delirium. Patients with dementia sleep less deeply and have reduced REM and increased awakening after sleep onset. Patients need constant reassurance and to be nursed in a lit room to minimize disorientation. Hypnotics may aggravate the situation. Drugs such as haloperidol 0.5–2.0mg or risperidone 0.5–1.0mg may be useful, particularly if given in the early evening, to pre-empt a restless period and give adequate time for the drug to take effect before settling for the night. **Note**: Risperidone should not be used if the patient has a history of cerebrovascular disease

Medications
- Steroids, especially if taken late in the day; bronchodilators; psychotropic agents; enervating antidepressants, e.g. fluoxetine; withdrawal from sedative hypnotics or analgesia

Environmental and other factors
- External noise and nocturnal disruption, e.g. during hospitalization
- Psychophysiological—conditional arousal response, poor sleep hygiene
- Sleep–wake schedule disorder—disruption of normal schedule, excessive napping during the day
- Use of caffeine, nicotine or alcohol may also contribute to sleep disturbances

Management
A full assessment must be carried out to define the individual's sleep characteristics and to address all potential reversible causes. Assessment methods can be divided into objective and subjective measurements. Subjective measurements include patient interview and/or the use of self-report sleep questionnaires or sleep diaries. Objective measures include polysomnography (PSM) or wrist actigraphy. The use of PSM is mainly indicated if an underlying physiological disturbance is suspected and will also depend upon the goals of treatment, the patient's clinical condition and local availability.

In the absence of any obviously reversible causes, the aim of treatment is to achieve enough restorative sleep to ensure daytime alertness, concentration and energy. Treatments can be divided into pharmacological and non-pharmacological interventions. There have been relatively few trials of these interventions in palliative populations and the evidence mainly comes from work on primary insomnia populations.

Non-pharmacological
Cognitive and behavioural interventions aim to improve sleep by altering poor sleep habits and tackling negative attitudes or beliefs about sleep. Excessive arousal in bed can be a frequent cause and effect of insomnia. Patients may need to undertake relaxing activities to distract themselves from the anxiety and the pressure to fall asleep, as well as changing their beliefs about sleep. An unpredictable sleep pattern needs to be managed by reinforcement of the rest–activity sleep–wake cycle as well as changing the way one reacts to this. Interventions include sleep hygiene measures, sleep restriction, stimulus control measures and sleep relaxation therapies

such as hypnosis and somatic imagery training, progressive muscle relaxation, psychotherapy, complementary therapy, i.e. aromatherapy and cognitive therapy. Cognitive–behavioural therapy includes a combination of both cognitive and behavioural interventions and is the mainstay of treatment for insomnia that is due wholly or in part to heightened cognitive or physiological arousal and poor sleep hygiene.

Pharmacological

Benzodiazepines and other drugs that act on benzodiazepine receptors such as cyclopyrrolone (Zopiclone) are the standard medications of choice in the treatment of transient or short-term insomnia.

Hypnotic medication is used frequently in palliative care and may enhance quality of life. The choice of hypnotic depends on several factors, including duration of effectiveness, rate of absorption and metabolism as well as the potential risks or side-effects. Nocturnal confusion may be induced, particularly in individuals with baseline cognitive dysfunction. Most are absorbed quickly, reaching peak concentrations within an hour or less. Non-benzodiazepine hypnotics have a very short half-life of about 1 hour. Temazepam, lorazepam and oxazepam have intermediate half-lives ranging from 8 to 15h in healthy adults, whereas diazepam is longer acting and is cleared more slowly. Chloral hydrate has modest short-term efficacy but is more toxic than benzodiazepines.

Sedating tricyclic antidepressants (e.g. amitriptyline) are often used but are associated with anticholinergic side-effects. Trazodone is a sedating heterocyclic with milder anticholinergic side-effects and a shorter half-life than most tricyclics and can be administered over a longer period.

Clomethiazole (chlormethiazole) is sometimes used. Sedative hypnotics in the elderly are associated with falls, cognitive impairment and worsening of nocturnal respiratory disturbance and should be used in low doses.

There is little current evidence to support the effectiveness of melatonin in secondary sleep disorders, although it is thought to be safe for short-term use.

Sleep disorders in families and carers

Palliative care also encompasses the needs of both families and other informal carers. Therefore attention needs to be directed to carers who may themselves experience chronic fragmented night-time sleep and yet still be expected to undertake daytime chores and care provision. Up to 95% of cancer caregivers report severe sleep problems.[3] These affect all aspects of sleep and may be associated with clinical depression.

---

3 Carter, P.A., Chang, B. L. (2000) Sleep and depression in cancer caregivers. *Cancer Nursing*, **23**(6): 410–15.

Palliative haematological aspects

Anaemia in chronic disorders

Anaemia is defined as a haemoglobin concentration in adults of less than 13.0g/dL in men and 11.5g/dL in women. Anaemia occurs commonly in chronic renal disease, endocrine diseases and connective tissue disorders. In the latter, various factors may contribute and commonly more than one is present. It is also a common problem, occurring in over 50% of patients with solid tumours and in most patients with haematological malignancies such as multiple myeloma and lymphoma.

Symptoms caused by anaemia include:
- Fatigue
- Weakness
- Breathlessness on exertion
- Impaired concentration
- Chest pain
- Exacerbation of congestive cardiac failure
- Low mood
- Loss of libido
- Anorexia

There are no specific criteria for the functional assessment of anaemia. However, randomized controlled trials of the management of anaemia in malignancy have used validated tools in assessing its effect on quality of life (QOL), e.g.:
- Cancer Linear Analogue Scale (CLAS)
- Functional Assessment of Cancer Therapy—Anaemia (FACT—An)

Causes of anaemia
- Reduced red cell production due to bone marrow infiltration:
  - multiple myeloma
  - prostate cancer
  - breast cancer
  - leukaemia
- Chemotherapy-induced bone marrow suppression
- Anaemia of chronic disease related to malignancy
- Malnutrition/malabsorption, e.g. post-gastrectomy:
  - vitamin B_{12} deficiency
  - folate deficiency
  - iron deficiency
- Blood loss:
  - gastrointestinal
  - haematuria
- Chronic renal failure
- Reduced red cell survival/haemolysis:
  - autoimmune haemolysis—lymphoproliferative disorders
  - physical haemolysis—microangiopathic haemolytic anaemia (MAHA) in some adenocarcinomas

- Anaemia of chronic disorder related to malignancy—a combination of effects:
  - suppressed erythropoietin production
  - impaired transferrin production
  - shortened red cell survival

Management of anaemia (📖 see Table 6l.1)
Investigate cause of anaemia where appropriate
Diagnostic indicators
- Reduced marrow production/bone marrow failure:
  - full blood count—pancytopenia and reduced reticulocytes
  - bone marrow examination—may show infiltration by non-haematological cells, e.g. prostatic or breast carcinoma, or hypocellular marrow post-chemotherapy
- Bleeding:
  - clinical—haematuria, melaena
  - acute—blood count and film: normochromic, normocytic anaemia, reticulocytosis and polychromasia
  - chronic—iron deficiency anaemia
- Malabsorption/malnutrition:
  - low serum vitamin B_{12}
  - reduced serum or red cell folate
  - reduced ferritin
- Haemolysis:
  - blood film: polychromasia; autoimmune—spherocytes; MAHA—red cell fragments (schistocytes); reticulocytosis
  - autoimmune—positive direct Coombs test
  - bilirubin—raised

Table 6l.1 Differentiation between iron deficiency anaemia and anaemia of chronic disease

	Iron deficiency anaemia	Anaemia of chronic disease
Blood film	Hypochromic microcytic	Normochromic or hypochromic
Red cell distribution width (RDW)	Increased	Microcytic ± Normal
Total iron-binding capacity (TIBC)	High	Normal/low
Plasma iron	Low	Low
Serum ferritin	Low	Normal/raised

N.B. The two causes can coexist.

Decrease bleeding risk

- Consider discontinuation of drugs that may increase risk of bleeding, e.g.:
  - aspirin
  - NSAIDs
  - anticoagulants
  - steroids
- Consider gastroprotection using:
  - proton pump inhibitors
  - H_2-receptor antagonists
  - prostaglandin analogues, e.g. misoprostol
- Give vitamin K in liver disease-related coagulopathies as evidenced by prolonged prothrombin time (PT). Vitamin K tablets (menadiol phosphate) 10mg p.o. daily for 1 week, then recheck PT
- Give tranexamic acid (antifibrinolytic agent) 1g p.o. t.d.s. or q.d.s. for mucosal bleeding. Tranexamic acid can also be given topically and as a mouthwash. (Use with care in bleeding from the bladder or prostate as clot formation is enhanced and subsequent urinary retention may become a problem.) Etamsylate may also be useful

Replace haematinic deficiencies

- Iron deficiency:
  - ferrous sulphate 200mg b.d. or t.d.s. (or Ferrograd 325mg p.o. daily) before food for 3 months
- Folate deficiency:
  - folic acid 5mg o.d.
- Vitamin B_{12} deficiency:
  - hydroxycobalamin 1000mcg IM every three months

Blood transfusion

Patients who are becoming terminally ill may receive blood transfusions inappropriately. The decision to transfuse should not be made on the basis of one haemoglobin result alone, but in the context of symptoms attributable to anaemia which are adversely affecting quality of life. It is important to document the clinical effect of the transfusion which will help in discussing the merits or otherwise of further transfusions. Blood transfusion helps about 75% of patients in terms of well-being, strength and breathlessness.

- Since 1998, all red cells have been leuco-depleted, therefore an in-line blood filter is not now required. One unit of leuco-depleted packed red cells (approximately 300mL) results in a rise in haemoglobin of 1g/dL
- The aim should be to transfuse up to 11–12g/dL but this will vary according to the individual clinical situation
- Patients at risk of pulmonary oedema should have furosemide cover (20mg p.o. with alternate units)
- Patients should be told that the beneficial effects may not be apparent for a day or two post-transfusion

Indications for blood transfusion in patients with palliative care needs

- Haemoglobin of less than 9g/dL (patients may benefit from transfusion at higher levels)
- Prognosis longer than two weeks
- Reasonable performance status (i.e. not predominantly bedbound) (ECOG >2)
- Presence of at least two of the following symptoms in association with Hb < 9g/dL:
  - breathlessness on exertion
  - weakness
  - angina
  - postural hypotension
  - worsening cardiac failure
  - worsening fatigue

Blood transfusion reactions

Acute life-threatening transfusion reactions are very rare; however, new symptoms or signs that occur during a transfusion must be taken seriously as they may herald a serious reaction. As it may not be possible to identify the cause of a severe reaction immediately, initial supportive management should generally cover all possible causes. These include:

- Acute haemolytic transfusion reaction
- Infusion of a bacterially contaminated unit
- Severe allergic reaction or anaphylaxis
- Fluid overload
- Transfusion-related acute lung injury (TRALI)
- Febrile non-haemolytic transfusion reaction

Acute haemolytic transfusion reaction

Incompatible Group A or B transfused red cells react with the patient's own anti-A or B antibodies. This results in acute renal failure, and can cause disseminated intravascular coagulation (DIC) The reaction can occur after only a few ml of blood have been transfused.

- **Symptoms:** acute onset of pain at venepuncture site, loins, chest
- **Signs:** fever, hypotension, tachycardia, oozing from venepuncture sites
- A similar picture is seen with the transfusion of bacterially contaminated red cells
- **Action:** If a severe acute reaction is suspected:
  - stop the transfusion, keep the IV line open with sodium chloride 0.9% infusion
  - monitor temperature, heart rate, BP, respiratory rate, urine output
  - recheck the patient's identification, the blood unit and documentation
  - inform the blood bank
  - further management will depend on the patient's developing clinical picture

Infusion of bacterially contaminated unit

This may cause haemolysis or clots within the blood bag. For this reason, visual inspection of every unit is part of the pre-transfusion check. Symptoms and signs are identical to acute haemolytic transfusion reaction. Treat as for acute haemolytic transfusion reaction in addition to:

- taking blood cultures
- sending the blood unit to microbiology

Major allergic reactions

Rare but life-threatening complications usually occur in the early part of a transfusion. These complications are more common with plasma-containing blood components, e.g. fresh-frozen plasma (FFP) or platelets.

- **Symptoms**: chest pain, breathlessness, nausea and abdominal pain
- **Signs**: hypotension, bronchospasm, periorbital and laryngeal oedema, vomiting, urticaria
- **Action**:
  - stop transfusion
  - high concentration O_2
  - chlorphenamine 10–20mg IV over 1–2 minutes
  - Hydrocortisone 100–200mg IV
  - Adrenaline 0.5–1mg (0.5–1mL of 1 in 1000) IM
  - Salbutamol 2.5–5mg by nebulizer
  - Maintain IV access

Fluid overload

More common in patients with a history of heart or renal disease, but any patient with advanced malignancy is susceptible. In these patients, each red cell unit should be given over 3–4h and a maximum of two units given per day. Clinical signs to be aware of:

- **Symptoms**: Breathlessness with basal crepitations
- **Signs**: BP may be raised initially, tachycardia, raised jugular venous pressure (JVP) may be present

- **Action**:
  - stop transfusion
  - high concentration O_2
  - furosemide 40mg IV

Transfusion-related acute lung injury (TRALI)
Usually caused by antibodies in donor's plasma that react strongly with the patient's leucocytes.
- **Symptoms**: Rapid onset of breathlessness and dry cough
- **Signs**: Chest X-ray shows bilateral infiltrates—'white-out'
- **Action**:
  - stop transfusion
  - give 100% O_2
  - seek expert advice and treat as adult respiratory distress syndrome (ARDS)

Febrile non-haemolytic transfusion reaction
Affects 1–2% of patients.
- **Symptoms and signs**: A rise in temperature <1.5°C from the baseline or an urticarial rash +/- rigors usually occurs towards the end of a transfusion or up to two hours after it is finished; BP and heart rate remain stable
- **Action**:
  - treat with paracetamol
  - give chlorphenamine 10mg p.o. or IV for rash
  - continue transfusion at a slower rate
  - observe for any deterioration

Iron overload is not often a concern in palliative care but if 50–75 units of red cells have been given, haemosiderosis may develop causing heart and liver dysfunction or failure of pancreatic endocrine function.

Contraindications to blood transfusion

- Patient refusal
- No symptomatic benefit from previous transfusion
- Patient moribund with life expectancy of days

Erythropoietin

- This is a hormone made by the kidney. It stimulates the production of red blood cells and is licensed for anaemia of chronic renal failure and for patients undergoing chemotherapy who are receiving platinum-containing chemotherapy (NICE guidance)
- It may also be effective in improving the chronic anaemia of cancer
- An injection of 150–300 units/kg SC three times a week for 4–6 weeks increases the Hb significantly in 50–60% of patients with cancer. The patients most likely to benefit include those with a low erythropoietin concentration, adequate bone marrow reserve and those who have an initial good response (i.e. an increase in Hb of >1g/dL within four weeks of starting treatment)
- The maximum benefit is achieved after about two months, which may be a factor limiting its usefulness in palliative care patients where prognosis is short
- Patients should be given iron supplements during erythropoietin therapy to maximize the response
- The haemoglobin level must be monitored weekly to ensure this does not increase above 12.0g/dL, because of the thrombotic risk

Complications

- Hypertension
- Thrombosis
- Iron deficiency, if not on iron supplements

Screening of donated blood products is inevitably becoming ever more stringent and blood transfusion may become justified only for the most needy. Erythropoietin may therefore become more commonly used. It is already used where appropriate for Jehovah's Witnesses.

Bleeding and haemorrhage

Bleeding occurs in about 20% of patients with advanced cancer and may contribute to death in 5%. Bleeding may be directly related to the cancer itself, e.g. local bleeding from fungating tumours, or indirectly related, e.g. peptic ulceration or nose bleeds secondary to treatment with NSAIDs or thrombocytopenia, respectively.

A systemic deterioration in a patient's condition may be mirrored by a decline in the haematological profile.

Obvious bleeding

- Oral mucosa or nose
- Gums
- Nasopharynx
- Haemoptysis
- Haematemesis
- Skin/muscle

Hidden bleeding

- Gastrointestinal—melaena, anaemia, (raised urea may be noted)
- Pulmonary—worsening breathlessness, pleural effusion
- Urogenital—macroscopic or microscopic haematuria
- Cerebral—headache, visual disturbance, change in neurology
- Gynaecological—vaginal bleeding

General management of bleeding

Where possible and when appropriate, attempt to correct haemostatic factors that contribute to a bleeding tendency.

The sight of blood can have a profound effect on patients and their carers. Relatives and patients who have coped calmly with a full range of demanding symptoms may become very distressed in the event of a bleed. If that bleed is significant there are few who are stoic enough not to be frightened. Explanation of what is happening, or what happened and the opportunity for fears to be expressed and listened to can be a very important part of professional supportive care in such circumstances.

Factors that contribute to bleeding

Platelets

Thrombocytopenia due to:
- Reduced marrow production:
  - marrow infiltration
  - myelosuppression following chemotherapy
- Increased consumption/utilization:
  - disseminated intravascular coagulation (DIC)
  - autoimmune
- Splenic pooling:
  - hypersplenism

Abnormal function

As seen in:
- Acute myeloid leukaemia
- Myelodysplasia
- Myeloproliferative disorders
- Paraproteinaemias, e.g. multiple myeloma
- Treatment with NSAIDs, aspirin
- Renal failure

Coagulation factors

High-level expression of tissue factor leading to:
- Extrinsic pathway activation
- Thrombin generation
- Consumption of clotting factors
- DIC

Metastatic liver disease

Results in:
- Reduced synthesis of vitamin K-dependent factors

DISSEMINATED INTRAVASCULAR COAGULATION (DIC)

Acute DIC is uncommon and presents as a mixture of thrombosis and bleeding. The skin may develop petechiae and purpura, and gangrene may occur in areas of end circulation such as the digits, nose and ear lobes. Bleeding may occur in areas of trauma such as at venepuncture sites or as haematuria in the presence of a catheter. Treatment includes platelet infusions, FFP and cryoprecipitate.

Chronic DIC (as measured by laboratory tests) is more common and may be asymptomatic but thrombotic symptoms of DVT, PE or migratory thrombophlebitis may occur. Treatment is usually with heparin (low molecular weight).

Laboratory investigations for DIC
- D-dimers—are more specific than fibrin degradation products (FDPs). A significant increase in D-dimers + prolonged PT, reduced fibrinogen, and thrombocytopenia are necessary for diagnosis (D-dimers are also increased in infection, impaired renal function, post-transfusion, malignancy and with increasing age)
- **Prothrombin time (PT)**—less sensitive, usually prolonged in acute DIC, but may be normal in chronic DIC
- **Activated partial thromboplastin time (APTT)**—less useful, as may be normal or shortened in chronic DIC
- **Platelets**—reduced or falling count found in acute DIC
- **Blood film**—may show red cell fragments (schistocytes)

THROMBOCYTOPENIA

Spontaneous bleeding due to thrombocytopenia is rare if the platelet count is >20 × 10^9/L but traumatic bleeding is problematic if the platelet count is less than 40 × 10^9/L. Sepsis will increase the bleeding tendency. If platelet function is abnormal, bleeding may occur at higher counts.

- A platelet transfusion may be considered if there is bleeding which is distressing. It will only raise the platelet count for a few days. This treatment should not be given routinely if there is no evidence of bleeding and the count is greater than 10 × 10^9/L. If the platelet count is less than 50 × 10^9/L and the patient is bleeding, platelets should be given
- A pool of platelets is derived from four units of donated blood and is approximately 300mL
- Platelets must be kept at room temperature and transfused within 30min, using a sterile administration set or a platelet infusion set. **Never** use an in-line filter
- The donor should be ABO compatible with the patient
- Occasional reactions with rigors and fever may occur .These respond to chlorphenamine 10mg IV and hydrocortisone 100mg IV

It is important to anticipate which patients are likely to require platelet transfusions and to decide the appropriateness prior to a crisis. The whole team should be involved in decisions concerning ongoing regular prophylactic transfusions and their withdrawal. With platelet counts of 10–20 × 10^9/L the risk of a major bleed is small, severe bleeding occurring mostly with counts less than 5 × 10^9/L.

Tranexamic acid (inhibits fibrinolysis) can be used to control mucosal bleeding due to thrombocytopenia:
- 1g orally t.d.s. or slow IV injection
- Mouthwash 1g every six hours for oral bleeding
- Topical tranexamic acid for superficial fungating tumours

On average, it takes two days of therapy to slow down bleeding and four days for bleeding to stop.

Blood products

These are less commonly used in the palliative care setting and close liaison with the haematology department is essential when considering administration. The list below outlines some products and their indications.

Indications for blood products

Fresh-frozen plasma (FFP)

- Disseminated intravascular coagulation
- Rapid correction of warfarin overdose
- Liver disease
- Coagulopathy due to massive blood loss

Cryoprecipitate

- In DIC when fibrinogen <1.0g/L
- For bleeding in cases of dysfibrinogenaemia

Bleeding directly related to cancer

Radiotherapy should be considered in patients with local bleeding caused by cancer, e.g. ulcerating skin tumours, lung cancer causing haemoptysis, gynaecological cancer causing vaginal bleeding and bladder/prostate cancer causing haematuria.

Specific situations

Nose bleeds

- Most nose bleeds are venous, and when arising from the anterior septum can often be stopped by pressure
- Silver nitrate caustic pencil can be applied to the bleeding point. The nose can be packed with calcium alginate rope (e.g. Kaltostat) or with ribbon gauze soaked in adrenaline (epinephrine 1:1000 1mg in 1mL).If the bleeding is more posterior, and continues into the nasopharynx, a Merocel nasal tampon may need to be inserted for 36 hours with antibiotic cover, or the nose packed with gauze impregnated with bismuth iodoform paraffin paste (BIPP) for three days. These should be performed by a clinician with previous experience, preferably by an ENT surgeon
- The ENT department may need to be contacted for further management with a balloon catheter or cauterization under local anaesthetic

Surface bleeding

The bleeding from tumour masses may respond well to radiotherapy.
Other measures include the following:

Physical
- Gauze applied with pressure for 10 min soaked in adrenaline
  (epinephrine) 1:1000 1mg in 1mL or tranexamic acid 500mg in 5mL:
  - silver nitrate sticks applied to bleeding points
  - haemostatic dressings, i.e. alginate, e.g. Kaltostat, Sorbsan

Drugs
- Topical:
  - sucralfate paste 2g (two 1g tablets crushed in 5mL KY jelly)
  - sucralfate suspension 2g in 10mL b.d. for mouth and rectum
  - tranexamic acid 5g in 50mL warm water b.d. for rectal bleeding
  - 1% alum solution for bladder
- Systemic:
  - antifibrinolytic, e.g. tranexamic acid 1.5g p.o. stat and 0.5–1g b.d.–t.d.s.
    p.o. or slow IV 0.5–1g t.d.s. **Do not use if DIC suspected**
  - haemostatic, e.g. etamsylate 500mg q.d.s. (restores platelet
    adhesiveness)

Haemoptysis

- One-third of patients with lung cancer develop haemoptysis, although the incidence of acute fatal bleeds is only 3%, of which some occur without warning
- The patient is more likely to die from suffocation secondary to the bleed than from the bleed itself. Bleeding due to cancer, is most commonly from a primary carcinoma of the bronchus. A massive haemoptysis is usually from a squamous-cell lung tumour lying centrally or causing cavitation. Metastases from carcinoma of the breast, colorectum, kidney and melanoma may also cause haemoptysis
- Infection in the chest and pulmonary emboli are other causes of haemoptysis
- A generalised clotting deficiency seen with thrombocytopaenia, hepatic insufficiency or warfarin therapy can also be contributory factors

Treatments for **non-acute haemorrhage** include oncological, systemic and local measures. If radiotherapy is inappropriate, coagulation should be enhanced with oral tranexamic acid 1g t.d.s. The risks of encouraging hypercoagulation need to be considered carefully in patients with a history of a stroke or ischaemic heart disease.

Erosion of a major artery can cause **acute haemorrhage,** which may be a rapidly terminal event. However, it may be possible to anticipate such an occurrence and appropriate medication and a red/green/blue towel to reduce the visual impact should be readily available. Relatives or others who witness such an event will need a great deal of support. If the haemoptysis is not immediately fatal, the aim of treatment is sedation of a shocked, frightened patient.

It *may* be appropriate to have emergency medication in the home to sedate the acutely bleeding patient, although such a strategy can only be arrived at after discussion with the family, carers and the patient's GP, and needs to be documented clearly.

Assessment

Consider the commonest causes:
- Tumour bleeding
- Clotting disorders
- Infection
- Pulmonary embolism

Treatment

- Treat any evidence or signs suggestive of infection
- Consider radiotherapy referral (not if multiple lung metastases) or brachytherapy, where the radiation sources are placed close to the tumour within the lungs
- Consider and treat other systemic causes of bleeding (see Chapter 15)
- Perform blood tests for clotting screen and platelets
- Give tranexamic acid 1g t.d.s. p.o.:
  - stop if no effect after 1 week
  - continue for 1 week after bleeding has stopped, then discontinue

- continue long term (500mg t.d.s.) only if bleeding recurs and it responds to a second course of treatment

Small bleeds can herald a larger massive haemorrhage; consider siting an IV cannula to administer emergency drugs.

Haematemesis

The incidence is 2% in patients with cancer and may be either directly associated with the cancer and/or secondary to gastroduodenal irritants such as NSAIDs, or aspirin. The management includes stopping NSAIDs if possible or changing to celecoxib (reduced effect on platelets) and adding a proton pump inhibitor or H_2-receptor antagonist; a gastroprotective agent such as sucralfate may also be useful.

Major bleeds

If the patient's condition is not stable, and he/she has a history of major haemorrhage or ongoing bleeding:
- Consider appropriateness of transfer to an acute medical/endoscopy unit
- Site an IV cannula to anticipate the need for emergency drugs
- Treat anxiety or distress as needed:
  - midazolam 2–5mg initially by slow IV titration (10mg diluted to 10mL with sodium chloride 0.9%)
- If no IV access, midazolam 5–10mg SC (give IM if shocked or vasoconstricted)

Rectal bleeding

This may be associated with local tumour (radiotherapy may be the treatment of choice to stop the bleeding) and/or radiotherapy. Bloody diarrhoea may occur acutely with pelvic radiotherapy which causes acute inflammation of the rectosigmoid mucosa, but this should be self-limiting. A predsol retention enema 20mg in 100mL o.d.–b.d. or prednisolone 5mg and sucralfate 3g in 15mL b.d. may help.

Bleeding from chronic ischaemic radiation proctitis may respond to tranexamic acid, etamsylate or sucralfate suspension given rectally.

Haematuria (📖 see Chapter 6g Genitourinary problems)

This may occur with carcinoma of the bladder or prostate or as a result of chronic radiation cystitis. Urinary infection will aggravate the situation. Tranexamic acid or etamsylate may be useful, although there is the risk of clot formation and urinary retention. Alum 50mL of a 1% solution can be useful if retained in the bladder via a catheter for 1 hour.

Massive terminal haemorrhage

Massive terminal haemorrhage occurs as a result of a major arterial haemorrhage and usually causes death in minutes. For patients who have undergone all possible treatment options, this inevitably terminal event should be treated palliatively, the main aim being comfort for the patient and support for the family.

It is usually associated with tumour erosion into the aorta or into the pulmonary artery (causing haematemesis or haemoptysis) or carotid or femoral artery (causing external bleeding). If a massive haemorrhage is unexpected, the only appropriate management may be to stay with the patient and attempt to comfort any distress.

Major haemorrhage may be preceded by smaller bleeds. Patients may have been receiving platelets and blood products, which have now been discontinued. If major haemorrhage is anticipated, it may be appropriate to warn family members of the possibility. Appropriate drugs, already drawn up in a syringe, should be kept available at the bedside to ensure fast administration. Red, blue or green towels (which mask the colour of blood) should be available to help control the spread of blood.

In the event of a massive bleed, the aim of treatment will be to rapidly sedate and relieve patient distress from what will, by definition, be the terminal event. Where possible, drugs should be given IV or else by deep IM injection.

Drug options

Midazolam

Midazolam 10mg SC, IV or bucally will sedate most patients. Heavy alcohol drinkers and patients on regular benzodiazepines may require larger doses.

Ketamine

The effect of ketamine is more predictable in palliative care patients than benzodiazepines and opioids, since the patient is unlikely to have been taking it regularly. Ketamine 150–250mg IV will rapidly sedate a patient dying from a terminal haemorrhage. If the IM route is deemed necessary, a larger dose of 500mg will be required.

Opioids

These are less recommended for the management of terminal haemorrhage for the following reasons:

- As a controlled drug, nurses may not be able to leave a dose by the bedside or to check doses quickly
- Variable doses will be required depending on how opioid-naïve the patient is
- Diamorphine needs to be dissolved, leading to further delay

Summary

- Midazolam 10–20mg IV, SC, IM or buccal
- Ketamine 150–250mg IV or 500mg IM
- Opioid dose will vary

Thromboembolism

It is over 130 years since Trousseau first noticed the association between cancer and thrombosis. Patients with cancer are at high risk of developing venous thromboembolism (VTE) and the risk increases as malignancy advances. Therefore, it follows that palliative care patients are extremely thrombogenic.

Studies have suggested that the incidence of deep vein thrombosis (DVT) may be as high 52% (with 33% of those being bilateral) in palliative care.

Thrombogenic risk

Virchow's triad describes the predisposing factors for VTE as:
- Stasis
- Endothelial perturbation
- Hypercoaguability

The following list suggests some of the reasons that patients with cancer are at such high risk.

Prothrombotic risk in cancer

- **Stasis**:
  - Immobility due to weakness, lethargy
  - Compression of vessels by tumour, e.g. pelvic disease
  - Extrinsic compression from oedematous legs
- **Endothelial perturbation:**
  - Recent surgery
  - Central venous access
  - Direct tumour invasion of vessel
- **Hypercoagulable state**:
  - Dehydration
  - Tissue factor/tumour procoagulant release
  - Increased platelet activation
  - DIC
  - Cytokine-related thrombotic changes
  - Prothombotic changes from certain chemotherapeutic agents

Deep vein thrombosis (DVT)

Signs and symptoms vary depending upon the severity of DVT. It should be suspected in those patients with a swollen, tender, warm, erythematous leg, although it is unreliable to make a firm clinical diagnosis on the basis of these findings alone. Some are asymptomatic, whilst extreme cases may lead to vascular insufficiency and gangrene. The risk of a pulmonary embolus from a distal DVT (i.e. below knee) is low; and only about 20% of calf vein thromboses progress to a proximal thrombosis.

Differential diagnosis
- Cellulitis
- Lymphoedema
- Oedema due to hypoproteinaemia
- Ruptured Baker's cyst

Diagnosis
It is not always practical to confirm the presence of a DVT if the patient is in the terminal stages of illness or to treat all patients with VTE. If a patient is not going to be anticoagulated there is little point in investigating a suspected thrombus. Anticoagulation carries risks as well as benefits and these should be weighed up on an individual basis first.
- Doppler ultrasound:
  - non-invasive; no ionizing radiation; easily repeatable
  - can be performed at the bedside if suitable equipment is available
  - accuracy is lower for non-occlusive iliac thrombus and calf vein assessment than ascending venography
- Venography:
  - invasive; involves ionizing radiation; contrast media is injected into a vein on the dorsum of the foot; low risk of allergic reaction
  - no longer the first-line investigation; useful when Doppler is inconclusive, for example in patients with large oedematous legs or with previous deep vein thrombosis
  - gives excellent visualization of all the leg veins
- Light reflection rheography:
  - non-invasive
  - can be done at bedside
  - high sensitivity but poor specificity and therefore not used greatly in clinical practice
  - cannot localize thrombus or distinguish intrinsic from extrinsic compression
- D-dimers:
  - use in cancer patients is limited due to high false-positive rate in malignancy
- Magnetic resonance angiography:
  - non-invasive
  - good at imaging leg vessels
  - use in palliative care patients is yet to be evaluated

Pulmonary embolus (PE)

Evidence from post-mortem studies suggests that pulmonary emboli are underdiagnosed clinically in the palliative care setting.

This may be due to several factors:
- Patient not well enough for investigation
- Other lung pathologies make radiological diagnosis problematic
- Concerns over anticoagulation in some patients
- Breathlessness assumed to be due to other causes

Most PEs occur as a complication of DVT in the legs or pelvis. The risk of PE from untreated DVT is estimated at 50% and the mortality rate of untreated PE at 30–40%. Most deaths from PE occur in the first hour.

Signs and symptoms

These will vary depending upon the extent of thrombus, the general condition of the patient, other respiratory/cardiovascular co-morbidity and whether chronic pulmonary emboli or an acute event has occurred.

In some patients pulmonary emboli may go unnoticed, causing mild breathlessness, whilst in more severe cases, sudden cardiovascular collapse and death occur. Features suggestive of pulmonary emboli include:
- Breathlessness and cough
- Haemoptysis
- Palpitations
- Chest pain

Clinical signs may vary and are useful if present, but absence of signs should not exclude the diagnosis if there is a strong clinical suspicion. Likewise many of the signs could be accounted for by other co-morbidities. Signs may include:
- Tachycardia
- Tachypnoea
- Atrial fibrillation
- Raised JVP
- Hypotension
- Loud P_2 heart sound
- Cyanosis
- Syncope

Investigations

It is important to decide whether an investigation is going to alter management and, if so, which test would be the most appropriate and best tolerated by the patient. A balance between the test most likely to confirm the diagnosis and that with the least disruption/burden to the patient may need to be considered. Several tests that may be done in the acute setting may be less appropriate near the end of life.

- Arterial blood gases:
  - painful and unlikely to give much useful information in presence of coexisting lung disease
- Pulse oximeter O_2 saturation
  - non-invasive, rapid result
- ECG
  - majority of ECGs are normal
  - most common abnormality is sinus tachycardia
  - $S_1Q_3T_3$ phenomenon rare
  - atrial fibrillation may be present
- D-dimers:
  - a negative result is helpful in excluding the diagnosis. A positive result does not confirm the diagnosis in the presence of malignancy, infection, increasing age or impaired renal function
- Chest X-ray
  - useful in considering other causes of breathlessness besides PE

Objective testing for PE
All imaging techniques have 499 their limitations and different degrees of burden on the patient:
- **Spiral CT**:
  - first-line investigation
  - requires large volume of IV contrast
  - gives assessment of pulmonary veins
  - other chest pathologies identified
  - can be used to assess lower limb veins and inferior vena cava (IVC) at the same time
- **Ventilation/Perfusion (V/Q) scan**:
  - usually well-tolerated procedure
  - use falling due to CT and pulmonary angiography
- **Pulmonary angiography**:
  - 'gold standard' investigation
  - invasive
  - complication rate 0.5%, mortality 0.1%
  - limited use in palliative care population
  - rarely used now with advent of CT pulmonary angiography
- **Magnetic resonance angiography**:
  - under evaluation
  - limited use in palliative population

Chronic venous thrombosis

Patients with hypercoagulability related to disseminated malignancy or with cancers obstructing veins may have chronic venous thrombosis requiring warfarin and/or low molecular weight heparin (LMWH). Migratory thrombophlebitis affecting superficial veins, which is largely associated with disseminated bronchogenic adenocarcinoma, may also cause venous and arterial clotting.

Treatment of VTE

Treatment goals should be to relieve symptoms and prevent further thrombotic events:
- **DVT**:
  - consider leg elevation
  - analgesia for swelling and tenderness (NSAIDs may interfere with the INR)
  - compression stockings if tolerated, ease the symptoms of venous hypertension
  - consider anticoagulation
  - venocaval filters may prevent a pulmonary embolism if recurrent DVTs are a problem despite anticoagulation, but are associated with painful engorgement of both lower limbs
- **PE**:
  - oxygen
  - opioids ± benzodiazepines for breathlessness and fear
  - consider anticoagulation

Recurrence of thrombotic episodes while on warfarin may be managed by increasing the dose to achieve an INR in the higher therapeutic range e.g. 3.0–4.0 (see p.505).If there are problems achieving a therapeutic range e.g. because of compliance, the necessity for medication which potentiates warfarin, poor nutrition, poor venous access, then consider long-term LMWH in therapeutic dose.This also eliminates the need for INR monitoring.Rarely, patients experiencing recurrent thrombotic episodes despite the above may require LMWH in addition to warfarin.Anticoagulation in a patient with advanced malignancy should be considered carefully prior to initiation. Palliative care patients are at a high risk of haemorrhage for several reasons:
- Presence of DIC
- Consumption of clotting factors
- Platelet dysfunction/thrombocytopenia
- Tumours may be vascular
- Liver metastases

Each patient should be considered on an individual basis taking into account the following:
- Prognosis
- Bleeding risk
- Ability to control symptoms and the patient's quality of life without anticoagulation
- Perceived burden of anticoagulation
- Patient's views

Local haematology department guidelines should be sought regarding anticoagulation. Traditionally in palliative care, patients were initially treated with LMWH and, depending on the clinical circumstances, considered for commencing warfarin at the same time. Once the INR was stable at a therapeutic dose, the LMWH would then be discontinued. Emerging evidence from three RCTs comparing warfarin with LMWH in the management of cancer-related VTE have suggested that LMWHs reduces the recurrence of VTE whilst anticoagulated by 50% without significant difference in bleeding complications. Within the palliative care setting long-term LMWH should be the first-line anticoagulant of choice.

Important!

Never commence anticoagulant therapy without first checking the INR or platelet count.

Warfarin in patients with cancer

Despite being the mainstay of long-term anticoagulation for VTE, extreme caution should be used when recommending warfarin. Several studies have demonstrated significant increases in rates of bleeding amongst cancer patients on warfarin (in the order of 20%). Therefore, more frequent monitoring of the International Normalized Ratio (INR) (which should be maintained between 2 and 3) is often needed in patients with cancer (i.e. every 2–3 days) to reduce the risk of bleeding (☐ see Table 6l.2).

Problems with using warfarin in patients with advanced cancer

- High risk of bleeding. Even higher if thrombocytopenia or liver metastases present
- Unpredictable metabolism of warfarin
- Interaction with other drugs
- Difficulty maintaining INR in therapeutic range
- Burden of repeated INR checks to optimize safety
- Progression of thrombus despite therapeutic INR in a proportion of patients

Rapid reversal of warfarin

Give 12–15mL/kg FFP, 1 unit 300mL—usually 3–4 units of fresh plasma and 10mg vitamin K by slow IV injection.

Low molecular weight heparin in patients with cancer

Although the mainstay of treatment of VTE in patients with cancer remains long-term anticoagulation with warfarin, this is likely to change. There is now level 1a evidence comparing long-term LMWH with warfarin in this patient group. LMWH has been shown to reduce the recurrence of VTE from 17% to 9% with no stastistical difference in bleeding when compared with warfarin.

LMWH may be of particular benefit in palliative care since there is no need to measure the INR, and the drug does not react with other medicines.

The progressive nature of advanced malignancy invariably heralds changing symptoms, which necessitate drug alterations. This is a particular area of risk in warfarinized patients, where drug interactions may increase the INR.

There have been concerns that the once-daily injection of LMWH is too invasive, burdensome and detrimental to patients' quality of life, while others would argue that this is less of a burden than the alternate-day INR checks that may be required to minimize the risk of warfarin-related haemorrhage.

A phenomenological study amongst palliative care patients receiving long-term LMWH suggests it is an acceptable intervention and does not have an adverse impact on quality of life.

LMWH is more costly than warfarin. However, this does not take into account costs of repeated blood monitoring and prolonged length of hospital stay whilst loading warfarin to therapeutic levels.

Potential benefits for LMWH
- Reliable pharmacokinetics
- Anticoagulant effect not altered by diet or concomitant drug use
- Fast onset of action
- Repeated blood test monitoring not required

At present, there are no guidelines defining which patients should receive LMWH for long-term anticoagulation. Each patient should be considered individually, but the following patients should be considered for LMWH rather than warfarin:
- Continued thrombosis despite the INR being within the therapeutic range
- Liver metastases
- Symptoms that are difficult to control adequately with regular medication
- Regular INR checks considered too great a burden
- Poor venous access for blood testing

VTE and brain metastases

The management of VTE in those patients with brain metastases is complicated and there is no consensus. Studies comparing the use of venacaval filters with anticoagulation, show that 40% of patients with filters may experience further thrombotic events and 7% of those anticoagulated may develop neurological deterioration from intracerebral bleeding. The role of LMWH in these patients is yet to be clarified.

Length of anticoagulation

A patient should remain anticoagulated as long as the prothrombotic risk leading to VTE persists. In cancer, the prothrombotic risk increases as disease advances and so anticoagulation should, in theory, continue indefinitely. The decision should be made taking into account the patient's views, effect of treatment, logistics of treatment and the complications. As the disease progresses and the bleeding tendency increases, stopping anticoagulation may be the lesser of two evils.

Table 6l.2 Target INR

Target INR	Indication
2.0–2.5	DVT prophylaxis
2.5	Treatment of DVT and PE (or recurrence in patients not on warfarin)
3.5	Recurrent DVT and PE in patients receiving warfarin Mechanical prosthetic heart valves

Developing a good relationship with haematology colleagues

- In order to provide the best possible care for patients with end-stage haematological disease, palliative care teams need to build close working relationships with colleagues in haematology
- Historically, this relationship has been challenging, as there has been a lack of understanding of the respective roles
- Many patients may benefit in terms of symptom control and the prolongation of life resulting from aggressive active haematological intervention (including invasive procedures and frequent infusion of blood products) even in the terminal stages. This may be difficult for palliative care teams, whose aim for dying patients is to control symptoms in the least burdensome manner
- The stereotypical prejudices inherent in both specialties are not helpful
- It is crucial for the benefit of patients that there are good working relationships between haematology and palliative care specialists, so that patients and their families can have access to and the support of both approaches, and are aware of all the issues and choices

There are reasons why palliative care involvement in haematological patients is challenging, as outlined below:

- There may be a misperception that palliative care teams only provide terminal care and therefore referrals should only be made when the patient is 'actively dying'
- Problems may have occurred previously with well intentioned but perhaps misguided palliative interventions, e.g. thrombocytopenic patients bleeding or myeloma patients developing renal failure after having been started on NSAIDs
- Communication issues. The palliative care team may inadvertently question the patient's knowledge and understanding of their illness and attitude to continuation of treatment, which might overtly or covertly be seen to undermine the haematology treatment plan
- Fear that the palliative care team will take over patients who have often been managed for many years by the haematology team
- It is important to fully appreciate that the haematology team may have looked after their patient through several near-death crises. The patients may have responded to previous treatments in extremis and, for instance, offering further chemotherapy may be totally appropriate
- During treatment and as disease progresses haematology patients can become very ill, very quickly. This may not be the terminal stage, however, as patients may respond to active support with antibiotics, fluids and blood products

In the haematology context it is often very difficult to identify when a patient is dying.

- Haematology colleagues need to be aware that palliative care specialists do not take over patients, or undermine their colleagues, or use medication to shorten the lives of patients
- Palliative care teams should work alongside haematology teams, amicably negotiating the treatment path with patients and families

Further reading

Books

Provan D., et al. (2009) *Oxford Handbook of Clinical Haematology* (3rd edn). Oxford: Oxford University Press.

Articles

Noble S (2008) Factors influencing hospice thromboprophylaxis policy; a qualitative study *Palliative Medicine* **22**:7:808–814

Psychiatric symptoms in palliative care

Adjustment disorders

Adjustment disorders are defined as a maladaptive reaction to an identifiable psychosocial stressor which occurs within three months of the onset of the stressor and which does not persist for longer than six months. Although the symptoms are not specified, the commonest presenting symptoms are depression and anxiety. Clinical presentations can include anger, bitterness and blaming others. A useful marker is that the patient with adjustment disorder feels bad about the situation, whereas patients with a depressive disorder feel bad about themselves.

Treatment

An adjustment disorder does not respond to antidepressants and generally improves as new levels of adaptation are reached. Certain interventions, such as problem-oriented psychotherapy, may be helpful. The symptoms may fluctuate in severity on a daily basis and patients can often be distracted from their distress. Beta-blockers or a short course of benzodiazepines can be helpful.

Anxiety

It is normal to be anxious in certain circumstances, many of which pertain in the palliative setting. The spectrum of anxiety ranges from 'normal' through to persistent and severe anxiety. Anxiety becomes a problem when its duration and severity exceed normal expectations. It may be acute or chronic. Anxiety is common in the terminally ill for various reasons, including the fear of uncontrolled symptoms and of being left alone to die.

Anxiety assessment
- Is it severe?
- Is it long-standing?
- Is it related to alcohol withdrawal?
- Is it situational?
- Is it related to a specific fear?
- Are the family anxious?[1]

Management involves assessing the patient for any reversible factors such as pain, or unfounded worries. Stimulant drugs or excessive alcohol intake or withdrawal may exacerbate the anxiety.

It is necessary to provide the time and opportunity for patients to express their worries and concerns and for these concerns to be addressed

---

1 Kaye P. (1999) *Decision Making in Palliative Care*, pp. 34–5. Northampton: EPL Publications.

honestly and clearly. Relaxation techniques and various complementary therapies may help, as may the controlled safe atmosphere of a hospice with professional carers.

It is important for all members of the palliative care team to be aware of the 'infectious' nature of anxiety, which can distress individual members of the palliative care team and, by default, the whole team. These situations are often predictable, and extra effort should be made to support staff during potentially stressful situations and to avoid being driven to extreme management decisions.

Pharmacological treatment of anxiety

Benzodiazepines

These are very useful drugs but have received a bad press because of their addictive potential, but used appropriately and at the correct dosages they can be very effective. They are traditionally divided into compounds which have more sedating effects and those which have more anxiolytic actions. However, there is considerable overlap on the anxiety/sedating spectrum.

They are useful to break the anxiety cycle, to restore sleep and to reduce the suffering of the situation where a patient feels that he/she is 'losing control'. They are not a substitute for taking the time to allow a patient to ventilate their fears.

- Diazepam: 1–5mg p.r.n., p.o.—diazepam has a long half-life and may therefore accumulate and be sedative
- Lorazepam: 1–2mg p.r.n., p.o. SL—lorazepam is short-acting, rapidly anxiolytic and less sedating than diazepam
- Midazolam: 5–10mg p.r.n., SC or buccal—midazolam is useful for emergency sedation

Drugs used for anxiety

Diazepam is an appropriate first-line benzodiazepine.

Lorazepam is shorter acting and (taken sublingually) has a faster onset of action; it is useful on a p.r.n. basis.

Midazolam can be used if a CSCI is required.

Propranolol is helpful, especially for controlling the somatic symptoms of anxiety, e.g. tremor and palpitations.

The anxiolytic effect of buspirone develops over 1–3 weeks, and it probably has little place in palliative care.

SSRIs can be used for panic attacks if benzodiazepines are ineffective.

Diazepam
Tabs: 2mg, 5mg, 10mg; oral solution: 2mg/5mL, 5mg/5mL

rectal tubes: 5mg/2.5mL, 10mg/2.5mL; supps: 10mg;

inj. (emulsion): 10mg/2mL (Diazemuls)—IV use only;

inj. (solution): 10mg/2mL—IM use

Blood levels increased by omeprazole (increased sedation).

Lorazepam
Tabs: 1mg, 2.5mg; Inj.: 4mg/1mL

Midazolam
Inj.: 2mg/1ml; 5mg/1ml

Sedative effect markedly enhanced by itraconazole, ketoconazole and possibly fluconazole.

Propranolol
Tabs: 10mg, 40mg, 80mg, 160mg; oral solution: 50mg/5mL

Antidepressants
Selective serotonin re-uptake inhibitor (SSRI) antidepressants such as paroxetine and citalopram (must not be used in those under 18 years of age) have less reported side-effects than the tricyclics and also have anxiolytic properties. However, care must be taken to avoid enervating SSRIs such as fluoxetine, which can initially increase anxiety. Complementary therapies, e.g. aromatherapy, and massage and specific interventions, for instance hypnosis, relaxation and imagery, may help increase the patient's sense of control.

Complex anxiety states with depression and psychosis may be more suitably treated with neuroleptics. The help of a psychiatric team should be obtained in managing such patients.

Depression

Estimates of the prevalence of depression in patients vary greatly, but it is probable that of those with advanced cancer at least 25% may develop a significant mood disorder. A review of 12 articles reported a range of depression rates from 3% to 69%. Certain types of cancer, such as pancreatic cancer, are associated with an increased incidence of depression.[3] A spectrum ranging from sadness to adjustment disorder to depressive illness is recognized. But there is concern that depression may be under-diagnosed. This may be due to a number of reasons, including a diurnal variation in symptoms such that it may be missed, social 'cover-up', or presentation with physical symptoms. One of the main difficulties is distinguishing depression from appropriate sadness at the end of life.

In the physically *healthy* population, depression is diagnosed if patients have a persistent low mood and at least four of the following symptoms which are present most of the day for the preceding two weeks:

1　Diminished interest or pleasure in all or almost all activities
2　Psychomotor retardation or agitation
3　Feelings of worthlessness or excessive and inappropriate guilt
4　Diminished ability to concentrate and think
5　Recurrent thoughts of death and suicide
6　Fatigue and loss of energy
7　Significant weight loss or gain
8　Insomnia or hypersomnia

In patients with advanced cancer, symptoms 6–8 are almost universal, and it is doubtful whether physical symptoms should be included at all when diagnosing depression in the terminally ill.

Atypical presentations of depression

- Irritability
- Agitation and anxiety symptoms
- Histrionic behaviour
- Hypochondriasis
- Psychotic features (delusions, paranoia) that are mood-congruent, e.g. content of delusions consistent with depressive thoughts

Pharmacological treatment of depression

There is little information concerning the effectiveness of antidepressant medication in terminally ill patients. There is, however, a body of evidence showing that under-treatment is common, with patients being prescribed antidepressants within the final six weeks of life, allowing little time for therapeutic benefit. Psychostimulants, which have a faster onset of action than classical antidepressants, are rarely used in this terminal situation despite some evidence of benefit. Being younger and having breast cancer increase the chance of being prescribed antidepressants.[2]

2 Breitban w., *et al.* (2004) Psychiatric Symptoms in Palliative Medicine In: Doyle D. H., et al. (eds) *Oxford Textbook of Palliative Medicine* (3rd edn). Oxford: Oxford University Press. pp 746–771

Think list

- Corticosteroids—may help mild depression and low mood by improving sense of well-being, but can also induce psychosis or depression in others. Starting low-dose dexamethasone, e.g. 4mg daily for a week followed by 2mg daily for a week, can elevate a patient's mood whilst waiting for a response to antidepressants
- Psychostimulants (methylphenidate or dexamfetamine)—particularly if prognosis <3 months
- ECT (electroconvulsive therapy)—response can be very rapid; very occasionally appropriate, e.g. severe depression developing during chemotherapy
- Pathological crying may respond to citalopram

Tricyclic antidepressants (TCAs)

TCAs may take several weeks to lift depression. They all have antimuscarinic properties to greater or lesser degrees and therefore may be associated with symptoms such as hypotension, dry mouth and difficulty in micturition. TCAs are not therefore recommended for the treatment of depression in advanced cancer. They can however be useful if associated with marked anxiety.

Selective serotonin re-uptake inhibitors (SSRIs)

For example:
- Citalopram 20mg o.d.
- Sertraline 50mg o.d.
- Fluoxetine 20mg o.d.

These drugs are less sedative than tricyclic antidepressants and have few antimuscarinic effects and low cardiotoxicity.

SSRIs may cause nausea, vomiting and headaches and extrapyramidal reactions can occur occasionally. Gastrointestinal side-effects are dose-related. There is little to choose between the SSRIs, but fluoxetine has a slower onset of action and may cause more agitation than other SSRIs: it is therefore not recommended as first line particularly in patients who are agitated.

- SSRIs may increase the risk of GI bleeding, especially in patients taking NSAIDs
- Serious reactions may develop with MAOIs and selegiline (serotonin syndrome)
- Increased serotonergic effects are seen with St John's Wort, which should be avoided by enquiring whether the patient is taking any non-prescribed medications
- Fluoxetine and fluvoxamine both increase the blood levels of carbamazepine and phenytoin (risk of toxicity)

- Use an SSRI unless other treatment is specifically indicated
- Dose escalation is not usually needed, so more rapid control of symptoms may be possible
- The side-effects of SSRIs are better tolerated than TCAs in ill patients with cancer

A trial of at least three weeks, and preferably six or more, is needed to properly assess response to an antidepressant. Discontinuation symptoms (withdrawal) will not usually occur if stopped within six weeks of starting.

Antidepressant discontinuation syndromes occur with both TCAs and SSRIs.

SSRI discontinuation symptoms include dizziness, light-headedness, insomnia, fatigue, anxiety/agitation, nausea, headache, and sensory disturbance. SSRIs should be withdrawn gradually when possible, using alternate-day dosing if needed.

Symptoms of withdrawal are more common with paroxetine (short half-life), and least common with fluoxetine (half-life of weeks).

Paroxetine
- Tabs: 20mg; liquid: 20mg/10mL
- Dose: 20mg mane p.o.—increase by weekly increments of 10mg as necessary to max. 50mg o.d.

Citalopram
- Tabs: 10, 20, 40mg; oral drops: 40mg/mL
- Dose: 20mg mane p.o.; max. 60mg o.d.

Sertraline—(useful in association with anxiety)
- Tabs: 50, 100mg
- Dose: 50mg mane p.o.; max. 200mg o.d.

Other antidepressant drugs
Venlafaxine is a serotonin and noradrenaline re-uptake inhibitor (SNRI). It causes less side-effects than the SSRIs but is contraindicated in uncontrolled hypertension and those at high risk of cardiac arrhythmia. The slow-release capsules are preferable as they seem to be tolerated better. Mirtazepine is a noradrenergic and specific serotonergic antidepressant (NaSSA) and is useful if there is marked anxiety/agitation. At lower doses the antihistaminic effect predominates producing sedation, which is reduced with higher doses when the noradrenergic transmission increases. Appetite may increase with subsequent weight gain which may be beneficial.

Venlafaxine
- Tabs: 37.5, 75mg
- Dose: 37.5mg b.d. p.o. increased to 75mg b.d.
- Caps: m/r 75, 150mg
- Dose: 75mg o.d. p.o. increased to 150mg o.d.
- Dose should be increased gradually to the usual dose 150mg, and higher according to response; maximum 375mg daily (225mg if m/r)

Mirtazepine
- Tabs (scored): 15, 30, 45mg
- Also available as oral solution and dispersible tablets
- Dose: 15mg nocte p.o. increased to 30mg nocte
- Dose should be increased gradually to usual dose 30mg, and higher according to response; maximum 45mg daily

St John's Wort
A number of patients may be taking St John's Wort as an antidepressant. It is not a licensed medication, and has a number of significant drug interactions:
- Increases serotonergic effects with SSRIs; therefore avoid
- Reduces anticoagulant effect of warfarin
- Reduces plasma levels of carbamazepine, phenytoin, phenobarbital (risk of fits)
- Reduces plasma levels of digoxin

Screening for depression

There are no universally accepted criteria for diagnosing depression in the terminally ill. In patients with advanced cancer, many of the symptoms of depression, e.g. changes in appetite, energy levels and sleep pattern, are common and there is still considerable controversy as to whether these physical symptoms should be included. Depressed mood, irritability, loss of interest in anything, feelings of worthlessness and lack of hope for the future are more important in this population.

Rating scales to measure depression are increasingly used. Such tools are not diagnostic and can only serve to indicate whether a patient has particular psychiatric symptoms suggestive of a diagnosis of depression. The decision should then be taken whether to treat for depression or to refer the patient for further assessment. The majority of rating scales consist of a number of symptoms or feelings. Patients indicate their own response and the person administering the scale calculates the scores.

Several instruments have been developed which define a threshold score for the predictability of depression. However, a defined cut-off threshold suitable for patients with early cancer or those receiving treatment may not be valid for patients with advanced disease receiving palliative care. Previous research has suggested that a scale developed for use in the post-natal period (the Edinburgh Depression Scale) may be useful for screening in palliative care. It does not include somatic symptoms but does include symptoms such as sadness, feelings of helplessness and thoughts of self-harm which may be particularly discriminatory in the palliative care population. Each item is scored from 0–3—the most negative response scoring highest. Recent research has found that a six-item Brief Edinburgh Depression Scale (BEDS)[3] with a score of 6 out of 18 gave a sensitivity of 72% and specificity of 83%.

3 Lloyd-Williams M., Shiels C., Dowrick C. (2007) The development of the Brief Edinburgh Depression Scale (BEDS) to screen for depression in patients with advanced cancer. *Journal of Affective Disorders*, **99**(1–3): 259–64.

BRIEF EDINBURGH DEPRESSION SCALE

Name

Please UNDERLINE the answer which comes closest to how you have felt IN THE PAST 7 DAYS, not just how you feel today

I have blamed myself unnecessarily when things went wrong:-
Yes, most of the time
Yes, some of the time
Not very often
No, never

I get a sort of frightened feeling as if something awful is about to happen
Very definitely and quite badly
Yes, but not too badly
A little, but it doesn't worry me
Not at all

Things have been getting on top of me
Most of the time and I haven't been able to cope at all
Yes, sometimes I haven't been coping as well as usual
No, most of the time I have coped quite well
No, I have been coping as well as ever

I have been so unhappy that I have had difficulty sleeping
Yes, most of the time
Yes, quite often
Not very often
No, not at all

I have felt sad or miserable
Yes most of the time
Yes, quite often
Not very often
No, not at all

The thought of harming myself has occurred to me
Yes, quite often
Sometimes
Hardly ever
Never

Confusional states

Delirium: An aetiologically, non-specific, global, cerebral dysfunction characterized by concurrent disturbance of level of consciousness, attention, thinking, perception, memory, psychomotor behaviour, emotion and sleep–wake cycle.

An acute confusional state (or delirium) is associated with mental clouding, leading to a disturbance of comprehension which is characterized by decreased attention, disorientation and cognitive impairment with poor short-term memory and concentration.

The prevalence of delirium may be as high as 85% for hospitalized terminally ill patients and is particularly common in elderly patients moved from a familiar environment. It may be exacerbated by deafness and poor vision.

While delirium is normally understood as a reversible process, there may not be time for it to improve in terminally ill patients. Occasionally, irreversible processes such as multiple organ failure cause delirium.

The diagnosis may be obvious with a rapid onset of altered behaviour and incoherent rambling speech. The symptoms may fluctuate and there may be insight. Severe delirium can progress to psychotic features with hallucinations and delusions.

The differential diagnosis includes dementia, which is a more chronic condition, is not associated with mental clouding and is irreversible. see p. 735.

It may be appropriate, if done sensitively, to carry out a simplified mini-mental score test to help management and to monitor clinical progress.

Mini-mental score

A test devised for the serial testing of cognitive mental state on a neuro-geriatric ward. A score of 20 or less was found in patients with dementia, delirium, schizophrenia or affective disorder.[5]

5 Folstein M. F., Folstein S. E., McHugh P. R. (1975) 'Mini-Mental State': a practical method for grading the cognitive state of patients for the clinician. *Journal of Psychiatric Research*, **12**: 189–98

Mini-mental state evaluation (MMSE) sample

Score	Section	Task
	Orientation	
5	e.g.	What is the date?
	Registration	
3	e.g.	Listen carefully. I am going to say three words. You say them back after I stop. Ready? Here they are... APPLE (pause), PENNY (pause), TABLE(pause). Now repeat those words back to me. [Repeat up to 5 times, but only score the first trial.]
	Language	
2	e.g.	What is this? [Point to a pencil or pen]
3	e.g.	Please read this and do what it says. [Show examinee the words on the stimulus form.] CLOSE YOUR EYES.
30	Total score	

This table is only a sample of the complete MMSE, which takes about 10–15 minutes, and requires some written material for the last test. The full MMSE can be purchased from Psychological Assessment Resource (PAR) Inc. by calling: (+1) (813) 968-3003

Score results

30–29	Normal
28–26	Borderline cognitive dysfunction.
25–18	Marked cognitive dysfunction – may be diagnosed as demented.
<17	Severe dysfunction – severe dementia.

Delirium and confusion

Treat reversible **cause** of confusion if possible.
   Consider:
- Hypercalcaemia
- Hypoglycaemia
- Hyponatraemia
- Renal failure
- Liver failure
- Drug-related causes
  - opioids
  - corticosteroids **and** withdrawal
  - alcohol and withdrawal
  - benzodiazepine **and** withdrawal
  - SSRI withdrawal
  - nicotine withdrawal
  - digoxin
  - lithium

NB benzodiazepines and phenothiazines accumulate in liver failure and opioids in renal failure
- Cerebral tumour, primary or secondary
- CVA or transient ischaemic attack (TIA)
- Anxiety/depression
- Infection
- Hypoxia
- Disorientation with move to hospital (in pre-existing dementia)
- Thiamine (vitamin B_1) deficiency
- Non-convulsive status epilepticus

The cause is often multifactorial, and symptoms such as pain or those associated with constipation or urinary retention may aggravate confusion.

Prescribing for delirium and confusional states
- Drugs should only be prescribed if necessary
- Night sedation should be given only after an attempt has been made to remove other causes of insomnia such as fear, noisy and unfamiliar surroundings, unrelieved pain, nocturia and stimulant medication such as steroids
- Reassurance and helping to orientate the patient and alleviate fear may be all that is required. The patient and family should be comforted by being told that the patient is not 'going mad', but that this is a temporary setback which is hopefully reversible. Daytime sedation should only be necessary if the patient is very distressed and not amenable to reassurance or is a danger to themselves or others
- Doses should be adjusted according to age and general condition, level of disturbance and likely tolerance
- Antipsychotics are considered to be the drugs of choice for delirium, haloperidol being the most commonly used
- The risk of extrapyramidal side-effects (EPSE) is greatest in the elderly, and with the older antipsychotics such as haloperidol and chlorpromazine. Newer drugs such as risperidone, olanzapine and promazine are better tolerated, but may not be adequate if rapid

control is needed (they are associated with an increased risk of stroke in elderly patients with dementia.)

- Chlorpromazine and levomepromazine are more sedative than haloperidol
- Benzodiazepines carry a risk of paradoxical agitation (disinhibition with worsening of behavioural disturbance) especially in the elderly. Used in conjunction with haloperidol, lorazepam improves the control of the acutely disturbed patient, but used alone is less effective than antipsychotics in delirium
- Most antipsychotics decrease the convulsive threshold, and may increase the risk of convulsions in susceptible patients, but the actual risk is undetermined

Benzodiazepines in agitation and restlessness

Although antipsychotics are considered the treatment of choice for delirium, agitation and restlessness in the patient with advanced cancer may often be primarily an anxiety state, with secondary cognitive impairment or clouded consciousness. In this condition, benzodiazepines may be more effective than antipsychotics. A knowledge of the previous psychological state of the patient is vital in determining this.

Alcohol withdrawal

The best treatment for alcohol withdrawal in palliative care is usually alcohol if the patient is able to swallow. However, in practice, patients who have been deteriorating over months have usually gradually reduced their alcohol intake.

Benzodiazepines are the drugs of choice in managing alcohol withdrawal symptoms and preventing agitation and seizures. Chlordiazepoxide is the benzodiazepine of choice but diazepam can also be used. Lorazepam should be used in severe liver disease. Clomethiazole may be used as an alternative to benzodiazepines.

Wernicke's encephalopathy (thiamine/vitamin B_1 deficiency) may be more common than anticipated in the terminally ill. The diagnosis can be confirmed by red blood cell (RBC) transketolase estimation. The diagnosis should be considered in any patient with a history of alcohol misuse who develops unexplained:

- Ophthalmoplegia
- Nystagmus
- Ataxia (not due to intoxication)
- Acute confusion (not due to intoxication)
- Memory disturbance
- Seizures
- Coma/unconsciousness

A presumptive diagnosis of Wernicke's encephalopathy should prompt treatment with high-dose parenteral B-complex vitamins.

Vitamin B preparation

Pabrinex (vitamins B and C)

- Inj.: pair of ampoules containing 10mL
- Dose: 1 pair of ampoules daily for seven days—for acute and severe vitamin B deficiency states

- Serious allergic reaction may rarely occur on IV administration (probably <1 in 250000, compared to incidence of 1–10% allergy with penicillin). Inject slowly over 10 minutes

Antipsychotics (□ see Table 6m.1)
Typical antipsychotics
Haloperidol
- Caps: 0.5mg; tabs: 1.5mg, 5mg; liquid: 2mg/1mL; inj.: 5mg/1mL
- Indometacin given with haloperidol can cause severe drowsiness.

Levomepromazine (methotrimeprazine)
- Tabs: 6mg, 25mg; susp.: 25mg/5mL; inj.: 25mg/1mL (Nozinan)
- 6mg tabs are available on a named patient basis only
- Oral bioavailability of levomepromazine is approx. 40%. Use half the daily oral dose by CSCI
- Avoid concurrent use with monoamine oxidase inhibitors (MAOIs)

Promazine
- Tabs: 25mg, 50mg; liquid: 25mg/5mL, 50mg/5mL; inj.: 50mg/1mL
- Useful for restlessness and agitation in the elderly

Atypical antipsychotics may be better tolerated than other antipsychotics and have a lower propensity than haloperidol for causing drug-induced movement disorders. They should be used with caution with cardiovascular disease, a history of epilepsy and in the elderly. Olanzapine and risperidone are associated with an increased risk of stroke in the elderly with dementia.

Risperidone
- Tabs: 0.5mg, 1mg, 2mg, 3mg, 4mg, 6mg; and dispersible tablets 0.5mg, 1mg, 2mg, 3mg, 4mg; liquid: 1mg/1mL
- Avoid in patients with cerebrovascular disease

Olanzapine
- Tabs: 2.5mg, 5mg, 7.5mg, 10mg; dispersible: 5mg, 10mg, 15mg, 20mg
- Dispersible tablets can be placed on the tongue to dissolve/disperse
- Avoid in patients with cerebrovascular disease

Quietiapine
- Tabs: 25mg, 100mg, 150mg, 200mg, 300mg

Benzodiazepines
Lorazepam
Lorazepam is shorter acting than diazepam, and is therefore safer in repeated doses; it can be given SC or sublingually for a more rapid effect and in uncooperative patients.
- Tabs: 1mg, 2.5mg; inj.: 4mg/1mL
- Dilute inj. with equal volume of water or sodium chloride 0.9% for IM use

Diazepam
- Tabs: 2mg, 5mg, 10mg; syrup: 2mg/5mL; rectal soln: 5mg/2.5mL, 10mg/2.5mL; supps: 10mg
- Blood levels increased by omeprazole (increased sedation)

Midazolam
- Inj.: 1mg/1mL, 2mg/1mL, 5mg/1mL. **Caution is needed**.
- Dose: 20–30mg/24h CSCI (max. 100mg/24h)
- Sedative effect markedly enhanced by itraconazole, ketoconazole and possibly fluconazole

Table 6m.1 Treatment of delirium and confusion with antipsychotics when no reversible causes diagnosed

Presentation	Non-elderly	Elderly
Confusion ± drowsiness, or where sedation undesirable/unnecessary	Non-sedative antipsychotic Haloperidol 1.5–3mg nocte or b.d. SC/CSCI (Risperidone 0.5–1mg b.d.) (Quetiapine 25mg o.d. to start)	Non-sedative antipsychotic with lower risk of extrapyramidal side-effects (EPSE) Risperidone 0.5mg nocte or b.d. p.o. Haloperidol 0.5–1mg nocte SC/CSCI.
Agitated confusion where sedative effects desired; mild–moderate agitation	Sedative antipsychotic Levomepromazine 25–50mg SC/CSCI/p.o. (Chlorpromazine 25–50mg b.d.–q.d.s. p.o.)	Sedative antipsychotic with lower risk of EPSE Promazine 25mg nocte or up to q.d.s. p.o. Levomepromazine 12.5–25mg/24h CSCI (Olanzapine 2.5mg nocte p.o.)
Acutely disturbed, violent or aggressive; at risk to themselves or others. Antipsychotic with proven safety record in repeated high doses for rapid titration; suitable for parenteral use*	Haloperidol 5mg SC/IM ± lorazepam 1–2mg SC/IM repeated after 20–30 minutes.	Haloperidol 2.5mg SC/IM ± lorazepam 0.5–1mg SC/IM repeated after 30 minutes

* Risperidone and olanzapine must be avoided in patients with a history of cerebrovascular disease/dementia.

Equivalent doses of antipsychotic and benzodiazepine medication

Occasionally patients are taking antipsychotic drugs or benzodiazepines on a long-term basis. The approximate equivalent doses are outlined in Table 6m.2, although, as ever, doses should be based on an overall assessment of the patient's individual needs. Switching antipsychotics or benzodiazepines, while not recommended, is sometimes required in the palliative care setting especially if the previous oral route is no longer available.

Table 6m.2 Benzodiazepine drug equivalence (an approximate guide)

Antipsychotic drug equivalence			
Antipsychotic drug	**Approximate equivalent daily dose**		
Chlorpromazine	100mg		
Haloperidol	2–3mg		
Levomepromazine	25–50mg		
Olanzapine	2.5–5mg		
Pimozide	2mg		
Quetiapine	25–150mg		
Risperidone	0.5–1mg		
Trifluoperazine	5mg		
	Equivalent dose anxiolytic/ sedative	**Approximate duration of action**	**Approximate subcutaneous dose over 24h**
Diazepam	5mg p.o. or p.r.	3h to 4 days	N/A
Clonazepam	0.25mg p.o.	6–24h	1mg
Midazolam	2.5mg SC	15mins to 4h	10mg
Lorazepam	0.5mg p.o.	7–8h (mean)	N/A
Temazepam	10mg p.o.	7–8h	N/A

These doses are approximate only. Cautious dosing advised in elderly/debilitated

Psychostimulants

Potential uses for psychostimulants:
- Depression
- Opioid-induced sedation or cognitive impairment
- Fatigue
- Cognitive impairment due to brain tumours
- Hypoactive delirium
- Hiccups

Psychostimulants for depression

Psychostimulants have been shown to be effective in depression in medically ill patients including the terminally ill, although they do not seem to be effective in primary depression. They are rarely prescribed for depression in the UK. They are useful because of their rapid onset, and are generally well tolerated. The beneficial effects of these drugs are reported to occur within 36–48h. Drug habituation is generally not a problem.

Methylphenidate appears to have been used more widely, but dexamfetamine is equally effective.

Doses of methylphenidate as low as 1.25mg daily have been used successfully in patients over 90 years old. Methylphenidate (average dose after titration 30mg daily) is as effective as imipramine 150mg o.d. in significantly reducing depressive and anxiety symptoms.

Psychostimulants have been used as adjuvants to reduce opioid-induced sedation and potentiate analgesia. It is not known whether this is due to a reduction in opioid-induced sedation, thus allowing dose escalation of the opioid, or to a direct potentiation of opioid analgesia.

Side-effects of psychostimulant drugs including agitation, dysphoria, insomnia, nightmares and hypomania have been reported.

Methylphenidate
- Tabs: 5, 10, 20mg
- Dose: 2.5–5mg b.d. p.o. (8.00am and 12 noon); increase every few days up to 20mg b.d. according to response

Dexamfetamine sulphate
- Tabs: 5mg
- Dose: 2.5–5mg o.d. p.o. (8.00am and 12 noon); increase every few days up to 20mg o.m. according to response

Restlessness/anguish (📖 see Chapter 16)

Spiritual distress (📖 see Chapter 9)

At the time of referral and transition to the palliative/terminal phase of an illness, many patients have an increased spiritual awareness. The concerns of these patients are often based on the existential questions:

• Who am I?
• What am I?
• Will I be remembered?
• How will I be remembered?

Patients experiencing emotional suffering often have 'Soul pain', but this may go unrecognized.

The integration of spiritual care into the palliative care team is therefore vital, to ensure that patients have the opportunity to disclose and discuss these concerns, which can cause great emotional distress. However, the spiritual needs are often not included in the assessment of the quality of life of terminally ill patients, and may not be identified by health professionals.

Suicide

Depression is increased in patients with terminal cancer and the incidence of suicide and thoughts of self-harm are increased in depressed patients. The incidence of suicide is therefore more common than previously believed.

Patients with cancer have twice the risk of committing suicide as the general population. Factors such as depression, advancing disease and hopelessness increase the risk of suicide. Other risk factors include actual suicidal thoughts, uncontrolled pain, exhaustion and fatigue, past suicidal attempts, substance abuse, recent bereavement, poor social support and family history of suicide. It is also thought that certain sites of cancer, i.e. oropharyngeal, lung, gastrointestinal, urogenital and breast, may be associated with an increase in the risk of suicide.

Patients with cancer tend to commit suicide by an overdose of analgesia or sedative drugs. Many doctors believe that if they enquire about suicidal intent, they may precipitate a suicide. Contrary to this belief, talking and sharing his/her thoughts of self-harm permits the patient to describe his/her feelings.

Suicidal ideation must not, however, be confused with patients who request death to be hastened—these patients may also be depressed, but may have other underlying fears e.g. of a painful or undignified death. (📖 See also Chapter 1 Euthanasia).

The initial assessment and evaluation of a patient with suicidal ideation should include the following:

- Establishment of rapport and an empathic approach
- Assessment of the patient's understanding of their illness and symptoms
- Assessment of their mental status
- Assessment of other factors, e.g. poor pain control
- Assessment of an external support system
- Establishment of their prior psychiatric history
- Assessment of their family history
- Recording of past suicide attempts or threats
- Assessment of suicidal thinking and plans
- Formulation of a treatment plan

Patients may require initial close supervision on a one–to-one basis. Careful attention should be paid to pain relief and relief of other distressing symptoms. It may be necessary to commence neuroleptic medication initially in addition to antidepressant medication. A psychiatric opinion should be obtained.

The patient's family and the palliative care team itself may need a lot of support.

Further reading

Books

Chochinov H., Breitbart W. (eds) (2000) *Handbook of Psychiatry in Palliative Medicine*. Oxford: Oxford University Press.

Doyle D. H., *et al* (eds) (2004) *Oxford Textbook of Palliative Medicine* (3rd edn). Oxford: Oxford University Press.

Kaye P. (1999) *Decision-making in Palliative Care*, pp. 34–5. Northampton: EPL Publications.

Kearney M. (2000) *A Place of Healing: Working with Suffering in Living and Dying*. Oxford: Oxford University Press.

Lloyd-Williams M. (2003) *Psychosocial Issues in Palliative Care*. Oxford: Oxford University Press.

Articles

Ahronheim J., *et al* (1996) Treatment of the dying in the acute care hospital: advanced dementia and metastatic cancer. *Archives of Internal Medicine*, **156**: 2094–100.

Block S. D. (2000) Assessing and managing depression in the terminally ill. *Annals of Internal Medicine*. **132**(3): 209–18.

Breitbart W., Jacobsen P. B. (1996) Psychiatric symptom management in terminal care. *Clinics in Geriatric Medicine*, **12**(2): 329–47.

Cox J., Holden J., Sagovsky R. (1987) Detection of postnatal depression: Development of the 10-item Edinburgh Postnatal Depression Scale. *British Journal of Psychiatry*, **150**: 782–6.

Folstein G. A., Folstein S. E., McHugh P. R. (1975) Mini Mental State. *Journal of Psychiatric Research*, **12**: 189–98.

Henderson M. (2007) Use of a clock-drawing test in a hospice population. *Palliative Medicine*, **21**: 559–565.

Kovach C., *et al* (1999) Assessment and treatment of discomfort for people with late stage dementia. *Journal of Pain and Symptom Management*, **18**: 412–19.

Laird M. (2005) The assessment and management of depression in the terminally ill. *European Journal of Palliative Care*, **12**(5): 101–4.

Lawrie I. (2004) How do palliative medicine physicians assess and manage depression? *Palliative Medicine*, **18**: 234–238.

Leonard M. (2008) Reversibility of delerium in terminally ill patients and predictors of mortality. *Palliative Medicine*, **22**(7): 848–854.

Lloyd-Williams M., Payne S. (2002) Can multidisciplinary guidelines improve the palliation of symptoms in the terminal phase of dementia. *International Journal of Palliative Nursing*, **8**: 370–5.

Lloyd-Williams M., Friedman T., Rudd N. (1999) A survey of antidepressant prescribing in the terminally ill. *Palliative Medicine*, **13**: 243–8.

Spiller J. A. (2006) Hypoactive delirium: assessing the extent of the problem for inpatient specialist palliative care. *Palliative Medicine*, **20**(1): 17–23.

Paediatric palliative care

There can be no Doubt that a perfect Cure of the Diseases of Children is as much desired by all, as any thing else whatsoever in the whole art of Physick.

Walter Harris, 1698

Who needs paediatric palliative care?

The emergence of a new specialty

- Advances in the treatment of life-threatening neonatal and paediatric conditions have dramatically improved survival rates over recent years
- One of the most striking reductions in mortality has been achieved for children with malignant conditions, although there remain certain forms of cancer for which the prognosis remains extremely poor
- Similarly, there is a range of non-malignant conditions which continue to be life-limiting, despite the advances outlined above
- The patient population in paediatric palliative care is quite different from that encountered in adult practice. Approximately 40–50% of children with palliative care needs have a malignancy
- The remainder have a variety of conditions including congenital abnormalities and neurodegenerative disorders
- Modern pharmacological and technical approaches now make it possible for some children, who would previously not have survived at all, to live longer, sometimes into adulthood. Many of these children have long illness trajectories which see them deteriorate slowly and inexorably toward a state of high dependency and disability
- It can be difficult to identify a point where treatment becomes exclusively palliative, and this presents a major challenge to service providers
- Many conditions are rare and the prognosis is often unpredictable, the child could die at any time or may live a number of years. These children often have multiple symptoms, requiring frequent medical intervention, in addition to complex psychological needs
- The parents and siblings of these children also need support in adjusting to the diagnosis and ongoing care of the child

Specialist paediatric palliative care services have recently been established in a number of centres throughout the world and focus variably on the three main care settings: home, hospice and hospital. Families will generally move between the various settings according to need, but it has become clear that where home care is offered as a realistic option, most families will wish to care for their child at home. Children's home care teams and outreach nurses are becoming more common, and are often able to take on a palliative care role providing support for children with life-limiting diseases and their families in their own homes.

In addition, children's hospices are also being established, providing an option for respite and terminal care. Specialist palliative care services for children in hospitals are not as widely available away from major centres, although adult palliative care teams are available for advice in many hospitals.

Much of the introductory material for this chapter has been produced by the Royal Children's Hospital, Melbourne Paediatric Palliative Care team.

The box below is taken from *A Guide to the Development of Children's Palliative Care* Services and lists numerous conditions that may affect the child in palliative care.[1]

- Conditions for which curative treatment is possible but may fail, e.g. leukaemia.
- Diseases where premature death is likely but intensive treatments may prolong good quality life, e.g. cystic fibrosis, muscular dystrophy.
- Progressive conditions where treatment is exclusively palliative and may extend for many years, e.g. mucopolysaccharidoses, other neurodegenerative conditions.
- Conditions, often with neurological impairment, causing weakness and susceptibility to complications, e.g. non-progressive CNS disease

Background

Children in the terminal phase of illness are known to suffer significantly from the inadequate recognition and treatment of symptoms, aggressive attempts at cure, fear and sadness. Any child's death is experienced as a profound loss by parents, siblings, their extended family and the wider community. Bereaved parents suffer intense grief and may be at increased risk of death themselves from both natural and unnatural causes.[2]

For those living in developed nations, child mortality has fallen to such an extent that the death of a child seems an utterly unnatural and devastating affront. It is now so uncommon as to create a sense of alienation for families who are caring for a dying child or whose child has died. This increases the importance of support for the family throughout the child's illness, from diagnosis and treatment through terminal care, to bereavement.

1 Association for Children with Life-threatening or Terminal Conditions and their Families and the Royal College of Paediatrics and Child Health (2003) *A Guide to the Development of Children's Palliative Care Services* (2nd edn). Bristol: ACT

2 Li J., Precht D. H., Mortensen P.B., Olsen J. (2003) Mortality in parents after death of a child in Denmark: a nationwide follow-up study. *Lancet*, **361**: 363–7.

Prevalence of UK paediatric palliative care needs[1]

In a district of 250 000 people with a population of 50 000 children aged <19yrs, in one year:
- 5 are likely to die from a life-limiting condition, of which 2 would be from cancer, 1 from heart disease and 2 from other life-limiting conditions.
- At the same time about 50 children would be suffering from a life-limiting condition and, of these, about half would have palliative care needs.

Provision of paediatric palliative care

The provision of paediatric palliative care is patchy and the structure of specialist teams variable. Before thinking about service provision, it may be helpful to consider what and who surrounds a family in this situation.

A large number of agencies and individuals may be involved in supporting children and families and although this is appropriate, there is the potential for confusion, intrusion and replication of services. It is often helpful to nominate a *key worker* who can coordinate the various services involved and act as a first point of call for families. Through effective communication, including regular meetings, a comprehensive management plan can be created for the child in question. But it is important that all the professionals involved are supported themselves, as this can be a demanding and unfamiliar area of practice. A specialist paediatric palliative care team can support the agencies and individuals involved in caring for the family. Such a team may include some or all of the following:

- Paediatric palliative care nurses (who may provide advice in both hospital and community settings)
- A specialist palliative care paediatrician
- Social worker
- Psychologist and or psychiatrist
- Chaplain

Sometimes, advice and support are also needed from other teams or professionals who have special expertise or knowledge regarding a particular condition. This is often necessary in cases where children have very rare conditions.

Differences between paediatric and adult palliative care

Developmental factors

An understanding of developmental issues is essential to the management of a child with palliative care needs. Infants and young children are completely dependent on the adults in their lives for providing care and protection. They also depend on others to make decisions on their behalf.

As children grow and develop, their capacity to care and decide for themselves increases. Indeed, the emergence of autonomy is a central developmental task of adolescence. In this way, care that is appropriate for a child of 11 may be inappropriate two years later as the need for independence, privacy and greater control grows. This can be difficult for both parents and healthcare professionals to accept. The natural desire to protect a child who is experiencing a devastating illness can lead to that child feeling stifled.

The relationship between development and illness is bidirectional. That is, the changing developmental status of the child influences the way in which they experience illness, and illness, in turn, influences the child's development. Chronic illness can delay development, but the life experience it brings may also make a child seem old beyond their years.

The child's developmental level will influence all aspects of palliative care, but the following issues are worth highlighting:
- Communication of wishes, fears and symptoms
- Understanding of illness and death
- Assessment of symptoms
- Management of symptoms
- Decision-making
- Importance of play as a means of understanding the world
- Importance of kindergarten and school

Approach to consultation

Developmental level and cognitive ability will vary widely and are not necessarily related to age, so an appraisal of the child's level of understanding will need to be made early in the consultation. While not unique to the paediatric setting, the child and family's previous experience with medical procedures and staff will strongly influence their attitude to professionals. Honest communication and the development of trust early in the course of the illness will provide a solid foundation on which to face the challenges of palliative care. Conversely, long-term intense treatment involving repeated hospitalization and painful procedures may make a child wary of health professionals. Therefore, consultation and communication style need to be highly flexible and adapted to each individual child and their family. A great deal of patience may be required.

Physiology/pharmacokinetics

These change as the child grows and develops. Neonates have a higher relative volume of distribution and lower clearance than adults, so the half-life of many drugs is prolonged. Conversely, infants and young children may metabolize certain drugs more quickly than adults. Children over six months of age, for example, may need higher doses of morphine than expected for their size.

Differences in family structure and function

Parents are socially and biologically invested with the responsibility of caring for and protecting their child. Consequently, the development of a fatal illness in the child leads many parents to feel they have failed in this important role. Denial is a common reaction and, despite advice to the contrary, parents may feel compelled to try everything and do anything to find a cure. This can be a difficult time for the child, the family and the staff caring for them. Staff may feel the child is being subjected to overly burdensome treatment and may also worry that the child is unable to talk about the reality of what is happening. Maintaining hope and a supportive presence while advocating strongly for the child's needs are important elements in managing such situations. A 'hope for the best, prepare for the worst' approach is often helpful.

Whilst the management of the patient is foremost, involving the family in decisions and information sharing is extremely important. Families will often have a great deal of knowledge about their child's medical condition and, in the case of a child with a rare disease, often know more about it than some professionals. In addition, many parents will have already been heavily involved in treatment decisions, and will expect this level of involvement to continue.

The structure of families in the UK may now include the natural parents, step-parents, partners, foster parents and siblings not directly related to the child. Organizing effective communication amongst these groups is sometimes challenging but is extremely important, particularly towards the end of life.

Siblings require special consideration in paediatric palliative care. They are almost universally distressed, but often feel unable to share this with their parents. Negative outcomes such as developmental regression, school failure and behavioural problems may be seen if the needs of siblings are not adequately addressed (see Chapter 17).

School

The centre of a child's day-to-day life is school, and any disruption of this routine can add to a child's sense of isolation and substantiate their feelings of being 'different' from their friends. Peer groups can be an enormous source of support for a child living with a life-limiting disease. For these reasons children often remain in school during treatment and even as death approaches. Keeping schools informed (with the permission of the parents/child) is important so that practical arrangements regarding the support required in school and flexibility of school hours can be discussed.

Medical staff can facilitate school attendance by scheduling elective and semi-elective treatments appropriately. For example, the child with bone marrow suppression who really wants to be at school for art on Tuesdays might benefit from having their regular blood transfusion on Monday. As death approaches, the school staff may need support. A plan for supporting staff and pupils through bereavement may also be helpful.

Illness trajectory

This will vary with the particular diagnosis. Often the palliative phase of care in children is much longer than for adults. Indeed, it may even extend from the time of diagnosis. There is also commonly a great deal of uncertainty surrounding the prognosis. Children in advanced states of disability and dependence are at high risk of dying from complications like respiratory infections but also have the potential to live many years. Families can find this extremely difficult to cope with, and they may experience negative thoughts and feelings about their situation and about their child.

Physical and emotional exhaustion, as well as concern for the child's suffering, may see them wishing it would all be over. Parents often feel alone with these thoughts, believing they are too terrible to share. The protracted nature of many illness trajectories presents challenges in planning support for the child and their family in terms of both symptom management and psychological support.

Ethical issues in paediatric palliative care

Medical ethics involves the application of ethical principles to medical practice and research.

As in adult palliative care, the most widely used framework for ethical decision-making involves the process of balancing four key principles:

1 **Autonomy**—the right to self-determination
2 **Non-maleficence**—the need to avoid harm
3 **Beneficence**—the ability to do good
4 **Justice**

In palliative care most dilemmas relate to end-of-life situations. In paediatric palliative care the inability of the child to act autonomously adds an extra dimension to the decision-making process.

Autonomy

- In order to act autonomously, one must act with intention and understanding and without controlling influences
- To act autonomously, individuals must demonstrate an understanding of their situation and the implications of their decisions
- They must also be able to communicate their decisions

Children represent a continuum in this regard, from the non-verbal infant to the adolescent striving for self-determination. Thus, a child's ability to make informed choices depends on his/her developmental level and life experience. For example, an eight-year-old child with a chronic illness may, through his/her own experience, and those of fellow patients be better positioned to participate in decision-making than an older child with no previous medical history.

Children may be able to make some decisions about their medical care even where major decisions are made by others. They may, for example, make choices regarding pain control and venepuncture sites. Empowering children in this way gives them a sense of control that impacts positively on their experience of care. Furthermore, even if not deemed sufficiently competent to act autonomously, a child's preferences and insights may guide decision-making by others and should be sought actively.

Decision-making in the palliative care setting requires:

- The ability to understand one's illness in physiological terms and to conceptualize death as an irreversible phenomenon
- The capacity to reason and consider future implications (formal operations stage of cognitive development)
- The ability to act autonomously and not acquiesce to the authority of doctors and parents.[3]

---

3 Leikin S. (1989) A proposal concerning decisions to forgo life-sustaining treatment for young people. *Journal of Pediatrics*, **115**: 17–22.

The Royal College of Paediatrics and Child Health (UK) describes four levels of child involvement in decision-making:
1 Being informed
2 Being consulted
3 Having views taken into account in decision-making
4 Being respected as the main decision-maker[4]

Age is not necessarily a good measure of capacity although an arbitrary distinction is drawn for legal purposes

Competence

Even young children have the right to be informed regarding decisions which affect their future. Both the Royal College of Paediatrics and Child Health and the American Academy of Pediatrics advocate strongly for the participation of children in decision-making to the extent that their ability allows.

Competence is assessed according to:
- Cognitive ability. This may be reflected in young patients' ability to provide a clinical history as well as their understanding of the condition, treatment options and the consequences of choosing one option over another. Other factors to consider include their level of schooling, verbal skills and demonstrated capacity to make decisions
- Presence or absence of disturbed thinking (e.g. in the setting of psychiatric disorder)

Treatment should be discussed with parents and child if appropriate, and ideally both will have an understanding of what is involved. Where this is not the case, providing more time for families to think about issues may help. In extreme circumstances a court of law can be asked to decide what is best.

Decision-making regarding life-sustaining treatment

Doctors, children and informed parents share the decision; with doctors taking the lead in judging the clinical factors and parents the lead in determining best interests more generally.[5]

Decisions are made on the grounds of benefit/burden proportionality. In order to justify a particular intervention, the expected benefits of that intervention must outweigh the burdens.

End-of-life decision-making is a collaborative process. It should involve the child (where possible), the family and all the health professionals involved in providing care to the child. An important underlying principle of the process is open communication between staff and families.

4 Royal College of Paediatrics and Child Health (1997) *Withholding or Withdrawing Life-Saving Treatment in Children: a framework for practice.* London: RCPCH.

5 British Medical Association (2001) *Withholding and Withdrawing Life-prolonging Medical Treatment. Guidance for Decision-making* (2nd edn). London: BMJ Books.

"Physicians should do more than offer a 'menu' of choices—they should recommend what they believe is the best option for the patient under the circumstances and give any reasons, based on medical, experiential, or moral factors, for such judgements.[6]"

The Royal College of Paediatrics and Child Health (RCPCH) outlines five circumstances under which withholding or withdrawing curative medical treatment may be considered:

- The child has been diagnosed as brain dead according to standard criteria
- Permanent vegetative state. These children have 'a permanent and irreversible lack of awareness of themselves and their surroundings and no ability to interact at any level with those around them'[6]
- 'No chance situation': life-sustaining treatment simply delays death without providing other benefits in terms of relief of suffering
- 'No purpose' situation: the child may be able to survive with treatment but the degree of mental or physical impairment would be so great that it would be unreasonable to ask the child to bear it
- The 'unbearable' situation. In the face of progressive, irreversible illness, the burden of further treatment is more than can be borne

A practical approach to decision-making[7]—questions to be answered

- Is this intervention going to cure the disease?
- Is this intervention going to prevent progression of the disease?
- What impact will the intervention have on the child's quality of life?
- Will the intervention improve the child's symptoms?
- Will the intervention make the child feel worse?
- How long will the child feel worse for?
- What will happen without the intervention?
- How will the intervention change the outcome?

Disagreement

Society invests parents with the responsibility of acting on behalf of their children. There are occasions however, where parents insist on what staff may view as inappropriate treatment. Conversely, parents may refuse treatment that is of potential benefit to the child. It is important that the best interests of the child are advocated for and that decision-making is shared between the family and the healthcare team.

Families often need time to absorb and process difficult information, and decision-making should be viewed as a process not an event. Most disagreements can usually be resolved by regular open and honest communication. Where conflict can not be resolved, it may be helpful to request a second opinion from an independent practitioner. It may also be beneficial to include other family members or cultural and religious leaders from the local community. In extreme circumstances where agreement can not be

6 American Academy of Paediatrics (1994) Guidelines on forgoing life-sustaining medical treatment. *Pediatrics*, **93**: 532–6.

7 Frager G. (1997) Palliative care and terminal care of children. *Child and Adolescent Psychiatric Clinics of North America*, **6**: 889–909.

reached despite the above interventions, it may be necessary to seek legal judgement.

Advance directives

Where children have an existing condition then a gradual or sudden deterioration may be anticipated. It is helpful for health professionals to assist families in planning for crises so that interventions considered unhelpful to the child are not initiated. Written documentation in the medical record as well as a letter for the family to have with them is required.

Advance directives should record:

- What has been discussed
- Who was present
- What decisions were made
- What the child and family's wishes are regarding various interventions
- Who should be called in case of a crisis

Provision of hydration and nutrition

- Food and fluid should always be offered if the child is able to take it by mouth
- Most authors consider the provision of nutrition and hydration by artificial means to be a medical intervention subject to the same assessment of benefits/burdens as any other
- The insertion of tubes into the gastrointestinal tract carries with it the burdens of discomfort and the potential for complications, and therefore needs to be justified on the grounds of the benefits it may provide to the patient
- Some argue, however, that the provision of food and fluid constitutes a basic component of humane care and can never be withdrawn or withheld
- In the paediatric setting, this concept is extended by the centrality of feeding to the parental role and the vulnerability of infants and small children
- Children in the terminal phase of illness will naturally cease eating and drinking as their requirements decrease, and it is not necessary in these circumstances to provide fluid and nutrition by artificial means

The situation faced by the family and staff is more problematic for children who have been kept alive for long periods prior to deterioration by gastrostomy or central venous feeding. Ethically there may be no difference between withdrawing treatment and not initiating potentially life saving treatment. Emotionally, however, it is often difficult for families not to feel guilty if they believe that by stopping artificial nutrition they are hastening their child's death. The effect of the provision or omission of artificial hydration and nutrition on the timing of death is uncertain. However, it is worth noting that dehydration may contribute to opioid toxicity, delirium and constipation and may require correction to alleviate these distressing clinical symptoms.

Medical ethics in different cultures

It is important to understand the limitations of Western ethics. The beliefs, values and conceptual frameworks used by other cultures must be considered when making decisions with families. The most appropriate source of information is the family itself, as there will be considerable variability within cultural groups.

Psychosocial needs in paediatric palliative care

Physical, emotional and spiritual needs cannot be addressed in isolation as each affects the other. For example, a child's pain can heighten parental anxiety and family distress may adversely affect pain control. A multi-disciplinary approach to palliative care is required and there is therefore the potential for a large number of individuals and services to become involved in the care of the child. Coordination of these professionals and the services each is providing is essential to avoid replication or omission, or disempowerment of the family. This can be achieved regular communication between team members and the appointment of a key worker for each child. This person may be a general practitioner, paediatrician, nurse or an allied health worker.

Providing emotional and psychological support for the sick child is as essential as providing relief of physical symptoms.

Communicating with children about death and dying

A child can live through anything so long as he or she is told the truth and is allowed to share with loved ones the natural feelings people have when they are suffering.

Herbert, 1996[8]

Parents may instinctively want to protect their children from 'bad news'. However, children very often know a great deal about their illness and prognosis. Children may not reveal what they know for fear of upsetting their parents, who then falsely assume their child knows very little. Children are very sensitive to discrepancies between verbal and non-verbal information. They readily sense distress in those around them and may feel anxious and isolated as a result. They may also generate fantasies to explain unusual behaviour in their parents (e.g. 'I have been bad', 'Mummy and Daddy don't love me any more'). These notions may be more frightening than death and dying to a young child. This is particularly true of younger children, who are naturally egocentric and believe that the world revolves around them, and hence, personalize other people's emotional and behavioural reactions.

• Parents' reluctance to talk to their child about dying usually stems from an erroneous belief that their child's concept of death is similar to that of an adult's, and their consequent desire to protect them from emotional pain

8 Herbert M. (1996) *Supporting Bereaved and Dying Children and their Parents.* Leicester: BPS Books.

- Younger children's greatest fear is usually around immobility and separation from loved ones during their illness and after. Opening up discussions about death can help allay these fears and provide the child with reassurance
- School-aged children frequently have worries about experiencing pain and can be greatly reassured by discussions about pain control.
  They may also ask questions about what will happen after their death, and can receive great comfort from religious or family beliefs.
- Just as parents and siblings need to plan the time they have left with the sick child in order to build memories and have as few regrets as possible, the dying child may also wish to prioritize the time left to do special activities or spend time with loved ones

Children very often ask staff questions about their illness and prognosis. When confronted by a difficult question, staff may be uncertain as to how best to respond. Questions often come unexpectedly, when the staff member is especially busy or distracted. Children generally know the answer to the question before they ask it. In this way the child who asks 'Am I dying?', may already know the answer. What they seek is a person who can be trusted to speak honestly with them. Responding with a question such as 'What makes you ask me that?' or 'What is it that makes you think you are going to die?' may elicit information on which to base a response. The real question may be something completely different. Of course children, just like adults, are very individual in how they respond, and while some children may ask plenty of questions and request lots of information, other children may wish to hear limited information. It is important to be guided by the child, and also to remind them that they can ask questions whenever they wish.

Supporting the sick child

These ideas mirror the supportive measures used in adult palliative care.

- Listen:
  - ask the child how he/she would like to be supported
  - find out exactly what it is the child wants to know
  - let the child set the pace
- Allow the child to make choices where possible
- Explain things in simple language appropriate to the child's development and cognitive ability
- Wherever possible answer questions honestly
- Answer the question that is being asked. Try not to burden the child with too much unsolicited information
- Children may find it easier to talk while drawing or doing some other activity. They may also find it helpful to talk in an abstract way, e.g. about a character in a story or during play with dolls
- Artwork, play, story writing, music and other creative activities may provide an outlet for emotion
- Normalize feelings of fear, anger and sadness
- Try not to dismiss a child's beliefs unless they are potentially damaging
- Model and encourage expression of emotion. Children need to know they can express their feelings without alienating those around them
- Provide physical contact and comfort
- Maintain routine to the greatest extent possible
- Involve the child's friends in visits. If this is not possible, encourage letters, photos, email, videos, etc. Discourage social isolation but do allow time for privacy

Recruit the child's school teacher to help—this may be helpful even where children are not able to attend school.[9]

9 Herbert M. (1996) *Supporting Bereaved and Dying Children and their Parents*. Leicester: BPS Books.

Supporting parents

Communicating difficult information to parents

The way in which difficult information is communicated is important and sets the stage for the working relationship between professionals and family. Health professionals need to be aware of how their own feelings of anxiety, sadness and impotence may influence this process. Most parents desire a realistic appraisal of their child's condition delivered empathically and with a sense of hope. Realistic hope can be offered in terms of ongoing support from the team, attention to symptoms and help to maximize the child's quality of life. In situations where the family is pursuing curative treatment, hope can be maintained by 'hoping for the best but preparing for the worst'.

How should difficult news be delivered?
- Empathically
- In person, face-to-face
- Allow plenty of time
- Establish what the parents know or suspect, e.g. 'How do you think things are going?'
- Allow the family to set the pace
- Respect silence and do not feel compelled to fill it
- Allow expression of emotion
- Avoid being evasive
- Offer to help inform other family members, for example siblings, grandparents
- Offer to meet again soon

What information should be given?
- Honest accurate information devoid of technical jargon
- Try to determine what the family wish to know, e.g. 'Are you the sort of person who likes to know everything or just the basic information?'
- Simple language—there will be time later to explore details
- Avoid ambiguous language such as 'We might lose the battle' or 'He's passed away'. The words 'death' or 'dying' should be used

A brief outline of the expected disease course should be given and expected symptoms mentioned. It may also be helpful for some families to understand what can be done for these symptoms. Many parents have not experienced the death of a relative or friend and may be frightened at the prospect of seeing someone die. Information about the bodily changes that accompany death may be helpful, and it is possible to be very reassuring about the process as, for most children who are managed carefully, it is very peaceful. Families may be worried about pain and distress or a final dramatic event. In most cases, however, the terminal phase is characterized by the progressive shut-down of the various organ systems.

Parental reaction to bad news

Parents are often so shocked on being told that their child is dying, even if this is confirmation of their own suspicions, that they can not assimilate any other information at that moment. It is important to slow the process down, provide multiple opportunities to speak with the family, repeat information where necessary and provide written information. Following the initial shock, parents may feel confused and overwhelmed. They may be frightened that they will not be able to cope with the child's physical care or be unable to control their emotions. Parents also experience feelings of uncertainty. They may have difficulty making sense of what is happening and are unsure of what to do first.

Denial occurs occasionally. For some parents it may be an adaptive defence and does not always need to be 'broken down'. In fact, great caution should be exercised in confronting denial. Where denial is impairing optimal care and family functioning, however, it may be helpful to gently challenge inconsistencies and explore underlying concerns. Asking a question like, 'Is there ever a time even for a few seconds where you worry things might not turn out the way you hope?', may provide a window of opportunity for the parent to work through the issues confronting them.

Anger may arise from fear and confusion, often as an expression of despair. Parents feel an enormous loss of power and control in their lives. Their sense of justice is rocked. The struggle to understand, make sense of the situation and control emotions can produce anger. This may be directed at staff. In managing angry parents, it is important:

- To acknowledge the anger, e.g. 'I can see you're very angry'
- Not to take it personally
- Not to be defensive
- To allow ventilation of the anger, 'Can you tell me more about what you're feeling?'
- Not to dismiss the complaint or try and explain the situation logically
- To set limits, 'I can see you are angry and I am willing to speak with you about it but I can not let you damage property/threaten me, etc.'

Guilt is another common reaction amongst parents of dying children. They may feel that they failed to recognize and respond effectively to the symptoms of the child's illness. They may feel responsible because the illness is inherited. They may experience 'survivor guilt', believing that children are not supposed to die before their parents. They may believe that their action or inaction somehow triggered the illness. Parents may externalize these feelings and blame others. Staff members occasionally find themselves unfairly blamed for a child's illness or death. This may feel hurtful, but it is important not to become defensive or allow this to impact on the care of the child. Any inclination to label the family as 'bad' should also be avoided.

What parents need to know

Explaining to parents that children often ask questions about their illness and prognosis provides a key opportunity for them to consider how they might deal with these themselves.

Planning in advance is helpful and a team approach, with parents forming part of the team, essential. Parents bring particular knowledge of their child as a unique individual. Staff bring knowledge of the literature in this area and experience with other families in similar circumstances.

Families need to know that:

- Children are generally more aware of their prognosis than those around them believe
- If a child does not ask questions or speak about his/her illness it does not mean that he/she is oblivious or indifferent. Children often protect parents by feigning ignorance—'mutual pretence'
- The anxiety generated by misinformation is potentially more harmful than any arising from the truth. Children may have all sorts of worries and fantasies, many of which an adult might not expect; e.g.: 'What will happen to the cat?', 'Will my school friends forget me?', 'Will somebody be with me?', 'Are mummy and daddy breaking up?', 'Are mummy and daddy cross with me?', 'Did I get sick because I was bad?', 'Will it hurt?' To a young child, abandonment and withdrawal of their parent's love may be more frightening than the notion of death because they have not yet acquired a full understanding of death. An environment of honesty provides the child with opportunities to share these worries. They need to feel they can trust those around them
- A dying child may be better able to cope with news of their impending death than their parents
- They are important role models. Children look to their parents for cues regarding the appropriate way of reacting to a given situation. While courage and calm will help reassure a child, it is also reasonable for parents to show their sadness. It is helpful for children to understand why their parents are upset so that they do not make incorrect assumptions. An honest explanation may be reassuring

In extreme cases where parents still insist that information is withheld but the child is clearly distressed by this approach, the health professional's duty is to the child.

While, in general, honesty is the best approach, it is important to recognize that not all children benefit from detailed information and not all parents feel able to communicate openly with their child. The best interests of the child are what is important. Cultural factors also require careful consideration.

Parents' needs and the role of the health professional

Information

Parents generally want information so that they know what to expect. They may also want to discuss treatment options and plans for symptom control. Parents say that full information allows them to make decisions and helps them plan for the remaining time they have with their child. In general, it is best to be open and honest as a trusting relationship between parents and healthcare workers provides a solid foundation for the challenges of palliative care. It is also helpful to regularly check that families are not being overwhelmed with too much information (e.g. 'I know this is a lot of information for you to hear all at once. We can talk in more detail a little bit later on if you would prefer').

Time to be listened to

Many parents want to discuss their situation with the many healthcare workers involved in their child's care. They may need to speak about their concerns, fears, hopes and expectations on numerous occasions to clarify and make sense of a world gone awry. The healthcare worker (whether it be a paediatrician, social worker or nurse) needs to provide time and opportunities for parents to share these concerns. By listening to the concerns of parents, providing guidance, affirming their skills and resources and staying with them, staff can make a major difference to how a family copes. It is important to remember that some parents do not wish to have such discussions and individual coping styles should be respected.

Control

Parents talk of losing control of their lives. The healthcare worker can assist parents to regain a sense of control by providing them with information, including them in discussions regarding care, allowing them to decide who is allowed to visit and when, and so on. Making decisions for (rather than with) a family can be deskilling and destructive. Parents need to be viewed as competent partners in their child's care.

Emotional support

Parents with a sick child grieve for the 'normal' child they no longer have. With this grief comes a range of strong feelings and emotions which add to the task of caring. Parents need acknowledgement, compassion, empathy and non-judgemental understanding. Spiritual support may or may not be part of a family's support system when their child becomes sick. The child's illness may cause parents to question their faith, renew their faith or explore new avenues. Spirituality includes, but is not restricted to, religion. Local clergy, ministers of all faiths and other spiritual leaders are available to help during this confusing time.

Amidst major changes to their routines and view of the world, the family may, however, try to hang on to some sense of normality. Health professionals can facilitate this by scheduling treatment around important activities and school attendance, and encouraging the family to maintain routines and activities.

Practical support

Parents need advice and guidance from various professionals in order to learn what is available to help them. Most parents would not know where to begin if they have had no previous experience. Therefore, liaison between the hospital and community team is a helpful step.

Medical equipment may be required as part of the child's care, either routinely or in an emergency. It is possible to have equipment items on loan from a hospital or community agency, e.g. a palliative care service. Health professionals including social workers, occupational therapists and physiotherapists may be needed to make assessments of the child's and family's needs.

Sibling needs

The needs of siblings are very similar to those of the dying child.[10]

Relationships within families and communication patterns are important factors in determining how siblings react to a brother or sister's illness. It may be easier for children to adapt to having a sick sibling in a family where it is usual to discuss matters openly and to share their feelings and emotions.

Physical symptoms may develop such as nausea, vomiting, diarrhoea, constipation, headache and aching limbs. Symptoms similar to those experienced by the sick sibling may also be reported. Behavioural changes may also occur, including unusual aggression, temper tantrums or withdrawal from family or friends, rudeness, bullying and demanding attention. Regression in the form of thumb-sucking, enuresis, toileting problems or school refusal may occur. Sleeping problems include a fear of the dark, nightmares, waking in the night and wanting to sleep in the parents' bed. Older children and adolescents may withdraw completely or indulge in risk-taking behaviour.

It is important to note that some siblings will experience none of the above.

Information

Parents should be encouraged to be honest with siblings and to provide them with information at a level appropriate to their developmental stage. This might include facts about the illness, what treatment is being given, and what to expect. They may need reassurance that they and their parents are not likely to become ill and that nothing they did or said caused the illness. Siblings may have concerns regarding their own health and if they are reporting symptoms may benefit from the reassurance of a thorough physical examination by their doctor.

Routine

Whilst difficult to maintain at a time of such upheaval, the familiar routines are important for a child's sense of security. This includes going to school, continuing with extracurricular activities and maintaining contact with his/her own peer group. Siblings may need to know that it is acceptable to have fun.

Emotional support

Siblings may try to protect their parents from added distress by not burdening them with their own worries. Many are known to suffer in silence. Unexpressed emotion may manifest as school failure, behavioural problems and physical symptoms. Siblings may also try to excel at school to 'cheer their parents up'. Feelings of resentment, jealousy, isolation, fear, guilt, anger and despair need to be explored, acknowledged and normalized. It is helpful if parents are able to dedicate special time to be with their well children. Some parents may need permission to do this as they feel guilty if they leave the sick child's side.

---

10 Goldman A. (1994) *Care of the Dying Child.* Oxford: Oxford University Press.

Contact with the sick child

Regular visits to the sick child in hospital allow siblings to see what is happening for themselves. It is important, however, that they are adequately prepared for what they might see, e.g. 'John is very sleepy. He might not be able to talk to you but he will know you are there. He has medicine running into his body through a tube in his…arm this doesn't hurt', etc. In the rare circumstance where siblings cannot visit, regular updates, videos and photos can be helpful. Siblings can feel included by sending drawings, favourite toys, photos and videos to their brother or sister.

Inclusion in the care of the sick child

Siblings may benefit from the opportunity to be included in the care of the sick child and in the family's experience. Children can help by taking a drink to the child, changing the channel on the TV, reading a story, playing games and taking the cat in to visit.

School

It is helpful if the sibling's school teachers are kept informed (with the family's permission) of the sick child's condition. Schools can also help by identifying one person to whom the sibling can go if they need help.

Community-based care

Most children who need palliative care will be looked after in, and by, their local community. It makes sense then that the community team is involved from early in the child's illness so that relationships are well established by the time the child's care needs increase. Resources available to families may include:

- General practitioner who will often know the child and family
- Community-based paediatrician
- Palliative care services
- Paediatric palliative care services
- Domiciliary nursing
- Respite
- Children's hospices
- Counselling
- Religious groups
- Family and friends
- Community agencies (which may offer family support and financial assistance)

Since children will often move between hospital and community settings, it is important that there is a collaborative approach to care and that communication flows easily and appropriately. The use of a key worker can facilitate such communication.

The nature of the care available in a particular situation will vary a great deal depending on the particular community services available. Services are changing rapidly and it is important to check on current service availability before planning community care. Non-evidence-based optimism or pessimism about the community service availability can cause much needless distress for the child and family.

Bereavement (📖 see Chapter 17)
Death and dying

- Most adult palliative care programmes become involved with patients towards the end of life
- In contrast, children's programmes aim to identify children close to the time of diagnosis and provide services and support to the family as they progress through the disease process and eventual death
- Most children and their families wish to spend as much time at home as possible, and many hope to be able to care for their child during the terminal phase provided adequate support is available
- Some families will find this task extremely difficult and will wish to return to a hospital or hospice environment close to the time of death
- This should not be viewed as a failure of home care

The dying process

Taken from *A Practical Guide to Paediatric Oncology Palliative Care*, Royal Children's Hospital, Brisbane, 1999.

The actual dying process is usually an orderly and undramatic progressive series of physical changes which are not medical emergencies requiring invasive interventions. Parents need to know that these physical changes are a normal part of the dying process. It is very important that families are well supported at this time. If the child is dying at home, 24-hour support from experienced staff who they know and trust can make an enormous difference. Home visits by the GP, domiciliary nurse and oncology liaison nurse, where appropriate, to assist with managing the child's symptoms, are greatly appreciated by the family. This is a very emotional and difficult time for the whole family.

Restlessness and agitation

Generally, the child will spend an increasing amount of time sleeping, in part due to progressive disease and changes in the body's metabolism, but this may also be due to progressive anaemia or sedation from opioids required for pain relief.

Some children remain alert and responsive until the moment of death. Others may become confused, semiconscious or unconscious for several hours or days. Restlessness and agitation during the terminal phase is not uncommon and may be due to increasing pain, hypoxia, nausea, fear and anxiety. Agitation may be the child's only way of communicating distress. A calm peaceful environment and the presence of parents and family will assist in relieving the child's anxiety. Speech may become increasingly difficult to understand and words confused. Even though the child may not be able to communicate, they may be aware of people around them. Hearing may well be the last sense to be lost and the family should be encouraged to talk to the dying child. They may like to play their child's favourite music, read stories or just sit with and touch their child so the child knows they are not alone.

If agitation continues then additional drugs may be needed (📖 see medication section 'Agitation' and 'Terminal restlessness', see pp. 568 and 644 for drugs and doses, respectively). Treatment is directed at inducing a degree of sedation appropriate for the individual child. At this stage oral medications may not be tolerated and alternative routes of medication are essential.

A continuous subcutaneous infusion of opioid, and, e.g. midazolam, in a syringe driver is effective in controlling pain, agitation and restlessness. For the child who is dying at home it is important that the treating hospital/hospice has dispensed (or made provision for the general practitioner to organize) a home care pack containing drugs that may be required during the terminal phase of care. This ensures drugs are available in the home if and when the child requires them. Without a home care pack there may be a considerable delay in getting those drugs required for symptom relief.

Doses of medication should be recorded for parents on a treatment sheet. Occasionally, haloperidol is required when the benzodiazepines are unsuccessful. Regular monitoring of effectiveness of medication is essential. Additional drugs can be added to the syringe driver if needed.

Noisy/rattly breathing

Excessive secretions or difficulty in clearing pharyngeal secretions will lead to noisy breathing. Generally this occurs during the terminal phase of the child's illness and is associated with a diminished conscious state. It can also be problematic for children with neurodegenerative diseases or brainstem lesions where swallowing is impaired. Positioning on the side or slightly head down will allow some postural drainage and this may be all that is required. Providing reassurance and explanation to the family is essential as the gurgling noise can be very distressing to the family, while the child is usually unaware and untroubled by the noise and sensation.

Anticholinergic drugs can be used to reduce the production of secretions, and a portable suction machine at home may be of benefit for children with chronic conditions or those who are unconscious (📖 see medication section 'Noisy breathing' for drugs and doses, p. 616).

Incontinence

There may be a relaxation of the muscles of the gastrointestinal and urinary tracts, resulting in incontinence of stool and urine. Therefore, it is important to discuss with parents this possibility and how they wish to manage incontinence. If the child is close to death parents are often reluctant for a catheter to be inserted to drain urine and may choose to use incontinence pads or disposable incontinence draw sheets. It is important for the family that their child's dignity is respected. Disposable draw sheets are also useful for incontinence diarrhoea.

Eye changes

The pupils of a dying person become fixed and dilated. The eyes may become sunken or bulging and glazed. Eye secretions can be removed with a warm damp cloth. If eyes are bulging, which can occur with neuroblastoma, the cornea should be protected and lubricated.

Circulatory and respiratory changes

As the heart slows and the heartbeat becomes irregular, circulation of blood to the extremities is decreased. The child's hands, feet and face may be cold, pale and cyanotic. The child may also sweat profusely and feel damp to touch. Parents may wish to change their child's clothes and keep them warm with a blanket. Respiration may be rapid, shallow and irregular, then may slow with periods of apnoea (Cheyne–Stokes breathing). This breathing pattern is distressing for parents and siblings to witness, and they need reassurance that it is a normal part of the dying process and that it is not distressing to the dying child.

It is important to inform parents that when death occurs the child may again be incontinent of urine and stool. There may also be ooze from the mouth and nose, particularly if they roll their child to undress and wash him/her. Parents who are not prepared will be distressed when this occurs.

In our efforts to achieve a peaceful death for the child, it is essential that symptoms are closely monitored and that there is ongoing assessment of the effectiveness of therapeutic interventions. Early detection of symptoms and appropriate intervention is crucial to achieve a pain-free and peaceful death for the child.

Staff support

The death of a child is a relatively unusual event, so that the modern paediatrician is more familiar with cure and prevention than with death and dying. While advances in medicine have led to happier outcomes for the majority of children, there remains a group for whom cure is impossible. The relative infrequency with which death occurs in childhood has implications for those caring for this group of children. Staff may feel a sense of failure and impotence. A lack of exposure to dying children may leave them feeling ill-equipped to support a child and family through this phase of their care. They may also have become very attached to the child and family and experience their own grief. All these responses are normal, but in the absence of adequate self-awareness and support, health professionals may, over time, become 'burnt out'.

Burn-out is 'the progressive loss of idealism, energy and purpose experienced by people in the helping professions as a result of the conditions of their work'.[11] This may manifest as excessive cynicism, a loss of interest in work and a sense of 'going through the motions'. Other features include fatigue, difficulty concentrating, depression, anxiety, insomnia, irritability and the inappropriate use of drugs or alcohol. The consequences for families are significant as staff affected in this way may:

11 Edelwich J., Brodsky A. (1980) *Burn-out: Stages of Disillusionment in the Helping Professions.* New York: Human Sciences PR.

- Avoid families or blame them for difficult situations
- Be unable to help families define treatment goals and make optimal decisions
- Experience physical signs of stress when seeing families

The quality of care may be compromised and families may become disenchanted with the health professional and seek help elsewhere, sometimes from inappropriate sources.

Risk factors

There are a number of risk factors for the development of behaviours and responses which may impact upon patient care and these can be categorized in the following way:

- Clinician-related:
  - identification with the family or situation
  - unresolved loss and grief in own past
  - fear of death and disability
  - psychiatric disorder
  - inability to tolerate uncertainty
- Family-related:
  - anger, depression
  - uncooperative families
  - family member is a health professional
  - complex or dysfunctional family dynamics
  - well known to staff (e.g. friends, relatives, colleagues)
  - intractable pain or difficult symptoms
- Situation-related:
  - family member/s are friends or relatives of the clinician
  - uncertainty/ambiguity
- Disagreement about goals of care:
  - patient/clinician
  - team
- Protracted hospitalization[12]

While it is common for health professionals to experience emotions such as anger and sadness in the course of clinical care,[13] it is important that these do not result in behaviours which could compromise the quality of that care. Recognition of the emotion helps control it to some extent as does accepting the normality of experiencing emotion. It may also be helpful to seek out a trusted colleague to whom you can talk.

12 Meier D. E., Back A. L., Morrison S. (2001) The inner life of physicians and care of the seriously ill. *Journal of the American Medical Association*, **286**: 3007–14.

13 Vachon M. L. S. (1995) Staff stress in hospice/palliative care: a review. *Palliative Medicine* **9**: 91–122.

Strategies for self-care

Stress amongst staff who provide palliative care for children, in any setting, is likely to be great, and the stresses involved in providing palliative care for children may affect the caregiver's ability to provide care in a sensitive and professional manner. Regular supervision and access to professional expertise by staff in areas where long-term relationships with patients and families are built up are important, and should ideally be written into job descriptions.[14]

There are a number of ways in which staff may be supported:

• Formal support through regular team meetings reduces conflict between staff members as long as open discussion is encouraged. This is dependent on the structure of the team and the quality of facilitation

• Formal support at an individual level is beneficial for some. It is particularly useful in circumstances where concerns can not be raised in the group context

• Informal peer support is generally regarded by staff as being most effective[15]

• Support from family and friends

• Maintaining perspective through involvement in outside activities. Formal supervision may assist in developing the self-awareness necessary to achieve this

• Education provides staff with the skills they require to overcome feelings of impotence. In a recent survey of resident medical officers in the United Kingdom, lack of training in the breaking of bad news was identified as a serious deficiency in their education[16]

The care of the dying child presents enormous challenges, but if done well has the potential to bring lasting benefits to both the family and the health professional.

---

14 Association for Children with Life-threatening or Terminal Conditions and their Families and the Royal College of Paediatrics and Child Health (2003) *A Guide to the Development of Children's Palliative Care Services* (2nd edn). Bristol: ACT.

15 Woolley H., Stein A., Forrest G. C., Baum J. D. (1989) Staff stress and job satisfaction at a children's hospice. *Archives of Disease in Childhood*, **64**: 114–18.

16 Dent A., Condon L., Blair P., Fleming P. (1996) A study of bereavement care after a sudden and unexpected death. *Archives of Disease in Childhood*, **74**: 522–6.

The Association for Children with Life Threatening or Terminal Conditions and their Families (ACT) Charter

The diverse needs of children have led to the development of a national association, ACT (Association for the Care of Children with Life-threatening or Terminal Conditions and their Families).

As a service to such children and families ACT has developed the following Charter.

- Every child shall be treated with dignity and respect and shall be afforded privacy whatever the child's physical or intellectual ability.
- Parents shall be acknowledged as the primary carers, and shall be centrally involved as partners in all care and decisions involving their child.
- Every child shall be given the opportunity to participate in decisions affecting his or her care, according to age and understanding
- Every family shall be given the opportunity of a consultation with a paediatric specialist who has a particular knowledge of the child's condition.
- Information shall be provided for the parents, and for the child and the siblings, according to age and understanding. The needs of other relatives shall also be addressed.
- An honest and open approach shall be the basis of all communication which shall be sensitive and appropriate to age and understanding.
- The family home shall remain the centre of caring whenever possible. All other care shall be provided by paediatric trained staff in a child-centred environment.
- Every child shall have access to education. Efforts shall be made to engage in other childhood activities.
- Every family shall be entitled to a named key worker who will enable the family to build up and maintain an appropriate support system.
- Every family shall have access to flexible respite care in their own home and in a home from home setting for the whole family, with appropriate paediatric nursing and medical support.
- Every family shall have access to expert, sensitive advice in procuring practical aids and financial support.
- Every family shall have access to paediatric nursing support in the home, when required.
- Every family shall have access to domestic help at times of stress at home.
- Bereavement support shall be offered to the whole family and be available for as long as required.

Drugs and doses

The following section is divided into the common symptoms experienced by very ill children and outlines a management strategy for each.

- Agitation
- Anorexia
- Bleeding
- Breathlessness
- Constipation
- Convulsions
- Cough
- Gastro-oesophageal reflux
- Gastrostomy care
- Hiccup
- Infection
- Mouthcare
- Muscle spasm
- Nausea and vomiting
- Noisy breathing
- Pain
- Other pain syndromes
- Psychological issues
- Raised intracranial pressure
- Skin
- Sleeplessness
- Sweating
- Terminal restlessness
- Ventilation at home
- **Emergency Drugs' Summary**

Introduction to drugs and doses

The approach to the care of a dying child and his/her family greatly influences the quality of their lives and the ability of the parents and siblings to cope with the child's death. Most symptoms are readily amenable to effective management. It is important, however, to adopt an individualized approach, taking into account the unique circumstances of each child and family.

Planning care

Medical assessment

- Make sure you are armed with as much information about the child and his family as possible
- Make sure you involve all the right people: this might include parents, siblings, grandparents and other carers. Whether you involve the child him/herself will depend on the child's age, understanding and state of health and the parents' wishes. It is often helpful to have another involved professional present, for example the district nurse in the community setting, so that someone else is fully aware of the discussion and can answer any questions the family might have after you have left
- Try and arrange things so that you are not in a hurry and are unlikely to be disturbed
- Be methodical: take a thorough history, and perform a full examination. Allow the child and parents time to voice their concerns as fully as possible

Explanations

- Explain symptoms and management options
- Identify any concerns the child or family may have and address these (e.g. concerns about the use of strong opioids)
- You may not have all the answers: if not, say so

Plans

- Identify, articulate and document the current goals of care
- Formulate a plan of action in consultation with the parents and/or child
- Listen to any concerns that arise from this and be prepared to compromise on a management plan if the parents/child want something different
- Ensure there is a plan for the exacerbation of current symptoms and the development of new ones. Knowledge of the child's condition will be important here and expertise may be required from sub-specialists
- Run over the plan at the end of the consultation in language the parents and/or the child can understand
- It may be helpful to write the plan down and give a copy to the family

Communication
- Families need access to advice and support around the clock: make sure family members/carers know how to contact professionals, particularly out of normal working hours
- Liaise with relevant professionals and carers—leave clear written instructions in medical records or contact the community team to discuss directly—many different healthcare professionals may be involved, particularly in the community, and it is important that everyone is aware of any changes in management
- A key worker, as advocated in the ACT charter, can be invaluable

Review
- Make a time/date when the management plan will be reviewed, and by whom

CHECKLIST
- Exploration
- Explanation
- Compromise
- Communication
- Review

Routes for drug administration
According to the bioavailability of the drug and patient preference, different routes of administration should be considered for each drug prescribed. These include:
- Oral
- Sublingual
- Buccal
- Nasal
- Intravenous
- Subcutaneous
- Transdermal
- Rectal
- Epidural/spinal

The syringe driver
A syringe driver is a small, portable, battery-driven infusion pump used to give continuous medication parenterally, usually over a 24h period. Syringe drivers can deliver medication intravenously (e.g. via a central venous catheter) or subcutaneously. This route of delivery is particularly suitable for children who are unable to tolerate oral medication or who require immediate control of difficult symptoms which are resistant to oral medication. Although it is a common route by which to administer medication at the end of life, it can also be used for short periods prior to this to gain control of difficult symptoms or when the oral route is impractical (e.g. persistent vomiting).

Indications for using a syringe driver

- Unable to swallow
- Unable to absorb oral medication (e.g. persistent vomiting, bowel obstruction)
- Refusing oral medication
- Unsatisfactory response to oral medication

Advantages of using this delivery system are:
- Continuous blood levels of medication
- Less requirement for needles
- Maintenance of independence
- The ability to deliver complex drug combinations safely

Providing they are compatible, combinations of drugs can be mixed together and given in the same syringe driver. In circumstances where high concentrations of drugs are required or the agents are unstable or incompatible, separate syringe drivers may be needed. As a general rule, it is advisable not to mix more than three drugs in any one syringe—check compatibility first.

A continuous infusion delivered via a patient controlled analgesia (PCA) system is an alternative to the syringe driver and has been used effectively in the postoperative setting by children as young as 7yrs. This device provides a background continuous infusion and allows the patient to administer bolus p.r.n. doses of analgesia by pressing a 'boost' button. The dose and number of p.r.n. doses available is preset and the device has a 'lockout' facility which prevents overdose.

Setting up a syringe driver (📖 see Chapter 4c)

Drug information

This document was written in July 2007. Whilst every effort has been made to ensure all information is accurate, it remains the responsibility of the prescriber to check this information against the most currently available data before administering any of the drugs in this document.

It is important to note that doses of the same medication may vary for different indications and this document should be consulted by symptom section rather than drug name.

Due to limitations of space, information regarding all side-effects and interactions for each drug are not included; further information regarding this should be sought from more detailed texts such as the *British National Formulary for Children*.

Many of the medications recommended in this text are not licensed for use in children, or for the indications, or via the routes suggested here. In 'general paediatrics' it is often necessary to prescribe medications 'off licence' and it is also very common in paediatric palliative care. In the UK, unlicensed use is permitted at the discretion of the prescriber, and is the prescriber's responsibility. The recommendations that follow are based on evidence where it is available as well as the experience of clinicians working in paediatric palliative care and pain management.

Agitation/delirium

Consider the following causes:
- Terminal restlessness
- Uncontrolled pain
- Medication (e.g. benzodiazepines, polypharmacy)
- Gastro-oesophageal reflux
- Urinary retention
- Constipation
- Dehydration
- Sepsis
- Cerebral causes: raised intracranial pressure, intracranial bleed
- Hypoxia
- Environmental irritation: too hot/cold/bright light
- Fear/anxiety
- Nausea
- Positioning

Terminal restlessness

Restlessness and agitation are not uncommon in the terminal phase of illness. Children with neurodegenerative conditions can become particularly agitated and, therefore, care needs to be taken to ensure that no remediable factors are missed. Families may need to be reassured that these symptoms are part of the dying process and, although difficult to witness, may not be causing distress to the child. (La See section on Terminal restlessness, p. 526.)

Uncontrolled pain

Take a careful history and fully examine the child before excluding pain. Remember common childhood causes such as toothache and otitis media. Children in chronic pain may not be as demonstrative as those in acute pain. Indeed, they may appear quiet and withdrawn. In children unable to communicate, ask the parents and carers how their child expresses pain. Look for facial expressions such as frowning and grimacing during examination and turning/mobilizing.

In the setting of uncontrolled pain, sedation does not address the underlying problem. Indeed, sedatives may render a child in pain unable to communicate this to those caring for them and therefore they should be used with caution.

Urinary retention

Children with neurodegenerative disease or those on opioids may have problems with retention of urine. Constipation may exacerbate this problem. Retention predisposes to urinary tract infection, which will add to the discomfort. If a urinary tract infection is suspected, consider sending an appropriate sample for analysis. Antibiotic treatment is likely to reduce any discomfort caused by infection. Retention may be relieved by gentle bladder massage or a warm bath. Bethanechol may also be helpful. Catheterization is only occasionally necessary and need not be permanent.

Constipation
Common causes include analgesia (particularly opioids), dehydration and immobility. Poor diet may be a contributory factor but may not be rectifiable. (☐ See section on Constipation, p. 584.)

Medication
Check drug chart for medications that may increase agitation.

Sepsis
Check temperature and examine for source of infection: wounds, Hickman lines and bladder are possible sites for consideration. Swab/send samples as appropriate, but first consider whether doing so will affect your management. Discuss whether treatment is appropriate/desirable with the child, their parents and other professionals involved. Sometimes treatment may be appropriate even in the terminal phase to control unpleasant symptoms. (☐ See section on Infection, p. 603.)

Cerebral causes
Raised intracranial pressure, intracranial bleeds. History and careful neurological examination may help with this diagnosis. Consider whether investigation is in the best interests of the child and whether it will influence management.

Hypoxia
Invasive tests should be avoided. Pulse oximetry may be helpful.

Environmental irritation
Too hot/cold, bright light.

Fear/anxiety
Discuss directly with the child if possible and appropriate. Children may have concerns that adults do not consider (e.g. they might be worried about pets or who is going to look after their parents). Explanations and reassurance are helpful if the child is able to identify and talk about what is worrying them. Children are often worried about being left alone, so make sure someone they trust is with them. Placing familiar objects near the child is also useful if they are not being nursed at home. Photos of family and friends, toys and stuffed animals are examples. Many children benefit from learning simple relaxation or guided imagery techniques. Anxiolytics may be necessary if other measures fail.

Nausea
Check the history and drug chart for likely causes and treat/adjust medication as appropriate. (☐ See section on Nausea p. 610)

Gastro-oesophageal reflux/indigestion
Common in very disabled children. They can also be a possibility in children taking steroids or undergoing chemotherapy/radiotherapy. (☐ See section on Gastro-oesophageal reflux, p. 598.)

Positioning
The child may simply not be comfortable, and this may be frustrating for a child unable to turn him/herself. It may be worth adjusting the child's position if you suspect this may be a problem. Aids and equipment should be checked to ensure they are not contributing to discomfort.

Delirium

Is characterized by:
- Disturbed consciousness and impaired attention
- Cognitive disturbances such as disorientation and memory impairment
- An acute or subacute onset and fluctuation throughout the day

Often there is a prodrome in the form of restlessness, sleep disturbance, irritability and anxiety. Early recognition and treatment are important.

Management

General measures

- Treat any reversible cause if possible and appropriate (make sure the child is not in pain)
- Nurse the child in a quiet and safe environment surrounded by familiar people and objects
- If other measures are unsuccessful, pharmacological intervention may be necessary
- Benzodiazepines are the most commonly used medication in this setting
- Many children with neurological disease will have been on benzodiazepines for muscle spasm or seizures, and will therefore need and tolerate higher doses
- Benzodiazepines are generally very effective, but occasionally a paradoxical increase in irritability may be seen
- Haloperidol is less frequently used but may also be helpful, and is not too sedating. It may cause extrapyramidal side-effects at higher doses
- Families may need to understand that the child may not be as responsive once medication is given, but that the priority is the child's comfort

Medication

The choice of medication will depend on the circumstance for which it is being prescribed, duration of action required and the location of care. Children experiencing brief periods of anxiety or panic attacks may benefit from a benzodiazepine that has a short half-life, such as midazolam or lorazepam. Children needing a longer duration of action may do better with diazepam or clonazepam.

In the community, lorazepam, midazolam and clonazepam may all be given via the buccal or sublingual routes and are easy for families to use. Levomepromazine may be an appropriate agent for children who also have nausea. Midazolam is the benzodiazepine of choice for use in a syringe driver. Both midazolam and levomepromazine are useful if deeper levels of sedation are required. Lorazepam or midazolam can be used in combination with haloperidol in severe agitation.

Lorazepam
- Short half-life
- Form:
  - tablets: 1mg (scored), 2.5mg
  - oral suspension: only available as 'special'
  - injection: 4mg/mL, 1mL ampoule
- Dose (sublingual, oral): all ages: 25–50 mcg/kg (max. 4mg/24h in adults)
- Injectable form can be given sublingually
- Most children will need no more than 0.5–1mg for a trial dose. Well absorbed sublingually (good for panic attacks) and parent/child has control
- **Contraindications and warnings**: severe pulmonary disease, sleep apnoea, coma, CNS depression. **Caution** in hepatic and renal failure
- Licence: tablets are licensed as premedication in children >5yrs. Injection not licensed in children <12yrs except for the treatment of status epilepticus

Clonazepam
- Long half-life
- Form:
  - drops: 2.5mg in 1mL (1 drop = 100mcg), named patient basis
  - tablets: 0.5mg and 2mg
  - oral liquid: 500 mcg in 5mL, 2mg in 5mL, 12.5mg in 5mL 'specials'
  - injection: 1mg/mL
- Dose (sublingual): all ages 10mcg/kg per dose (max 500mcg) bd/tds
- If necessary, increase by 10–25% every 2–3 days to max. 0.1–0.2mg/kg per day
- Prescribe as number of drops. Count drops onto a spoon before administering. Irritability and aggression are not uncommon, in which case the drug should be withdrawn
- Increased secretions may occur in infants and young children
- Licence: tablets and injections are licensed for use in children but not for this indication

Midazolam
- Intranasal route may be unpleasant but has a fast onset of action (5–15 minutes). Tastes bitter when given orally but can be mixed with juice or chocolate sauce
- Very short half-life
- Max. effect in 30–60min. Duration 2h
- Form:
  - injection: 1mg in 1mL, 50mL vial; 2mg in 1mL, 5mL amp; 5mg in 1mL, 2mL, 5mL and 10mL amps
  - injection may be given orally, sublingually, intranasally or rectally
  - oral liquid: 2.5mg in 1mL only available as 'special'
  - buccal liquid: 10mg/mL, 5mL, 25mL 'special'

- Single doses:
  - intravenous/subcutaneous: 1month–18yrs: 100mcg/kg
  - sublingual/buccal: >1month–18yrs: 500mcg/kg (max. 10mg)
  - intranasal: >1month–18yrs: 200–300mcg/kg (max. 10mg)
    NB: Important: drop dose into alternate nostrils over 15 seconds.
  - rectal: >1month–18yrs: 500–750 mcg/kg
- Continuous infusion: >1month–18yrs: start at 2.5mg/24h (**NB**: this is **not** a per kg dose)
- Titrate to effect. There is considerable inter-individual variability in the dose required and doses of up to 40mg/24h have been used in palliative care. If high doses are needed, consider trying a different agent
- **Contraindications, caution and warnings**: caution with pulmonary disease, hepatic and renal dysfunction (reduce dose), severe fluid/ electrolyte imbalance and congestive cardiac failure
- Avoid rapid withdrawal after prolonged treatment
- Licence: injection licensed for sedation in intensive care, for induction of anaesthesia and conscious sedation in children. Other routes and indications not licensed

Diazepam
- Long half-life
- Form:
  - tablets: 2mg, 5mg, 10mg
  - oral solution: 2mg in 5mL and 5mg in 5mL
  - injection (solution and emulsion): 5mg in 1mL
  - rectal tubes: 2mg in 1mL, 2.5mg tube, 5mg tube; 4mg in 1mL: 10mg tube
- Dose (oral):
  - 1 month–12yrs: 50–100mcg/kg per dose b.d.
  - >12yrs: 2.5–5mg b.d.
- Licence: rectal preparation is licensed for use in children >1yr with severe agitation. Other forms not licensed for agitation per se

Other medication
Haloperidol
- Form:
  - tablets: 500mcg, 1.5mg, 5mg, 10mg, 20mg
  - capsules: 500 mcg
  - oral liquid: 1mg in 1mL; 2mg in 1mL; 1mg in 5 mL; 5mg in 5mL, 10mg in 5mL 'specials
  - injection: 5mg in 1mL, 1mL ampoule; 10mg in 1mL, 1mL and 2mL amps
- Dose (oral):
  - 2–12yrs: 10–25 mcg/kg b.d. (max. 10mg/24h)
  - >12yrs: 250mcg–15mg b.d. (max. 30mg/24h)
- Dose (subcutaneous):
  - 2–12 yrs: 10–25 mcg/kg b.d.
  - >12 yrs: 0.25–5mg b.d
- **Contraindications and warnings**: bone marrow suppression, phaeochromocytoma
- Licence: injection not licensed for use in children

Levomepromazine
- Form:
  - tablets: 25mg, 6mg-named patient
  - injection: 25mg in 1mL, 1mL ampoule
- Dose: (SC/IV continuous infusion):
  - all ages: 0.35–3mg/kg per 24h then titrate to response (max. adult dose 200mg/24hrs)
- **Contraindications and warnings**: parkinsonism, postural hypotension, antihypertensive medication, epilepsy, hypothyroidism, myasthenia gravis
- May reduce seizure threshold
- Sedating, especially in SC doses exceeding 1mg/kg per 24h in children under 12 yrs or 25mg/24h in children over 12 yrs
- Can be used subcutaneously but may cause inflammation at injection site
- Licence: Licensed for this indication in children

Anorexia

Poor appetite and weight loss are common in children with terminal illness, particularly towards the end of life. This causes a great deal of anxiety amongst many parents and carers because:

- They may consider one of their main caring roles is to keep their child well-fed
- They often perceive eating as a road to recovery
- Acceptance that their child doesn't want to eat may go hand in hand with acceptance that the terminal phase is approaching

Consider reversible causes

- Oral candidiasis
- Pain (in mouth or elsewhere)
- Gastro-oesophogeal reflux
- Nausea/vomiting
- Constipation
- Medication

Management

General measures

- Explanation and discussion with the family may be helpful. Listen to parents' concerns and reassure as appropriate. It may be helpful for families to understand that as the child becomes less mobile and as the body winds down, the child's need for fluid and food diminishes
- Provide small meals on small plates. The child may prefer to snack through the day rather than sit down to a meal
- Make food less effort to eat (e.g. by providing mashed meals or wholesome soups, ice cream and rice pudding)
- Offer 'favourite' meals
- Offer supplementary high-calorie/high-protein drinks
- Try not to make an issue out of mealtimes
- Low-dose steroids will stimulate the appetite but will not change the course of the disease and may have harmful side-effects. They are almost never given for this indication

Bleeding

Management

General measures

- Consider a platelet transfusion if bleeding is problematic and related to low platelet count in a child with a reasonable prognosis where a transfusion would improve quality of life
- Unfortunately, there are few options for dealing effectively with large bleeds in the palliative stages, focus should instead be on anticipation and relief of anxiety and pain
- If bleeding is likely, explain this to the parents and prepare a management plan
- If a significant bleed is a possibility then benzodiazepines should be readily available (see below) and the use of dark towels and blankets may be helpful.

Medication

Bleeding gums

Use a soft toothbrush if possible. If not, avoid brushes altogether. Consider gentle regular antibacterial mouthwash to prevent secondary infection. Absorbable haemostatic agents such as Gelfoam may be useful.

Tranexamic acid

An antifibrinolytic agent that will help to stabilize blood clots and reduce oozing from the mouth and other mucosal surfaces. Commence treatment at the onset of bleeding and continue for 72h after bleeding has stopped.

- Form:
  - tablets: 500mg
  - liquid: 500mg in 5mL 'special'
  - injection: 100mg in 1mL, 5mL amp.
- Should read: Dose (mouthwash): use undiluted preparation for injection and apply to bleeding point or dilute preparation for infection 1:1 for oral use and mouthwash.
- Dose (mouthwash): use undiluted preparation for injection and apply to bleeding point or dilute preparation for injection 1:1 for oral use and mouthwash
- Dose (oral): 1month–18yrs: 25mg/kg t.d.s.
- **Caution**: reduce dose in renal failure; do not use in children with haematuria because of the risk of clot retention
- Licence: licensed for use in children

Small bleeds

Tranexamic acid
See oral dose above

Topical adrenaline
- Form: 1:1000 solution
- Small external bleeds: soak gauze, apply directly to bleeding point

Sorbsan dressing
- Haemostatic dressing: apply directly to the bleeding point

Vitamin K
Consider in liver dysfunction with coagulation abnormalities.
- Form:
  - tablets: 10mg
  - Konakion MM Paediatric: 10mg/mL, 0.2mL ampoule for oral, IM or IV use
  - Konakion MM: 10mg/mL, 1mL ampoule for IV injection or infusion only
- Dose (oral/IM/IV):
  - < 12 yrs: 300mcg/kg once (maximum 10mg)
  - >12 yrs: 10mg once
- **Caution**: reduce dose in liver impairment; reports of anaphylactoid reactions
- Licence: licensed for use in children for warfarin reversal

Vaginal bleeding
- May respond to oral progesterone

Catastrophic haemorrhage

An anxiolytic or sedative drug such as midazolam or diamorphine is useful, as a large haemorrhage is likely to be very frightening if the patient is conscious. If haemorrhage is likely then an anxiolytic in a suitable form (e.g. subcutaneous or buccal) should be readily available, and all carers/staff should be aware of how to administer it. A rapid onset of action may be desirable, so provision should be made for parenteral administration. For example:

Midazolam
- Form:
  - injection: 10mg in 2mL
- Dose (SC/IV stat):
  - 1–12 years: 0.05–0.1mg/kg as a single dose
  - >12 years: 2mg as a single dose
- Dose may need to be repeated

Terminal haemorrhage may not always be painful and the 'traditional' use of diamorphine in this instance may not be appropriate. However, some bleeds are undoubtedly painful and diamorphine should be available if this is a possibility.

Diamorphine
Dose (SC) stat:

Age	Dose
1–3 months	20mcg/kg
3–6 months	25–50mcg/kg
6–12 months	75mcg/kg
>12 months	75–100mcg/kg
12–18 yrs	2.5–5mg

Breathlessness

Dyspnoea, like pain, is a subjective symptom and may not correlate with objective signs.

Consider causes and treat reversible factors as appropriate:

- Anaemia
- Airway obstruction
- Anxiety
- Ascites causing elevated diaphragm
- Bronchospasm
- Cerebral tumours
- Chest pain (musculoskeletal or pleuritic)
- Congenital heart disease
- Cystic fibrosis
- Infection
- Metabolic disorders, including uraemia
- Raised intracranial pressure
- Respiratory muscle dysfunction, e.g. neurodegenerative disorders
- Primary or secondary tumours within lung fields or abdomen causing elevated diaphragm.
- Pleural effusion/pneumothorax*/haemothorax
- Pulmonary fibrosis
- Superior vena cava (SVC) obstruction*
- Increased secretions
- Pulmonary oedema
- Pulmonary embolism*
- Pericardial effusion*

*These are **medical emergencies** that may require specialist intervention. Swift treatment of these conditions can significantly reduce symptoms.

Management

General measures

- Anxiety is likely to be an associated feature. Try reassurance, relaxation techniques, distraction and anxiolytics where necessary
- Provide a flow of fresh air—fan/window
- Try not to overcrowd the room
- Optimize position
- Excess secretions may respond to gentle physiotherapy and suction

Oxygen

May be helpful in hypoxic patients but is not without consequences (e.g. wearing a mask can be uncomfortable and interfere with the ability of the child to be close to parents and carers. Equipment can also compromise mobility). The benefits of this intervention need to outweigh the burdens.

Children often refuse masks but may tolerate nasal specs. Consider humidifying oxygen which will dry the mouth less.

Caution is needed in circumstances where chronic hypercapnia has left the child dependent on hypoxic respiratory drive. Too much oxygen will result in hypoventilation, so titrate carefully.

Medication
The choice of medication will depend on the underlying cause. Bronchospasm will respond to a bronchodilator. Anxiety that is unresponsive to reassurance, distraction or relaxation techniques may require treatment with a benzodiazepine. Excessive secretions may respond to physiotherapy and/or mucolytic agents. Opioids, however, are generally very effective.

Bronchodilators
Salbutamol
May be helpful if bronchospasm present. Salbutamol may exacerbate anxiety.
- Form:
  - nebulized solution: 2.5mg in 2.5mL; 5mg in 2.5mL
  - inhaled form: 100mcg/dose
- Dose (nebulized):
  - 6 months–5yrs: 2.5mg t.d.s./q.d.s.
  - 5–12yrs: 2.5–5mg t.d.s./q.d.s.
  - >12 yrs: 5mg t.d.s./q.d.s.
- Dose (inhaled):
  - all ages: 1–2 puffs, 4–6 times a day (a spacer device should be used to improve delivery)

There is some evidence that small babies do not respond to salbutamol because of receptor immaturity and it is advisable to use ipratropium first in those aged <1yr.
- Licence: licensed for use in children

Ipratropium
May be helpful if bronchospasm present.
- Form:
  - nebulized solution: 250mcg in 1mL, 500mcg in 2mL
  - inhaled form: 20mcg/dose and 40mcg/dose
- Dose (nebulized):
  - <5 yrs: 125–250mcg t.d.s.–q.d.s. (max 1mg/24h)
  - 5–12yrs: 250mcg t.d.s.–q.d.s. (max 1mg/24h)
  - >12yrs: 500mcg t.d.s.–q.d.s.
- Dose (inhaled):
  - <5yrs: 125–250mcg/dose t.d.s.–q.d.s. Max 1 mg daily
  - 6–12yrs: 250mcg/dose t.d.s.–q.d.s. Max 1mg daily
- Licence: licensed for use in children

Morphine
Effective in treating dyspnoea, although there may be no measurable effect on respiratory rate or oximetry. Morphine reduces anxiety, pain and pulmonary artery pressure. Begin with half the paediatric analgesic dose and titrate to effect (☐ See section on Pain, p. 618).

Benzodiazepines
Many children will be frightened by dyspnoea. Benzodiazepines may be helpful in addition to relaxation techniques and guided imagery. The choice of ben-

zodiazepine will depend on the circumstance for which it is being prescribed. Children experiencing brief periods of anxiety or panic attacks in association with dyspnoea may benefit from a benzodiazepine with a very short half-life, such as midazolam, given buccally or subcutaneously. Sublingual lorazepam is another option for panic attacks or anxiety related to dyspnoea. Children needing a longer duration of action may do better with diazepam, clonazepam or a subcutaneous midazolam infusion.

Diazepam
- Form:
  - tablets: 2mg, 5mg, 10mg
  - oral solution: 2mg in 5mL and 5mg in 5mL
  - injection (solution and emulsion): 5mg in 1mL
  - rectal tubes: 2mg in 1mL: 2.5mg tube, 5mg tube; 4mg in 1mL: 10mg tube
- Dose (oral):
  - 1 month–1 yr: 50mcg/kg b.d.
  - 1–4yrs: 500mcg-3mg b.d.
  - 5–12 yrs: 1.5-10mg b.d.
  - >12 yrs: 2-10mg b.d.
- **Contraindications and warnings**: acute porphyria. Potential for dependency. Can affect respiration if given IV or rectally
- Licence: not licensed for this indication in children

Lorazepam
- Form:
  - tablets: 1mg (scored), 2.5mg
  - oral suspension only available as 'special'
  - injection: 4mg in 1mL, 1mL ampoule
- Dose (sublingual, oral):
  - all ages: 25–50mcg/kg (max. dose in adults 4mg/24h)
- Most children will not need more than 0.5–1mg for trial dose. Well absorbed sublingually (good for panic attacks) and child has control
- **Contraindications and warnings**: severe pulmonary disease, sleep apnoea, coma, CNS depression.
- **Caution** in hepatic and renal failure children >5 years
- Licence: tablets licensed as premedication in children >5 yrs. Injection not licensed in children <12yrs except for treatment of status epilepticus

Clonazepam
- Form:
  - drops: 2.5mg in 1mL (1 drop = 100mcg). Named patient basis
  - tablets: 0.5mg, 2mg
  - injection: 1mg in 1mL
  - oral liquid: 500 mcg in 5mL, 2mg in 5mL, 12.5mg in 5mL 'specials'

- Dose (sublingual):
  - all ages: 10mcg/kg per dose (max 500mcg bd/tds)
  - if necessary, increase by 10–25% every 2–3 days to max: 100mcg/kg/day
- Long half-life
- Prescribe as number of drops. Count drops onto spoon before administering
- Irritability and aggression not uncommon, in which case the drug should be withdrawn. Increased secretions may occur in infants and young children
- Offers the advantage of sublingual absorption and droplet administration
- Licence: tablets and injections licensed for use in children but not for this indication

Midazolam

Intranasal route may be unpleasant but has a fast onset of action (5–15 minutes). Tastes bitter when given orally but can be mixed with juice or chocolate sauce.

- Max. effect in 30–60min. Duration 2h
- Form:
  - injection: 1mg in 1mL, 50mL vial; 2mg in 1mL, 5mL amp; 5mg/in 1mL, 2mL, 5mL, 10mL amps
  - injection may be given orally, sublingually, intranasally or rectally
  - oral syrup only available as 'special': 2.5mg/mL
  - buccal liquid: 10mg/mL, 5mL; 25mL 'special'
- *Single doses*:
  - intravenous/subcutaneous: >1month–18yrs: 100mcg/kg
  - sublingual/buccal: >1month–18yrs: 500mcg/kg (max. 10mg)
  - intranasal: >1month–18yrs: 200–300mcg/kg (max 10mg).
    NB: Important: drop dose into alternate nostrils over 15 seconds.
  - rectal: >1month–18yrs: 500–750 mcg/kg
- *Continuous IV/SC infusion*: >1month–18yrs: start at 2.5mg/24h (**NB**: this is **not** a per kg dose)
- Titrate to effect. There is considerable inter-individual variability in the dose required and doses of up to 40mg/24h have been used in palliative care. If high doses are needed, consider trying a different agent
- **Contraindications and warnings**: caution with pulmonary disease, hepatic and renal dysfunction (reduce dose), severe fluid/electrolyte imbalance and congestive cardiac failure. Avoid rapid withdrawal after prolonged treatment
- Licence: injection licensed for sedation in intensive care, induction of anaesthesia and conscious sedation in children. Other routes and indications not licensed

Dexamethasone

May be helpful in circumstances such as bronchospasm, bronchial obstruction, lymphangitis carcinomatosa, SVCO and raised intracranial pressure. Administration requires careful consideration as steroids may produce potentially distressing side-effects in children if given for more than a few days. To avoid this, it is preferable to prescribe short courses (3–5 days) of steroids. These can be repeated if necessary.

- Form:
  - tablets: 500mcg and 2mg
  - oral solution: 2mg in 5mL
  - injection: 4mg in 1mL, 1mL; can be given orally
- Dose (oral):
  - 1 month–18yrs: 100mcg/kg b.d.
- Dose (SC/IV)
  - can be given in as single doses or as a continuous infusion
- Higher doses may be needed in SVCO (consult paediatric oncologist)
- If no effect after 3–5 days, stop steroids (no need to tail off dose)
- Do not give after midday as steroids can affect night-time sleep
- Co-prescribing: consider antacids and anti-thrush treatment
- **Contraindications and warnings: caution** in renal disease, cardiac disease and cystic fibrosis. Avoid in cardiac insufficiency
- Licence: not licensed for this indication in children

Radiotherapy

In cases where dyspnoea is secondary to malignant chest disease, radiotherapy should be considered, although the burden of treatment needs to be weighed against the potential benefits. It is more likely to be beneficial if tumour bulk is close to the major airways rather than distal to them. Radiotherapy also has an important role in managing breathlessness secondary to SVC obstruction, carrying the added advantage of controlling haemoptysis—which even in small volumes can be upsetting for the child and family.

Constipation

Prophylaxis and early intervention are important in managing this distressing symptom. A laxative should always be considered when opioids are commenced.

- What are the child's usual bowel habits?—children vary a lot; what is constipation for one may be a normal pattern for another
- Has there been a change in the usual pattern?

Consider cause

- Inactivity
- Metabolic: dehydration; hypercalcaemia; hypokalaemia
- Cystic fibrosis
- Reduced oral intake
- Spinal cord/cauda equina compression
- Bowel obstruction
- Fear of pain on defaecation: secondary to hard stools, rectal/anal grazes and tears
- Drugs: opioids; anticholinergics; anticonvulsants; vincristine chemotherapy
- Social: shy about using toilets away from home, not knowing where the toilets are, etc. Liaise with parents

Management

General measures

- Check for bowel obstruction, faecal impaction and rectal/anal grazes/ tears (NB conduct a rectal examination only if absolutely necessary)
- Consider the underlying cause and address it if appropriate/possible
- Increase fluid intake where possible and appropriate
- If parenterally fed consider altering the feed
- Increase mobility if possible
- Optimize access to the toilet
- Encourage regular toileting, especially after meals
- Try oral medication first, then proceed to rectal preparations if necessary

Medication

Many children with non-malignant conditions will have been on laxatives for some time. Parents often know which laxatives are most effective for their child.

It is generally helpful to use a combination of a stimulant laxative (e.g. senna, bisacodyl, docusate or sodium picosulphate) and a softening agent (e.g. Movicol, magnesium hydroxide). Combined preparations are available (e.g. co-danthramer and co-danthrusate) for use in adult palliative care but are less frequently used in paediatrics. As second-line agents, prokinetic agents such as metoclopramide may be helpful. (See section on Nausea and vomiting, p. 610 for dose). Movicol (polyethylene glycol) is an iso-osmotic laxative, better tolerated than older osmotic laxatives and increasingly considered the laxative of choice in children. If constipation is morphine-related and resistant to the usual measures, it may be helpful to change to another opioid such as fentanyl.

Polyethylene glycol
Stool softener
- Form:
  - powder sachets
  - mix each sachet with approximately 60mL water or squash
- Dose (oral): (Movicol Paediatric Plain)
  - maintenance therapy in >2yrs: 1–2 sachets/day
  - in impaction/severe constipation

number of sachets/day	2–4yrs	5–11yrs
Day 1	2 sachets	4 sachets
Day 2	4 sachets	6 sachets
Day 3	4 sachets	8 sachets
Day 4	6 sachets	10 sachets
Day 5	6 sachets	12 sachets
Day 6	8 sachets	12 sachets
Day 7	8 sachets	12 sachets

- License: not licensed for faecal impaction in children <5yrs or for chronic constipation in children <2yrs

Bisacodyl
- Form:
  - tablets: 5mg
  - suppository: 5mg, 10mg
- Dose (oral/rectal):
  - give tablets at night, suppositories in the morning
  - 1 month–10yrs: 5mg o.d.
  - >10yrs: 10mg o.d.
  - higher doses may be necessary
- Acts in 12h orally, in 20–60 minutes rectally
- Stimulant laxative

Senna
- Form:
  - syrup: 7.5mg in 5mL
  - tablets: 7.5mg
  - granules: 15mg in 5mL
- Dose (oral):
  - <2yrs: syrup 0.5mL/kg o.d.
  - 2–6yrs: syrup 2.5–5mL o.d.
  - 6–12yrs: syrup 5–10mL or 1–2 tablets o.d.
  - >12yrs: syrup 10–20mL or 2–4 tablets o.d.
  - for granules use ½ the syrup dose
- Stimulant laxative
- Acts in 8–12h
- Often used in combination with lactulose
- Licence: Syrup licensed in children >2yrs, tablets not recommended in children <6yrs

Co-danthramer
- Form:
  - suspension: dantron 25mg/poloxamer 200mg in 5 mL; dantron 75mg/poloxamer 1g in 5 mL (Forte)
  - capsule: dantron 25mg/poloxamer 200mg; dantron 37.5mg/poloxamer 500mg (Forte)
- Dose (oral):
  - only for use in terminally ill children
  - <12yrs: 2.5–5mL of the 25/200mg strength suspension or 1–2 (25/200mg strength) capsules o.d.–b.d.
  - >12yrs: 5–10mL of the 25/200mg strength suspension or 1–2 (25/200mg strength) capsules o.d.–b.d., titrate as needed
- Combined stimulant (dantron)/softener (poloxamer) laxative
- Acts in 8–12h
- Makes urine red (inform carers)
- Can cause superficial burns in children who are incontinent and/or in nappies
- **Avoid** in acute respiratory depression, paralytic ileus, liver disease and moderate to severe renal impairment
- Licence: only licensed for use in terminally ill children

Docusate sodium
- Form:
  - elixir: 12.5mg in 5mL; 50mg in 5mL. Dilute with milk or orange juice
  - capsule: 100mg
  - enemas: Fletchers' Enemette: 90mg in 5mL; Norgalax microenema: 120mg in 10g
- Dose (oral):
  - 6 months–12yrs: 2.5mg/kg t.d.s.
  - >12yrs: 100mg t.d.s.
- Dose (rectal):
  - <3yrs: 2.5mL Fletchers' Enemette
  - >3yrs: 5mL Fletchers' Enemette
- Softener and stimulant
- Acts in 24–48h
- Licence: capsule not licensed for children. Norgalax enema licensed for children >12yrs. Fletchers Enemette licensed for children >3yrs

Lactulose
Lactulose is not very effective in opioid-induced constipation.
- Form:
  - solution: lactulose 3.1–3.7g/5ml with other ketoses
- Dose (oral):
  - <1yr: 2.5mL b.d.
  - 1–5yrs: 5mL b.d.
  - 5–10yrs: 10mL b.d.
  - >10yrs: 15mL b.d.
- Mild osmotic laxative, which is very sweet to taste and can cause bloating
- Acts in 48h
- May cause colic

- Titrate dose up as required
- Can be disguised in fruit juice, milk or water
- Licence: Licensed for use in children

Magnesium hydroxide
Stool softener
- Form:
  - liquid: 415mg in 5mL
- Dose (oral):
  - <3yrs not recommended
  - >3yrs 5–10mL nocte (adult 30–45mL nocte)

Sodium picosulfate
- Form:
  - sachet: 10mg sachets contain sodium picosulfate 10mg + magnesium citrate powder
  - sodium picosulfate liquid: 5mg in 5mL
- Dose (oral) sachet:
  - 1–2yrs: ¼ sachet o.d.
  - 2–4yrs: ½ sachet o.d.
  - 4–9yrs: ½–1sachet o.d.
  - >9yrs: 1 sachet o.d.
- Dose (oral) liquid:
  - 2–5yrs: 2.5mL nocte
  - 5–10yrs: 2.5–5mL nocte
  - >10yrs: 5–15mL nocte
- Effective within 2–3 h
- Drink plenty of water before and after administration
- **Warning**: can cause dehydration and electrolyte disturbance
- **Caution** in children with impaired renal or cardiac function
  Licence: Licensed for use in children >1yr

Arachis oil enema
- Form:
  - enema 130mL arachis oil BP
- Dose (rectal):
  - 3–7yrs: {1/3}–½ of the enema
  - 7–12yrs: ½–¾ of the enema
  - >12yrs: ¾–1 of the enema
- Use as required
- Faecal softener
- **Contraindications and warnings**: hypersensitivity to arachis oil or peanuts.
- Licence: licensed for children >3 yrs

Sodium citrate enema
- Form:
  - micro-enema 450mg sodium citrate/75mg sodium laurylsulphate/5mg sorbic acid in 5mL (Relaxit). Other combinations available, but not licensed for children under 3yrs

- Dose (rectal):
  - 1 enema (when using in children <3yrs insert only half nozzle length)
- Osmotic laxative
- Licence: licensed for children >3 yrs

Phosphate enema
- Form:
  - enema sodium acid phosphate 21.4g/sodium phosphate 9.4g in 118mL (Fleet)
  - other combinations available
- Dose (rectal):
  - 3–7yrs: $\frac{1}{3}$ –$\frac{1}{2}$ enema
  - 7–12yrs: $\frac{1}{2}$–$\frac{3}{4}$ enema
  - >12yrs: $\frac{3}{4}$–1 enema
- Osmotic laxative
- Licence: licensed for children >3 yrs

Convulsions

Convulsions are most commonly seen in the palliative care setting in children with neurodegenerative disorders or intracranial malignancies.

Children with neurodegenerative disorders will often already be on multiple anticonvulsant medications and their parents/carers will be knowledgeable about recognizing and treating fits. For these children fits are often variable in type and may become frequent, severe and more difficult to control towards the end of life.

Children with intracranial malignancy will not necessarily develop fits. However, for those who do, it is a frightening new symptom for the child and carers to learn how to manage. If fits are likely then prophylactic anticonvulsants should be considered and parents warned about what to expect. They should be given a clear plan of what to do in the event of a convulsion. The mainstay of medical treatment, a benzodiazepine (lorazepam, midazolam or diazepam), should be readily available with clear instructions as to how and when it should be administered.

Not all fits are grand mal: more subtle behaviours (e.g. grimacing or coughing) may also represent seizure activity. These may not require treatment if they are not troubling the child.

Investigation and treatment of persistent fitting should be tailored to the child's stage of illness and discussion will be required with the appropriate medical teams and the family.

Consider causes and treat as appropriate

The emergence, or increasing frequency/severity, of fits may be caused by worsening disease, but other potentially reversible factors should be considered:

- Hypoglycaemia
- Electrolyte imbalance
- Sub-therapeutic anticonvulsant medication
- Infection, e.g. UTI
- Raised intracranial pressure/other intracranial pathology

Management

- Not all fits require treatment
- Where treatment is required, the choice of anticonvulsant depends on the type of fit. Advice from the paediatric unit where the child is being managed should be sought
- Single agent therapy is ideal. Where children are already on multiple medications, reducing the number of different anticonvulsants may improve seizure control
- Withdrawal or addition of anticonvulsants should be done cautiously as most agents need to be tailed off or titrated down
- Relatively higher doses of anticonvulsants are required for children <3yrs because of a higher metabolic rate and more efficient drug clearance
- In difficult cases a SC infusion of midazolam or phenobarbital may be used to enable a child to stay at home. Clonazepam can be used as an alternative to midazolam

The management of seizures will depend on the goals of care at the time. A child who is enjoying a reasonable quality of life and is in the early stages of a life-limiting illness should be treated as any other. Children in the terminal phase of illness should be kept comfortable, and this will include reasonable efforts to abort the seizure.

Acute management of a fit
- Place the child on his side in a place where he cannot fall or be injured
- If the fit lasts longer than 5min, prepare to give rectal diazepam (avoid the SC or IM routes where possible) or sublingual/intranasal lorazepam or midazolam

Medication
Diazepam
- Dose (rectal):
  - <1 month: 1.25–2.5mg
  - 1 month–2 yrs: 5mg
  - 2–12 yrs: 5–10mg
  - >12 yrs: 12mg
- If the fit shows no signs of abating once the diazepam has been fetched and prepared, give the required dose
- Wait five minutes
- If the fit continues, the dose may be repeated
- If the fit continues after two doses of rectal diazepam, phenytoin, phenobarbital or rectal paraldehyde will be required

Alternative medication
Midazolam
- Dose (buccal):
  - 0–6 months: 300mcg/kg
  - 6 months–5 yrs: 2.5mg
  - 5–10 yrs: 7.5mg
  - 10–18 yrs: 10mg
- Dose (intranasal):
  - 200–300mcg/kg (dropped into alternate nostrils over 15 seconds). (Max. 10mg)

Clonazepam
- Form:
  - Drops: 2.5mg in 1mL (1 drop = 100mcg). Only available as named patient
- Dose (sublingual):
  - all ages: 10mcg/kg per dose (max 500mcg)
- Prescribe as number of drops. Count drops onto spoon before administering
- Titrate up according to response
- Irritability and aggression are not uncommon, in which case the drug should be withdrawn. Increased secretions may occur in infants and young children

Lorazepam
- Dose (sublingual) 100mcg/kg single dose
- Dose may be repeated after 10 minutes if convulsion continues

Maintenance treatment

Medications used for emergency management of seizures do not have a prolonged effect, and if fitting is likely to be an ongoing problem, maintenance treatment is indicated. In most cases management is straightforward and successful. For the minority, fits are persistent and difficult to control, but even the most persistent fits can usually be controlled in the home environment provided there is good multi-disciplinary support. The administration of antiepileptics for children with no oral route (or other enteral route such as a PEG) becomes more of a challenge. If a permanent intravenous route is available then phenytoin can be administered via this route. Carbamazepine can be given rectally. Other alternatives are phenobarbital, midazolam and clonazepam which can all be given by subcutaneous infusion, but they are relatively sedative compared to the other medications mentioned. Rectal paraldehyde may also be helpful.

Provision should be made for breakthrough seizures, which may be managed with rectal diazepam, buccal intranasal or subcutaneous midazolam, or rectal paraldehyde.

Clonazepam
- Form:
  - injection: 1mg in 1mL
- Dose (IV bolus over 30 seconds)
  - 50mcg/kg (max 1mg)
- Dose (continuous IV or SC infusion):
  - start at 10mcg/kg per 24h and titrate to effect. Doses up to 60mcg/kg have been used

Midazolam
- Form:
  - injection: 1mg in 1mL, 50mL vial; 2mg in 1mL, 5mL amp; 5mg in 1mL, 2mL, 5mL, 10mL amps
  - injection may be used for oral, sublingual, rectal and intranasal routes
- Starting dose (continuous IV or SC infusion):
  - <5kg: 1mcg/kg/min (max 5mcg)
  - >5kg: 5mg/24h and titrate to effect

Phenobarbital
Can be given orally or as a continuous subcutaneous infusion and has anticonvulsant and anxiolytic properties.
- Form:
  - injection 60mg in 1mL. 200mg in 1mL available as 'special'
- Dose (IV loading dose):
  - >1 month: 15mg/kg over 5 minutes. Single dose or loading dose, no faster than 1mg/kg per min

- Maintenance dose (IV/SC continuous infusion or as oral doses):
  - commence 24h after loading dose
  - 1 month–12yrs: 5–10mg/kg per 24h
  - >12yrs: 600mg/24h
- Review dose after one week as drug induces its own metabolism
- Requires separate syringe driver (does not mix)

Paraldehyde
- Form:
  - injection 100% (5mL ampoule)
  - also available as already diluted 'special'
- Dose (rectal):
  - 1–3 months: 0.5mL single dose
  - 3–6 months: 1mL single dose
  - 6 months–1year: 1.5mL single dose
  - 1–2years: 2mL single dose
  - 2–5years: 3–4mL single dose
  - 5–18years: 5–10mL single dose
  - Dilute twofold with olive oil or sunflower oil or dilute 1:10 with 0.9% sodium chloride
- Incompatible with most plastics so use immediately
- Do not give intramuscularly
- Licence: not licensed for use in children

Cough

Coughing can be a distressing symptom for child and carers alike if it is impacting on sleep, play and eating. If persistent it can precipitate pain, vomiting and seizure activity in the predisposed child. The primary aim should always be to treat underlying causes but if this is not possible or is more of a burden than benefit, cough suppressants can be used.

Consider causes and treat reversible factors if appropriate:
- Infection
- Bronchospasm
- Gastro-oesophageal reflux
- Aspiration
- Drug-induced (e.g. ACE inhibitors)/treatment related (e.g. total body irradiation)
- Malignant bronchial obstruction/lung metastases
- Heart failure
- Secretions
- Cystic fibrosis
- Subclinical seizures

Management
General measures
- Keep child as upright as possible
- Raise head of bed: Use blocks under head end of cot/bed or pillows
- Consider physiotherapy, suction for children with secretions. Modified physiotherapy is the mainstay of treatment for children with thick secretions
- Consider a trial of humidified air/oxygen
- Trial of nebulized saline

Medication
The choice of medication will depend upon the underlying cause. A dry throat may respond to simple linctus. Bronchospasm will respond to bronchodilator therapy. If the underlying cause cannot be reversed, a suppressant such as an opioid will be required.

Simple linctus
This may be helpful if the cough is exacerbated by a dry throat.
- Form:
  - linctus: paediatric preparation (0.625% citric acid monohydrate); adult preparation (2.5% citric acid monohydrate)
- Dose (oral):
  - 1 month–12yrs: paediatric preparation 5–10mL t.d.s.–q.d.s.
  - >12yrs: adult preparation 5–10mL t.d.s.–q.d.s.
- Licence: licensed for children and adults (appropriate preparation)

Codeine linctus
Very constipating: laxatives should always be prescribed
- Form:
  - linctus: paediatric preparation: codeine phosphate 3mg in 5mL; adult preparation: 15mg in 5mL
- Dose (oral):
  - 1–5yrs: 5mL paediatric preparation t.d.s.–q.d.s.
  - 5–12 yrs: 2.5–5mL adult preparation t.d.s.–q.d.s.
- Licence: not licensed for use in children under 1yr

Dihydrocodeine tartrate
- Form:
  - tablet: 30mg
  - liquid: 10mg in 5mL
- Dose (oral):
  - 1–4yrs: 500mcg/kg, 4–6h
  - 4–12yrs: 500mcg–1mg/kg, 4–6h
  - >12yrs: 30mg, 4–6h
- Very constipating: laxatives should always be prescribed
- **Contraindications and warnings**: avoid or reduce dose in moderate/severe renal failure, chronic liver disease and hypothyroidism. Avoid in respiratory depression, cystic fibrosis, head injury and raised intracranial pressure
- Licence: not licensed for this indication

Morphine linctus
- Form:
  - solution: 10mg in 5mL
- Dose:
  - start with half the paediatric analgesic dose (📖 See section on Pain, p. 620) and titrate to effect
- Licence: not licensed for this indication

Bronchodilators
Cough can be a manifestation of hyperreactive airways and a trial of nebulized salbutamol/ipratropium may be helpful.

Salbutamol
- Form:
  - nebulizer solution: 2.5mg in 2.5mL, 5mg in 2.5mL, 5mg in 1mL (other preparations available, see appropriate text)
  - inhaled form: 100mcg/dose
- Dose (nebulized):
  - 6 months–5yrs: 2.5mg t.d.s.–q.d.s.
  - 5–12yrs: 2.5–5mg t.d.s.–q.d.s.
  - >12yrs: 5mg t.d.s.–q.d.s
- Dose (inhaled):
  - all ages: 1–2 puffs 4–6 times a day (a spacer device should be used to improve delivery)
- May induce mild tachycardia, nervousness, tremor or hypokalaemia
- Interactions: see appropriate text
- Licence: licensed for use in children

Ipratropium bromide
- Form:
  - nebulizer solution: 250mcg/mL, 500mcg in 2mL
  - inhaled form: 20mcg/dose and 40mcg/dose
- Dose (nebulized):
  - <1yr: 125mcg t.d.s.–q.d.s.
  - 1–5yrs: 250mcg t.d.s.–q.d.s.
  - 5–12yrs: 500mcg t.d.s.–q.d.s.
  - >12yrs: 500mcg t.d.s.–q.d.s.
- Dose (inhaled):
  - <6 yrs: 20mcg/dose t.d.s.–q.d.s.
  - 6–12yrs: 20–40mcg/dose t.d.s.–q.d.s.
- Licence: licensed for use in children

Mucolytics

May be helpful if secretions are thick. Agents like acetylcysteine and dornase-alfa may be used in patients with cystic fibrosis who have thick secretions. However, their use should be discussed with the child's paediatrician.

Normal saline
- Dose (nebulized):
  - all ages: 2.5–5mL p.r.n.
- May induce cough reflex in some cases

Gastro-oesophageal reflux

Many neurologically impaired children suffer with gastro-oesophageal reflux. Consider reflux if the child refuses food, vomits, has dysphagia, abnormal movements (Sandiffer's syndrome or extensor posturing), cough, intractable hiccups, aspiration pneumonia or is irritable when supine.

Management

General measures
- Check for overfeeding
- If nasogastric/gastrostomy-fed, consider changing regimen from large bolus to smaller, more frequent volumes. Continuous feeding is another option
- Thicken feeds
- Ensure optimal posture for feeds
- Adjust posture overnight to keep child more upright: use blocks under cot/bed, or use pillows
- Surgery can be considered in children with a longer prognosis Gastrostomy and fundoplication is effective in 80% but is not without complications. Gastrostomy alone will increase the likelihood of reflux as will nasogastric feeding
- Postpyloric tube feeding is a better option than nasogastric tube feeding

Medication

Antacids
To be really effective antacids should be given four-hourly. This may limit their usefulness.

Gaviscon
- Form:
  - tablets: sodium alginate 500mg, 100mg potassium bicarbonate
  - suspension: sodium alginate 500mg, potassium bicarbonate 100mg/5mL
  - Dual Infant sachets: sodium alginate 225mg, magnesium alginate 87.5mg with colloidal silica and mannitol per dose (dose = half sachet)
- Dose (oral):
  - Birth–2yrs: ½–1 Dual Infant sachet (do not use other preparations with feeds. Max 6 times in 24hrs)
  - 2–12yrs: 2.5–5 mL liquid or 1 tablet after meals and at bedtime
  - >12yrs: 5–10 mL or 1–2 tablets after meals and at bedtime
- Can cause constipation
- Licence: liquid and tablets licensed for use in children over 12yrs, for children <12yrs on medical advice only. Infant sachets licensed for infants and young children but, for children under 1yr, only under medical supervision

Lansoprazole

As effective as omeprazole but FasTabs dissolve better in water and do not block tubes as readily.

- Form:
  - orodispersable 'FasTab' tablet: 15mg, 30mg
  - suspension: 30mg/sachet
- Dose (oral):
  - <30kg: 0.5—1mg/kg (max 15mg) once daily in morning
  - >30kg: 15–30mg once daily in morning.
- Fastabs can be divided before mixing with water for enteral feeding tubes
- Suspension is not suitable for administration through feeding tubes
- **Contraindications and warnings**: **caution** in patients with hepatic impairment
- Licence: not licensed for children

Omeprazole

Is the drug of choice for reflux oesophagitis. It is more effective than ranitidine and has a good safety profile. Individuals vary in their response and doses will need to be titrated to achieve effective acid suppression. It easily blocks feeding tubes, therefore for a child who is enterally fed dissolve in sodium bicarbonate (see below) or consider lansoprazole as an alternative.

- Form:
  - capsule: 10mg, 20mg, 40mg
  - MUPS dispersible tablets: 10mg, 20mg, 40mg
  - tablets: 10mg, 20mg, 40mg
  - intravenous infusion: 40mg vial
  - intravenous injection: 40mg vial
- Dose (oral):
  - 1 month–2yrs: 700mcg–3mg/kg o.d.—round up to nearest capsule size, (max 20mg)
  - 10–20kg: 10–20mg o.d.
  - >20kg: 20–40mg o.d./b.d.
- Capsules can be opened and the granules mixed in an acidic drink
- If capsules are to be opened and given via gastrostomy or NG tube disperse in 10mL of 8.4% sodium bicarbonate and flush well afterwards (omeprazole readily blocks tubes)
- Tablets can be dispersed in water or mixed with fruit juice or with yoghurt
- **Contraindications and warnings**: **caution** in patients with hepatic impairment
- Interactions: see appropriate text
- Licence: licensed for use in children >2yrs with severe ulcerating reflux oesophagitis

Ranitidine

- Form:
  - injection: 50mg in 2mL
  - tablets: 150mg, 300mg; effervescent tablets 150mg, 300mg
  - liquid: 15mg in 1mL

- Dose (oral):
  - 1–6 months: 1mg/kg t.d.s.; max. 3mg/kg per day
  - 6 months–3years: 2–4mg/kg b.d.
  - 3–12 years: 2–4mg/kg (max 150mg) b.d. Can increase to 5mg/kg (max 300mg) in severe gastro-oesophageal reflux disease
  - 12–18 years: 150mg b.d. or 300mg o.n. Can double the dose for up to 12 weeks in moderate to severe gastro-oesophageal reflux disease
- Dose (IV)
  - 1 month–18 years: 1mg/kg (max 50mg) every 6–8 hours

Gastrostomy care

Children with life-limiting illnesses commonly have gastrostomy tubes in situ, either a PEG (percutaneous endoscopic gastrostomy) or MIC-KEY (Medical Innovations Corporation UK Gastrostomy Button). These allow feeding in the presence of disordered swallowing and ease the administration of medication.

Considerations
- Daily cleaning of the skin around the stoma site will help prevent irritation and infection
- Formation of granulation tissue is reduced by the regular rotation of the tube by 360° daily
- Ensure all connections and tubings are comfortable for the child and not in a position where they can be easily pulled at or dislodged

Blockage
- Gastrostomy tubes block easily. They should be flushed before and after all feeds and medications. Some drugs are notorious for causing blockages and alternatives should be considered (e.g. lansoprazole instead of omeprazole)
- If blocked, flushing with a large (50mL) syringe of pineapple juice may help dissolve the blockage. If not successful Pancrex V (a pancreatic enzyme) can be instilled into the tube for 30 minutes

Granulation tissue
- Apply topical steroid-based, antifungal cream (e.g. Tri-Adcortyl) twice daily for up to 10 days
- May need second course, but prolonged use not advised
- If not resolving, swab and exclude infection

Infection
- Indicated by erythema, swelling, tenderness and oozing around the tubing. Swab before treating
- Fucidin cream topically may be sufficient
- Consider systemic antibiotics

Dislodged tubes
- Most families will keep spare Mic-Keys or gastrostomy tubes with them which are easily replaced. If not available, a size 12G Foley catheter can be used to keep the stoma patent until stocks are found.

Infection at the end of life

Management of infection at the end of life needs careful consideration, and if possible, forward planning. This avoids decisions being made in a crisis and may spare the child from intrusive and futile interventions. Discussing and recording a preferred course of action with the parents, and where appropriate the child, in advance of the terminal phase is ideal. Such plans should always be open for further discussion and revision should this be necessary. Treating infection, even at the end of life should always be considered in terms of benefit and burden. For example, if antibiotics reduce symptoms and make the child more comfortable, the benefits may outweigh the burden of the treatment. Each case must be considered on an individual basis.

Mouthcare

A painful mouth can cause anorexia, discomfort and difficulties eating. It can also make it difficult for the child to take oral medication. Good mouthcare can significantly enhance quality of life for children in the palliative care setting.

A general examination should always include inspection of the mouth as oral problems are readily overlooked but can usually be easily managed.

Consider cause and treat as appropriate

- Oral candidiasis
- Dry mouth
- Ulcers
- Bleeding gums
- Dental caries
- Impacted teeth
- Gum hyperplasia
- Medications, e.g. morphine, antidepressants, antihistamines or anticholinergics

Management

General measures

- If using oxygen, try humidifying it or using nasal prongs
- Keep mouth clean and moist
- Rinse mouth after vomiting
- If possible, brush teeth, gums and tongue and other mucous membranes two or three times a day with a soft toothbrush
- Clear a coated tongue by gently brushing with a soft tooth brush, or by using effervescent vitamin C
- Sucking pineapple chunks will help maintain a clean mouth but avoid if there is ulceration in the mouth because of pain and mucosal break down with pineapple
- If the mouth is too painful to brush, regularly clean with pink sponges dipped in water or mouthwash, particularly after eating or drinking
- Avoid preparations containing alcohol
- Try water sprays or atomizers
- Ice chips may be helpful
- Artificial saliva: a number of preparations are available
- Moisten lips with petroleum jelly or lip balm
- Refer to dentist if appropriate, consider a specialist dentist for children with severe neurodisability

Medication

Oral candidiasis may present as classic white plaques or less commonly as atrophic candidiasis with a red glossy tongue. Remember that candidiasis may extend beyond the line of vision to the oesophagus.

Nystatin

- Form:
  - pastilles: 100 000 units
  - oral solution: 100 000 units in 1mL
- Dose (oral):
  - 1 month–18yrs: 1mL or 1 pastille, 6hr
  - for oesophageal candida in the immunocompromised: 5mL, 6hr

- The child should not eat or drink for 20 minutes after taking nystatin
- Continue 48h after clinical cure to prevent relapse
- Licence: licensed for children

Miconazole oral gel
- Form:
  - oral gel: 24mg in 1mL
- Dose (topical to inside of mouth, then swallow):
  - birth–1 month: 1–2mL b.d.
  - 1 month–2yrs: 2.5mL b.d.
  - 2–6yrs: 5mL b.d.
  - >6yrs: 5mL q.d.s.
  - Licence: licensed for children >1month

Fluconazole
- Form:
  - capsules: 50mg, 150mg, 200mg
  - oral suspension: 50mg in 5mL; 200mg in 5mL
  - also available IV
- Dose (oral):
  - 1 month–12 yrs: 3mg/kg for 14 days
  - >12 yrs: 50mg o.d. for 14 days (max 100mg o.d.)
- **Contraindications and warnings**: reduce dose in renal impairment. Co-administration with terfenadine contraindicated, interacts with several drugs: see other texts. May cause haematological and biochemical abnormalities particularly in children with HIV or malignancies
- Licence: licensed for use in children

Ulcers/mucositis

- Often related to neutropenia resulting from high-dose chemotherapy or radiotherapy
- Mouthwash, type will depend on the severity of the mucositis. Chlorhexidine 0.2% (swished for one minute or swabbed three times daily) is generally adequate for those children with mild to moderate mucositis. Hydrogen peroxide mouth rinse (diluted 1 in 8 with water or saline and used two to three times daily) may need to be used in addition to chlorhexidine in children with severe mucositis
- An antifungal agent (see above) should be used. This should be given 20–30 minutes after chlorhexidine
- Mucositis can be extremely painful and analgesia appropriate to the degree of pain should be given. For children with severe mucositis, opioid analgesia may be required

Aphthous ulcers

Adcortyl in orabase
- Form:
  - oral paste
- Dose (topical):
  - all ages: apply thin layer to affected area b.d.–q.d.s.

Choline salicylate (Bonjela)
- Form:
  - clear gel
- Dose (topical):
  - >4 months: ¼ inch (about 0.6 cm) of gel up to six times daily; may sting initially

Bleeding gums
📖 See section on Bleeding, p. 576.

Muscle spasm

Muscle spasm, commonly experienced by children with neurodegenerative conditions, can cause significant pain and distress. It may also interfere with positioning and activities. Spasms themselves cause pain leading to further spasms, and a distressing cycle of symptoms can evolve. Muscle spasms may be difficult to distinguish from movement disorders or convulsions and therefore a good history and examination are imperative.

Management

General measures

- Early involvement of physiotherapy and occupational therapy teams is invaluable for advice on moving, handling, positioning and seating, and is essential to prevent the problem worsening
- Long-standing contractures in a child with a relatively long prognosis can inhibit daily caring and may be managed surgically or with botulinum toxin injection. This should be assessed by an orthopaedic surgeon and can now be done under local anaesthetic
- Discussion with a paediatric neurologist may also be helpful.
- Baclofen and benzodiazepines are the most commonly used drugs, with dantrolene and tizanidine being increasingly used by paediatric neurologists
- More invasive techniques, such as intrathecal baclofen pumps, may be considered if the benefits outweigh the burdens of the initial surgery and the necessary follow-up
- While it is generally possible to reduce muscle spasm, it may not be possible to abolish it altogether

Caution

- High tone and muscle spasm may be the only things that allow a child to sit or stand. Therefore, treating spasms will require careful assessment as it may impact on the child's mobility and also on their independence.
- Many of the effective drug therapies may also cause significant sedation

Medication

Analgesia (see section on Pain, p. 618).

Baclofen

- Form:
  - tablet: 10mg
  - liquid: 5mg in 5mL
  - also available as intrathecal injection for specialist use: see below
- Starting dose (oral):
  - >1yr–12yrs: 2.5mg t.d.s.
  - >12yrs: 5mg t.d.s.
  - increase dose every three days to maintenance dose

- Maintenance dose (oral):
  - 1yr–2yrs: 5–10mg b.d.
  - 2–6yrs: 10–15mg b.d.
  - 6–10yrs: 15–30mg b.d.
  - >12yrs: 10–20mg t.d.s.
- Baclofen can also be used intrathecally as a continuous infusion into the lumbar intrathecal space via an indwelling catheter and SC pump. The rate of infusion can be altered according to the child's clinical needs at different times of day
- **Contraindications, cautions and warnings**: may cause drowsiness and hypotonia. Avoid rapid withdrawal. Use with caution in epilepsy. See other texts for interactions
- Doses should be reduced in renal impairment
- Licence: licensed for oral use in children >1yr

Diazepam
- Form:
  - tablets: 2mg, 5mg, 10mg
  - oral solution: 2mg in 5mL and 5mg in 5mL
  - suppositories: 10mg; and rectal tubes: 2mg in 1mL: 2.5mg tube, 5mg tube; 4mg in 1ml: 10mg tube
- Dose (oral):
  - 1 month–5yrs: 50–100 mcg/kg b.d.–q.d.s.
  - 5–12yrs: 2.5–5mg b.d.–q.d.s.
  - >12 yrs: 5–15mg b.d.
- May cause sedation
- Licence: tablets and liquid licensed for use in cerebral spasticity and control of muscle spasm in tetany

Dantrolene
- Form:
  - capsules: 25mg, 100mg
- Dose (oral):
  - starting dose:
  - 1 month–12yrs: 500mcg/kg o.d.
  - >12yrs: 25mg o.d.
- Titration: increase dose frequency to t.d.s. then q.d.s. at seven-day intervals. If response unsatisfactory continue increasing the dose in increments of 500mcg/kg in children <12yrs and 25mg in those >12yrs until maximum dose reached
- Maximum dose:
  - 1 month–12yrs: 2mg/kg (or 100mg total) q.d.s.
  - >12yrs: 100mg q.d.s.
- **Contraindications and warnings**: hepatic impairment. **Caution** with cardiovascular/respiratory disease. Monitor liver function
- Licence: not licensed for this indication in children

Nausea and vomiting (Fig. 7.1, Table 7.1)

Consider cause
- Obstruction: gastric outflow/bowel
- Constipation
- Uraemia/deranged electrolytes/hypercalcaemia
- Raised intracranial pressure
- Upper gastrointestinal tract irritation
- Anxiety
- Cough
- Pain
- Drugs: opioids, chemotherapy, carbamazepine, NSAIDs
- Intercurrent illness, e.g. gastroenteritis, urinary tract infection

Management

General measures
- Treat the underlying cause if possible
- Ensure optimal pain management
- Avoid strong food smells and perfumes—may antagonize nausea
- Keep meals small and remove leftover food quickly

Medication

- Give an appropriate antiemetic according to suspected cause (see below), if this is ineffective or the cause is unclear, a phenothiazine such as levomepromazine will usually be effective
- Levomepromazine is an effective antiemetic with anticholinergic, antihistaminergic and antidopaminergic actions
- Non-oral routes should be used if a child is vomiting (e.g. subcutaneous, parenteral or rectal routes) until symptoms are under control when the oral route can be re-established
- Review: if treatment is not successful, reconsider cause

Opioid-induced nausea and vomiting

Opioid-induced nausea is mediated predominantly via dopaminergic pathways. Haloperidol is a dopamine antagonist which acts centrally. It is more potent in this action than metoclopramide. Metoclopramide is a dopamine antagonist and acts on both the CTZ and the gastrointestinal tract (prokinetic action). Like haloperidol, it may cause dystonic side-effects, although these can be managed with benztropine. Domperidone is available for oral administration and does not cross the blood–brain barrier. Therefore, this means it is less effective than metoclopramide and haloperidol but that it is also less likely to cause extrapyramidal side-effects. Dexamethasone may be a useful adjuvant agent. Levomepromazine has antidopaminergic activity in addition to its anticholinergic and antihistamine properties.

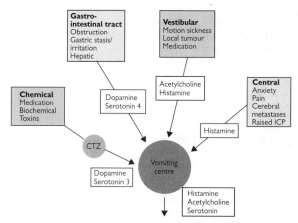

Fig. 7.1 Suspected causes of nausea and vomiting and suggested receptors/neurotransmitters involved.

Table 7.1 Receptor site affinities of antiemetics*

	D_2 antagonist	H_1 antagonist	ACh antagonist	5-HT$_3$ antagonist
Metoclopramide	++	0	0	(+)
Ondansetron	0	0	0	+++
Cyclizine	0	++	++	0
Hyoscine hydrobromide	0	0	+++	0
Haloperidol	+++	0	0	0
Prochlorperazine	++	+	0	0
Chlorpromazine	++	++	+	0
Levomepromazine	++	+++	++	0

D_2 = dopamine; H_1 = histamine 1'; ACh = muscarinic, cholinergic; 5-HT$_3$ = serotonin group 3.
*Adapted from Twycross R, Back I. (1998) Nausea and vomiting in advanced cancer. *European Journal of Palliative Care*, **5**: 39–45.

Haloperidol
- Form:
  - tablet: 500mcg, 1.5mg, 5mg, 10mg, 20mg
  - capsule: 500mcg
  - oral liquid: 1mg in 1mL, 2mg in 1mL, 1mg in 5mL, 5mg in 5mL, 10mg in 5mL 'specials'
  - injection: 5mg in 1mL, 1mL amps; 10mg in 1mL, 2mL amps
- Dose (oral):
  - 1 month–12yrs: 12.5–50mcg/kg b.d.
  - >12yrs: 500mcg–2mg b.d.–t.d.s.
- Dose (SC):
  - all ages: 25–85mcg/kg over 24h
- Licence: injection not licensed for use in children

Metoclopramide
- Form:
  - tablet: 10mg
  - syrup/oral solution: 5mg in 5mL
  - paediatric liquid: 1mg in 1mL
  - injection: 5mg in 1mL, 2mL ampoule
- Dose (oral/slow IV/SC):
  - 1 month–1 yr (less than 10kg): 100mcg/kg b.d. (max 1mg)
  - 1–3 yrs (10–14kg): 1mg b.d.–t.d.s.
  - 3–5 yrs (15–19kg): 2mg b.d.–t.d.s.
  - 5–9 yrs (20–29kg): 2.5mg t.d.s.
  - 9–18 yrs (30–60kg): 5mg t.d.s.
  - 15–18 yrs (over 60kg): 10mg t.d.s.
- Dystonic reactions can occur with any dose, but the risk increases with dose: reverse with benztropine or procyclidine
- Use with **caution** if intestinal obstruction suspected: if colic develops, reduce dose or stop altogether
- **Caution**: in moderate renal failure use 75% dose, in severe renal impairment use 25–50% dose. Reduce dose in severe liver disease.
- Licence: licensed for use in children

Levomepromazine
- Form:
  - tablet: 25mg, 6mg named patient
  - injection: 25mg in 1mL, 1mL ampoule
- Dose (oral):
  - 2–12yrs: 0.1–1mg/kg (max 25mg) o.d.–b.d.
  - >12yrs: 6.25–25mg o.d.–b.d.
- Dose (SC/IV continuous infusion):
  - all ages: 0.1–0.25mg/kg per 24h (max. 25mg/24h)
- Highly sedative in higher doses (SC dose >1mg/kg per 24h)
- May reduce seizure threshold
- Postural hypotension especially if used with opioids
- Little experience in very small children
- **Caution**: parkinsonism, postural hypotension, antihypertensive medication, epilepsy, hypothyroidism, myasthenia gravis
- Licence: not licensed for use as antiemetic in children

Domperidone
Less effective than metoclopramide, but has a reduced risk of dystonic side-effects. May be an alternative for a patient who has responded well to metoclopramide but experienced dystonic side-effects.
- Form:
  - tablet: 10mg
  - suspension: 5mg in 5mL
  - suppositories: 30mg
- Dose (oral):
  - <35kg: 250–500mcg/kg t.d.s. to q.d.s. (max 2.4mg/kg/24h)
  - >35kg: 10–20mg t.d.s. to q.d.s. (max 80mg/24h)
- Dose (rectal):
  - 15–35kg: 30mg b.d.
  - >35kg: 60mg b.d.
- Use with **caution** if intestinal obstruction suspected: if colic develops, reduce dose or stop altogether
- Licence: only licensed for use in children with nausea and vomiting secondary to radiotherapy/chemotherapy

Chemotherapy/radiotherapy-induced nausea and vomiting

$5-HT_3$ antagonists (e.g. ondansetron) are very effective in relieving nausea and vomiting associated with chemotherapy. Since they are constipating, adjuvant laxatives may be necessary. In refractory cases dexamethasone can be used as a second-line agent, in combination. Levomepromazine is recommended as the third-line agent. High-dose metoclopramide is used in some centres.

Ondansetron
- Form:
  - tablet: 4mg, 8mg
  - tablet (melt): 4mg, 8mg
  - oral solution: 4mg in 5mL
  - injection: 2mg in 1mL, 2mL and 4mL ampoules
- Dose (oral):
  - 1m–12yrs: 4mg b.d.–t.d.s.
  - >12yrs: 8mg b.d.–t.d.s.
- Dose (IV over 2–5 minutes):
  - 1 month–12yrs: $5mg/m^2$ (max. 8mg) b.d.–t.d.s.
  - >12yrs: 8mg b.d.–t.d.s.
- Ondansetron has been used as continuous IV/SC infusion in palliative circumstances:
- Dose (continuous infusion)
  - 1 month–12years: $5–15mg/m^2$ per 24h (max 24mg)
  - 12–18 years: 24mg/24h
- Consider co-prescribing a laxative (ondansetron is constipating)
- Licence: licensed for post-chemotherapy nausea and vomiting

Dexamethasone
Caution is required when treating children with steroids. Side-effects include weight gain, and distressing behavioural and emotional changes if steroids are used for more than a few days. For this reason it is preferable

to prescribe steroids in short courses (3–5 days) and to repeat courses if necessary.
- Form:
  - tablet: 500mcg; 2mg
  - oral solution: 2mg in 5mL
  - injection: 4mg in 1mL; can be given orally
- Dose (oral, IV):
  - <1yr: 250mcg t.d.s.
  - 1–5yrs: 1–2mg t.d.s.
  - 6–12yrs: 2–4mg t.d.s.
  - >12yrs: 4mg t.d.s.
- Co-prescribing: consider antacids and anti-thrush treatment
- **Caution**: renal disease, cardiac disease or cystic fibrosis. Avoid in children with cardiac insufficiency
- Licence: not licensed for use as an antiemetic in children

Levomepromazine
- Form:
  - tablet: 25mg, 6mg named patient
  - injection: 25mg in 1mL, 1mL ampoule
- Dose (oral):
  - 2–12yrs: 0.1–1mg/kg (max. 25mg) o.d.–b.d.
  - >12yrs: 6.25–25mg o.d.–b.d.
- Dose (SC/IV continuous infusion):
  - all ages: 0.1–0.25mg/kg per 24h (max. 25mg/24h)
- Highly sedative in higher doses. (SC dose >1mg/kg per 24h)
- May reduce seizure threshold
- Postural hypotension especially if used with opioids
- No experience in very small children
- **Caution**: parkinsonism, postural hypotension, antihypertensive medication, epilepsy, hypothyroidism, myasthenia gravis
- Licence: not licensed for use as an antiemetic in children

Raised intracranial pressure

Cyclizine

Possesses anticholinergic and antihistamine activity. Where raised intracranial pressure is a major factor in generating nausea and vomiting, cyclizine is often helpful. Drowsiness is a common side-effect but may be desirable in some circumstances.

Cyclizine can be given subcutaneously, and although it does have the potential to crystallize in syringe drivers, this is an uncommon problem in practice. It may cause redness at the infusion site.
- Form:
  - tablets: 50mg
  - injection: 50mg/mL, 1mL amp.
  - suppositories: 12.5mg, 25mg, 50mg, 100mg ('special')
- Dose (slow IV bolus):
  - >1 month: 500 mcg–1mg/kg t.d.s. max. single dose <6 years: 25mg >6 years 50mg

- Dose (IV/SC continuous infusion):
  - <2yrs: 3mg/kg per 24h
  - 2–5yrs: 50mg/24h
  - 6–12yrs: 75mg/24h
  - >12yrs: 150mg/24h
- Dose (oral/rectal):
  - <2yrs: 1mg/kg t.d.s.
  - 2–5yrs: 12.5mg t.d.s.
  - 6–12yrs: 25mg t.d.s.
  - >12yrs: 50mg t.d.s.
- Tablets may be crushed
- **Caution**: hepatic and renal failure, epilepsy, heart failure
- **Side-effects**: dry mouth, drowsiness, blurred vision, headache, urinary retention, restlessness, insomnia, hallucinations
- Cyclizine is compatible with drugs most commonly used subcutaneously including diamorphine
- Incompatible with sodium chloride 0.9% solution, mix with water for injection
- Licence: tablets licensed for use in children >6 yrs. Injection not licensed for use in children

Dexamethasone

Dexamethasone has the potential to improve nausea in such cases because, in addition to being an effective antiemetic agent, it may also directly impact on raised intracranial pressure by reducing oedema. Caution is required when treating children with steroids. Side-effects include weight gain, and distressing behavioural and emotional changes can occur with prolonged steroids use, so it is important to weigh the benefits against the burdens. It is preferable to prescribe steroids in short courses (3–5 days) and to repeat courses if necessary. Monitoring blood/urinary glucose may be necessary, and is advised in prolonged courses. Try to avoid prescribing after 3pm as may affect sleep.

- Form:
  - tablets: 500mcg; 2mg
  - oral solution: 2mg in 5mL
  - injection: 4mg in 1mL; can be given orally
- Dose (oral/IV)
  - <1yr: 250–500mcg b.d.
  - 1–5yrs: 1mg b.d.
  - 6–12yrs: 2mg b.d.
  - >12yrs: 4mg b.d.
- Co-prescribing: consider antacids and anti-thrush treatment
- **Caution**: renal disease, cardiac disease or cystic fibrosis. **Avoid** in cardiac insufficiency
- Licence: not licensed for use as antiemetic in children

Noisy breathing

Excessive respiratory secretions more often cause distress to parents and carers than to the child. Reassurance may be all that is required. But pharmacological intervention may be warranted where the child is distressed. Suction may be helpful, although it is not always available.

Drug treatment is more effective when started before or immediately after the secretions are evident.

Antisecretory agents may cause drowsiness and anticholinergic side-effects: glycopyrronium has fewer CNS side-effects than hyoscine hydrobromide because it does not cross the blood–brain barrier. Sometimes, however, a sedative effect may be desirable.

Management

Medication

Glycopyrronium bromide
- Form:
  - injection: 200mcg in 1mL; 1mL, 3mL ampoules
  - tablets: 1mg, 2mg; named patient basis only
- Dose (IV/SC):
  - 1 month–18yrs: 4–8mcg/kg (max. 200mcg) t.d.s.–q.d.s.
- Dose (continuous SC infusion):
  - 1 month–18yrs: 10–40mcg/kg per 24h (max. adult dose 1200mcg/24h)
- Dose (oral):
  - 1 month–18yrs: 40–100mcg/kg t.d.s.–q.d.s.
- **Contraindications and warnings**: see appropriate text
- Compatible with morphine and midazolam
- Licence: not licensed for this indication in children

Hyoscine hydrobromide
- Form:
  - self-adhesive patch; drug released at a rate of 1mg over 72h
  - injection: 400mcg in 1mL amp.; 600mcg in 1mL amp.
- Dose (topical):
  - **caution** in children with intracranial malignancy: it may cause agitation. Patches may inflame skin, hence rotation of sites is advised
  - 1month–3yrs: ¼ patch over three days
  - 3–9yrs: ½ patch over three days
  - >10yrs: one patch over three days
- Hyoscine patches can be cut or cover portion to prevent contact with the skin
- Dose (SC, IV):
- Single dose given over 2–3 minutes:
  - 1–12yrs: 10mcg/kg q.d.s.
  - >12 yrs (>40kg): 400mcg q.d.s.
- Subcutaneous continuous infusion:
  - all ages: 40–60mcg/kg per 24h (max. dose 2400mcg/24h)
- Licence: transdermal preparation licensed for use in children >10yrs for motion sickness

Pain

- Adequate pain control can be achieved for the vast majority of children, but requires careful attention to recognition, assessment, treatment and review
- Assessment should include a careful history and examination to elucidate the exact nature and likely cause(s) of pain so that the most effective management can be initiated
- Assessment should include discussion with parents/carers and staff as well as the child if possible
- A number of pain assessment tools are available to aid diagnosis and monitor pain and the analgesic effect
- Assessment of pain in children, particularly young infants and non-verbal children, may be difficult
- Pain may be under-diagnosed and therefore inadequately treated in children, particularly those who are unable to communicate readily
- Pain is closely associated with fear and anxiety

Recognizing pain in children with communication difficulties:
- Discuss with family/carers who know the child well
- Look for signs, including: crying, becoming withdrawn, increased flexion or extension, hypersensitivity, frowning/grimacing on passive movement, poor sleep, increasing frequency of fits

Management

General measures

- Management should include reducing stress/anxiety as far as possible as well as analgesic measures
- Analgesics should be used in conjunction with non-pharmacological techniques
- Explanations and discussion often help to reduce anxiety
- A calm, quiet environment may help to reduce anxiety
- Distraction is a useful tool but should not replace consideration of pharmacological intervention
- A formal record of pain scores is helpful when introducing a new intervention, particularly when many carers are involved or when the child's communication is limited. Such a record may reassure or indicate that further measures are required, and allows comparison between different interventions to be made in a robust manner
- Carefully recording all information in medical records on a regular basis is essential to enable anyone who consults the records to easily recognize changes and assess the success of previous interventions

Medication

Choosing an analgesic:
- For mild to moderate pain, it is usual to start by using a non-opioid analgesic on a p.r.n. basis, progressing to regular use
- Some non-opioid analgesics may be used in conjunction with one another or in conjunction with opioids for added analgesic effect (📖 see below)
- If non-opioid analgesics do not control pain effectively then opioid analgesics will usually be helpful

- The oral route is preferred and adequate pain relief can be achieved using this route for most children
- In the palliative care setting where pain is constant, analgesics should be given regularly rather than p.r.n.
- Weak opioids like codeine have a dose limitation. Strong opioids do not, and the dose should be titrated until effective analgesia is achieved or side-effects prevent further escalation. If side-effects are problematic these can be treated with other medication, or the opioid can be changed to a different preparation with a different side-effect profile
- If a patient is having regular analgesia of any kind, it is important to prescribe additional p.r.n. analgesia for breakthrough pain
- Once stable, it may be possible to change to a slow-release form of medication
- Discuss the management plan with the family. If opioids are to be used, a careful explanation is required so that families are prepared for drowsiness, understand that laxatives are necessary and are reassured about issues relating to addiction and dependence
- Plan for exacerbations and crises. Make sure appropriate medications and plans for their use are available to the family. This may include parenteral forms of medication for children on oral opioids
- All analgesic regimens should be regularly reviewed, particularly during titration
- Seek advice from appropriately skilled staff if you are unsure or analgesia is not quickly achieved

Non-opioid analgesics for mild/moderate pain

Paracetamol
- Form:
  - tablets: 500mg; dispersible tablet: 120mg, 500mg
  - oral solution: 120mg in 5mL
  - oral suspension: 120mg in 5mL; 250mg in 5mL
  - suppositories: 60mg, 125mg, 250mg, 500mg; other strengths available as 'special'
  - injection:10mg/mL: 50mL, 100mL vials
- Dose (oral):
  - 1 month–12 yrs: 15mg/kg t.d.s.–q.d.s.
  - >12 yrs: 500mg–1g q.d.s. (see British National Formulary for Children)
- Dose (rectal):
  - birth–1 month: 20mg/kg max. t.d.s.
  - 1 month–12yrs: 20mg/kg t.d.s.–q.d.s. (max. 90mg/kg per 24h or 4g/24h)
  - >12yrs: 500mg–1g t.d.s.–q.d.s. (max. 90mg/kg per 24h or 4g/24h)

- Dose (IV):
  - <10kg: 7.5mg/kg over 15min., 4–6h (max. 30mg/kg per 24h)
  - 10–50kg: 15mg/kg over 15min., 4–6h (max. 60mg/kg per 24h)
  - >50kg: 1g over 15min. 4–6h (max 4g in 24h)
- **Contraindications and warnings**: dose-related toxicity in hepatic failure; in moderate renal failure (creatinine clearance 10–50mL/min per 1.73m^2) the minimum interval between doses is 6h. In severe renal failure (creatinine clearance <10mL/min per 1.73m^2) the minimum interval is 8h. Significantly removed by haemodialysis but not by CAPD
- May provide additional analgesia in combination with opioids
- Licence: licensed for analgesic use in children

Non-steroidal anti-inflammatory drugs (NSAIDs)

- Possess analgesic and antipyretic properties
- Are particularly useful for bone pain
- Individuals may respond better to one agent than another
- Should not be given to children with thrombocytopenia or with coagulation disorders
- Can be combined with paracetamol or opioids for additive analgesia
- If GI side-effects are likely, it may be useful to prescribe antacids and/or a proton pump inhibitor

Ibuprofen
- Form:
  - tablets: 200mg, 400mg, 600mg
  - tablet (slow release): 800mg
  - capsule (modified release): 300mg
  - liquid: 100mg/5mL
  - granules: 600mg/sachet
- Dose (oral):
  - 1 month–12yrs: 5mg/kg t.d.s.–q.d.s. (30mg/kg per 24h to a max. 2.4g/24h)
  - >12yrs: 200–600mg t.d.s.–q.d.s. (max. 2.4g/24h)
- **Cautions**: avoid if peptic ulcer or history of; risk of GI bleeding if coagulation defects (ibuprofen considered safer than other NSAIDs); avoid if hypersensitivity to other NSAIDs or aspirin. Caution needed in renal, cardiac or hepatic impairment and asthma
- Licence: granules and 800mg slow-release tablet not licensed for children. Liquid and immediate-release tablets not licensed for <3months or <5kg

Diclofenac
- Form:
  - tablets: (enteric coated) 25mg, 50mg; (dispersible) 50mg; (modified release) 75mg, 100mg
  - capsules: (modified release) 75mg, 100mg
  - suppositories: 12.5mg, 25mg, 50mg, 100mg
  - injection: 25mg in 1mL as 3mL ampoule

- Dose (oral/rectal):
  - 6 months–18yrs: 300mcg–1mg/kg t.d.s. (max. 3mg/kg per 24h to max. 150mg/24h)
  - Dose (deep IM* or IV) IV must be further diluted and given over 30–120 minutes. *Intramuscular injections not recommended in children. Consider all alternative agents/routes
  - >6 months: 300mcg–1mg/kg o.d.–b.d. (max. 3mg/kg per 24h to max. 150mg/24h)
- **Cautions and contraindications**: avoid if peptic ulcer present or history of one; avoid if hypersensitivity to other NSAIDs or aspirin. Caution needed in renal, cardiac or hepatic impairment and asthma. Avoid suppositories if there is ulceration of lower bowel/anus. Avoid IV use if concurrent NSAID or anticoagulant therapy
- Licence: 25mg + 50mg tablets and 12.5mg + 25mg suppositories licensed for chronic arthritis in children >1yr. Other preparations are not licensed for use in children

Opioid analgesics for moderate/severe pain

- Usually commenced when non-opioid analgesics have been tried and have not been fully effective or if pain is severe at presentation
- Always co-prescribe a regular laxative: opioids can be expected to cause constipation and it is better to prevent this from the outset

Other side-effects which should be anticipated and promptly managed are:

- Drowsiness: usually wears off after 3–5 days. Families may need forewarning as they may interpret drowsiness as a severe decline in the child's condition
- Nausea and vomiting (🕮 see section on Nausea and vomiting, p. 610)
- Pruritus: topical measures and antihistamines. Ondansetron may be effective
- Urinary retention: Check that constipation is not a contributory factor. Bethanechol may be helpful. Catheterization is required infrequently
- Respiratory depression: this is very unlikely if the dose is titrated appropriately. Naloxone will reverse respiratory depression, but this may be at the cost of analgesic effect if not administered carefully
- Euphoria, dysphoria
- Nightmares: a night-time dose of haloperidol may be useful
- Physical dependence: opioids should be weaned and not ceased abruptly or a withdrawal reaction may occur
- Tolerance: this is the need for escalating doses to achieve the same therapeutic effect. It is managed by increasing the dose. Families may need to be reassured that tolerance is rare and does not necessarily imply disease progression

Weak opioids
Codeine phosphate
- Form:
  - tablets: 15mg, 30mg, 60mg
  - syrup: 25mg in 5mL
  - linctus: 15mg in 5mL; 3mg in 5mL

- injection: 60mg in 1mL (for IM use, never give IV), 1mL amp.; 10mg/mL, 30mg/mL 1mL amps 'specials'
- suppositories (specials): 1mg, 2mg, 3mg, 5mg, 6mg, 10mg, 15mg, 30mg
- Dose (oral/rectal/IM*):
  - birth–12yrs: 500mcg–1mg/kg, 4–6h (max. 240mg/24h)
  - >12yrs: 30–60mg, 4–6h (max. 240mg/24h)
  - *Intramuscular injections not recommended in children. Consider all alternative agents/routes
- Constipation common: prescribe laxatives prophylactically
- **Cautions, contraindications and warnings**: little experience in young children, avoid in children <3 months. Avoid in renal impairment. Use with caution in hepatic impairment
- Licence: licensed for children >1yr

Dihydrocodeine tartrate
- Form:
  - tablets: 30mg
  - liquid: 10mg in 5mL
  - injection: 50mg in 1mL
- Dose (oral/SC):
  - 1–4yrs: 500mcg/kg, 4–6h
  - 4–12yrs: 500mcg–1mg/kg, 4–6h
  - >12yr: 30mg, 4–6h
- Constipation common: prescribe laxatives prophylactically
- **Cautions, contraindications and warnings**: avoid or reduce dose in moderate/severe renal failure, chronic liver disease and hypothyroidism. Avoid in respiratory depression, cystic fibrosis, head injury and raised intracranial pressure
- Licence: licensed for use in children >4yrs

Tramadol
Synthetic version of codeine with twice the potency of codeine and one-fifth the potency of morphine. Less constipating than codeine.
- Form:
  - capsule: 50mg
  - tablet: 50mg
  - orodispersable tablet: 50mg
  - injection: 50mg in 1mL
  - modified release: 100mg, 150mg, 200mg, 300mg, 400mg
- Dose (oral):
  - >12yr: 50–100mg, 4–6h (max 400mg/day)
- **Cautions, contraindications and warnings**: See under Morphine sulphate, p. 622
- Licence: licensed for use in children >12yrs

Strong opioids
Morphine sulphate
- Form:
  - tablets: 10mg, 20mg, 50mg
  - tablets/capsules (modified release): 5mg, 10mg, 15mg, 20mg, 30mg, 50mg, 60mg, 90mg, 100mg, 120mg, 150mg, 200mg

- granules for suspension (modified release): 20mg, 30mg, 60mg, 100mg, 200mg sachets
- oral solution: 10mg in 5mL; 100mg in 5mL
- injection also available but diamorphine is preferable for this purpose (📖 see Diamorphine hydrochloride)
- suppositories: 10mg, 15mg, 20mg, 30mg. 5mg is available as special
- Starting dose (oral/rectal):
  - 1–12yrs: 200–400mcg/kg, 4h
  - >12yrs: 5–20mg, 4h
- Starting dose (SC/IV stat):
  - 1–12yrs: 100–200mcg/kg, 4 h
  - >12 yrs: 2.5–10mg/dose, 4h
- Starting dose (continuous infusion):
  - >1yr: 10–15mcg/kg per hour
- **NB In children from 6 months–5 years morphine is metabolized more rapidly than in adults, in children <6 months less rapidly**
- Prescribing regimen:
  - always prescribe breakthrough doses (total dose/24h ÷ by 6)
  - if pain not controlled increase dose by 25–50%
  - use 4h dosing until pain well controlled, then convert to m/r preparation and prescribe 12h (total dose/24h ÷ by 2)
  - slow-release preparations normally given b.d. may need to be given t.d.s. in some children
  - keep required dose under constant review and adjust to give optimum pain control
- **Contraindications and warnings**: avoid in paralytic ileus, acute respiratory depression and liver disease. Caution needed in raised intracranial pressure, head injury, biliary colic, hypothyroidism. Reduce dose in renal failure: use 75% in moderate renal failure (creatinine clearance 10–50mL/min per 1.73m^2) and 50% in severe renal failure (creatinine clearance <10mL/min per 1.73m^2)
- Licence: Sevredol tablets licensed in children >3yrs. M×L capsules not licensed in children <1 year. Oramorph is unlicensed in children <1yr: 5mg suppositories are not licensed

Diamorphine hydrochloride
- Form:
  - injection: 5mg, 10mg, 30mg, 100mg, 500mg
  - tablets: 10mg, but no advantage over morphine sulphate and only one dose available
  - diamorphine is more potent than morphine. Diamorphine is metabolized to morphine but is more water-soluble and therefore considered more convenient for SC and IV injection
- Dose (intravenous):
  - all ages: 12.5–25mcg/kg per hour continuous IV infusion
- Dose (subcutaneous):
  - All ages: 20–100mcg/kg per hour continuous SC infusion

- Conversion:
  - The dose of parenteral diamorphine is one-third the dose of oral morphine, so if converting directly from oral dose: total dose morphine sulphate over 24h ÷ by 3.
- **Contraindications, cautions and warnings**: paralytic ileus and phaeochromocytoma. Avoid in head injury or raised intracranial pressure. Caution in acute respiratory failure and biliary colic. Reduce dose by 50% in severe renal impairment
- Licence: injection form licensed for children with terminal illness

Fentanyl
Fentanyl is less sedating and less constipating than morphine, but it is more difficult to adjust the dose in response to unstable pain when used transdermally. Unless contraindicated, it is generally better to stabilize the pain using an oral or parenteral opioid before changing to fentanyl patches.

- Form:
  - patches: for transdermal absorption over 72h: 12mcg/h, 25mcg/h, 50mcg/h, 75mcg/h, 100mcg/h
  - lozenge: for buccal use: 200mcg, 400mcg, 600mcg, 800mcg, 1200mcg, 1600mcg
  - injection form available but should be used by those with specific experience in paediatric pain medicine
- Dose (transdermal):
  - all ages: Table 7.2 shows the conversion from total daily dose of oral morphine sulphate to fentanyl dose:

Table 7.2 Conversion of oral morphine sulphate to fentanyl patch dose

Oral morphine (total daily dose) (mg/24h)	70–135mg	135–224mg	225–314mg	315–404mg	405–494mg
Fentanyl patch mcg/h	25	50	75	100	125

Converting from oral morphine sulphate:
- Continue oral morphine preparation for up to 12h after first fentanyl patch applied as patch will take 6–12h to reach therapeutic levels
- Wait 24–48h after application before evaluating analgesic effect or changing dose
- Always provide p.r.n. doses of oral morphine for breakthrough pain
- Use new area of skin with each patch change
- Avoid exposure of patch to excessive heat (sunbathing; hot-water bottle, etc.) as heat will increase absorption
- Dose (buccal):
  - useful for incident and breakthrough pain
  - dose not related to background analgesic dose, therefore start with 200mcg lozenge and adjust dose according to response
- Although fentanyl may be less constipating than morphine, a laxative should be co-prescribed

- **Contraindications and warnings**: 📖 see Diamorphine (p. 623). Fentanyl is less problematic in renal failure than diamorphine
- Licence: lozenges and transdermal preparation unlicensed for use in children

Buprenorphine

Buprenorphine is available in both patch and sublingual formulations. Its advantage over fentanyl is the lower morphine equivalency at which "BuTrans" patches can be used. Buprenorphine is a partial mu-agonist and has a ceiling dose—in practice this is rarely an issue. Theoretically, buprenorphine can block opioid receptors to the effects of other major opioids, and therefore it should not be used at high dose alongside these.

- Form:
  - "BuTrans" patches: for transdermal absorption over 7 days: 5mcg/h, 10mcg/h, 20mcg/h
  - "Transtec patches": for transdermal absorption over 4 days: 35mcg/h, 52.5mcg/h, 70mcg/h
  - tablet: for sublingual use: 200mcg, 400mcg
  - injection form available, but should be used by those with specific experience in paediatric pain medicine
- Dose (transdermal):
  - all ages: start at 5 mcg/h if opioid naïve and titrate after at least 72h. Dose can be adjusted at 3-day intervals using a patch of the next strength or 2 patches of the same strength. Maximum of 2 patches at one time recommended by manufacturers
  - if not opioid naïve, convert using morphine equivalency (60 times potency of morphine)
  - **Contraindications and warnings**: 📖 see Diamorphine, p. 623
  - Licence: tablets and transdermal preparation unlicensed in children

Oxycodone

- Form:
  - Capsules: 5mg, 10mg, 20mg
  - Liquid: 5mg in 5mL; concentrate: 10mg in 1mL
  - Tablets, modified release: 5mg, 10mg, 20mg, 40mg, 80mg
- Dose (oral):
  - **For opioid-naïve patients:**
  - 2–12yrs: 0.2mg/kg immediate release preparation 4 h
  - >12 yrs: 5–10mg immediate release preparation 4 h
  - **For children already on opioids:**
  - conversion ratio from morphine to oxycodone is 2:1 (i.e. total daily dose of oxycodone is half the total daily dose of morphine)
  - alternatively: to determine dose of oxycodone, divide total morphine dose by 12 and give up to 4-hourly
  - convert to long-acting preparation when stable
- **Contraindications**: acute respiratory depression, paralytic ileus, liver disease, moderate to severe renal failure
- Other opioids such as hydromorphone and methadone are available, but their use should be discussed with a paediatric pain or palliative care specialist.

Pain syndromes and adjuvant therapy

Bone pain

Radiotherapy

- Useful for discrete bone metastases
- May be given as a short course or single dose
- Effective treatment with minimal side-effects

Non-steroidal anti-inflammatory drugs (NSAIDs)

When used in combination with opioids, NSAIDS may lower the dose of opioid required for effective analgesia. Common choices are:

Ibuprofen

- Form:
  - tablets: 200mg, 400mg, 600mg
  - tablet (slow release): 800mg
  - capsule (modified release): 300mg
  - liquid: 100mg in 5mL
  - granules: 600mg/sachet
- Dose (oral):
  - 1 month–12yrs: 5mg/kg t.d.s.–q.d.s. (max. 30mg/kg per 24h to max. 2.4g/24h)
  - >12yrs: 200–600mg t.d.s.–q.d.s. (max. 2.4g/24h)
- **Cautions**: avoid if peptic ulcer or history of; risk of gastrointestinal bleeding in patients with coagulation defects (ibuprofen considered safer than other NSAIDs); avoid if hypersensitivity to other NSAIDs or aspirin. Caution in renal, cardiac or hepatic impairment and asthma
- Licence: granules and 800mg slow-release tablet not licensed for children. Liquid and immediate-release tablets are not licensed for children <3months or <5kg

Diclofenac

- Form:
  - tablet: (enteric coated) 25mg, 50mg; (dispersible) 50mg; (modified release) 75mg, 100mg
  - capsules: (modified release) 75mg, 100mg
  - suppositories: 12.5mg, 25mg, 50mg, 100mg
  - injection: 25mg in 1mL, as 3mL ampoule
- Dose (oral/rectal):
  - 6 months–18yrs: 300mcg–1mg/kg t.d.s. (max. 3mg/kg per 24h to max. 150mg/24h)
- Dose (deep IM* or IV: IV must be further diluted and given over 30–120 minutes). ***NB**: Intramuscular injections not recommended in children: consider all alternative agents/routes
  - >6 months: 300mcg–1mg/kg o.d.–b.d. (max. 3mg/kg per 24h to max. 150mg/24h)

- **Cautions, contraindications and warnings**: avoid if peptic ulcer or history of; avoid in patients with hypersensitivity to other NSAIDs or aspirin. Caution in renal, cardiac or hepatic impairment and asthma. Avoid suppositories if lower bowel/anus is ulcerated. Avoid IV use if patient is on concurrent NSAID or anticoagulant therapy
- Licence: 25mg and 50mg tablets and 12.5mg and 25mg suppositories licensed for chronic arthritis in children >1yr. Other preparations not licensed for use in children

Selective COX-2 inhibitors

These are not widely used because of the associated risk of cardiovascular and cerebrovascular disease. COX-2 (cyclo-oxygenase 2) inhibitors such as celecoxib are equianalgesic when compared with non-selective NSAIDs. They offer certain advantages in that the risk of gastrointestinal bleeding is reduced, and they have no effect on platelet function.

Bisphosphonates

Bisphosphonates have been shown to reduce bone pain related to both malignant and non-malignant causes in adults. They have been used in children. Seek advice before using.

'Resistant' and neuropathic pain

Most pain can be controlled with adequate doses of opioid medication, and much of what is regarded as 'resistant' pain can be managed with a dose increase or an alternative route of delivery (e.g. parenteral, spinal) or opioid switch (changing to an alternative strong opioid).

In some instances, however, adding an adjuvant agent which targets a particular pain mechanism or pathway may be helpful. Neuropathic pain has particular features including a lancinating or burning quality, shock-like features or associated paraesthesiae.

Furthermore, antidepressants or antiepileptic medications may be a useful addition to the regimen where these features are present. The choice between the two classes of drug will depend on the child's other symptoms. For example, a child with sleeping difficulties might benefit from a tricyclic antidepressant, whereas one with a coexistent seizure disorder will benefit from an anticonvulsant.

Tricyclic antidepressants

Tricyclic antidepressants can enhance opioid-induced analgesia and improve sleep.

Amitriptyline

- Form:
  - tablets: 10mg, 25mg, 50mg
  - oral solution: 25mg in 5mL; 50mg in 5mL
- Dose (oral):
  - 1–18yrs: 0.5–1mg/kg nocte
- Starting dose should be at the lower end of the range, then increased by 25% every four days until max. dose (2mg/kg per day) reached or side-effects preclude further titration. Full analgesic effect may not be seen for two weeks
- **Contraindications and warnings**: see imipramine
- Licence: not licensed for treatment of neuropathic pain in children

Imipramine
- Form:
  - tablets: 10mg, 25mg
- Dose (oral):
  - >1 month: 200–400mcg/kg nocte
  - titrate (50% increase every three days) up to 1–3mg/kg nocte
- **Contraindications and warnings**: acute porphyria; hepatic impairment
- **Caution** with cardiac disease (monitor ECG at doses >150mg/day)
- Do not use for 3 weeks after discontinuing MAOIs
- Interactions and side-effects: see other texts for full information
- Causes antimuscarinic effects: sedation, cardiac arrhythmias and lowers seizure threshold
- Licence: not licensed for neuropathic pain in children

Anticonvulsants

Carbamazepine
- Form:
  - tablets (immediate release): 100mg, 200mg, 400mg; chewable tablets 100mg, 200mg
  - tablets (modified release): 200mg, 400mg
  - oral liquid: 100mg in 5mL
  - suppositories: 125mg, 250mg
- Dose (oral):
  - 1 month–12yrs: start with 2.5mg/kg b.d.; increase by 2.5mg/kg b.d. at weekly intervals to a maximum of 10mg/kg b.d.
  - >12yrs: 200–400mg b.d.–t.d.s.
- The medication should be started at the lower end of the dose range and slowly titrated until therapeutic levels are achieved, symptoms are relieved or side-effects are limiting (e.g. ataxia, drowsiness, nausea.) Titrating slowly minimizes side-effects
- The suspension is absorbed faster than tablets. This might, therefore, necessitate dividing the total daily dose of suspension into three or four doses in order to maintain therapeutic levels
- **Contraindications and warnings**: A–V conduction abnormalities, history of bone marrow depression, intermittent porphyria, MAOIs within previous two weeks, sensitivity to tricyclics. Reduce dose in those with advanced liver disease. Numerous drug interactions—see other texts for full information
- Licence: licensed for use in children

Gabapentin
- Form:
  - capsules: 100mg, 300mg, 400mg
- Dose (oral):
  - all ages: start at 10mg/kg once daily for four days then b.d. for four days then t.d.s.
  - adjust dose according to response. Max. daily dose in adults is 1.8g/24h
  - capsules can be opened and the contents added to small volumes of fluid or food

- **Contraindications, cautions and warnings**: avoid abrupt withdrawal. Caution in renal failure: reduce frequency of doses
- Side-effects are much reduced if dose is titrated slowly as above
- Licence: licensed for children >6yrs for epilepsy

Ketamine

Ketamine is a useful adjuvant agent for patients with neuropathic pain because of its action on NMDA receptors. It has a tendency to cause agitation and hallucinations in higher doses. Seek specialist advice before using.

Nerve blocks, spinal administration and other neuroanaesthetic approaches

May be helpful for children who do not respond to any of the above measures, or for whom regular medication is practically difficult or poorly tolerated. Commonly used drugs used for these purposes are opiate analgesics and anaesthetic agents, or a combination of the two. Availability of such interventions varies widely across the world, and early consultation with your local anaesthetic team is advisable before options are discussed with the patient/parents. Spinal infusions can be managed in the community if appropriately trained staff members are available. If this is not possible, single-dose epidural/spinal analgesia may be a more practical alternative and would allow some assessment of whether a continuous infusion is likely to be beneficial in the longer term.

Pain associated with tumour-related oedema

Including pain related to intracranial tumours and nerve plexus compression.

Steroids

- Should be used with caution in children
- Short courses (up to five days) can be very effective for this type of pain
- Potential problems include insomnia, mood and behaviour changes, and in longer-term use rapid weight gain and body image changes and reduced mobility caused by proximal myopathy. Dyspepsia can be anticipated and prophylaxis should be prescribed
- Give entire dose before midday to reduce the likelihood of sleep disturbance at night

Dexamethasone

- Form:
  - tablets: 500mcg, 2mg
  - oral solution: 2mg in 5mL
  - injection: 4mg in 1mL can be given orally
- Dose (oral/SC/IV):
  - <1yr: 0.25–0.5mg b.d.
  - 1–5yrs: 1mg b.d.
  - 6–11yrs: 2mg b.d.
  - >12yrs: 4mg b.d.
- Higher doses are needed for those children with raised intracranial pressure or spinal cord compression
- **Contraindications and warnings**: caution in patients with renal disease, cardiac disease or cystic fibrosis. Avoid in cases of cardiac insufficiency
- Licence: licensed for use in children for symptoms associated with brain tumours but not specifically for nerve pain

Painful procedures

- If a procedure is likely to cause discomfort take preventive action!
- Explain all procedures to parents and children as appropriate to reduce anxiety
- Undertake procedures in friendly if not familiar surroundings
- Have parents/carers or the nurse who know the child best present.
- Use anaesthetic creams and distraction techniques appropriate to the age of the child
- Benzodiazepines are often employed in small doses *in conjunction with analgesia* for more difficult procedures, e.g. midazolam given buccally, IV or intranasally gives light sedation and some amnesia

Midazolam

- Oral:
  - 1month–12yr: 500mcg/kg. Max. 15mg
- Buccal/intranasal:
  - 1month–12 yr: 200–300mcg/kg half the dose should be dropped into each nostril over 15 seconds. Max. 10mg

Nitrous oxide
- Inhaled nitrous oxide has analgesic and amnesic properties but is non-sedating, so is generally used in co-operative children aged five years or older. Careful supervision is required

Ketamine
- Ketamine is another useful agent but requires careful supervision by trained staff and is usually started in an inpatient setting. We suggest contacting the nearest specialist palliative care team for further advice.

Psychological issues—anxiety and depression

Management

General measures

- Provide an environment and the opportunity for the child to raise his/her concerns and fears
- Children often find relaxation techniques, such as guided imagery, very helpful
- Complementary therapies (for example, music therapy) may be useful, particularly in non-verbal children
- Counselling and complementary therapies should ideally also be available to parents/primary carers
- Formal psychotherapeutic techniques may be also be helpful

Anxiety

Medication

- Medication should be use in combination with non-pharmacological techniques
- Anxiety may be a manifestation of depression, in which case an antidepressant may be more appropriate
- The choice of benzodiazepine will depend on the circumstance for which it is being prescribed. Children experiencing brief periods of anxiety or panic attacks may benefit from a benzodiazepine with a short half-life, such as midazolam, given buccally or subcutaneously. Sublingual lorazepam is another option for short-lived anxiety, panic attacks or anxiety related to dyspnoea. Those children who need a longer duration of action may prefer diazepam

Midazolam

Injection may be diluted in sodium chloride 0.9% or glucose 5% for buccal and intranasal routes. Tastes bitter when given orally but can be mixed with juice or chocolate sauce. Intranasal route may be unpleasant but has a fast onset of action (5–15 minutes)

- Form:
  - injection: 1mg in 1mL, 50mL vial; 2mg in 1mL, 5mL amp; 5mg in mL in 2mL, 5mL, 10mL amps
  - buccal liquid: 10mg/mL, 5mL, 25mL 'special'
  - oral liquid: 2.5mg in 1mL; only available as special
- Single doses:
  - Oral: 1 month–18 yrs: 500mcg/kg (max. 20mg) 30 mins prior to procedure
  - Buccal: 6 months–10 yrs: 200–300mcg/kg; >10 yrs: 6mg
  - Intranasal: 1 month–18yrs: 200–300mcg/kg (max. 10mg)
  - Rectal: 1 month–18 yrs: 300–500mcg/kg 15–30 mins prior to procedure
  - Intravenous: 1 month–5 yrs: 50–100mcg/kg; 6–12 yrs: 25–50mcg/kg; >12 yrs: 2.5mg
- Continuous intravenous/subcutaneous infusion: >1month–18yrs: 2.5mg/24h (**NB**: this is **not** a per kg dose)
- Titrate to effect

- **Contraindications, caution and warnings**: caution with pulmonary disease, hepatic and renal dysfunction (reduce dose), severe fluid/electrolyte imbalance and congestive cardiac failure. Avoid rapid withdrawal after prolonged treatment
- Licence: licensed for sedation in intensive care and for induction of anaesthesia. Other routes and indications not licensed

Clonazepam
- Form:
  - drops: 2.5mg in 1mL (1 drop = 100mcg), named patient
  - tablets: 0.5mg, 2mg
  - injection: 1mg in 1mL (1mL ampoule)
  - oral liquid 500mcg in 5mL, 2mg in 5mL, 12.5mg in 5mL 'special'
- Dose (sublingual):
  - all ages: 10mcg/kg per dose (max 500mcg) bd–tds
  - If necessary, increase by 10–25% every 2–3 days to max. 100mcg/kg per day
  - Prescribe as number of drops. Count drops onto spoon before administering
- Irritability and aggression not uncommon, in which case drug should be withdrawn. Increased secretions may occur in infants and young children

Lorazepam
- Form:
  - tablets: 1mg (scored), 2.5mg
  - suspension: only available as special
  - injection: 4mg in 1mL, 1mL ampoule
- Dose (sublingual, oral):
  - all ages: 25–50mcg/kg single dose (max. 4mg in adults in 24h)
  - most children will not need more than 0.5–1mg for trial dose
- Well absorbed sublingually (good for panic attacks) and child has control
- Injection can also be given sublingually
- **Contraindications, caution and warnings**: severe pulmonary disease, sleep apnoea, coma, CNS depression. Caution in hepatic and renal failure
- Licence: tablets licensed as pre-medication in children >5yrs. Injection is not licensed for use in children <12yrs except for the treatment of status epilepticus

Diazepam
- Form:
  - tablets: 2mg, 5mg, 10mg
  - oral solution: 2mg in 5mL and 5mg in 5mL
  - injection (solution and emulsion): 5mg in 1mL
  - suppositories: 10mg
  - rectal tubes: 2mg in 1mL, 2.5mg tube, 5mg tube; 4mg in 1mL: 10mg tube
- Dose (oral):
  - 1 month–12yrs: 50–100mcg/kg b.d.–q.d.s.
  - >12yrs: 2.5–5mg b.d–q.d.s.
- Potential for dependency in prolonged courses
- Licence: rectal preparation is licensed for use in children >1yr with severe anxiety. Tablets and liquid licensed for night terrors and sleep-walking

Depression

A survey in 1999 by the Office for National Statistics reported a 4% incidence of clinically significant emotional disorders in children (aged 5–15yrs) in the general population of the UK. The incidence of depression in terminally ill children is unknown, but it is likely that for many it remains unrecognized and untreated.

The clinical picture will depend on the age and developmental stage of the child, but the expected features of depressed mood—anhedonia, social withdrawal and disturbed sleep and appetite—may be present. The diagnosis is less dependent on somatic symptomatology because of the coexistence of illness.

Diagnosis may be difficult: trust the instincts of parents and carers and consult a child psychologist at an early stage.

Fluoxetine
- Form:
  - Capsules: 20mg, 60mg
  - Liquid: 20mg in 5mL
- Dose (oral):
  - 6–18yrs: 10mg o.d. increase slowly to 20mg
- Contraindications and warnings: avoid in hepatic or renal insufficiency. Lowers seizure threshold. Do not use with, or within two weeks of taking MAOIs
- Interactions: see appropriate text
- Licence: not licensed for use in children

Amitriptyline
Although tricyclic antidepressants no longer constitute the first-line management of depression in children, amitriptyline may be an appropriate choice in circumstances where neuropathic pain and disturbed sleep coexist.
- Form:
  - tablets: 10mg, 25mg, 50mg
  - oral solution: 25mg in 5mL; 50mg in 5mL
- Dose (oral):
  - all ages: 0.5–1mg/kg nocte
  - start at lower end of dose range and increase by 25% every 2–3 days until maximum dose (2mg/kg per day) reached or side-effects preclude further dose increase. Full effect may not be seen for two weeks
- **Contraindications and warnings**: see imipramine
- Licence: not licensed for treatment of neuropathic pain in children

Imipramine
- Form:
  - tablets: 10mg, 25mg
- *Starting dose (oral):*
  - 6–7yrs: 25mg nocte
  - 8–11yrs: 25–50mg nocte
  - 12–18yrs: 25mg t.d.s. or 75mg nocte
- *Maintenance dose (oral):*
  - 12–18yrs only: increase stepwise to 150–200mg daily in divided doses in first seven days. Continue until definite improvement then gradually reduce dose to long-term maintenance dose of 50–100mg daily
- **Contraindications, cautions and warnings**: acute porphyria and hepatic impairment. Caution in cardiac disease. Do not use with, or within two weeks of taking MAOIs. Lowers seizure threshold
- Interactions: see appropriate text
- Licence: not licensed for this indication in children
- **NB:** The Committee on Safety of Medicines has advised that citalopram, escitalopram, paroxetine, sertraline, venlafaxine and fluvoxamine are contraindicated in children <18yrs

Raised intracranial pressure

Consider raised intracranial pressure if the child shows evidence of:
- Confusion
- Personality change
- Drowsiness
- Vomiting
- Headache (especially on waking)
- Focal neurology

Management

General measures

- Investigation should be considered only if it will contribute to management decisions
- Reduction of tumour bulk may improve symptoms, e.g. cranial irradiation and chemotherapy
- In some circumstances a ventricular shunt may be helpful
- Symptomatic management may include analgesia ([] see section on Pain, p. 620), antiemetics and steroids. The antiemetic of choice is cyclizine

Medication

Dexamethasone

Caution is required when using steroids in children. Side-effects, including behavioural and emotional changes and sleep disturbance, may occur, and in longer-term use weight gain and proximal myopathy are also likely. For this reason it is preferable to prescribe steroids in short courses (3–5 days) and to repeat courses if necessary.

- Form:
  - tablet: 500mcg, 2mg
  - oral solution: 2mg in 5mL
  - injection: 4mg in 1mL; can be given orally
- Dose (oral/IV over 3–5 minutes):
  - <35kg: 20mg loading dose, 4mg/3h for 3 days; 4mg/6h for 1 day; 2mg/6h for 4 days; decrease by 1mg daily
  - >35kg: 25mg loading dose, 4mg/2h for 3 days; 4mg/4h for 1 day; 4mg/6h for 4 days; decrease by 2mg daily
- Dose (SC):
  - can also be given in equivalent doses SC as single doses, or as continuous infusion over 24h
  - if no effect after 3–5 days, stop steroids (no need to tail off)
  - co-prescribing: consider antacids and anti-thrush treatment
- **Contraindications, caution and warnings**: caution if renal disease, cardiac disease or cystic fibrosis. Avoid in cardiac insufficiency
- Licence: licensed for use in children but not as antiemetic

Cyclizine
- Form:
  - tablets: 50mg (tablets may be crushed)
  - injection: 50mg/mL (1mL)
  - suppositories: 12.5mg, 25mg, 50mg, 100mg ('special')
- Dose (IV stat):
  - >1month: 500mcg–1mg/kg t.d.s. Max. single dose <6 yrs: 25mg, >6yrs: 50 mg
- Dose: SC/IV continuous infusion:
  - 1month–2yrs: 3mg/kg per 24h
  - 2–5yrs: 50mg/24h
  - 6–12yrs: 75mg/24h
  - >12yrs: 150mg/24h
- Dose: oral/rectal:
  - <2yr: 1mg/kg t.d.s.
  - 2–5yrs: 12.5mg t.d.s.
  - 6–12yrs: 25mg t.d.s.
  - >12yrs: 50mg t.d.s.
- **Caution**: hepatic and renal failure, epilepsy, heart failure
- Side-effects: dry mouth, drowsiness, blurred vision, headache, urinary retention, restlessness, insomnia, hallucinations
- Cyclizine is compatible with drugs most commonly used SC, including diamorphine
- Incompatible with sodium chloride 0.9% solution
- Licence: tablets licensed for use in children aged over 6 yrs. Inj. not licensed for use in children
- Avoid in high concentrations with high concentrations of oxycodone (see page 625)

Skin

Management

General measures

- Like adults, children with terminal illnesses have skin that is susceptible to breakdown with poor healing abilities
- Good nursing care is required to predict and prevent problems, which once established may be difficult to treat
- Frequent and appropriate turning is essential to avoid pressure areas breaking down
- The use of suitable mattresses and mobility aids should be considered
- Consult the tissue-viability nurse if available
- Dressing changes can be very painful. Consider the use of a short-acting analgesic such as buccal diamorphine, entonox and/or topical anaesthetic agents such as lidocaine (📖 see also section on Procedural pain, p. 630)

Medication

- At-risk areas:
  - protect with Opsite, Tegaderm or Cutifilm
- Broken areas:
  - use Duoderm, Spyrosorb
- Infection:
  - send swab for culture. Use Intrasite gel, Iodosorb paste covered with Opsite or Tegaderm and consider antibiotics
- Cavities:
  - pack with Kaltostat or Sorbsan
- Fungating tumours and odour:
  - use topical metronidazole gel, oral metronidazole, charcoal dressings or honey and sugar
- Painful ulcers:
  - consider anaesthetic preparations, e.g. lidocaine/prilocaine (EmLa cream) or a topical morphine gel

- Associated cellulites or discharge:
  - consider antibiotics (oral is usually sufficient)

📖 See also adult section on Skin, p. 381.

Sleeplessness

Disturbed sleep has a major impact upon the child and family's quality of life. Adequate sleep may be the difference between a family's ability to cope with the stresses placed upon them or not.

Many children with neurodisability have poor sleep patterns related to underlying brain maldevelopment or associated problems such as seizures, reflux, visual impairment or medication.

Management

General measures

- Address the child's fears and concerns
- Consider the sleep pattern: the child may be sleeping a lot in the day and may be reversing the day/night pattern. It may be appropriate to keep the child awake more in the day or to provide extra stimulation during the day—this will depend on the child's stage of illness. The child may be unaware of when he is expected to sleep if intervention is needed around the clock
- Optimize bedtime routine: bath if possible, story, hot drink if appropriate, lights low
- Increase exposure to light in the mornings
- Consider complementary therapies to aid relaxation
- Try and disturb the child as little as possible during the night: this may mean re-scheduling medications

Medication

Melatonin

- Melatonin helps children to fall asleep faster and in some may increase the length of sleep.
- Form:
  - tablets: 1mg, 2mg, 3mg
  - tablets (sustained release): 1.5mg, 3mg
- Dose (oral):
  - initial dose: 2–3mg, 30–60min before bedtime.
  - increase to 4–6mg after 1–2 weeks
  - Maximum dose: 10mg generally accepted (though higher doses have been used)
- **Contraindications and warnings**: avoid in endocrine disorders. Has been associated with seizures
- Licence: not licensed for use in children

Temazepam

- Form:
  - tablets: 10mg, 20mg
  - oral solution: 10mg in 5mL
- Dose (oral):
  - 1 month–12yrs: 1mg/kg nocte (max 20mg)
  - >12yrs: 10–20mg nocte
- **Contraindications, caution and warnings**: caution in severe liver disease. Avoid in CNS depression and acute pulmonary insufficiency
- Interactions: see appropriate text
- Licence: not licensed for use in children

Chloral hydrate
- Form:
  - oral solution: elixir paediatric chloral mixture BP 2000: 500mg in 5mL; 'special'
  - chloral elixir paediatric BP 200mg in 5mL, 'special'
  - suppositories: 25mg, 50mg, 60mg, 100mg, 200mg, 500mg only available as 'specials'
  - tablets: chloral betaine 707mg (= chloral hydrate 414mg)
- Dose (oral/rectal):
  - 1 month–12yrs: 30–50mg/kg (max. 1g) nocte
  - >12yrs: 0.5–1g nocte
- **Contraindications, caution and warnings**: avoid in liver disease and severe renal failure. Caution in cardiac disease, respiratory insufficiency, porphyria and gastritis. Avoid prolonged administration and abrupt withdrawal
- Licence: unlicensed for use in children

Promethazine hydrochloride
- Form:
  - tablets: 10mg, 25mg
  - elixir: 5mg in 5mL
  - injection: 25mg in 1mL, as 1mL ampoule
- Dose (oral):
  - <1yr: 5–10mg nocte
  - 1–5yrs: 10–20mg nocte
  - 6–12yrs: 20–25mg nocte
  - >12yrs: 25–50mg nocte
- May be useful in mild cases
  - **Contraindications and warnings**: porphyria; CNS depression; hypersensitivity to phenothiazines. Do not use with, or within two weeks of taking MAOIs
- Licence: licensed for use in children >2yrs

Sweating

Consider cause
- Disease, e.g. malignant pyrexia, lymphoma, neuroblastoma
- Drugs, e.g. opioids, amitriptyline, chemotherapy
- Infection

Management

General measures
- Disease-modifying treatment may improve sweating if it is part of a malignant syndrome
- Fan, cotton clothing, skin care
- Encourage plenty of fluids to avoid dehydration

Medication
Paracetamol
- Form:
  - tablets: 500mg; dispersible tablets: 120mg and 500mg
  - oral solution: 120mg in 5mL
  - oral suspension: 120mg in 5mL; 250mg in 5mL
  - suppositories: 60mg, 125mg, 250mg, 500mg; other strengths available as 'specials'
  - injection: 10mg/mL, 50mL, 100mL
- Dose (oral):
  - Birth–3 months: 20mg/kg, 6–8h. (max. 60mg/kg per 24h)
  - 3 months–1yr: 60–120mg, 4–6h (max. 90mg/kg per 24h)
  - 1–5yrs: 120–250mg, 4–6h (max. 90mg/kg per 24h)
  - 6–12yrs: 250–500mg, 4–6h (max. 90mg/kg per 24h or 4g/24h)
  - >12yrs: 500mg–1g, 4–6h (max. 90mg/kg per 24h or 4g/24h)
- Dose (rectal):
  - Birth–1 month: 20mg/kg max. t.d.s.
  - 1 month–12yrs: 20mg/kg t.d.s.–q.d.s. (max. 90mg/kg per 24h or 4g/24h)
  - >12yrs: 500mg–1g t.d.s.–q.d.s. (max. 90mg/kg per 24h or 4g/24h)
- Dose (IV):
  - <10kg: 7.5mg/kg over 15min, 4–6h (max. 30mg/kg per 24h)
  - 10–50kg: 15mg/kg over 15min, 4–6h (max. 60mg/kg per 24h)
  - >50kg: 1g over 15min, 4–6h (max. 4g/24h)
- **Contraindications and warnings**: dose-related toxicity in hepatic failure; in moderate renal failure (creatinine clearance 10–50mL/min per 1.73m^2) the minimum interval between doses is 6h. In severe renal failure (creatinine clearance < 10mL/min per 1.73m^2) the minimum interval is 8h. Significantly removed by haemodialysis but not by CAPD
- Licence: licensed for antipyretic and analgesic use in children >3months

Naproxen
- Form:
  - tablets: 250mg, 375mg, 500mg
- Dose (oral):
  - >1 month: 5–15mg/kg b.d. (max. 1g/24h)
- **Contraindications, caution and warnings**: Contraindicated if known hypersensitivity to aspirin or other NSAIDs. Caution in asthma and cardiac, hepatic or renal failure; avoid if creatinine clearance < 20mL/min per 1.73m^2. Extreme caution if current or previous history of peptic ulceration
- Licence: not licensed for use in children for this indication

Other

Dantrolene, steroids and H_2-receptor antagonists have also been used with some success in adults.

Terminal restlessness

Restlessness and agitation are not uncommon during the terminal phase. Nursing the child in a calm, peaceful and preferably familiar environment is helpful, as is having a parent or other trusted adult present. Supporting the parents and carers at this point is fundamental, and helpful support will impact on the child indirectly. From the child's perspective, it is important to exclude poorly controlled pain/other symptoms or inadequate positioning as a cause of distress. Hypoxia may also be a factor.

Supporting and nursing a family in this circumstance is extremely challenging, particularly for staff who have established strong bonds. It is important for staff to actively seek their preferred support in order to optimize their ability to function effectively during care-giving and to protect coping mechanisms for the future.

The choice of medication to alleviate the restlessness will depend on the clinical circumstances. Midazolam is very effective and can be given via a continuous subcutaneous infusion combined with other medication such as diamorphine as necessary. Levomepromazine is also compatible with these medications and is an appropriate choice for children who have coexistent nausea.

Medication

Midazolam

Injection may be diluted in sodium chloride 0.9% or glucose 5% for oral, buccal and intranasal routes. Tastes bitter when given orally but can be mixed with juice or chocolate sauce. Intranasal route may be unpleasant but has a fast onset of action (5–15 minutes). Drop dose into alternate nostrils over 15 seconds.

- Form:
  - injection: 1mg in 1mL, 50mL vial; 2mg in 1mL, 5mL amp.; 5mg in 1mL, 2mL, 5mL and 10mL amps
  - buccal liquid: 10mg/mL, 5mL, 25mL 'special'
  - oral syrup: 2.5mg/mL, 'special'
- Single doses:
  - intravenous/subcutaneous: >1month–18yrs: 100mcg/kg
  - buccal/sublingual: >1month–18yrs: 500mcg/kg (max. 10mg)
  - intranasal: >1month–18yrs: 200–300mcg/kg (max. 10mg)
  - rectal: >1month–18yrs: 500–700mcg/kg
- Continuous intravenous/subcutaneous infusion:
  - 1 month–18 yrs: 300mcg–1000mcg/kg/24h. Doses of up to 40mg/24h have been necessary. If high doses required consider changing to a different agent
  - well absorbed subcutaneously
- Midazolam is compatible in a syringe driver with morphine, diamorphine, cyclizine and other commonly used drugs
- **Contraindications, caution and warnings**: caution with pulmonary disease, hepatic and renal dysfunction (reduce dose), severe fluid/electrolyte imbalance and congestive cardiac failure. Avoid rapid withdrawal after prolonged treatment
- Midazolam raises seizure threshold, making it a good choice for children likely to fit

- Licence: licensed for sedation in intensive care and for induction of anaesthesia in children >7yrs. Other routes and indications not licensed

Clonazepam
- Form:
  - drops: 2.5mg/mL (1 drop = 0.1mg), named patient basis
  - tablets: 0.5mg, 2mg
  - injection: 1mg in 1mL, 1mL ampoule
  - oral liquid: 500mcg in 5mL, 2mg in 5mL, 12.5mg in 5mL 'specials'
- Dose (sublingual):
  - all ages: 10mcg/kg per dose (max 500mcg)
  - if necessary, increase dose by 10–25% every 2–3 days to max. 100mcg/kg per day
  - prescribe as number of drops. Count drops onto spoon before administering
- Irritability and aggression are not uncommon, in which case drug should be withdrawn. Increased secretions may occur in infants and young children
- Licence: not licensed for this indication

Levomepromazine
- Form:
  - tablet: 25mg and 6mg
  - injection: 25mg in mL, 1mL ampoule
- Dose (continuous SC/IV infusion):
  - all ages: 0.5–1mg/kg per 24h. Titrate to effect (max. adult dose 200mg/24h)
- Also acts as antiemetic
- May lower seizure threshold
- Can be used in conjunction with midazolam
- Highly sedative in higher doses (SC dose >1mg/kg per 24h)
- Postural hypotension especially if used with opioids
- Little experience in very small children
- **Caution**: parkinsonism, postural hypotension, antihypertensive medication, epilepsy, hypothyroidism, myasthenia gravis
- Licence: not licensed for use as an antiemetic in children

Ventilation at home

Increasing numbers of children with life-limiting or life-threatening illnesses are accessing home ventilation. Most commonly, these children have neuromuscular diseases (e.g. Duchenne muscular dystrophy). Ventilation may also be required for children with craniofacial abnormalities, spinal injuries and congenital central hypoventilation syndrome (Ondine's curse).

Levels of ventilation

Nocturnal ventilation

Most children will start with ventilatory support overnight, this may be:

- Continuous Positive airway pressure (CPAP) via a face or nasal mask
- Positive pressure ventilation (PPV), delivered via a face or nasal mask or via a tracheostomy

24h ventilation

- Children may continue to use CPAP or PPV via their mask system, but a tracheostomy may be more practical if ventilation is a long-term option
- The commonest home ventilation devices encountered in the UK are the Nippead Ventilator and the Breas Ventilator. Children requiring such support usually have respiratory home support teams who can offer advice if difficulties are encountered with the machines
- During acute exacerbations of illness increased ventilation may be required, necessitating alterations in the duration or pressures of ventilation. Consultation and continued communication with a respiratory physician is essential when caring for such children at home

General measures

- Feelings of claustrophobia are common when nocturnal ventilation is first experienced. Thus, adequate explanation and reassurance is essential. Different masks exist with differing fixings that may allow the child some input into the decision-making process
- The masks are tight fitting and can become uncomfortable, particularly if the child is hot or sweating. Ensure that the environmental temperature and humidification are appropriate
- Pressure marks are common, and care is needed to prevent skin breakdown. Consider gauze over the ears and DuoDerm under the edge of the mask
- Water may accumulate in the tubing, causing the ventilator to alarm. This can be removed easily by suction or the tubing can be changed before seeking further advice
- Ventilators either have an inbuilt battery backup or else a separate battery pack for use in an emergency. These usually last 2–3h. Alternatives should always be available and those caring for a child should be appropriately trained to provide care during a power cut.

Emergency drugs' summary

The following information is given as a rough guide for quick reference only (Tables 7.3–7.7).

Many of the following drugs, doses or indications are unlicensed for use in children.

Table 7.3 Analgesics

Drug	Route	1month–1yr	2–12 yrs	12–18 yrs	Notes
Morphine	p.o./p.r.	100mcg/kg	200–400mcg/kg	10–15mg	4h starting doses
Diamorphine	CSCI	20–100mcg/kg/h	20–100mcg/kg/h	20–100mcg/kg/h	24h starting dose
	SC/IV stat	5–15mcg/kg[†]	5–15mcg/kg[†]	2.5–5mg	4-h as needed
Ibuprofen	p.o.	5mg/kg	5mg/kg	200–600mg	t.d.s.–q.d.s. Max. 2.4g/day

[†]These are very small doses. Recommendations in BNF:
1–3 months: 20mcg/kg 6 hourly
3–6 months: 25–50mcg/kg 6 hourly
6–12 months: 75mcg/kg 4 hourly
1–12 years: 75–100mcg/kg 4 hourly

Table 7.4 Antiemetics

Drug	Route	1 month–2yr	2–12yrs	12–18 yrs	Notes
Cyclizine	p.o./p.r.	1mg/kg t.d.s.	2–5yrs: 12.5mg t.d.s.	25–50mg t.d.s.	
Cyclizine	SC/iv continuous infusion	3mg/kg per 24h	2–5yrs: 50mg/24h 6–12yrs: 75mg/24h	150mg/24h (max.)	
Cyclizine	iv stat	500mcg–1mg/kg t.d.s. (max. 25mg)	500mcg–1mg/kg tds. <6yrs: max 25mg >6yrs: max 50mg	>12yrs: 50mg (t.d.s)	Give slowly over 3–5 minutes
Haloperidol	p.o.	12.5–50mcg/kg b.d.	12.5–50mcg/kg b.d.	0.5–2mg b.d.–t.d.s.	Increased risk of extrapyramidal side-effects in children lowers fit threshold.
Ondansetron	iv	5mg/m² b.d.–t.d.s. (max. 8mg)	5mg/m² b.d.–t.d.s. (max. 8mg)	8mg b.d.–t.d.s	Give over 3–5min. Can be given as continuous infusion
Ondansetron	p.o.	1mg b.d.–t.d.s –4mg	2–4yrs: 4mg b.d.–t.d.s. 4–12yrs: 4mg b.d.–t.d.s	8mg b.d.–t.d.s	
Metoclopramide	p.o./IM/slow IV/SC	100–170mcg/kg t.d.s.	100–170mcg/kg t.d.s.	100–170mcg/kg t.d.s.	Increased risk of extrapyramidal side-effects in children
Levomepromazine	p.o.		0.1–1mg/kg o.d.–b.d.	6.25–25mg o.d–b.d.	Very sedating in doses over 1mg/kg/24 h
Levomepromazine	SC/iv continuous infusion	0.1–0.25mg/kg (max. 25mg/24h)	0.1–0.25mg/kg (max. 25mg/24h)	0.1–0.25mg/kg (max. 25mg/24h)	

Table 7.5 Sedatives

Drug	Route	<1yr	1–12 yrs	12–18 yrs	Notes
Diazepam	p.o./p.r.	50–100mcg/kg per dose	50–100mcg/kg per dose	2.5–5mg b.d.	Repeated as needed
Lorazepam	p.o./sublingual	25–50 mcg/kg per dose	25–50mcg/kg per dose	25–50mcg/kg per dose	Max 4mg in 24 h
> Midazolam	CSCI SC/iv stat Buccal stat	1 month–18yrs: 2.5mg/24h 1 month–18yrs: 100mcg/kg 1 month–18yrs: 500mcg/kg (max 10mg)			

Table 7.6 Antisialogogue (for death rattle)

Drug	Route	2–18 yrs	Notes
Hyoscine hydrobromide	SC stat	1–12yrs: 10mcg/kg>12yrs (>40kg): 400mcg	Repeat every 4h as needed Sedating
Hyoscine hydrobromide	CSCI	40–60mcg/kg per 24h	Max dose 2400mcg/24h
Gycopyrronium	SC/iv stat	1month–18yrs: 4–8mcg/kg	Repeat every 6–8h as needed Doses for drooling much lower, max. 200mcg/dose
Gycopyrronium	CSCI	1month–18yrs: 10–40mcg/kg per 24hr	Max adult dose 1200mg/24h

Table 7.7 Average weights for healthy children

Age	Mean weight (kg)	% Adult dose
Newborn	3.5	12.5
6months	8	22
1yr	10	25
3yrs	15	33
5yrs	20	40
7yrs	25	50
12yrs	40	75
Adult male	70	100
Adult female	60	100

NB: weight in stones × 6 equals weight in kg.

The percentage adult dose should only be used as a rough guide when paediatric doses in mg/kg are not available.

Further reading

Books

Bluebond-Langner M. (1978) *The Private Worlds of Dying Children*. Princeton: Princeton University Press.

BNF (2007) *BNF for Children* (3rd edn). London: BMJ publishing group, RPS publishing and RCPCH.

Goldman A. (1994) *Care of the Dying Child*. Oxford: Oxford University Press.

Goldman A., Hain R., Liben S. (2006) *Oxford Textbook of Palliative Care for Children*. Oxford: Oxford University Press.

Herbert, M. (1996) *Supporting Bereaved and Dying Children and their Parents*. Leicester: BPS Books.

Jassah S. S. (2006) *Basic Symptom Control in Paediatric Palliative Care: The Rainbow Children's Hospice Guidelines* (6th edn). Loughborough: Rainbow Children's Hospice.

Lidstone V., *et al.* (2006) *Paediatric Palliative Care Guidelines*. (2nd edn) London: The South West London and the Surrey, West Sussex and Hampshire and Sussex Cancer Networks.

Orloff S., Huff S. (2004) *Homecare for Seriously Ill Children: A Manual for Parents*. Alexandria: CHI.

Royal Children's Hospital, Brisbane (1999) *A Practical Guide to Paediatric Oncology Palliative Care*. Brisbane: Royal Children's Hospital.

Royal College of Paediatrics and Child Health (2003) *Medicines for Children* (2nd edn). London: RCPCH.

Royal College of Paediatrics and Child Health (2004) *Withholding or Withdrawing Life-saving Treatment in Children* (2nd edn). London: RCPCH.

Articles

Leikin S. (1989) A proposal concerning decisions to forgo life-sustaining treatment for young people. *Journal of Pediatrics*, **115**: 17–22.

Liben S., Papadatou D., Wolfe J. (2008) Paediatric palliative care: challenges and emerging ideas. *Lancet*, **371**: 852–64.

Waechter E. H. (1971) Children's awareness of fatal illness. *American Journal of Nursing*, **7**: 1168–72.

Palliative care in non-malignant disease

Introduction

The majority of patients in the UK (over 90%) receiving specialist palliative in-patient care services have cancer. There is increasing recognition of the unmet need in patients with other progressive, incurable, non-malignant diagnoses which has been highlighted by recent publications. The Departments of Health in the UK are striving to redress this balance, dictating that all the patients with end-stage illness should have access to the services offered by multidisciplinary palliative care teams.

Specialist palliative care inpatient units have traditionally been wary about taking responsibility for patients in whom the prognosis is uncertain, with the fear that precious resources would become overburdened by patients with longer term chronic illness. Studies in motor neurone disease (MND), however, showed that patients did not 'block' specialist beds any more than any other patients, and most hospices now accept patients with MND and other progressive neurological diseases into their programmes. It was perhaps the emergence of AIDS in the mid-1980s that made all specialist units take notice of a group of dying patients for whom they felt obliged to take some responsibility.

Patients with end-stage non-malignant disease suffer from as many distressing symptoms as those with cancer. Despite this, there remains a lack of confidence in looking after patients with less familiar illnesses. This may partly stem from the fact that the dying phase is often different from that seen in cancer. It has been noted that the trajectories of illness fall into four general patterns.[1] Patients dying from cancer often have a plateau phase during which they tend to deteriorate gradually over time until the final three months of life, and usually it becomes obvious when the terminal phase is entered and when treatment and interventions can be aimed more at comfort. Patients dying from organ failure such as chronic heart or lung disease, on the other hand, are often deteriorating over a somewhat longer period, interspersed by acute episodes that may be better managed within a hospital environment, where acute care management is both appropriate and readily available. Patients with dementia and general frailty, however, generally have poor function from much earlier in the trajectory, and their care needs reflect this increased dependency. The fourth group is made up of people who suffer sudden, unexpected death.

This may highlight educational and training issues, but does not mean that the palliative care team should take over the role of other specialist teams. Rather they should work alongside specialists in the other fields, ensuring

1 Lunney J. R., et al. (2003) Patterns of functional decline at the end of life. *Journal of the American Medical Association*, **289**: 2387–92.

that the principles of palliative care are upheld and that patients and their families receive optimal treatment.

The percentage of the population over 65 years has increased and will continue to do so. The main causes of death are organ failure such as heart disease, cerebrovascular and neurological disorders and chronic respiratory disease making up approximately one-third of deaths, dementia, debility and frailty forming a further third and cancer making up one-quarter of deaths. Sudden death accounts for the final twelfth.[2] Palliative care teams will need to find a way to deliver appropriate care to all patients regardless of diagnosis. To this end, there is a higher percentage of patients with non-malignant disease in the hospice movement in the USA (20–30%) and there is evidence that this trend is increasing in the UK, particularly within hospital specialist palliative care services.

With increasing dialogue, partnership, research and funding, the vision of providing services where they are needed should be a realistic aim.

Prognosis in non-cancer

Several attempts have been made to develop prognostic indicators for non-cancer patients, in an attempt to plan the best palliative care for this diverse group. As with cancer prognostic schemes, a search has been made to find one or more measurable indices which could correlate with survival. However, the approach using a combination of functional ability and specific laboratory parameters seems to be the most fruitful so far. The Gold Standards Framework and the Royal College of General Practitioners have developed the Prognostic Indicator Guidance which is helpful.[2]

Palliative care in non-malignant respiratory disease

Introduction

- The course of chronic respiratory disease is often marked by slow, inexorable decline with prolonged periods of disabling dyspnoea, reducing exercise tolerance, recurrent hospital admissions and of premature death
- Symptoms in the late stages of disease can often be worse than those in patients with advanced lung cancer
- Patients also experience loss of dignity, social isolation and psychological problems, with increasing dependency on family and carers. Thus, a holistic approach to management is crucial
- Regardless of diagnosis, the needs of the dying patient should be met by palliative care services
- Barriers to the provision of excellent holistic end-of-life care include the highly unpredictable disease trajectories of non-malignant respiratory diseases and the failure to appreciate that these disorders are life-threatening

The potential requirement for palliative care in end-stage pulmonary disease

Respiratory disease accounted for 153 168 of 632 062 (24.2%) deaths in the United Kingdom in 1999 (Table 8a.1):

Table 8a.1 Deaths from respiratory disease in 1999

Condition	Deaths (%)
All respiratory disease	153 168 cases (100)
Pneumonia and TB	67 591 cases (44.1)
Cancer	35 879 cases (23.4)
Progressive non-malignant causes	39 939 cases (25.1)
COPD + asthma	(21.0)
Pulmonary circulatory disease	(4.1)
Pneumoconiosis	(0.8)
Cystic fibrosis	(0.1)
Sarcoidosis	(0.07)
Others (congenital, foreign body, etc.)	9759 cases (6.4)

It is predicted that chronic obstructive pulmonary disease (COPD) will be the third leading cause of death globally by 2020. Research into symptomatology, survival, appropriate care and utilization of services is needed if the needs of this population are to be met.

Terminal symptoms, quality of life, and survival of patients with end-stage pulmonary disease

Symptoms presenting in the final weeks and months of life include dyspnoea, cough, fever, haemoptysis, stridor and chest wall pain—a similar picture to symptoms experienced by patients with lung cancer.

The inability to predict disease trajectory in patients with non-malignant terminal disease makes end-of-life decisions difficult. Studies indicate that quality of life is at least as poor as those suffering from malignant lung disease.

Symptom pathophysiology and assessment

Less than 5% of patients with non-malignant disease die in hospices compared to at least 20% of lung cancer patients. More palliative care services are available to cancer patients.

Dyspnoea

Dyspnoea can be defined as difficult, uncomfortable or laboured breathing, or, when an individual feels the need for more air. It is the most frequently experienced symptom in those with end-stage respiratory disease and is multifactorial in origin.

Not clearly understood, the mechanism of dyspnoea has been described as a mismatch between central motor activity and incoming afferent information from chemo- and mechanoreceptors. A person's emotional state, personality and cognitive function also influence its perception.

A good history and examination is invaluable. (📖 See Chapter 6e.)

Recurrent aspiration

This is often a feature in the development of respiratory failure. There may be a bulbar cause, e.g. MND, CVA, or there may be repeated micro-aspiration leading to bronchiectasis.

The right main bronchus is the most direct path to the lungs, leading more commonly to right lower lobe infections. Diagnosis can be made clinically, on CXR or on barium swallow.

Treatment includes:
- Nursing in a semi-recumbent position
- Speech and language therapy assessment
- Thickened foods and fluid
- Nasogastric tube
- Treatment of the associated pneumonia with antibiotics and physiotherapy

Management of end-stage respiratory disease

The end-stage is not easy to recognize but usually comprises:
- Persistent dyspnoea despite maximal therapy
- Poor mobility and loss of independence
- Increased frequency of hospital admission
- Decreased improvements with repeated admission
- Expressions of fear, anxiety
- Panic attacks
- Concerns expressed about dying

Drugs for dyspnoea

Anxiolytics

Anxiety can exacerbate breathlessness. Clinical experience suggests that low-dose anxiolytics (diazepam) can result in improvements despite a lack of evidence.

Antidepressants

Tricyclic antidepressants and serotonin selective re-uptake inhibitors have been shown to be beneficial.

Oral opioids

- Site of action may be central (brainstem) or peripheral lung receptors, or they may help by decreasing anxiety. Opioids can cause serious side-effects such as CO_2 retention, nausea, drowsiness and respiratory depression, so care is needed
- A trial of opioid in COPD patients without CO_2 retention is appropriate with close monitoring
- Low doses and small increments should be used, e.g. 2.5mg morphine elixir 4 hourly
- Subcutaneous diamorphine can be used in patients unable to swallow
- In the terminal phase, opioid therapy is justified for the treatment of dyspnoea even in the presence of CO_2 retention

Mucolytics

N-Acetylcysteine can be used, as can steam inhalers and nebulized saline.

Palliative oxygen therapy

A significant proportion of patients will have resting hypoxia, although its degree may not correlate with the level of dyspnoea. Symptoms may be improved by oxygen. Even in the absence of hypoxia, oxygen may relieve dyspnoea in COPD patients.

Non-pharmacological measures

General

- Vaccinations—influenza and pneumococcal
- General nursing care—fan, open windows, regular repositioning, relief of constipation
- Good nutrition
- Physiotherapy—forced expiratory technique, controlled coughing, chest percussion
- Psychological support—aims to improve communication, recognize the impact of anxiety and depression, reduce delays in end-of-life

decision-making, provide strategies to relieve symptoms and maximize quality of life
- Pulmonary rehabilitation—participants enrol in a programme designed to optimize functional status and reduce symptoms through self-management education and training, psychosocial support and nutritional counselling
- Controlled breathing techniques—e.g. pursed lip/slow expiration
- Non-invasive mechanical ventilation—shown to decrease the need for intubation
- Lung reduction surgery—initial benefit in FEV_1, but lasts only 3–4 years
- Lung transplantation—emphysema is the most common indication

COPD

Pharmacological treatments

Bronchodilators
- Beta-2 agonists, e.g. salbutamol
- Anticholinergic agents (may aggravate prostatism or glaucoma), e.g. ipratropium bromide
- Inhaled bronchodilators ± spacers should be used where possible as nebulizers deliver medication less efficiently

Inhaled/oral steroids

These benefit 15–20% of patients with stable COPD. As such, a trial with steroids is indicated, where at least a 20% increase in FEV_1 would justify their continued use.

Theophylline

The pharmacokinetics of theophylline are unstable and there is a narrow therapeutic range. However, if used judiciously, it may have a place in COPD management.

Oxygen
- Has a definite place in the management of selected hypoxic patients
- Usually employed overnight, followed by intermittent daytime use through to continuous use
- Care needs to be taken where headaches, drowsiness or confusion appear, indicating potential carbon dioxide retention

Long-term oxygen therapy (LTOT)

This can extend life expectancy if administered for 12–15h per day, although there is a lack of evidence to support an increased quality of life.

Indications for LTOT:
- PaO_2 <7.3kPa when breathing air
- $PaCO_2$ may be normal or >6.0kPa
- Two measurements separated by 4 weeks when clinically stable
- Clinical stability = no exacerbations or peripheral oedema for four weeks
- FEV_1 <1.5L and FVC <2.0L
- Non-smokers
- PaO_2 between 7.3 and 8.0kPa, together with secondary polycythaemia, peripheral oedema or pulmonary hypertension
- Nocturnal hypoxia (SaO_2 below 90% for >30% of the night)
- Interstitial lung disease or pulmonary hypertension where PaO_2 <8kPa
- Palliation of terminal disease

Interstitial/fibrotic lung disease

These include:
- Idiopathic fibrotic disorders, e.g. idiopathic pulmonary fibrosis, autoimmune pulmonary fibrosis
- Connective tissue disorders, e.g. systemic lupus erythematosus (SLE), rheumatoid arthritis, scleroderma
- Drug-induced diseases, e.g. nitrofurantoin, amiodarone, gold, radiation
- Occupational, e.g. silicosis, asbestosis, farmer's lung
- Primary unclassified, e.g. sarcoidosis, amyloidosis, AIDS, adult respiratory distress syndrome (ARDS)

These conditions are, however, rare.

Treatment includes immunosuppressants such as steroids, cyclophosphamide, azathioprine and penicillamine with variable success.

Neuromuscular, restrictive and chest wall diseases

These cause respiratory muscle weakness or loss of compliance in the respiratory cage. Muscular function can be affected at various sites, from the spinal cord to the muscles themselves.

Features that characterize some of these conditions include:
- Increased ventilatory drive with inadequate ventilatory response
- Sleep disorders
- Unbalanced weakness of spinal and thoracic muscles leading to kyphoscoliosis
- Bulbar incoordination
- Diaphragmatic paralysis
- Pulmonary embolism

Supportive treatments
- Oxygen
- Antibiotics
- Physiotherapy
- Techniques to clear secretions
- Inspiratory muscle training
- Beta-2 agonists

Ventilatory support
This can include:
• Rocking beds
• Abdominal pneumatic belts
• Negative pressure body ventilators
• Non-invasive positive pressure ventilation
• Nasal continuous positive airways pressure

There have been many advances in this field, but many patients still choose to refuse such invasive treatments.

Bronchiectasis

Survival of patients has improved markedly with the advent of antibiotic therapy. Conditions associated with bronchiectasis include:
• Cystic fibrosis
• HIV infection
• Rheumatoid arthritis
• Infection, inflammation
• Bronchopulmonary sequestration
• Allergic bronchopulmonary aspergillosis
• Alpha1-antitrypsin deficiency
• Congenital cartilage deficiency
• Immunodeficiency
• Yellow nail syndrome
• Bronchial obstruction
• Unilateral hyperlucent lung

Diagnosis is usually made by high-resolution CT scanning.
Treatment involves:
• Antimicrobial drugs—directed by sputum microbiology, usually treated for longer periods
• Bronchodilator therapy
• Chest physiotherapy
• Nebulized recombinant human deoxyribonuclease
• Anti-inflammatory treatment
• Supplemental oxygen
• Immunoglobulin administration/enzyme replacement
• Surgery
• Management of haemoptysis
• Management of halitosis—e.g. broad-spectrum antibiotics, mouth and gum care

Cystic fibrosis

• Affects 1 in 2500 newborns
• Marked by alteration in ion and water transport across epithelial cells resulting in recurrent pulmonary infection, bronchiectasis, lung fibrosis and pancreatic insufficiency
• Most care takes place in specialized units with home support teams trained in the principles of palliative care

HIV-associated

Pulmonary complications:

- Bacterial, e.g. *Streptococcus pneumoniae*, *Pseudomonas aeruginosa*
- Mycobacterium, e.g. *M. tuberculosis*, M. avian complex
- Fungi, e.g. *Pneumocystis jiroveci* (formerly known as *Pneumocystis carinii*), *Cryptococcus neoformans*
- Viruses, e.g. cytomegalovirus
- Parasites e.g. *Toxoplasma gondii*
- Malignancies, e.g. Kaposi's sarcoma, non-Hodgkin's lymphoma
- Interstitial pneumonitis, e.g. lymphocytic pneumonitis
- Other, e.g. COPD, pulmonary hypertension

Tuberculosis

Recurrent reactivation results in severe pulmonary scarring, cavitation and secondary aspergillosis infection. If left unchecked, tuberculosis then results in respiratory failure, recurrent bacterial infection and massive haemoptysis.

Chronic bronchitis and emphysema

These conditions cause 80% of cases of pulmonary hypertension. Treatment usually involves:

- Oxygen
- Non-invasive ventilation
- Beta-2 agonists
- Diuretics in the management of fluid retention in the acute phase of cor pulmonale
- The use of pulmonary vasodilators is of doubtful significance

Obstructive pulmonary hypertension

- This is often caused by repetitive, silent pulmonary embolism. Other causes include vasculitis, sickle-cell anaemia and infective endocarditis
- Treatment can involve anticoagulation, and occasionally pulmonary thromboendarterectomy or the insertion of an inferior vena caval filter

Primary pulmonary hypertension

- Of unknown aetiology
- Symptoms can include progressive dyspnoea, decreased exercise tolerance, central chest pain and syncope
- Occasionally it is associated with haemoptysis, fluid accumulation and sudden death
- Treatment involves oxygen, anticoagulation and vasodilators such as hydralazine and nifedipine

Pulmonary embolism (📖 see Chapter 6l)

There is an increased incidence of thromboembolism in dependent, hospitalized patients.

- The triad of venous stasis, alteration in coagulation and vascular injury are fundamental in the pathogenesis
- Should be suspected with symptoms of dyspnoea, pleuritic pain and haemoptysis
- 40% of high-risk patients with proximal DVTs are asymptomatic when pulmonary embolism occurs

Investigation includes:

- Arterial blood gas (not commonly available in palliative inpatient units)
- ECG
- CXR
- Doppler ultrasonography/contrast venography
- V/Q scan
- Angiography
- Enhanced spiral CT scan

Prevention involves adequate hydration, promotion of mobility, the avoidance of venous obstruction, compression stockings and low molecular weight heparin (LMWH).

Treatment usually involves heparinization with LMWH and consideration of warfarinization, or vena-caval filters.

For patients with metastatic malignancy there is increasing evidence that warfarin is not as effective as LMWH. (📖 See Chapter 6l.)

Pneumothorax and pleural disease

Pathogenesis includes spontaneous and iatrogenic causes. Treatment usually involves intercostal tube drainage if appropriate, or oxygen, analgesia and opiates in the terminally ill.

- Causes of pleural effusion are multiple but include infection, cardiac failure, hypoalbuminaemia and renal impairment
- Treatment may consist of intermittent aspiration ± chemical pleurodesis
- Localized pleural pain may be secondary to rib fracture, infection or pneumothorax. It may respond to normal analgesia, or may require a local anaesthetic intercostal nerve block

Respiratory terminal care and palliative sedation

During the terminal phase, simple measures are important:

- Constant draught from fan or open window
- Regular sips of water
- Sitting upright

In the terminal stages, the emphasis changes from active interventions to supportive and symptomatic measures:

- Non-invasive ventilatory support and active physiotherapy may be withdrawn
- Drugs for palliating symptoms are often unavoidable
- The oral route should be used where possible, but failing this, drugs may be given by the subcutaneous route

The 'rattle' associated with loose respiratory secretions, although probably not distressing to the patient, may be addressed by re-positioning, or by the use of hyoscine hydrobromide or glycopyrronium bromide.

- As many patients approaching death with end-stage respiratory disease will have uncontrolled dyspnoea, sedation and opioid use should not be withheld because of an inappropriate fear of respiratory depression
- Options include benzodiazepines or opioids. The risks and benefits must be carefully considered and the justification for sedation clearly defined. Such decisions are often made by teams rather than individuals, and it is appropriate that patients and families are fully involved in the decision-making process

Further reading

Books

Ahmedzai S. (1998) Palliation of respiratory symptoms. In *Oxford Textbook of Palliative Medicine* (2nd edn) (ed. D. Doyle, G. Hanks, N. MacDonald). Oxford: Oxford University Press.

Ahmedzai S., Muers M. (eds) (2005) *Supportive Care in Respiratory Disease*. Oxford: Oxford University Press.

Back I. (2001) *Palliative Medicine Handbook* (3rd edn). Cardiff: BPM Books.

Davis C. L. Percy G. (2006) Breathlessness, cough and other respiratory problems. In *ABC of Palliative Care* (ed. M. Fallon, G. Hanks) 2nd edn. Oxford: Blackwell.

Doyle D., *et al* (eds). (2004) *Oxford Textbook of Palliative Medicine* (3rd edn). Oxford: Oxford University Press.

Fallon M. (ed.) *ABC of Palliative Care*. London: BMJ Books.

Watson M., Lucas C., Hoy A. (2003) *Adult Palliative Care Guidance* (2nd edn). London: The South West London and the Surrey, West Sussex and Hampshire Cancer Networks.

Wilcock A. (1997) *Dyspnoea*. In *Tutorials in Palliative Medicine* (ed. P. Kaye), pp. 211–33. Northampton: EPL Publications.

Articles

Elkington H., *et al.* (2005) The healthcare needs of chronic obstructive pulmonary disease patients in the last year of life. *Palliative Medicine*, **19**(6): 485–91.

Freeman D, Price D. (2006) ABC of chronic obstructive pulmonary disease. Primary care and palliative care. *British Medical Journal*, **333**(7560): 188–90.

Rocker G. M., *et al.* (2007) Advanced chronic obstructive pulmonary disease: innovative approaches to palliation. *Journal of Palliative Medicine*, **10**(3): 783–97.

Seamark D. A., *et al.* (2007) Palliative care in chronic obstructive pulmonary disease: a review for clinicians. *Journal of the Royal Society of Medicine* **100**(5): 225–33.

Solano J. P., *et al.* (2006) A comparison of symptom prevalence in far advanced cancer, AIDS, heart disease, chronic obstructive pulmonary disease and renal disease. *Journal of Pain and Symptom Management*, **31**(1): 58–69.

Heart failure

Definition

Chronic heart failure is a progressive, fatal syndrome and is the final common pathway of many cardiovascular diseases. The European Society of Cardiology defines heart failure as the presence of symptoms of heart failure at rest or during exercise, and objective evidence of cardiac dysfunction (usually on echocardiography).

Incidence

Heart failure is the only major cardiovascular disease with increasing incidence. It is predominantly a disease of old age (mean 75 years). There are 67,000 new cases per annum in the UK.[1] A diagnosis of heart failure has huge cost implications: patients with heart failure occupy up to 2% of all inpatient bed days and account for up to 2% of NHS costs (most of which are hospital not community).

Prognosis

An estimated 5% of all deaths in the UK (24000 per annum) are from heart failure. (Death certification explicitly discourages doctors from recording heart failure as a cause of death—the true number is probably much higher). Some 40% of patients die within one year of diagnosis; 50% of patients with heart failure die suddenly; and 25% without worsening of their heart failure symptoms. This can occur at any stage of the disease. There are no reliable prognostic models either for poor overall prognosis or sudden death.

Relevant pathology and physiology

Coronary artery disease and hypertension are the commonest causes of heart failure. The direct insult is of mechanical pump failure; however this initiates an ongoing, complex cascade of haemodynamic, metabolic, neuroendocrine and renal dysfunction that is the syndrome of chronic heart failure.

Clinical features (Table 8b.1)

Breathlessness and fatigue are the classic symptoms of heart failure. Orthopnoea is a sensitive 'measure' of fluid overload.

Fluid retention causes not only breathlessness, cough and dependent oedema, but also anorexia, nausea, abdominal bloating and pain.

---

1 Allender S., et al. (2007) Coronary heart disease statistics: (15th edn). London: BHF.

Other common symptoms which are poorly recognized and therefore frequently not treated include:

• Pain (common, severe, prolonged and distressing). Probably due to a combination of angina, liver capsule distension, lower limb swelling and co-morbid disease, e.g. arthritis
• Anxiety and depression (severe in one-third of hospitalized patients). Depression adversely affects mortality and hospital readmission[2]
• Disordered sleep
• Memory loss and confusion
• Anorexia, nausea, vomiting and constipation
• Weight loss (usually mild, but severe cachexia is a poor prognostic sign)
• Loss of libido

Poor information, communication and understanding for patients are widespread and contribute to psychological morbidity.

Significant functional impairment in activities of daily living and social isolation are common, long before the end of life. Despite this there is poor access to social and therapy services. The pattern of functional decline is slow, compared to the classic patient with cancer who exhibits a precipitous decline approximately five months before death.[3]

Disease burden

The burden of chronic heart failure has physical, psychological and social dimensions. These needs have been demonstrated to be prevalent, severe, prolonged and usually unrecognized and unrelieved.

The disparity in symptom control and support offered to those dying from heart failure compared to cancer is described tellingly by those who have lost a parent to each illness.

Table 8b.1 New York Heart Association (NYHA) functional classification (summary)

Class	Symptoms
I	Heart disease present, but no undue dyspnoea
II	Comfortable at rest; dyspnoea on ordinary activities
III	Less than ordinary activity causes dyspnoea, which is limiting
IV	Dyspnoea present at rest; all activity causes discomfort

2 Jiang W., *et al.* (2001) Relationship of depression to increased risk of mortality and rehospitalization in patients with congestive heart failure. *Archives of Internal Medicine*, **161**(15): 1849–56.

3 Teno J. M., *et al.* (2001) Dying trajectory in the last year of life: does cancer trajectory fit other diseases? *Journal of Palliative Medicine*, **4**(4): 457–64.

Management
Disease-specific management
Education of patients and carers, including dietary (salt intake, alcohol, weight), smoking and exercise advice.

The cornerstones of drug treatment are angiotensin-converting enzyme (ACE) inhibitors and beta-blockers. They both improve symptoms and slow disease progression. Diuretics are used to control fluid overload. Angiotensin-II antagonists, spironolactone and digoxin are used where appropriate.

Symptom management
1 Ensure specific heart failure treatments are optimal. This is the first step in achieving good symptom control. Diuretics may need quite frequent dose changes to control fluid overload. Avoid over-diuresis which may cause dizziness, nausea, poor sleep and fatigue.
2 Avoid, where possible, drugs which may worsen cardiac function. These include some drugs commonly prescribed in cancer palliative care practice. (☐ See Table 8b.2).

Table 8b.2 Key drugs to avoid in heart failure patients

Drugs	Reason for avoidance
Non-steroidal anti-inflammatory (NSAID)	Salt and water retention and worsen renal function
Tricyclic antidepressants	Cardiotoxic
Lithium	Salt and water retention
Cyclizine	Probably cardiotoxic
Steroids	Water retention
Progestogens	Water retention
Flecainide/mexiletine	Depress myocardial function

3 Actively seek out and manage other likely symptoms. Bear in mind the likely causes of symptoms in a patient with heart failure and their renal function.
   - **pain**: follow the WHO ladder. Avoid NSAIDs and alter opioid dosing schedules as per renal function
   - **nausea**: try haloperidol for a biochemical cause and metoclopramide for gastric stasis
   - **anxiety and depression**: treat conventionally (with or without drugs). Newer classes of antidepressant such as sertraline (an SSRI) and mirtazepine are safer than tricyclics. Both of these are less likely to affect cardiac conduction, cause postural hypotension or interact with other drugs
   - **breathlessness management**: may include correction of anaemia, low-dose opioids and the non-pharmacological approaches used in respiratory rehabilitation and lung cancer management

• **adopt a palliative approach:** to psychological, social, spiritual, information and communication needs, actively pursuing and managing identified needs. Patients and carers may need help to manage the uncertainty of a future with a high chance of sudden death

End-of-life care

Diagnosing dying in heart failure is extremely difficult. Here, the disease trajectory is of a steady decline punctuated by unexpected sudden death.

Features suggested as characterizing a subgroup of patients with a poor prognosis are:[4]

• Previous admissions with worsening heart failure
• No identifiable reversible precipitant
• Optimum tolerated conventional drugs
• Deteriorating renal function
• Failure to respond soon after admission to changes in vasodilators or diuretics

In these patients, invasive treatments and monitoring should be reviewed and emphasis on palliation should predominate. Discontinuing cardiac drugs may be appropriate (📖 see table 8b.3). When a patient is clearly dying, the use of a guideline such as the Liverpool care pathway for the dying patient[5] is recommended.

Table 8b.3 Heart failure drugs discontinuation strategy

Continue drugs for short-term benefit (morbidity)	Weigh up advantages/ disadvantages of continuing drugs with medium-term benefits (morbidity/mortality)	Discontinue drugs with only long-term benefit (mortality)
• Loop and thiazide diuretics	ACE inhibiter/A2A	Statins
	Beta-blockers	Digoxin
• Digoxin/beta-blockers in AF	Spironolactone	in sinus rhythm
• Antianginals		
	Drugs for co-morbidities: hypoglycaemics antihypertensives thyroxine warfarin	

A2A = angiotensin-II antagonist. Adapted from SWLS&PCG/SWLCN.

Decreasingly important for symptom control GIBBS (2006)

➤

4 Ellershaw J., Ward C. (2003) Care of the dying patients: the last hours or days of life. *British Medical Journal*, **326**: 30–4.

5 www.mcpcil.org.uk/liverpool_care_pathway.

Implantable cardioverter defibrillator (ICD)

- If the patient has an implantable cardioverter defibrillator (ICD) in place it is important to consider and, where appropriate, discuss with the patient and family when would be an appropriate time for a technician to switch this off. In an emergency situation an ICD can be deactivated by applying a large magnet to the area of the chest overlying the ICD

Useful resources

- British Heart Foundation (2007) discussion document on 'Implantable cardioverter defibrillators in patients who are reaching the end of life' (www.bhf.org.uk)
- www.heartrhythmcharity.org.uk/html/icd_deactivation.html

Models of care

Although chronic heart failure is increasingly being managed across the community/hospital interface by multiprofessional heart failure teams, most patients currently never see a heart failure specialist. These teams should aim to address the disease management and supportive and palliative care needs of the majority of patients with heart failure. The minority of patients with extraordinary palliative needs may need to have direct involvement from specialist palliative care services, often in collaboration with active heart failure team management. Mutual support and education, plus joint management by heart failure and specialist palliative care teams should be objectives for the future.

Diuretics

Furosemide is less effective when given orally rather than parenterally in heart failure, cirrhosis and probably any hypoalbuminaemic state. It is more affected by food intake than bumetanide, which may be better absorbed orally than furosemide. Continuous infusion of furosemide may be given IV and has been given by CSCI. Spironolactone is used for ascites, particularly when associated with liver metastases, steroid-induced fluid retention and possibly heart failure. Metolazone, a weak thiazide diuretic, can be used alone but it is also synergistic with furosemide.

Further reading

Books

Johnson M., Lehman R. (2006) *Heart Failure and Palliative Care*. Oxford: Radcliffe Publishing.

Symptom control guidelines and key information in end-stage heart failure (2008) South West London Supportive and Palliative Care Group and South West London Cardiac Network

Articles

Gibbs J. S. R., et al. (2002) Living with and dying from heart failure: the rôle of palliative care. *Heart*, **88** (Suppl. 2): ii36–ii39.

Goldstein N.E., et al. (2004) Management of implantable cardioverter defibrillators in end-of-life care. *Annals of Internal Medicine*, **141**: 835–8.

Harding R. (2008) Meeting the communication and information needs of Chronic Heart Failure patients. *Journal of Pain and Symptom Management*, **36**(2): 149–156.

Nicol E.D. (2008) NHS heart failure survey: a survey of acute heart failure admission in England Wales and N. Ireland. *Heart*, **94**: 172–177.

Remme W., Swedberg K. (2001) Task force for the diagnosis and treatment of chronic heart failure. *European Heart Journal*, **22**(17): 1527–60.

Ward C. (2002) The need for palliative care in the management of heart failure. *Heart*, **87**(3): 294–8.

Palliative care in non-malignant neurological disease

Multiple sclerosis (MS)

There are an estimated 80 000 to 90 000 people with multiple sclerosis in the UK. In the majority (70–80%), the course of the disease is relapsing and remitting in nature at the onset. Half of these patients will enter a progressive phase within 10 years (secondary progressive MS). In a smaller group of patients the disease is progressive from the onset (~15%). In a population of patients with MS approximately 20–30% have marked paraparesis, hemiparesis or paraplegia, 15% are wheelchair-bound and 5% have severe cognitive impairment. It is estimated that only about 25% of patients who are severely disabled are alive at 10 years.

Death is commonly due to various secondary complications of MS (e.g. aspiration pneumonia, pulmonary embolus). If a sudden neurological deterioration occurs, precipitating factors such as infection should be sought. If there is no resolution of symptoms, a course of steroids is usually given, which has a high chance of improving symptoms for a further year or so.

Symptom management

Immobility

Walking is usually affected if the disease is progressive, via a combination of weakness, spasticity, fatigue, disuse, pain, cerebellar ataxia and sensory loss, particularly proprioception. Immobility inevitably becomes difficult towards the end of life, leading to many problems, which need to be addressed by the majority of members of the multidisciplinary team.

Pain

Chronic pain may be present in 60–80% of patients and some studies have shown inadequate control in 40% of them, with significant adverse effects on their quality of life. Neuropathic pain, which may present as a persistent burning discomfort often affecting the lower limbs, is usually treated with standard agents for neuropathic pain such as the tricyclic antidepressants and pregabalin.

Trigeminal neuralgia is a common paroxysmal pain and is classically treated with carbamazepine. Gabapentin has also been used.

Neurosurgical procedures such as percutaneous denervation may be considered, although this may leave the patient with paraesthesiae.

Lhermitte's sign is a syndrome of intermittent burning sensations or 'electric shocks' occurring on neck flexion. It is probably due to demyelination in the posterior columns of the spinal cord, and can occur in up to two-thirds of patients at some time during the course of the disease. It is often self-limiting but, if persistent, a cervical collar and carbamazepine may be needed.

Musculoskeletal pain is common, particularly back pain, and results from prolonged immobility, poor posture and gait abnormalities. It is probably caused by a combination of spasticity leading to muscular pain and abnormal stresses resulting in mechanical pain. Osteoporosis should also be considered and treated as appropriate. Simple analgesics or NSAIDs can be prescribed. Physiotherapy is needed to improve poor posture and to ensure that correct seating and wheelchair adaptations are provided. Passive and active exercises, TENS, massage as well as acupuncture may also be helpful.

The use of cannabinoids for symptomatic pain relief and reduction of spasticity in MS is still discussed. While there is mainly no objective benefit, there is an unmistakable subjective benefit from cannabis treatment.

Spasticity

Increased muscle tone occurs in the majority of patients with MS. It may cause difficulty with function of the affected limb, painful muscle spasms and, when severe, difficulty in nursing care. Neurophysiotherapists teach patients and their carers stretching techniques for shortened spastic muscles and passive joint exercises to maintain movement, which should be carried out regularly. Splints may be used and TENS may alleviate the frequency of painful muscle spasms and improve sleep. Aggravating factors such as urinary tract infections, pressure sores and constipation should be avoided and/or treated.

Baclofen can be built up slowly by 5mg every few days starting from 5mg t.d.s. up to a maximum of 80mg daily. Transient neuropsychiatric and gastrointestinal symptoms may occur. Reduction of baclofen should be gradual to avoid fits or hallucinations. Intrathecal baclofen can be used for severe spasticity and muscle spasms if they are affecting quality of life and have proved unresponsive to other therapies.

Benzodiazepines such as diazepam can be given at night if painful spasms disturb sleep.

Dantrolene is less sedating than other muscle relaxants but can further weaken muscles and is therefore often reserved for those patients who are wheelchair-bound. Liver function should be monitored.

Tizanidine, an alternative to baclofen, is associated with less muscle weakness than baclofen or diazepam. The starting dose is 2mg increased every 3–4 days in 2mg increments up to 24mg daily in divided doses. It can cause sedation and dry mouth, and liver function should be monitored for the first four months. Gabapentin is an alternative.

Intramuscular botulinum toxin can be effective for focal spasticity that interferes with hygiene or nursing care. It is generally only used when maintenance of function is less important, and should always be accompanied by a physiotherapy regime of passive stretching.

Tenotomies (surgical release of tendons) or other nerve blocks—most commonly obturator, perineal, adductor, or pudendal—may be needed.

Ataxia and tremor

Feeding, correct seating and head control can be very difficult. The role of the occupational therapist is crucial. There is some evidence, although minimal, for the benefits of propranolol and clonazepam. Severe tremor can be treated with stereotactic thalamotomy, but with initial benefit only. Other techniques of deep brain stimulation may be promising.

Urinary system

Assessment and treatment is important in order to improve symptoms and to minimize complications such as pressure atrophy of the kidneys, urinary tract infections and skin breakdown secondary to incontinence. Incontinence can lead to profound embarrassment and social isolation. Adequate fluid intake, bladder emptying (particularly if residual volume is more than 100mL) and treatment of infection are the principal priorities.

Hyperreflexia of the bladder is associated with a low capacity bladder and possible symptoms of mild urgency, frequency and incontinence. Treatment is usually with anticholinergic drugs such as oxybutinin or tolterodine. Incomplete bladder emptying, induced by these drugs, may require intermittent self-catheterization. Nocturnal incontinence may be relieved with desmopressin nasal spray 10–40mcg at night. If the overactive bladder is resistant to conventional management, transvesical phenol capsaicin may provide some benefit.

Bladder hypotonia and sphincter dyssynergia (sphincter contracts when voiding) results in incomplete emptying, of which the patient may be unaware. Catheterization will be needed. Intermittent catheterization is associated with less risk of UTI than a permanent indwelling catheter. However, the latter may be needed if all other methods fail to fully empty the bladder frequently enough to avoid problems. Even with a permanent catheter, an anticholinergic may still be needed for bladder spasm and urinary bypassing. If all else fails a urinary diversion may be the only viable option.

Constipation

Constipation is common due in large degree to delayed gut transit time, immobility and anticholinergic medication. Adequate dietary fibre and fluid intake are important, and regular oral laxatives or suppositories/enemas are frequently needed.

Fatigue

Fatigue is severe and disabling in the majority of patients, reflecting muscle weakness and sleep interruption (e.g. from nocturia or spasms). It presents as overwhelming tiredness which is not relieved by exercise or rest. It does not necessarily directly correlate with mood disturbance or the severity of the MS.

Precipitants such as exposure to hot baths and hot weather should be avoided. Amantadine and modafinil offer modest benefit. Explanation, reassurance and advice on modification of lifestyle, such as pacing activities, taking rest periods and gentle exercise, are essential. High-dose aspirin may have a modest effect on fatigue in MS.

Mood/cognitive disturbance

Clinical depression is common in MS. The estimated lifetime risk of developing depression is 50% and the risk of suicide is 7.5 times that of the healthy population. Depression is contributed to by many factors including the breakdown in family relationships, public embarrassment, social isolation and other losses of work, money, sexual abilities and confidence.

Antidepressants should be selected according to their side-effect profile; for example, a tricyclic antidepressant might be used if an overactive bladder and additional neuropathic pain are a problem. Conversely, an SSRI which is less sedating than a tricyclic would be preferable if the patient feels fatigued. Pseudobulbar affect (pathological laughing and crying), which occurs in up to 10% of patients, may be treated with dextromethorphan and quinidine. SSRIs may also be effective.

There is some degree of cognitive impairment in 50–60% of patients. The most common deficits relate to short-term memory, attention and speed of processing information and impaired learning. Personality and behaviour may change. Moderate to severe dementia is seen in 10% of patients with long-standing MS. Treatment with donepezil and cognitive rehabilitation may give some benefit.

Multiple sclerosis is usually only managed in late advanced-stage disease by specialist palliative care teams, although they may have an earlier role in providing respite. The principles of palliative care apply through the illness trajectory and should aim to provide the best and most acceptable quality of life for the individual. Therefore, good symptom control and support for families are paramount.

Further reading

Articles

Ben-Zacharia A. B., Lublin F. D. (2001) Palliative care in patients with multiple sclerosis. *Neurologic Clinics*, **19**(1): 801–27.

Elman L. B., *et al.* (2007) Palliative care in amyotrophic lateral sclerosis, Parkinson's disease, and multiple sclerosis. *Journal of Palliative Medicine*, **10**(2): 433–57.

Gibson J., Frank A. O. (2003) Supporting individuals with disabling multiple sclerosis. *Journal of the Royal Society of Medicine*, **96**(5): 256–7.

Parkinson's disease

Parkinson's Disease (PD) is the commonest neurodegenerative disease, after Alzheimer's disease, with an estimated incidence of 2/1000. It affects just under 1% of people over the age of 65 years. PD is probably not one disease but several with common clinical features.

Criteria for the diagnosis of Parkinson's disease

Bradykinesia (slowness and progressive decrease of amplitude of movement) plus at least one of the following:

- Tremor (frequently 'pill rolling')
- Rigidity (often cogwheeling in nature), or
- Disorders of posture (flexion of neck and trunk)
- Disorders of balance (loss of righting reflexes)
- Disorders of gait (short steps, shuffling, festination and freezing)

Classical pathological lesions seen in PD include loss of dopaminergic neurones in the substantia nigra and locus coerulus with formation of Lewy bodies in the cytoplasm. Degeneration of the nigrostriatal pathway leads to depletion of the neurotransmitter dopamine.

The aetiology is unknown, although neurotoxins such as 1-methyl-4-phenyl-1,2,3,6-tetrahydropyridine (MPTP), pesticides and herbicides have been linked to causation. First-degree relatives have a two- to threefold risk of developing PD.

Management

Research is underway into transplantation of human and animal fetal cells, allogeneic stem cells or retinal dopaminergic cells, and therapy with nerve growth factors.

Surgical options, such as subthalamic nucleus (STN) lesions, may be effective for disabling dyskinesias (abnormal, involuntary movements), relieving rigidity and tremor. Alternatively, deep brain stimulation using implantable electrodes and a pacemaker-like generator may be used, allowing flexibility to modify the response and reduce side-effects.

The mainstay of management is the pharmacological control of symptoms with the aim of achieving optimal quality of life. Patients with PD should be monitored by doctors and teams specializing in PD, who should be alerted if there are any changes to the basic clinical pattern; any reversible factors adversely affecting the PD should be pursued and subtle changes in medication advised, where appropriate.

Motor symptoms

Levodopa preparations

Dopamine does not cross the blood–brain barrier (BBB). To circumvent this problem, levodopa, which is able to cross the BBB, is used. Levodopa is converted to dopamine by the enzyme aromatic-L-amino-acid decarboxylase. The striatum is thus provided with the essential dopamine. However, the presence of too much dopamine outside the blood–brain barrier causes side-effects such as nausea. To circumvent this problem, inhibitors of the converting enzyme, which do not cross the BBB, are given to reduce peripheral dopamine. Carbidopa and benserazide are used in this way and combined with levodopa as the preparations Sinemet and Madopar, respectively.

These compounds are available as modified-release and immediate-release preparations. They are also available in a dispersible form to aid administration with an oral syringe or through a nasogastric or gastrostomy tube where necessary. The timing of medication and dose are individualized, some patients benefiting from a 'kick start' dose in the mornings and others by avoiding late-night medication which may interfere with sleep. Others benefit from long-acting medication at night to reduce painful stiffness. Any changes in dose should be undertaken slowly, allowing several weeks for the change in regimen to stabilize. The drugs should never be withdrawn unless severe side-effects develop, since withdrawal may render patients unable to move, swallow and adequately protect their airway.

Unfortunately, the efficacy of levodopa is marred by unwanted actions that become progressively more prominent with advancing disease. These patients may develop severe drug-induced dyskinesia, often alternating with sudden unpredictable loss of mobility (that is, freezing and hesitancy).

Dopamine agonists

These act directly on dopamine receptors and include bromocriptine, pergolide, ropinerole, pramipexole and cabergoline. Lisuride is rarely used in the UK. The new dopamine agonist rotigotine is available as a transdermal patch. However, they are more likely than levodopa to cause dopaminergic side-effects such as nausea, vomiting, drowsiness, hallucinations and confusion and should be titrated up slowly; cover with domperidone may be needed to treat the nausea.

Apomorphine is usually administered subcutaneously, either as boluses or as a continuous infusion using a portable minipump. Its rapid onset of action can 'rescue' patients from sudden 'off' periods. This drug is most commonly reserved for patients experiencing severe and frequent motor fluctuations despite adequate trials with other oral medications. Domperidone is needed for three days prior to starting treatment to prevent nausea. Painful nodules which ulcerate may develop and sites of injection should be changed daily. Apomorphine treatment should be guided by a specialist in PD.

Drugs that delay the breakdown of levodopa

Entacapone and tolcapone delay levodopa breakdown by inhibiting the enzyme catechol-O-methyl transferase (COMT). It usually relieves motor fluctuations and allows dose reduction of levodopa-containing drugs.

Anticholinergics

These are sometimes effective for tremor but not bradykinesia and rigidity. Dry mouth, urinary retention, drowsiness and confusion often limit their usefulness.

Glutamate inhibitors (e.g. amantadine)

Amantadine may help rigidity and bradykinesia. It can be useful as an adjunctive therapy and may be beneficial in reducing levodopa-induced dyskinesias. Common side-effects include peripheral oedema, livedo reticularis and hallucinations. It is sometimes used as an infusion before or after an operation, when patients are unable to take the regular drugs.

Monoamine oxidase type B selective inhibitor (selegeline, rasagiline)

This inhibitor boosts the dopamine available in the brain by reducing its metabolism, and may be useful symptomatically. It seems that rasagiline has a neuroprotective role. Selegeline is available as both an oral and a buccal melt preparation.

Other general measures for management of motor symptoms include input from members of the multidisciplinary team, particularly the physiotherapist, occupational therapist, speech therapist and dietician.

Nausea and vomiting

This may be due to drug treatment for PD or for another unrelated reason. Neuroleptics should not be used, in particular haloperidol, metoclopramide and prochlorperazine. (Most phenothiazines should be avoided since they may aggravate PD, except for clozapine and quetiapine which do not have extrapyramidal side-effects.) The safest drug to use is domperidone which can be given orally or rectally. A 5-HT$_3$ inhibitor such as ondansetron is also well tolerated and may even relief psychosis.

Depression

This may occur in 40% of patients with PD. It is not known whether it is an inherent feature of PD or secondary to the disability caused by PD. Therapy should start with a selective serotonin re-uptake inhibitor (SSRI) in a low dose. However, it may worsen symptoms of PD and can cause postural hypotension. Mirtazapine has proved helpful in relieving depression and anxiety and reducing tremor. Tricyclic antidepressants are less used because of their cognitive side-effects.

Constipation

This may be caused by a lack of adequate neurotransmitter in the myenteric plexus. Advice on diet, adequate fluids and exercise should be given. Aperients are usually needed.

Swallowing difficulties

The ability to take food, chew and swallow may vary during the day, especially in more advanced disease. A speech and language therapist may be able to analyse the cause of the difficulty and to provide useful advice. A dietician may be required to advise on diet. The occupational therapist can also help by providing appropriate feeding implements. Special seating and head and neck supports may be required.

Patients often lose a significant amount of weight in late-stage PD, since the severe dyskinesias use up a significant amount of calorific energy. Feeding difficulties are often associated with periods of motor disability. Patients may choose to use their good functional moments to attend to activities of daily living (ADL) or to pursue what they want to do, rather than wasting these precious moments on eating. They should be advised to eat little and often to make efficient use of time and energy intake.

A deterioration of PD can be triggered by minimal dehydration and patients should be encouraged to drink adequately, especially in hot weather. High calorific drinks and other nutritional additives are useful to supplement an often inadequate diet.

Urinary urgency and nocturia

Urinary urgency may be helped with drugs such as tolterodine, oxybutynin and trospium. Severe distressing nocturia may be helped by a nocturnal dose of desmopressin, but care should be taken to ensure that hyponatraemia and congestive cardiac failure are not induced by this treatment.

Postural hypotension

Patients should be given general advice on rising carefully from a lying or sitting position. It may be helpful to raise the head of the bed and some patients may tolerate compression stockings. If symptoms are severe, fludrocortisone may be needed. If dizziness is experienced, encourage the patient to take a full glass of water with medication, especially with the first dose of the day.

Sleep

Sleep disorders occur in 70–80% of patients with PD and are distressing for patients and carers alike. The patient may be awoken by motor fluctuations; they may wake up and be unable to move and any effort to turn may cause painful muscle spasms; painful neck extension and leg cramp may occur. Attempts should be made to maintain nocturnal levels of levodopa, including avoiding high protein meals in the late evening (amino acids compete with dopamine for receptor sites) and by giving domperidone in the evenings (if needed) to avoid a delay in gastric emptying. Restless leg syndrome (RLS), characterized by an urge to move the legs, with painful cramps, paraesthesiae and a burning sensation in the calves may be relieved by standard levodopa therapy and dopamine agonists.

Amantadine and selegeline are stimulant and should be avoided if at all possible in the evenings. If PD is associated with dementia a reversal of the sleep–wake cycle may occur. Short-acting hypnotics can be used if necessary. Hallucinations and panic attacks may also keep patients awake at night, which may be due to dopamine agonists and other antiparkinsonian medication therapy. (☐ See the Confusion/hallucinations section, p. 518).

Communication

Difficulties in communication can be very distressing, especially if the patient is cognitively intact but has unpredictable episodes of being unable to communicate adequately. As with other symptoms in PD, it may worsen in stressful situations. Impaired emotional expression (mask-like facies), so characteristic of PD, impairs the very important non-verbal aspects of communication and should be recognized. Speech therapists can be helpful in improving symptoms.

Dementia

May occur in up to 40% of patients. The deficiency of acetylcholine has provided a rationale for the use of acetylcholine esterase inhibitors. Modest improvement is seen with donepezil and rivastigmine.

Confusion/hallucinations

This may occur as part of the PD itself or as a result of medication. Nocturnal hallucinations are a particular problem but may improve if medication is avoided just prior to sleep. Patients will sometimes tolerate a degree of hallucinosis provided that the other features of the disease, such as motor disability, are reasonably well controlled. The newer antipsychotic agents such as clozapine (beware agranulocytosis), risperidone or olanzapine may help, although they should be avoided if there is cerebrovascular disease. Quetiapine is a very useful medication and may be the drug of choice in this regard, but for some is too sedating. Antimuscarinics should be avoided if possible. All medication may have to be reduced if symptoms persist. The anti-dementia drugs—such as donepezil, rivastigmine, galantamine and memantine—are proving very effective in suppressing drug-induced hallucinations and confusion.

Pain

Pain is a feature of PD and may be relieved by treating the stiffness with levodopa or dopamine agonists. Pain of a sensory nature often occurs in PD and should be treated appropriately. It is important to remember that patients, if demented, may not be able to communicate the presence of pain. Opioids should be used as appropriate while recognizing the increased risk of constipation.

Anxiety

This occurs in 40% of patients but in over 90% of depressed patients with PD. Symptoms of PD such as tremor and dyskinesia often worsen in situations induced by anxiety or emotional excitement (even by watching a television programme). Although a benzodiazepine may help, it may result in muscle weakness and falls due to loss of muscle tone. Very small doses such as diazepam 1mg b.d. or lorazepam can be effective, therefore the dosage should be carefully titrated from this low start dose.

The terminal phase

PD may worsen with infection, dehydration or other illnesses. Any reversible factors should be corrected where appropriate alongside the management of the PD itself, preferably in a specialist centre. Care and consideration needs to be given to continuing on the antiparkinsonian drugs for as long as possible in order to keep patients as comfortable as possible and able to communicate and swallow. However, if the patient develops distressing side-effects from the medication, withdrawal of therapy may be in the patient's best interests.

All patients should be encouraged, with help from the family and professionals, to discuss their attitudes and wishes for the management of acute life-threatening medical problems that may occur, such as pneumonia. An advance decision may be helpful in ascertaining patients' wishes for interventions (see Chapter 19a Legal and Professional Standards of Care).

Multiple system atrophy (MSA)

MSA, a progressive neurodegenerative disorder, results in autonomic dysfunction in addition to parkinsonian and, at times, cerebellar features. It is not hereditary and affects adults usually in the fourth or fifth decade. Post-mortem studies of patients diagnosed with PD indicate that between 10 and 25% had multiple system atrophy. It is poorly responsive to levodopa. The mean survival is nine years. As with PD, a multidisciplinary approach is essential.

Progressive supranuclear palsy (PSP)

PSP is the most common cause of an atypical parkinsonian syndrome with dementia. It occurs more commonly in men than women, with a peak incidence in the early 60s. PSP comprises postural instability associated with parkinsonism, vertical gaze palsy, bradyphrenia and progressive subcortical dementia. Patients are limited in their ability to move their eyes downwards on request, although the eyes are able to move downwards reflexly, such as when a patient is asked to stare at a stationary object and the head is gently rotated backwards.

Limited upwards eye movement is also common in PSP, but is not diagnostic. Within one year of diagnosis the majority of patients have frequent falls, are slow in performing ADLs (bradykinesia) and have speech difficulties. Some 25% are confined to a wheelchair by one year following diagnosis, increasing to 70% by four years. The mean duration of the illness is 4–6 years, though this is often shorter in older patients. PSP worsens usually with respiratory tract infections, hence antibiotic treatment should be given. Some patients who are referred to the ICU and intubated manage to recover with physical restitution.

Further reading

Articles

Bunting-Perry L. K. (2006) Palliative care in Parkinson's disease: implications for neuroscience nursing. *Journal of Neuroscience Nursing*, **38**(2): 106–13.

Clarke C. E. (2007) Parkinson's disease. *British Medical Journal*, **335**(7617): 441–5.

De Simone G., *et al.* (2006) Atropine drops for drooling: a randomized controlled trial. *Palliative Medicine*, **20**(7): 665–71.

Global Parkinson's Disease Survey (GPDS) Steering Committee (2002) Factors impacting on quality of life in Parkinson's disease: results from an international survey. *Movement Disorders*, **17**(1): 60–7.

Horstink M., *et al.* (2006) Review of the therapeutic management of Parkinson's disease. Report of a joint task force of the European Federation of Neurological Societies (EFNS) and the Movement Disorder Society—European Section (MDS-ES). Part II: Late (complicated) Parkinson's disease. *European Journal of Neurology*, **13**(11): 1186–202.

Olanow C. W. (2001) An algorithm (decision tree) for the management of Parkinson's Disease: treatment guidelines. *Neurology*, **26**(11, Suppl. 5): S1–S88.

Rascol O., *et al.* (2002) Treatment interventions for Parkinson's Disease: an evidence-based assessment. *Lancet*, **359**(9317): 1589–98.

Scott S. (2002) *Swallowing Problems and Parkinson's*. PDS Information Sheet 52. London: PDS.

Voelker R. (2006) Parkinson's disease guidelines, aid diagnosis, management. *Journal of the American Medical Association*, **10**(295): 2126–8.

Motor neurone disease

> When I wake each morning I decide...
> This can be a good day or a bad day—my choice.
> I can be happy or sad—my choice.
> I can complain or I can cope—my choice.
> Life can be a chore or a challenge—my choice.
> I can take from life or give to life—my choice.
> If all things are possible,
> How I deal with those possibilities is—my choice.
>
> Steve Shackel, diagnosed with MND (alternatively referred to as 'amyo-
> trophic lateral sclerosis' (ALS))[1]

Motor neurone disease (MND) is a family of diseases of unknown aetiology in which there is progressive degeneration of upper and/or lower
motor neurones, leading to wasting of muscles and weakness. The average survival is 40% at five years, although older patients presenting predominantly with bulbar signs may have a worse prognosis and conversely,
younger patients with largely lower motor neurone involvement may have
a better than average prognosis. The mean age of onset is 56 years.

Upper motor neurone involvement leads to generalized spasticity,
hyperreflexia, pathologic reflexes and often emotional lability (i.e. pseudobulbar affect).

Lower motor neurone involvement leads to weakness, muscle wasting, reduced muscle tone, hyporeflexia and fasciculation.

Involvement of bulbar innervated muscles leads to dysarthria and
dysphagia. The third, fourth and sixth cranial nerves and those of the lower
segments of the spinal cord are usually spared, such that eye movements,
bladder, bowel and sexual function are generally unaffected. Furthermore
intellect, memory, sight and hearing are also usually preserved.

Symptoms in MND are often similar to those in patients with cancer and
include:
- Weakness (100%)
- Constipation (65%)
- Pain (50–60%)
- Cough (50–60%)
- Insomnia (40–50%)
- Breathlessness (40–50%)
- Dribbling (30–40%)
- Anxiety and depression

In addition, problems related to mobility, communication and psychosocial
issues, both for the patient and their families, must be addressed, necessitating a fully multidisciplinary approach.

---

1 http://home.goulburn.net.au/~shack

Management

Extensive research has been conducted into stem-cell transplantation, autologous mesenchymal stem cells and allogeneic haemopoietic stem cells, but the therapeutic potential remains uncertain.

Riluzole, the only drug approved for the treatment of ALS slows the disease progression and extends survival and tracheotomy-free life by an average of 3 months.

Symptoms

Weakness

Attention to individual needs for maximum comfort is crucial in order to prevent pain and other problems such as contractures and joint dislocation. The role of the physiotherapist is important, not only for the patient but also to educate and advise relatives. Although it is important to maintain muscle function and to keep joints mobile, overenthusiastic physiotherapy may tire the patient and be counterproductive.

Insomnia

It is important to ascertain the cause of insomnia, which may range from pain and depression to the overwhelming anxieties of choking and the fear of dying. There is a general reluctance to prescribe night sedatives to patients with MND for fear of respiratory depression. In practice this rarely happens, and is insignificant in relation to the morbidity associated with chronic fatigue.

Respiratory insufficiency

Hypoventilation develops due to diaphragmatic and intercostal muscle weakness. The symptoms of respiratory insufficiency are dyspnoea, day-time sleepiness and weak cough. Non-invasive positive pressure ventilation (NIPPV) has been shown to improve quality of life and prolong survival. Bilevel positive air pressure (BiPAP) reduces the breathing work by regulating the positive end-expiratory pressure in response to the patient's initial breaths. Generally, it is initially used during sleep time. Respiratory infections should be treated, and a cough-assist device can be used to clear secretions.

Pseudobulbar affect

Pseudobulbar affect which is also know as 'uncontrolled laughing or crying' is present in up to 50% of patients. The patient and the family find this symptom quite disturbing. A selective serotonin re-uptake inhibitor (SSRI) might be effective as early as 48 hours after beginning the therapy. Amitriptyline may also provide some improvement.

Pain

Management of the cause of pain
- Stiff joints—careful positioning/physiotherapy
- Inflammation—NSAID
- Joint pains—Intra-articular steroid injections
- Muscle cramp—quinine sulphate (quinine in tonic water)
- Muscle spasm—diazepam/baclofen
- Skin pressure—regular turning/turning beds, analgesic ladder

Neuropathic pain is not a common feature of MND per se. However, patients may complain of pain associated with sensory disturbance, in which case tricyclic antidepressants may help.

The use of opioids in MND

There has been a reluctance to prescribe opioids for fear of causing respiratory depression in patients whose lung function may already be compromised. However, one study showed that over 80% of patients had been treated with morphine without detriment.

Dysphagia

A speech therapist will help in analysing the exact cause of dysphagia in order to recommend specific techniques to aid swallowing. Spasticity of the tongue causing difficulty in propelling a food bolus to the pharynx is a common cause.

Ice packs applied to the neck or chips of ice placed in the mouth may result in relaxation of the tongue and ease swallowing.

The subject of artificial feeding via a gastrostomy tube should be discussed with the patient and the advantages and disadvantages outlined. In end-stage disease, tube feeding may not necessarily prolong life. However, earlier in the disease, particularly if the patient is ambulant, gastrostomy feeding may slow the inevitable weight loss and its associated weakness and depression.

The dietician will advise on food consistency and general nutritional requirements, and the speech therapist on the timing of endoscopic percutaneous gastrostomy tube insertion.

Dysarthria

The speech therapist should be involved early on to teach the patient various techniques relevant to his/her own special needs. Various aids are available and include Lightwriters with or without synthesized voice function. Other computerized systems are available from specialized centres, including electronic equipment, telephone devices and communication boards which may be adapted to the physical abilities of the individual patient. It is essential to plan ahead since motor function may deteriorate rapidly.

Breathlessness

This is due to diaphragmatic and respiratory muscle weakness. The physiotherapist may suggest breathing techniques and help with chest drainage if appropriate. Antibiotics may be useful in controlling symptoms but if the patient is in a terminal stage they may be inappropriate, serving only to prolong dying.

Nocturnal hypoventilation is characterized by poor sleep and nightmares, early morning headaches and daytime tiredness with subsequent impaired concentration. In early stage disease, it may be appropriate to consider some form of limited ventilatory assistance, such as NIPPV, to aid respiration at night-time. As breathing becomes weaker, this form of ventilation may continue during the day.

Patients must be fully informed of the pros and cons of assisted ventilation. More invasive ventilation through a tracheostomy is generally not used in the UK. The wishes of patients for respiratory support should be discussed well in advance of acute problems arising. Patients with MND may die suddenly and unexpectedly with respiratory failure.

Choking

The normal reflexes which protect the airway are impaired so that swallowing food or saliva may result in choking. Although it is a common fear, patients rarely, if ever, die as a result of choking. Speech therapists may help by advising different techniques for protecting the airway such as chewing carefully and slowly, breathing in, swallowing and then deliberately coughing. This technique serves to clear the larynx and to minimize the possibility of choking.

Some patients find suction to the upper airways useful. For others it is avoided, since it not only causes trauma, fright and discomfort but may also be very distressing for the relatives to witness.

The Motor Neurone Disease Association (MNDA) supplies a box known as a Breathing Space Kit which provides support for patients and carers. It is a small box with two drawers which contain drugs prescribed by the GP. One side may contain rectal diazepam for the family to administer in an emergency and the other side, drugs such as diamorphine, hyoscine and diazepam, for the doctor or nurse to give.

The multidisciplinary team

All members of the team will have been involved in the care of a patient with MND at some time. These include the neurologist, physiotherapist, occupational therapist, speech therapist, dietician, case manager, GP, district nurse, social worker, palliative physician, palliative home care team and of course, the family or carer.

The MNDA provides an invaluable service not only in terms of liaising, supporting and educating patients and carers but also in facilitating the loan of equipment and helping financially.

Further reading

Book

Oliver D., Borasio G., Walsh D. (2006) *Palliative Care in Amyotrophic Lateral Sclerosis: from diagnosis to barearement* (2nd ed). Oxford: Oxford University Press.

Articles

Dawson S., Kristjanson L. (2003) Mapping the journey: family carer's perceptions of issues related to end stage care of individuals with Muscular Dystrophy or Motor Neurone Disease. *Journal of Palliative Care*, **19**(1): 36–42.

Leigh N., *et al.* (2001) Motor neurone disease. *European Journal of Palliative Care*, **8**(1): 10–12.

McDermott C., Shaw P. (2008) Diagnosis and management of motor neurone disease. *British Medical Journal*, **336**: 658–62.

Mitchell J. D., Borasio G. D. (2007) Amyotrophic lateral sclerosis. *Lancet* **369**: 2031–44.

MNDA. (2006) Nutritional management in MND/ALS patients: An evidence based review. London: MNDA

Oliver D. (1998) Opioid medication in the palliative care of motor neurone disease. *Palliative Medicine*, **12**(2): 113–15.

Polkey M. I., *et al.* (1999) Ethical and clinical issues in the use of home non-invasive mechanical ventilation for the palliation of breathlessness in motor neurone disease. *Thorax*, **54**(4): 367–71.

Neurological complications of AIDS

Prevalence: up to 65%.

AIDS dementia complex

- A syndrome of progressive cognitive loss with motor and behavioural dysfunction in HIV-infected patients
- Clinical features: apathy, social withdrawal, impaired concentration, slowing of speech and movement, unsteady gait, can progress to being bedridden with tetraparesis, urinary and faecal incontinence
- Investigations:
  - need to exclude opportunistic infection with toxoplasmosis or CMV
  - CT scan—cerebral atrophy and ventricular enlargement
  - MRI scan—white matter abnormality
- Management: antiretroviral drugs may improve the symptoms and prolong survival

Vacuolar myelopathy

- Aetiology: unclear but vacuolization of the white matter in spinal cord is seen at post-mortem
- Clinical features: progressive weakness, spasticity and ataxia, as well as urinary and faecal incontinence
- Management: no current treatment

Peripheral neuropathy

- Distal symmetrical polyneuropathy is the most common feature and may occur in 10–30% of cases. It is characterized by a symmetrical distal painful sensory loss which is associated with weight loss and dementia
- Management: trial of amitriptyline, gabapentin, pregabalin
- Inflammatory demyelinating neuropathy is characterized by progressive weakness and loss of tendon reflexes. It is usually mild
- Inflammatory polyradiculopathy can be due to CMV infection and is characterized by a progressive distal weakness, sensory problems and incontinence
- Management: consider corticosteroids and immunoglobulins
- Cranial nerve neuropathy, can involve the facial nerve

HIV-associated myopathy

Symptoms are progressive with symmetrical painless weakness of the proximal limbs and facial muscles.

- Investigations: electromyography (EMG), muscle biopsy
- Management: consider corticosteroids and plasmapheresis

Opportunistic infections of the CNS

- Common organisms: *Toxoplasmosis gondii*, *Cryptococcus neoformans*, JC (John Cunningham) virus, CMV
- Clinical features: headache, confusion, fever, seizures, focal signs
- Investigations: CT scan, MRI scan, lumbar puncture—CSF analysis

- Management:
  - Cerebral toxoplasmosis—pyrimethamine and sulfadiazine
  - Cryptococcal meningitis—amphotericin B
  - Progressive multifocal leucoencephalopathy (JC virus)—there is no effective treatment
  - CMV infection—ganciclovir

Further reading

Articles

National Institutes of Health. http://www.ninds.nih.gov/disorders/aids/aids.htm.

Stephenson J., et al. (2000) HIV-related brain impairment from palliative care to rehabilitation. *International Journal of Palliative Nursing*, **6**: 6–11.

Creutzfeldt–Jakob disease (CJD)

CJD is a rare degenerative disorder of the central nervous system. Prion proteins occur naturally, but it is the abnormal development and accumulation of rogue prion proteins in brain cells that leads to the development of CJD.

The most common form of the disease, accounting for 80% of all cases, is **sporadic**, presenting as a rapidly progressive multifocal dementia with poor memory and cognition, impaired balance and mobility, myoclonic jerks, slurred speech and visual problems. The incidence of sporadic CJD is 0.5–1 new case/million population per year.

Inherited prion disease, accounting for around 10% of cases, is due to autosomal dominant inheritance of a genetically mutated prion protein. The clinical course of inherited forms is usually more protracted than other forms.

Acquired prion disease occurs when rogue proteins have inadvertently been introduced into the individual (e.g. secondary to treatment with human-derived growth hormone, following the transplant of infected organs such as corneas, or the inadvertent use of contaminated neurosurgical instruments).

Variant (vCJD) was first described in 1996 and has been linked to the UK Bovine Spongiform Encephalopathy (BSE) epidemic of the 1980s. The median age at onset is younger than for patients with the sporadic disease, at 26 years. Common early features are dysphoria, withdrawal, anxiety and hallucinations, with subsequent neurological decline. The time course is longer than for sporadic disease (14.5 months mean duration compared with 4 months).

Unpublished research into the palliative care of patients with CJD has shown that many patients are being cared for by specialist palliative care services, and also that the key issues in their care include managing agitation and movement disorders, impaired communication and the dilemmas associated with end-of-life decisions. Frequently, there is a high level of distress amongst those emotionally close to the patient, in keeping with the younger age of patients, the distressing nature of the illness and its high media profile.

Following the death of a patient, the case should be discussed with the coroner, who may require a post mortem. As with any coroner's case, a post mortem can be carried out without permission from the next of kin which may cause great distress, particularly with some cultural/religious groups who will need a great deal of support at this time. All post mortems for CJD are usually carried out in designated neuropathology institutions. Following removal of the brain and spinal cord, families are able to view the body again if they wish. There is usually no visual evidence that the body has been tampered with. The brain and spinal tissue are then sent to the CJD Surveillance Unit where a formal tissue diagnosis may take months. The Unit has information for relatives and handles the situation sensitively, organizing the return of body parts to the family's funeral director for cremation or burial when the tests are completed.

Further reading

Articles

Bailey B., *et al.* Creuzfeldt-Jakob disease: extending palliative care nursing knowledge. *International Journal of Palliative Nursing*, **6**: 131–9.

Brown P. (2001) Bovine Spongiform Encephalopathy and variant CJD. *British Medical Journal*, **322**: 841–4.

Meek J. (1998) A case study: team support for a patient with CJD. *Community Nurse*, **4**: 27–8.

Spencer M., Knight R., Will R. (2002) First hundred cases of variant CJD: retrospective case note review of early psychiatric and neurological features. *British Medical Journal*, **324**: 1479–82.

Useful contacts

Multiple Sclerosis Resource Centre
7 Peartree Business Centre
Peartree Road
Stanway
Colchester
Essex CO3 5JN
Tel: 01206 505444
Freephone: 0800 783 0518
E-mail: themsrc@yahoo.com
Website: http://www.msrc.co.uk
Also provides a 24-h MS telephone counselling service: 0800 783 0518

Multiple Sclerosis Society
MS National Centre
372 Edgware Road
London NW2 6ND
Tel: 020 8438 0700
MS Helpline: Freephone 0808 800 8000, 9am–9pm
E-mail: info@mssociety.org.uk
Website: http://www.mssociety.org.uk
Provides information, support and practical help to anyone affected by MS and to those working with them. Also provides respite care centres and holiday homes.

Motor Neurone Disease Association
PO Box 246
Northampton NN1 2PR
Tel: 01604 250505
Fax: 01604 638289/624726
Helpline: 08457 626262
E-mail: enquiries@mndassociation.org
Website: http://www.mndassociation.org
Links to other sites and documents can be accessed through this site.

The National C-JD Surveillance Unit
Western General Hospital
Crewe Road
Edinburgh EH4 2XU
Telephone: 0131 537 2128
Website: http://www.cjd.ed.ac.uk

NHS National Prion Clinic
Box 98
National Hospital for Neurology and Neurosurgery
Queen Square
London WCIN 3BG
Tel: 020 7405 0755
E-mail: help.prion@st-marys.nhs.uk
Website: http://www.uclh.nhs.uk

Renal failure

Introduction

Renal failure is an important cause of death. As obesity and diabetes increase so does the incidence of chronic renal disease and end-stage renal failure. The importance of palliative care for patients with renal disease is that although there have been many advances in management in the form of dialysis and transplantation, there will nevertheless be those who enter the terminal phase for a variety of reasons and they require expert care.

Causes of death in renal failure are related to pre-existing comorbidity:

- Cardiac causes (over 50%), including myocardial infarction, heart failure due to fluid overload and electrolyte disorder-induced arrhythmias
- Peripheral vascular disease with associated sepsis and gangrene
- Cerebrovascular disease, including stroke
- Infection (20%), including dialysis and transplant-related infection
- Cancer
- Stopping dialysis

Decisions regarding dialysis

The speed of development of renal failure will clearly influence the decisions that a patient and their doctors will make about whether to start dialysis. Communication is, as ever, the key factor in arriving at satisfactory decisions. The quality of life immediately prior to the diagnosis of renal failure will be crucial. It is only the person living that life who can make judgements as to its quality. However, he or she will need the best prediction of potential for improvement to make decisions.

Renal failure is best measured by the estimated glomerular filtration rate (eGFR), as this is a more direct measure of renal function than the serum creatinine level, previously used (Table 8d.1).

Table 8d.1 Degree of renal failure*

	GFR (mL/min)	Serum creatinine (mmol/L)
Mild	20–50	150–300
Moderate	10–20	300–700
Severe	<10	>700

*This corresponds approximately with the US classification of chronic kidney disease (CKD) stages 3–5.

Symptom control in renal failure

As with palliative care for other illnesses, the management of the disease and concurrent symptom control should not be mutually exclusive. Unpleasant symptoms experienced by patients in renal failure should be palliated whether or not active dialysis is being offered. Symptoms include:

• Pain
• Fatigue/weakness
• Pruritis
• Anorexia
• Sleep disturbance
• Anxiety
• Dyspnoea
• Nausea
• Restless legs
• Depression

The principles of symptom control remain the same as with cancer and other non-cancer diagnoses. The aim must be to determine the cause of the symptom prior to treatment. Any other approach fails to make the best use of the therapeutics available.

Causes of pain in renal failure

• Concurrent comorbidity is common and may include diabetic neuropathy, peripheral vascular disease, arthritis and pressure sores
• Primary renal disease is less common but may include adult polycystic kidney disease and renal calculi
• Complications of renal failure such as renal osteodystrophy, gout, calciphylaxis and dialysis amyloid arthropathy
• Infection, including septic arthritis, peritonitis following peritoneal dialysis and discitis with epidural abscess
• Dialysis-related pain, such as 'steal syndrome' from AV fistulae, cramp, headache, abdominal pain with peritoneal dialysis.

Analgesic usage in renal failure

The absorption, metabolism and renal clearance of opioids are complex in renal failure. Individual opioids are affected by renal failure in different ways. Additional factors must also be considered if the patient is receiving dialysis. However, it is possible to ensure adequate analgesia if opioids are carefully selected and titrated.

Factors associated with altered handling of drugs in renal failure

- Oral absorption of drugs may be reduced because of vomiting, diarrhoea and gastrointestinal oedema
- Changes in hydration may affect the distribution of drugs in the body, leading to excessive drug levels
- Loss of plasma protein-binding capacity may occur due to uraemia. This may increase the plasma levels of drugs that are highly protein-bound, e.g. diazepam
- Increased permeability of the blood–brain barrier may occur, which may exaggerate the unwanted CNS effects associated with certain drugs

Analgesics

- **Paracetamol** is safe in renal failure but should be reduced to 3g every 24h if the patient has severe renal impairment. Paracetamol is dialysed by haemodialysis but not by peritoneal dialysis.
- **Codeine** should be avoided because of reports of profound toxicity, which may be delayed and can occur after trivial doses.
- **Non-steroidal anti-inflammatory drugs (NSAIDs)** should be avoided, if possible, in patients with any degree of renal impairment, although this counsel of perfection may not necessarily be appropriate in the palliative care setting. Where appropriate, sulindac is the NSAID of choice as it is reported to have renal-sparing effects. These effects are lost with doses above 100mg twice daily.
- **Morphine** (and its prodrug **diamorphine**) should be used with caution for chronic use in renal failure due to the accumulation of neurotoxic, active metabolites. The use of other opioids is generally preferred. If used, long-acting preparations should be avoided and the patient closely monitored for toxicity. Both morphine and its metabolites can be removed by dialysis, but 'rebound' can occur as drugs and metabolites re-equilibrate between the CNS and plasma and can lead to unpredictable analgesia and sedation.

- **Hydromorphone** has been reportedly used safely in patients with renal failure, but caution is still advised because the 3-glucuronide metabolite is neuroexcitatory and can accumulate. Dose reduction and careful titration is advised. Hydromorphone has also been used safely in patients receiving haemodialysis, but dose reduction and careful monitoring are required. It is water-soluble, and has a small volume of distribution and a low molecular weight, and studies have shown that plasma levels decrease to 60% of the pre-dialysis levels during treatment

- **Oxycodone** undergoes hepatic metabolism, but up to 19% is excreted unchanged in the urine. Toxicity caused by the accumulation of both the parent compound and its metabolites has been reported in renal failure. If used in patients in renal impairment, then dose reduction and careful titration is advised. Although oxycodone has a large volume of distribution, it is only 50% protein-bound and is water-soluble, making it likely to be dialysable. However, pharmacokinetic data on its use in dialysis is lacking, and other opioids should be used in its place, where possible.

- **Fentanyl** is mainly metabolized in the liver to inactive metabolites, and is therefore considered to be relatively safe in renal impairment. Although there are some reports of the parent compound accumulating in renal failure, its clinical effect is unclear. Fentanyl is not dialysable because of high protein binding and a high volume of distribution, so dose adjustment is not necessary for patients on dialysis. However, it may adsorb on to one type of filter, and specialist advice should be sought before use.

- **Alfentanil** is also highly protein-bound and metabolized in the liver. Because it has a short serum half-life it can be used for breakthrough pain and procedures. It can also be used very effectively via a SC syringe driver or as an intranasal spray. It is considered by many to be the opioid of choice in the end-of-life care of patients in renal failure. Alfentanil 1mg is equipotent to morphine 15mg.

- **Buprenorphine** appears to be a relatively safe opioid for use in renal failure. One study compared buprenorphine kinetics between healthy patients and those with renal failure (all dialysis-dependent with creatinine clearances of less than 5mL/min). It found that buprenorphine clearances and dose-corrected plasma concentrations were similar in the two groups but metabolites were increased in the group of patients with renal failure. Another study, which measured only buprenorphine (not its metabolites) over a 3-hour sampling period, reported that the disposition of buprenorphine was similar in patients with end-stage renal failure compared to healthy controls. The patients in renal failure showed no clinical evidence of sedation or respiratory depression. The effects of haemodialysis on transdermal buprenorphine have been studied in a case series of 10 patients. Elevated levels of buprenorphine or norbuprenorphine were *not* found. Furthermore, haemodialysis did not affect buprenorphine levels, leading to stable analgesic effects during therapy.

- **Methadone** undergoes hepatic metabolism, and its metabolites appear to be inactive. The parent compound and its metabolites are mainly excreted in the gut, and so methadone is considered to be a relatively safe drug in renal impairment. Methadone is not dialysable, and therefore no dose adjustments are required.

Other symptoms in renal failure

As with pain management, other symptom control measures demand careful assessment of the causes. The specific hazards of drug usage in renal failure must be considered.

The early stages of chronic kidney disease are notoriously asymptomatic; however, patients with stages 3–5 will experience unpleasant symptoms:

- CKD 3 (GFR 30–59mL/min): fatigue due to anaemia, muscle cramps
- CKD 4 (GFR 15–29mL/min): above plus nausea, oedema, anorexia, insomnia, poor concentration, neuropathy
- CKD 5 (GFR <15mL/min): above plus headache, pruritis, encephalopathy leading to death

Fatigue, daytime somnolence and weakness

These symptoms are common in patients in renal failure. The causes are usually multiple and include anaemia due to a low erythropoietin level and iron deficiency, poor nutrition, inadequate dialysis, biochemical disturbances, insomnia, depression and immobility because of uncontrolled pain. Severe fatigue can also be a feature of the immediate post-dialysis period, due probably to rapid changes in fluid volume, blood pressure and electrolytes.

Management

Depends on the likely prognosis. Non-drug measures include anaemia correction, improved nutrition, physiotherapy, a good night's sleep and increased social supportive care. Drug measures include the use of better analgesia, erythropoietin, iron, electrolyte correction and antidepressants.

Anorexia and weight loss

Has parallels with cancer and cardiac cachexia. It is due to fundamental metabolic changes and is part of the symptomatic spiral experienced in end-stage disease. Only some causes are correctable. Protein malnutrition may occur, especially in dialysing patients.

Other factors include:

- Chronic nausea
- Altered taste
- Dry mouth
- Gastric stasis due to diabetic neuropathy or opioids
- Constipation
- Social isolation
- Depression
- Abdominal discomfort in peritoneal dialysis (PD) patients.

Management

Includes:

- Attention to improved nutrition
- Treatment of oral infections, especially candida
- Trial of metoclopramide as a prokinetic antinausea drug
- Treatment of depression

Appetite stimulation with corticosteroids may temporarily improve appetite but is likely to exacerbate muscle wasting and fluid retention in the medium and longer term.

Pruritis

Has an incidence of over 50% in patients with end-stage renal disease, whether they are being dialysed or not. The pathophysiology seems to be both complex and multifactorial. Pruritis is transmitted via mechanisms similar to those for pain. However, other factors are also likely to be in operation in some patients, such as the local mast-cell release of histamine and cytokines, peripheral neuropathy and secondary hyperparathyroidism.

Management

In general, pruritis is usually less problematical after dialysis. Nutritional factors, anaemia as well as calcium and phosphate disturbance are general correctable causes which may help. Avoidance of dry skin and excessive hot baths and reduction of alcohol intake are all worth trying. Short, clean fingernails will reduce secondary infection following scratching. Topical capsaicin cream and tacrolimus ointment have both been advocated, but topical steroids are unhelpful. Specific measures include ultraviolet B phototherapy, which is effective but burdensome. Gabapentin and thalidomide have both been shown to be helpful. However, the former requires dose reduction (300mg on alternate days for a GFR <15mL/min) and the latter may be difficult to obtain and also be too sedative. Antihistamines are frequently prescribed with little objective evidence of benefit.

Nausea

Present in between 25 and 33% of patients. The cause may be due to rising levels of blood urea, but it may also be due to other non-renal causes such as medication, constipation, delayed gastric emptying due to diabetic neuropathy and fluid and electrolyte changes. As ever, the best treatment is to define and correct the cause if at all possible. In general, the standard antiemetics used in palliative care can be used in renal failure at normal dosage. However, caution is always required for untoward side-effects such as extra-pyramidal syndromes, constipation and hypotension. (📖 See Chapter 6b.)

Restless legs syndrome (RLS)

This is an unpleasant 'crawling' sensation felt in the legs. It is more common at night and may be relieved by movement. It occurs in 2–15% of the general population, but may occur in up to 30% of patients in renal failure. It is thought to be connected with dopaminergic dysfunction, iron metabolism and, possibly, uraemic neuropathy. RLS may be worse with anaemia, low ferritin and PTH levels as well as medication such as tricyclics, caffeine and neuroleptics. It is associated with pruritis, diabetes and the elderly.

Management

Management with adequate dialysis may help, as will treating anaemia and withdrawing offending medication. Specific drug treatment includes dopamine agonists such as pramipexole, ropinirole, pergolide and cabergoline, but they may all cause sleepiness and require slow titration. Benzodiazepines such as clonazepam at night are useful, as are opioids and gabapentin. Both the latter will require dose modification in patients in renal failure.

Calciphylaxis and muscle cramps

These are two other common symptoms of end-stage renal failure. The former is a very painful skin ulceration due to subcutaneous and small artery calcification. It carries a poor prognosis and requires careful management with both analgesia and explanation. The high incidence of cramps is due to water and electrolyte imbalance. This may be correctable by adjustment of the dialysis regime, but in end-of-life care, both quinine and vitamin E are useful.

Other symptoms

Include dyspnoea, depression, insomnia, anxiety and constipation and can be treated as with any palliative care patient. If the cause can be found then specific treatment can be given.

Formulary

Dose reduction of commonly used drugs in renal failure

DRUG Creat. GFR	Mild 150-300 20-50ml/min	Moderate 300-700 10-20ml/min	Severe >700µmol/L <10ml/min
Paracetamol	ND	ND	reduce to 1g 8h
NSAIDs	ND	Avoid if possible	Avoid unless on dialysis
WEAK OPIOIDS			
Co-codamol			
Co-dydramol	ND	6 tab in 24h	4 tab in 24h
Tramadol	ND	50-100mg 12h	50mg 12h
STRONG OPIOODS			
Alfentanil	ND	ND	ND
Buprenorphine	ND	ND	ND
Diamorphine	75% of ND	2.5-5mg 4h	2.5mg SC 8h*
Fentanyl	ND	75% of ND *	50% of ND*
Hydromorphone	ND	1.3mg	1.3mg *
Methadone	ND	ND	50% of ND
Morphine	75% of ND	2.5-5mg 4h	1.25-2.5mg 4h
Oxycodone	ND	ND	Avoid unless on dialysis
ANTI-EMETICS			
Cyclizine	ND	ND	ND
Domperidone	ND	ND	caution
Haloperidol	ND	ND	caution (may accumulate)
Levomepromazine	ND	ND	caution
Metoclopramide	ND	ND	avoid
Ondansetron	ND	ND	ND
ANTICHOLINERGICS			
Hyoscine Butylbromide	ND	ND	ND
Hyoscine Hydrobromide	ND	ND	ND
CENTRAL NERVOUS SYSTEM MODULATORS			
Amitriptyline	ND	ND	ND
Baclofen	5mg t.d.s.	5mg b.d.	5mg.o.d.
Benzodiazepines. Start with small doses. Increased cerebral sensitivity			
Citalopram	ND	ND	ND (caution)
Fluoxetine	ND	ND or alternate days	ND or alternate days
Gabapentin	300mg b.d.	300mg o.d.	300mg alternate days
Mirtazepine	ND	ND	15mg daily
Paroxetine	ND	20mg o.d.	20mg o.d.

*titrate
ND normal dose
With permission from Andrew Hoy

General considerations

As with the application of palliative care principles to any non-cancer illness, the philosophy that has proved helpful in the past has been to place the patient at the centre of all decision-making. Adaptations may well be required for the specific application of symptom management techniques to end-stage renal failure, not least the modification of drug dosage where renal excretion is important. Any palliative care specialist healthcare professional will need to learn from their colleagues in renal medicine, as well as contribute to innovative thinking in the care of this difficult group of patients.

Further reading

Books

Ashley C., Currie A. (eds) (2004) *The Renal Drug Handbook* (2nd edn). Oxford: Radcliffe Medical Press.

Broadbent A., Khor K., Heaney A. (2003) Palliation and chronic renal failure: opioid and other palliative medications—dosage guidelines. *Progress in Palliative Care*, **11**(4): 183–1901.

Brown E., Chambers J., Eggeling C. (2007) *End of Life Care in Nephrology*. Oxford: Oxford University Press.

Articles

Farrell A., Rich A. (2000). Analgesic use in patients with renal failure. *European Journal of Palliative Care*, **7**(6): 201–5.

Kirkham S. R., Pugh R. (1995) Opioid analgesia in uraemic patients. *Lancet*, **345**(8958): 1185. (Letter)

Filitz J., *et al.* (2006) Effects of intermittent haemodialysis on buprenorphine and norbuprenorphine plasma concentrations in chronic pain patients treated with transdermal buprenorphine. *European Journal of Pain*, **10**: 743–8.

Laegreid I., Hallan S. (2008) Renal failure in palliative care patients. *European Journal of Palliative Care* **15**(2): 58–62.

Robson P. (2004). The use of opioids in palliative care patients with renal failure. *CME Cancer Medicine*, **2**(2): 40–8.

AIDS in adults

Introduction

The acquired immunodeficiency syndrome (AIDS) is a cluster of clinical conditions that inevitably occur in a person infected by the human immunodeficiency virus (HIV). As this virus attacks and weakens the cellular immune system the infected person develops an increasing number of infections, often from weak but opportunistic micro-organisms. The virus also directly attacks various body tissues, resulting in chronic diarrhoea, severe weight loss, painful peripheral neuropathy, progressive dementia or profound pancytopenia. In the advanced stages of HIV infection, there is also an increasing incidence of malignancies such as Kaposi's sarcoma and non-Hodgkin's lymphomas, which were previously uncommon.

HIV principally affects the T-lymphocytes, resulting in impaired cell-mediated immunity. Certain lymphocytes (T4 cells) have a surface protein (CD4) which has a high affinity for HIV. The CD4 count declines with advancing disease and increasing immunodeficiency. Counts below 200/microlitre are associated with a high risk of developing opportunistic infection. The viral load is high following the initial infection and then declines as the immune system partially recovers after about 12 weeks. It remains at a low level for a variable length of time and then increases again with the collapse of the immune system.

Historical background

There has been much heated debate about the origins of AIDS. It is now widely accepted that the virus originated via the SIV (simian immunodeficiency virus) that infects other primates. AIDS was initially recognized in the gay community in the USA during the early 1980s; however, it soon became apparent that this was just the tip of a growing world pandemic. Transmission is through contact with blood or other body fluids infected with HIV. Those most vulnerable to HIV infection are therefore persons with multiple sexual partners, intravenous drug users, babies of infected mothers, persons receiving blood transfusions and health professionals who sustain needlestick injuries.

Complexity

The course of the illness is unpredictable, the presentation is variable and, even though antiretroviral drugs (ARVs) can prolong life by many years, death from AIDS is inevitable. Added to this complex clinical picture is the emotional, social and economic impact that this pandemic is having, especially in Sub-Saharan Africa. Fear, stigma, rejection, repeated bereavement and conflicting messages accompany this disease. With the rising death rate, declining life expectancy, prolonged suffering and economic disruption that is occurring as a direct result of AIDS, this condition is the single greatest health challenge to our world in the twenty-first century. Providing antiretroviral treatment in a responsible, effective and sustainable manner in the long term is going to require major changes in healthcare.

Statistics

The confusing and sometimes conflicting statistics that are presented tend to muddle rather than help, at a time when we need clear reasoning and constructive planning for the future. What is certain is that this pandemic is very large and is growing rapidly. Despite all the recent preventive strategies and medical advances, it is showing no signs of abating. By 2006, the WHO estimated that 40 million people worldwide were infected. The vast majority of these live in Sub-Saharan Africa where it is estimated that 1 in 5 adults is infected.

Worldwide there were 4.3 million new HIV infections and 2.9 million deaths due to AIDS during 2006. Even in the UK, where it is estimated that more than 88 000 people are HIV-positive, the number of infections has continued to rise despite the introduction of ARVs. AIDS is also spreading rapidly in Asia and South America.

Clinical features

AIDS has replaced syphilis and tuberculosis as the great mimic. It may present in such a myriad of ways that it should be considered as a possibility in any patient of any age with almost any complaint anywhere in the world. There are, however, a number of clinical presentations that are typical and even some that are diagnostic of AIDS. Loss of weight of more than 10%, diarrhoea or fevers lasting more than a month, generalized lymphadenopathy, especially including the submental and epitrochlear nodes, are very suggestive. Herpes zoster in a young adult, dry itchy skin and small darkly pigmented itchy bumps would also raise the suspicions of any health worker in an endemic area. Kaposi's sarcoma, cryptococcal meningitis and cerebral lymphoma are pathognomonic.

The classification devised by the WHO is a useful way of staging the illness clinically, especially when CD4 counts and viral loads are unavailable (📖 see Table 8e.1).

Table 8e.1 WHO clinical staging of HIV/AIDS (modified)

	Clinical stage			
	Seroconversion (1)	Early (2)	Intermediate (3)	Late (4)
Feature				
Activity	Normal	Rests occasionally	Rests for <50% of day	Rests for >50% of day
Weight loss	No	<10%	>10%	Wasted/ cachectic
Fever	Mild in 50%	Occasional	>1/12	>1/12
Diarrhoea		Occasional	>1/12	>1/12
Respiratory infections		URTIs Pneumonia Pleural effusion	Recurrent pneumonia Chronic otitis media	Pneumocystis carinii pneumonia (PCP)
Pulmonary TB			Miliary Lower lobes Mediastinal nodes	Extensive bilateral Resistant
Other TB				Pericardial Peritoneum Spine/bone Meningitis
Skin		Shingles H. simplex Dry Itchy papules Tinea corporis	Severe shingles Pellagra Stevens– Johnson syndrome Vaginal thrush	Persistent genital ulcers

Table 8e.1 WHO clinical staging of HIV/AIDS (modified) (*Continued*)

	Clinical stage			
	Seroconversion (1)	Early (2)	Intermediate (3)	Late (4)
Mouth		Aphthous ulcers Reiter's syndrome Gingivitis	Oral thrush Progressive gingivitis	Oesophageal thrush
CNS		Bell's palsy Guillain–Barré syndrome		Painful feet Paraplegia 25% dementia Cryptococcal meningitis Toxoplasmosis
Cancer				Kaposi's sarcoma Invasive cancer of the cervix Lymphoma
Lymph nodes	Generalized	Generalized	Generalized	Generalized or absent

Natural history

Following infection by HIV, the natural progression of this illness is very variable. For many, there are few symptoms initially and it is only after several years of relatively normal health that the typical clinical features of AIDS become apparent. In others, the initial seroconversion may be more pronounced, with fever, body pains, headache, ulceration of the mucosa of the mouth and genitalia, a maculopapular rash as well as hepato-splenomegaly and generalized lymphadenopathy. These symptoms usually resolve spontaneously over a few weeks. During this phase the person may, however, develop Bell's palsy or Guillain–Barré syndrome, indicating early neurological involvement.

After about 12 weeks the body reaches a steady state with a partial recovery of the immune system and a decline in the number of circulating viral particles. Now follows a phase of clinical latency where the only clinical signs may be of a generalized lymphadenopathy and occasional episodes of sweating, especially at night.

While a small proportion of infected people may progress rapidly to full-blown AIDS within one or two years, in the majority AIDS takes eight to ten years to develop. A few individuals progress very slowly and may be still alive after 20 years, even without ARVs.

As the immune system begins to become exhausted, the person becomes susceptible to a wide range of infections including recurrent upper respiratory tract infections, pneumonia, tuberculosis, a wide variety of intestinal micro-organisms, cryptococcal meningitis, herpes zoster and monilial infections of the mouth, vagina and oesophagus. The emergence of extreme drug-resistant tuberculosis in many parts of the world is a very worrying development as this poses a threat to everyone, whether HIV+ or not.

The variability of the resilience of the immune system together with the potentially fatal nature of some of the infections, make it difficult to estimate the prognosis of an individual.

The effects and limitations of highly active antiretroviral therapy (HAART)

The advent of highly active antiretroviral therapy (HAART) has radically changed the prospects for many people with AIDS. An emaciated person who appears to be beyond all help may start rapidly improving on ARVs. This has been nicknamed the 'Lazarus syndrome'. In Europe and North America, numerous hospices and hospital wards dedicated to caring for dying AIDS patients have been able to empty their beds and concentrate on other forms of care.

ARVs are the best available form of palliation for AIDS at present. The decision when to start ARVs and which combination to use may at first seem complex. The key to success is for the affected person and the doctor to negotiate the most suitable timing of the start of ARVs and the most suitable combination.

Good stories are a very effective way of explaining the use of ARVs and getting the right message across to less well-developed and educated communities, e.g.:[1]

Imagine you are hiking through the bushveld and enjoying the birdlife and the game. But, in the distance, you see a lion stalking you. You aren't too worried because you have a gun. But there are only two bullets in the gun, so you need to be quite sure about the best time to shoot. If you shoot too soon there is a good chance that you will miss the lion, and that the explosion will chase away all the wildlife. If you leave it too late the lion may be on top of you before you can take aim.

The lion represents AIDS and the distance between you and the lion shows how strong your immune system is—the closer the lion the weaker your immune system. The gun with the two bullets is your antiretroviral therapy, which you need to learn how to use properly so that you don't hurt yourself. The sound of the gun being fired represents the potential side-effects of the antiretroviral therapy—a real nuisance if the lion is far away, but the last thing you'd worry about when the lion is getting close!

The decision to start ARVs must not be hurried, they need to be used responsibly.[2] Time needs to be taken to help the person understand the various options and the need for strict adherence as fully as possible:
• Treatment needs to be taken for life
• It is very important to choose the first treatment regimen carefully as it is the one most likely to have the best results

---

1 Orrell C., Wilson D. (2003) The art of HAART: a practical approach to antiretroviral therapy. *CME*, 21(6): 306–12.

2 Brechtl J. R., Breitbart W., Galietta M., *et al.* (2001) The use of highly active anti-retroviral therapy (HAART) in patients with advanced HIV infection: impact on medical, palliative care, and quality of life outcomes. *Journal of Pain and Symptom Management*, 21: 41–51.

- Once the virus has been exposed to ARVs, subsequent regimens are less likely to give good results
- The start of ARVs should be delayed until the CD4 count is below 350/microlitre, or the symptoms of the infection are very troublesome. The exact timing of initiating ARVs is still hotly debated, but according to the WHO and other authorities (IAPAC—International Association of Physicians in AIDS Care) a cut-off point of 350 is currently international best practice
- Social and psychological problems, especially depression, need to be resolved where possible before starting ARVs, otherwise these will make adherence difficult
- The choice of drugs is growing rapidly. The inexperienced clinician should ask for advice from someone experienced with using ARVs
- In an effort to make the decision as simple as possible, the WHO is recommending fixed combinations in a similar way to the TB regimens: see www.who.int/hiv/pub/prev_care/draft/en/
- Efavirenz or nevirapine (NNRTIs) should be used in combination with zidovudine and lamivudine or stavudine and lamivudine (NRTIs from different categories) (☐ see Table 8e.2). If they are available, tenofovir (TDF) and emtricitabine (FTC) are currently the best agents to use in combination with the NNRTIs for first-line therapy—firstly because of their low risk of mitochondrial toxicity, and secondly because their long half-lives make once-a-day dosing possible and reduces the risk of resistance and virological failure

Table 8e.2 Classification of antiretroviral drugs*

Category I (NRTIs)	Category II (NRTIs)	Category III (NRTI)	Category IV (NNRTIs)	Category V (PIs)
Stavudine (d4T)	Didanosine (ddl)	Abacavir (ABC)	Nevirapine (NVP)	Nelfinavir (NFV)
Zidovudine (AZT)	Lamivudine (3TC)		Efavirenz[†] (EFV)	Indinavir/RTV (IDV)
				Lopinavir/RTV (combination)
				Ritonavir (RTV)[‡]

NRTI = nucleoside reverse transcriptase inhibitor
NNRTI = non-nucleoside reverse transcriptase inhibitor
PI = protease inhibitor
*For initiation of therapy in an ARV-naïve patient use two NRTIs (one from category I and one from category II) together with one NNRTI (category IV)
[†]EFV is teratogenic
[‡]RTV is most often used in combination with another PI at a low dose of 100mg twice daily. Here it is used as a P450 inhibitor to boost the levels of the combined PI. It is not a useful antiretroviral agent at this low dose. In adults, it is rarely used as an antiretroviral in its own right (600mg twice daily) due to increased adverse events (e.g. diarrhoea)

- The immunocompromised person who develops TB presents the clinician with an additional dilemma, as ARVs do not combine well with the standard anti-TB drugs. Where possible, the TB should be treated first. When the CD4 count is, however, <350, ARVs should preferably be added after 2 months of TB treatment and when the CD4 is <50, after 2 weeks of TB treatment. Close attention should, however, be paid to drug toxicity and drug interactions.
- The initial euphoria about ARVs is now abating somewhat as the problem of viral resistance to many of the drugs becomes apparent. Already 10% of new infections in Europe are resistant to at least one drug. Strict adherence (>97%) to complex drug regimens is needed to suppress the replication of the virus. Poor adherence leads to resistant strains developing rapidly, with resultant treatment failure and disease progression. Although minor side-effects such as rashes are common, usually appearing soon after initiating treatment, these can be managed symptomatically. Serious side-effects, such as lactic acidosis, may occur on d4T, ddI or rarely on AZT, and may be fatal if not detected early

Initial small, well-controlled trials of ARVs have been shown to be very effective in some African countries. Patients adhere to their drugs as well as patients in Europe and America. The distribution of ARVs on a large scale, however, is likely to overwhelm the already over-extended primary health services in countries such as South Africa unless there is a massive injection of funds into the health system. The cost of the drugs needed to cope with this pandemic is large, but even more will be needed to build up the infrastructure and improve the capacity of the hospitals and health centres to provide the treatment and monitor patients. The vast distances and poor public transport services in rural areas will limit access to ARVs for many patients.

Many large companies now have workplace ARV programmes where there is a strong focus on education and prevention of HIV, healthy living and eventually provision of ARVs when indicated. They have realized that it is better to keep their skilled staff healthy rather than constantly to recruit and retrain new workers.

The 'brain drain' of skilled doctors and nurses from developing countries to various places such as Canada, Australia, the UK and the Middle East is compounding the difficulties. The Melbourne Manifesto on the recruitment of health professionals, adopted at the World Rural Health Conference in May 2002, needs to be taken seriously. See http://www.globalfamilydoctor.com/aboutwonca/working-groups/rural_training/melbourne_manifesto.htm

The role of palliative care

As mentioned, current ARVs do not cure AIDS, but merely delay its natural progress. For many years to come the vast majority of infected people in the world will not have access to such drugs, some who are able to obtain them will not respond well or will be unable to adhere to the strict regimens required to suppress the virus. In the foreseeable future we will still be faced with millions of people, dying slowly of AIDS, who will need effective palliative care. Such care should have the same focus as palliative care in other situations, namely promoting quality of life, excellent symptom control, effective communication and appropriate support for both patient and family. Fear and stigma can make this a very difficult task, as does the challenge of not overlooking potentially curable infections.

Pain

Pain is common and often undertreated. Surveys have shown that up to 98% of advanced AIDS sufferers will have significant pain.

- Headache is a frequent symptom and cryptococcal meningitis (CM) and tuberculous meningitis (TBM) need to be excluded as these are treatable if diagnosed early. CM may be associated with raised intracranial pressure and the resulting severe headache can be relieved by daily serial lumbar punctures (LPs), draining off 15–20mL of CSF with great care. Focal signs may indicate a space-occupying lesion. If possible a scan should be done to confirm the diagnosis. In Africa toxoplasmosis is the commonest cause
- Severe sensory neuropathies are present in 30% of patients. Most are due to direct damage to peripheral nerves by the virus, but some may occur from the toxic effects of anti-TB treatment or ARVs (ddC, d4T and ddl)
- Herpes zoster may occur early in the course of the illness and may be severe with persisting post-herpetic neuralgia
- Persisting mouth and genital ulcerations are common and are very debilitating. Once again, treatable conditions such as candida and sexually transmitted infections (STIs) should be sought. Chronic ulceration due to persisting herpes simplex can be very frustrating, but some good results are reported from resource-poor areas in Africa where aciclovir tablets are crushed and applied topically
- Painful swallowing (odynophagia) may be due to oesophageal candidiasis, acid reflux and TB, which are treatable, or due to infection by cytomegalovirus (CMV) or Kaposi's sarcoma (KS), which often respond poorly to treatment
- Abdominal pain occurs in 20% of patients and may be due to many different causes. Patients with abdominal pain should be approached like all other patients. Surgical emergencies should be referred appropriately, lactic acidosis or pancreatitis due to ARVs (ddl, ddC and d4T) ruled out, infections such as salmonella, shigella or TB treated and effective analgesia provided for all
- Muscle and joint pains are also common. The same approach applies: identify treatable infections and conditions and provide effective analgesia for all. Pyrazinamide, used to treat TB, commonly causes severe arthralgia

Follow the principles of pain management: 'By mouth', 'By the ladder', 'By the clock' with careful follow-up and review. (💭 See Chapter 6a.)

The biggest challenge in poorly resourced areas is making morphine and other effective drugs available and accessible. Great progress has been made in Uganda with the introduction of appropriate legislation allowing the distribution of morphine at clinic level. In Zimbabwe, trained palliative care nurses are able to prescribe morphine. Other developing countries need to follow their example.

Diarrhoea

Recurrent and persisting diarrhoea may be present in more than 50% of patients with advanced AIDS. In places with poor sanitation, good hygiene has been shown to reduce this percentage significantly. Many of the patients with chronic diarrhoea will have an identifiable infection. The presence of fever or of blood in the stool should be investigated for a treatable cause. In areas that are resource-poor, a short empirical trial of metronidazole and co-trimoxazole may be tried. In order to reduce the frequency of diarrhoea to manageable levels, loperamide or morphine should be titrated up to an effective dose. Trying to cope with profuse diarrhoea with a lack of proper sanitation and/or easily accessible running water is a reality for most affected families in many areas in Third World countries. This places an extra burden and risk on already overwhelmed families. Chronic diarrhoea needs to be taken just as seriously as pain.

Fever

Sweating and fever are frequent throughout the course of AIDS. It may be part of the immune response or it may indicate the onset of yet another opportunistic infection. Careful assessment for possible treatable causes such as pneumonia, malaria or TB needs to be made. Extra fluids and antipyretics can be given until any possible treatable cause is identified.

Neurological

See 📖 p. 692.

Skin problems

Almost all patients with AIDS will have some kind of skin problem:

- Dry skin and itching are frequent. Excessive bathing, especially in warm water, should be discouraged. Aqueous cream can be used as a soap substitute. Soft white paraffin or UEA with 10% urea can be applied twice a day to the whole body. Judicious use of appropriate steroid creams and oral antihistamines (especially H_1 blockers) may bring relief of itching
- Itching may also be caused by 'Itchy bump disease' (pruritic papular eruption). This is very common in Africa and is a group of conditions causing inflamed, very itchy papules that leave small darkly pigmented bumps on the limbs and trunk
- Seborrhoeic dermatitis and psoriasis are common and should be treated appropriately
- Scabies should be considered in any patient with itching. It may present in the usual form of red itchy papules with burrows in the web spaces of the fingers and around the anogenital area. Occasionally scabies may present in a scaly, less itchy form (hyperkeratotic scabies) on the scalp, hands and trunk. Large thick crusts on the body with cracking may also be due to scabies
- Multiple purple–brown nodules of varying size scattered all over the body, especially on the face and in the mouth, are characteristic of Kaposi's sarcoma. It may occur at any stage of the illness and although it is often slowly progressive at first, it may spread to involve

internal organs and be rapidly fatal. Pain and dyspnoea are then often present and may be controlled with morphine. Palliative radiotherapy, intralesional chemotherapy and topical cryotherapy can be tried, especially if the patient is still reasonably well (CD4 >200/microlitre)

Emotional and mental symptoms

The diagnosis of being HIV-positive presents the infected person not only with the prospect of a fatal illness but also the stigma associated with AIDS. Many strong emotions crowd the mind including:

- Fear of rejection by others
- Fear of infecting others
- Anger and a sense of betrayal
- Sense of shame for having contracted the disease
- Sorrow in anticipation of the loss of everything
- Worry about how to cope and how one's children will survive

It is little wonder that anxiety and depression are common throughout the course of the illness, especially shortly after diagnosis and again as the symptoms of advanced AIDS become apparent. Family and community support, however, can help the infected person come to terms with the situation. Without support, the HIV-positive person may lose hope. Suicide then becomes a strong possibility.

Support groups for people living with AIDS have proved very effective in Africa in countering the despair and hardship that so often accompany this illness. Many HIV-positive people have become involved in caring for those who are sick at home, looking after the infants left behind and comforting the grieving. Some have been brave enough to speak out in public and have been very effective in breaking down stigma and prejudice. This has never been easy and at times it has been dangerous, kindling the wrath of an already outraged community.

Being a neurotropic virus, over 80% of people with AIDS will show some cognitive impairment, while 25% will go on to develop HIV-associated dementia or psychosis. Most are apathetic and withdrawn, while a few may become delirious and agitated, requiring sedation.

Nutrition

While good nutrition is essential for maintaining an adequate immune system, great care needs to be taken to ensure that the role of particular diets, such as the use of garlic, lemon juice and olive oil, is not seen as an alternative to effective medical care. The sick have always been vulnerable to exploitation by quacks and 'snake oil' salesmen. While vitamins and other micronutrients have their place, 'a round pill' should not replace 'a square meal'.

Where possible, six small balanced meals a day should be encouraged. Increased energy can be obtained by adding sugar, vegetable oil, peanut butter, eggs or dried milk powder to the local staple food. Alcohol should be avoided.

In the underprivileged areas of developing countries, both vegetable gardening and small-scale subsistence farming needs to be encouraged, as a means of survival and for the sense of well-being they encourage.

Social issues

The young adult is the main age group affected by the AIDS pandemic. Young adults may be the main 'bread-winners' and the parents of small children. Their deaths have a devastating effect on the community. In developing countries, the loss of income, the multiple bereavements, the growing orphan population, the child-headed households and children who have to leave school to care for dying parents and siblings are all causing great economic and emotional suffering.

Impact on Africa

In a survey of affected households in South Africa in 2002, it was found that 45% had an income of less than $150 a month, 57% had no running water inside their homes and 25% had no toilet. The plight of children is desperate. It was found that 22% of children under 15 years had lost at least one parent and 50% of children often went to bed hungry. The sick family members required care for extended periods, often as long as 12 months. Twenty per cent were too weak to wash and 16% were incontinent. The average life expectancy in South Africa has dropped by 10 years.

(SA Health Review 2002)[3]

Despite some countries having child support grants and disability pensions, multiple administrative obstacles may prevent access to these funds. The capacity of the health and social welfare services to cope in most Sub-Saharan countries is being stretched to the limits.

Spiritual issues

Fear, discrimination, stigma, rejection and isolation have added to the burden of those affected and infected by HIV/AIDS. While community organizations and religious groups are playing a role in helping those in need, the perception that AIDS sufferers have 'only themselves to blame' is still prevalent and will take much wisdom and compassion to overcome.

Health professionals need to be aware of the way different communities perceive illness and misfortune. In Africa, there is a common perception that some conditions are 'natural' while others are not. Unfamiliar illnesses or conditions that are not easily cured may be attributed to evil influences of 'sorcerers' or the jealousy of neighbours. In addition to seeking help from health professionals at a hospital or clinic for the symptoms of the disease, the affected person will consult a traditional healer to discover the person responsible for the misfortune. The 'victim' will also expect to be given some means of protection from this evil.

An example of this is the common interpretation for the persistently painful feet of the peripheral neuropathy that so often accompanies AIDS. This will be interpreted as being caused by an enemy who has sprinkled 'poison' just outside the front gate of the home of the affected person. Unless the poison can be neutralized there will be no lasting cure.

Great care is needed in dealing with spiritual issues, especially if there are cultural and language differences between the ill person and the healthcare worker. A helpful approach is for the health professional to admit his/her ignorance of the beliefs and customs of the community and to ask the ill person or the family for help in understanding their needs.

Medico-legal issues

AIDS is a minefield of medico-legal issues. The right to confidentiality, the concerns of the public and the fears of the health professionals have caused many heated debates and even several court cases. The way information is entered into medical records and on death certificates has needed to be revised and improved. Disclosure even to another health worker must be on a legitimate 'need to know' basis and only after proper informed consent has been gained (□ see section Death Certification, p.996).

Laws relating to employment, dismissal and benefits need to be reviewed. When others are at risk, especially within a family, the infected individual needs to be helped and encouraged to disclose their HIV status.

Communities also need to deal with the issues of HIV-positive children attending community schools. Proper education and the introduction of universal precautions have helped to allay the fears of parents in most cases.

All health workers are exposed to the risk of needlestick injuries. Therefore, prophylactic drugs, appropriate laboratory investigations, supportive counselling and a clear written policy of the process to be followed should be in place.

Care during the dying phase

The transition from fighting against a terminal illness to preparing for death is never easy, especially when the person is young. In addition, the opportunistic infections are often treatable. Thus both doctor and patient may remain focused on cure. Families find it equally difficult to let go. However, a time comes sooner or later when, despite all efforts, recovery does not take place. The same approach is needed to care for patients dying from AIDS as for those dying with cancer. The medication regimen should be simplified to only those drugs needed to provide good symptom control. This may include stopping ARVs and even anti-TB treatment. As long as the person is no longer sputum-positive for TB, there is little risk to others. It may be prudent to continue antifungals and agents for herpes simplex.

Treatment and ongoing prophylaxis for CMV retinitis may also be important, especially if retinal lesions are near the optic nerve or fovea. Some 50% of patients develop progressive sight deterioration within 2–3 weeks of stopping treatment.

Home-based care in developing countries has become a practical alternative to overcrowded public hospitals. With the support of established hospices, community groups have taken on the task of supporting affected families. Unfortunately, some families may perceive discharge from hospital as inappropriate. They are likely to take the ill person to another hospital for readmission and the unnecessary repeat of all investigations.

Bereavement and AIDS

Loss and grief are difficult to deal with at the best of times. Friends, neighbours and family members usually rally round and help to bear the burden of coping without the lost loved one. In developing countries, the multiple deaths of the AIDS epidemic are leaving the survivors with little support. It is not uncommon for an elderly widow, who has been struggling to survive on her small pension, to find herself having to care for six or seven grandchildren whose parents have died one by one in a short space of time. In this state of 'distracted grief' there is little time for anything other than survival. The stigma of AIDS creates further barriers within the wider community.

Frustrations, fears and compassion fatigue

Despite the warnings and predictions of the scale and complexity of the AIDS epidemic in the late 1980s, most health services in developing countries were ill prepared for the numbers of sick and dying patients that began to crowd hospitals and clinics in the 1990s. In South Africa, this dramatic rise began in 1997. Wards in public hospitals became overcrowded with emaciated men and women with chronic diarrhoea and persisting cough. More than 50% of deaths in the adult wards could be directly attributed to AIDS, while in the paediatric wards the figure was closer to 85% in some areas.

Advances

The identification of the causative organism, accurate diagnostic testing, HAART and the initial development of vaccines and microbicides against this virus are some of the advances that have taken place. Although there is a long way to go yet before we can even begin to consider that AIDS is under control, the future looks a lot brighter than it did ten years ago.

The challenge

AIDS is no longer just a disease, it is a human rights issue.
Nelson Mandela, November 2003.

Many international funders have made treatment possible in developing countries, the most well known are UNAIDS, PEPFAR (President's Emergency Plan For AIDS Relief—a US initiative) and Bill and Belinda Gates' Foundation. Sadly, however, the WHO's '3x5' campaign—aiming to have placed three million people on ARVs by 2005—never reached its target. In South Africa for instance, less than 20% of patients in need of ARVs are currently receiving them. It is clear that in order to achieve the WHO millennium development goal Target 7: 'To have halted by 2015 and begun to reverse the spread of HIV/AIDS', more than the money for the drugs will be required: the entire infrastructure of health services in developing countries will need supporting.

Resources
The following are a small selection of internet sites with information on AIDS:
Africa Alive—a forum for sharing ideas and strategies
Website: http://www.africaalive.org

AIDS Education Global Information System—a wide range of HIV/AIDS related topics
Website: http://www.aegis.com

Aidsmap—The British HIV Association
Website: http://www.aidsmap.com/

Medscape—a web site of educational activities
Web site: http://www.hiv.medscape.com/

Further reading

Books
O'Neill J., Selwyn P., Schietinger H. (eds) (2003) *A Clinical Guide on Supportive and Palliative Care for people with HIV/AIDS. Washington: US Dept of Health and Human Services.* (The guide is available as a free download from www.hab.hrsa.gov.)

Wilson D., et al. (eds) (2003) *Handbook of HIV Medicine.* Oxford: Oxford University Press.

Articles
Cameron D. (2002) Saving the history of the defeated and the lost—ethical dilemmas in the midst of the AIDS epidemic. *South African Family Practice,* **25**(4): 15–18.

Fassin D., Schneider H. (2003) The politics of AIDS in South Africa: beyond the controversies. *British Medical Journal,* **326**: 495–7.

Gallant J., et al. (2006) Efficacy and safety of tenofovir DF (TDF), emtricitabine (FTC) and efavirenz (EFV) compared to fixed dose zidovudine/lamivudine (CBV) and EFV through 96 weeks in antiretroviral treatment-naïve patients. Oral abstract session: *AIDS 2006—XVI International AIDS Conference;* Abstract no. TUPE0064.

Gazzard B. (2006) British HIV Association guidelines for the treatment of HIV-infetal adults with antiretroviral therapy. *HIV Medicine*, **7**: 487–503.

Jayasuriya A., *et al.* (2007) Twenty-five years of HIV management. *Journal of the Royal Society of Medicine*. **100**(8): 363–6.

Norval D. A. (2004) Symptoms and sites of pain experienced by AIDS patients. *South African Medical Journal*, **94**: 450–4.

Orrell C., Wilson D. (2003) The art of HAART: a practical approach to antiretroviral therapy. *CME*, **21**(6): 306–12.

Palliation in the care of the elderly[1]

Old age is associated with disease, it does not cause it.

The large majority of the population over the age of 85 years live at home; 20% live in nursing homes. Elderly patients with palliative care needs often have a constellation of complex and chronic requirements including:

- Management of physical and psychological symptoms of both acute and chronic illnesses
- Appropriate therapeutic interventions that can preserve function and independence and help patients maintain quality of life
- Clear communication on the usual course of illness so that they and their family members can make appropriate arrangements
- Recognition and management of caregiver stress

Elderly people in the UK may receive palliative care in a number of settings, including:
- At home with the care of a GP and community team
- In a residential or nursing home with support from a GP and nursing staff
- In a community hospital
- On a care-of–the-elderly unit/facility
- In an acute hospital

Background

- While a child born in 1900 could expect to live fewer than 50 years, life expectancy for a child born in 2010 is expected to increase to 86 years for a girl and 79 years for a boy.[2] The implication for increasing input from supportive and palliative care is clear
- In developed nations, the overwhelming majority of deaths occur in elderly patients suffering from multiple coexisting and progressive chronic diseases
- Some studies suggest that elderly patients are excluded from life-prolonging interventions even if they might be appropriate. This may be due to *de facto* rationing based on age rather than an emphasis on individualizing the goals of care. Specialist care-of-the-elderly teams are skilled at devising goals of care that are appropriate for an individual's particular needs
- Data suggests that elderly patients receive less pain medication than younger persons for both chronic and acute pain. Chronic pain syndromes

1 Meier D., Monias A. (2004) Palliative medicine and care of the elderly. In *Oxford Textbook of Palliative Medicine* (3rd edn) (ed. D. Doyle, *et al.*), pp. 935–944. Oxford: Oxford University Press.

2 Field M. J., Cassel C. K. (1997) Approaching death: Improving care at the end of life. Washington, DC: National Academies Press.

such as arthritis, and other musculoskeletal problems affect 25–50% of the community-dwelling elderly and are also typically under-treated

Carer burden

- The tremendous growth in the number of people over 65 years of age with chronic health problems challenges both national and personal resources
- In the UK, the duration of caring for an elderly relative can often exceed ten years
- Caregiving in general is not valued in western societies, where sometimes those involved in full-time caring can be made to feel that life is passing them by
- A large proportion of carers have financial difficulties

Risks to the carer include:

- Physical risks
  - increased mortality—many of the carers are themselves elderly and vulnerable
  - development of particular conditions, such as musculoskeletal diseases through lifting and handling
- Emotional risks
  - major depression, and associated comorbidities
- Social risks
  - isolation and loss of contact with friends and social circle. Close to 90% of carers say they need more help in caring for their loved ones in one or more of the following areas, including:
    - personal care
    - nursing
    - transportation
    - loss of income
    - loss of status within society

How can we address the needs of an elderly, frail and depressed woman who is shortly to be bereaved, and who through the course of caring for her demented husband over many years has lost contact with any support network of friends or family?

Medical goal-setting in the care of the elderly with chronic illness (Table 8f.1)

Table 8f.1 A checklist for palliative care throughout the course of chronic illness in the elderly

Early	Middle	Late
Discuss diagnosis, prognosis and course of disease	Assess efficacy of disease-modifying therapy Access appropriate support	Discuss changing goals of care with patient and family
Discuss disease-modifying therapies Manage comorbidities	Review course of disease	Confirm previous Advance Directives
Discuss goals of care, hopes and expectations	Reassess goals of care and expectations	Actively manage symptoms
Discuss advance care planning	Confirm Advance Directives and ensure a healthcare proxy is appointed	Review financial resources and needs
Advise financial planning/consultation with a social worker for future needs	Recommend physio/occupational therapies to preserve function and promote socialization Review behavioural and pharmacological symptom control	Review long-term care needs and discuss options
Inform patient and family about support groups Inquire about desire for spiritual support	Treat mood disorders Suggest support groups for patient and caregiver	Consider if palliative care needs are being well met in current care setting
Review behavioural and pharmacological symptom control	Offer social and emotional support to caregivers	Consider referral/planning to ensure peaceful death
Treat mood disorders	Review long-term care options and resource needs	Assess spiritual needs Offer respite care

Reproduced from Oxford Textbook of Palliative Medicine.[3]

3 Meier D., Monias A. (2004) Palliative medicine and care of the elderly. In *Oxford Textbook of Palliative Medicine* (3th edn) (ed. D. Doyle, *et al.*), pp. 935–944. Oxford: Oxford University Press.

Early in illness

Healthcare professionals should discuss goals of care with their patients. These goals may change as the disease progresses but may include:

- Prolonging life
- Preserving autonomy and independence
- Maintaining social activities
- Forming a plan for advanced stages of disease
- Staying at home

Mid-disease

The middle disease period is characterized by:

- Increased medical needs
- Declining function
- Loss of independence, and increased dependence on caregivers for assistance in basic activities of daily living. For example, patients with dementia require increased supervision, while patients with Parkinson's disease, heart failure or rheumatological diseases may need more help with ambulation

Patient needs

- Treatment for physical symptoms of chronic disease such as pain, dyspnoea, anorexia, nausea, vomiting, changes in bowel habit and insomnia which may become prominent during this phase of disease. These symptoms should be effectively treated as outlined in other chapters

Caregiver needs

- Help in supervision of the patient, the lack of which results in great caregiver stress, leading to unnecessary consideration of nursing home placement
- Information about local resources for adult day care, respite care, home care services and support groups
- Help to maintain physical, financial and emotional strength for the tasks ahead by providing opportunities to discuss and address their particular difficulties
- Where appropriate, encouragement of a regular rotating schedule of respite support from family and friends

Home needs

- Home evaluation for adaptive devices such as raised toilet seats, shower seats and other equipment

Late in disease of chronic illness

In the later stages of disease, the goals may shift to providing maximum comfort and security.

Patient needs

- To be treated as an individual, and as a person with particular characteristics and needs
- Careful attention to symptom control as, particularly in the last few months of life, patients may lose the ability to complain of pain and other symptoms (e.g. pain is often under-treated in end-stage dementia.)

- Ensuring that their wishes, fears and concerns, as far as possible, are discussed and addressed
- Ensure enjoyment of life as much as possible
- At this stage of disease, mortality is 50% at six months, and the goals of care shift to minimize suffering and maximize quality of life, according to the values and expressed wishes of the patient
- Physicians should discuss the merits, or otherwise, of continuing routine procedures with the patient and carers

Carer needs
- Patients in end-stage chronic disease may be bed or chair-bound. They can become completely dependent on caregivers for feeding, toileting, bathing and dressing and are often incontinent, which can be extremely distressing both for the patient and the carer
- As patients deteriorate carers can enter a chronic state of loss as they witness their relative's physical and mental deterioration. Recognition of the loneliness and pain of such a state can bring important comfort and help
- Due to increased care demands and exhaustion, the patient's family may benefit from respite admissions to allow the patient's choice to stay at home long term to be achieved

Placement needs
- It is important that efforts are made to find out where a patient would prefer to die, and where possible to ensure that this decision is, as far as possible, respected
- Patients who reside in a nursing home and want to remain there in the comfort and security of familiar surroundings may not want to be transferred routinely to the hospital for intercurrent illness or for symptoms that can be managed in the nursing home. 'Do not transfer' instructions should be discussed with the patient, family and staff where possible, and, if appropriate, to prevent an emergency move to an acute setting when the patient's condition deteriorates
- No one place is the ideal setting for terminal care for every person, as physical, emotional and social resources will all need to be balanced in the selection of place of care

Ageism and the care of the elderly

Ageist attitudes can inhibit the quality of palliative care available to elderly patients. Such attitudes may be displayed overtly or covertly:
- In hospitals— 'a disproportionate percentage of patients who are left waiting on trolleys for admission in the UK are elderly'
- By doctors and nurses—'He is too old to benefit from a hip replacement'
- By relatives—'Granny wouldn't want to be told about her disease'
- By the elderly themselves—'Why should anyone bother with me? I've had my day'

Common issues in palliative care of the elderly

Physical issues

Infection

- The late stages of many terminal illnesses are commonly complicated by life-threatening infections
- Immobility, malnutrition, incontinence, lung aspiration and decreased immunity increase the risk of pneumonia, cellulitis, decubitus ulcers, urinary tract infections and sepsis
- Decreased ability to express oneself and atypical presentation may lead to delayed recognition of infections
- Palliative care should focus on reducing the risk factors for infection by providing patients with good skin care, ambulation training and aspiration precautions
- As with all other treatments, the risks and benefits of antibiotic therapy need to be weighed

Pressure ulcers

- Many patients who are bedbound, incontinent and poorly nourished do not develop decubitus ulcers. This is due, in large measure, to the quality of care provided
- Those who do develop ulcers often do so in spite of excellent care
- The appearance of an ulcer may be a marker of deteriorating physical condition rather than a sign of poor medical or nursing care
- Use of pressure-relieving mattresses and cushions prior to the development of skin problems and good nursing care are the mainstays in preventing ulcers
- In the terminal phase, care should focus on relieving pain and limiting odour, not on ulcer cure
  - analgesia should be provided prior to all dressing changes
  - odour can be controlled with topical metronidazole gel, or silver sulfadiazine, or charcoal dressings
- Although the development of decubitus ulcers is not an independent risk factor for death, the presence of a pressure wound is a marker of advanced stage disease and poor prognosis

Pain

Treatment of pain in the elderly generally follows the same guidelines as in younger adults. Studies on clinical pain perception indicate that pain from headache and visceral pain decrease in the elderly, but musculoskeletal, leg and foot pain are more commonly reported by the elderly.

> Pain is undertreated in the elderly.

Concomitant diseases that are likely to cause chronic pain have a higher prevalence in the elderly and often exist alongside the major cause of pain, i.e. the development of bowel cancer will not prevent a patient from continuing to suffer the pain of rheumatoid arthritis.

Therefore a careful assessment of the actual cause of the patient's pain(s) is essential.

Nausea and vomiting

Common causes of nausea and vomiting in the elderly include:
- Drug reactions, including opioids
- Gastroparesis due to autonomic system dysfunction (especially caused by diabetes)
- Constipation

Management of nausea and vomiting in the elderly is the same as for younger patients, with particular attention being paid to possible side-effects from antiemetic medication. ('Start low, go slow.')

Constipation

Constipation is a nearly universal complaint of elderly patients. Over half of the elderly living in the community give a history of constipation. Risk factors include:
- immobility
- female gender
- depression
- chronic diseases
- common medications, e.g. opioids, calcium, iron, calcium channel blockers, tricyclic antidepressants and diuretics

Management

A patient who presents with a history of constipation should be given a rectal examination to exclude faecal impaction. (📖 See Chapter 6b.)

Diarrhoea

If patients are bedbound this symptom can be particularly exhausting and demeaning to patients and caregivers. A pattern of diarrhoea following a period of constipation often signifies overflow incontinence.

The incidence of *Clostridium difficile* enterocolitis has been highlighted recently as a common cause of diarrhoea in the elderly, particularly after the use of antibiotics (for Management 📖 see Chapter 6b.)

Cough

Common non-malignant causes of chronic cough in the elderly include oesophageal reflux disease, COPD and heart failure, and should be treated accordingly. Cough can also be a result of medications such as ACE inhibitors.

Dizziness

- Dizziness is a common complaint in elderly patients with chronic disease and may reflect a wide variety of physical problems
- The key to good management is a clear assessment, diagnosis and appropriate treatment of the underlying cause
- Secondary prevention is also important, reducing the risks of falls through education, and risk assessment of the patient's home.

Oral symptoms

Elderly patients are particularly prone to developing mouth problems arising as a result of denture problems, medication, mouth dryness and fungal infections.

- Infection should be treated appropriately and patients and caregivers instructed on oral hygiene
- Medications are the most common cause of dry mouth in elderly patients and should be kept under constant review
- When symptoms are not relieved with sips of water or ice, artificial saliva or commercial preparations containing mucin may provide relief

Falls

All patients who have had a fall should have a full history, examination and appropriate investigations looking for reversible causes whether or not they have a terminal illness. The consequences of the fall, e.g. hip fracture, subdural bleed, etc. will need managing on an individual basis according to clinical frailty and patient's wishes.

Assessment should include the following.

Blood pressure

Postural hypotension should be assessed by measuring the blood pressure both lying and standing. If there is a significant blood pressure drop on standing, reversible possibilities should be sought such as medication (e.g. diuretics, antihypertensives, antimuscarinics, beta-blockers, phenothiazines, withdrawal of steroids), anaemia, dehydration, insufficient adrenocortical function, etc. Patients should be advised to rise slowly from a lying/sitting position, to sleep propped up with pillows and to consider support hosiery. If no obviously reversible cause is found, treatment with fludrocortisone 0.05–0.1mg o.d. may be appropriate.

Medication review

Consider reducing or stopping:

- Hypotensive drugs: antimuscarinics, beta-blockers, phenothiazines, etc.
- Sedative drugs: benzodiazepines, opioid analgesics etc.
- Anticonvulsants (ataxia)
- Corticosteroids (proximal myopathy)

Neurological assessment:

- Spinal cord compression
- Cerebellar dysfunction
- Parkinson's disease or extrapyramidal symptoms
- Long tract signs suggestive of hemiparesis, etc.
- History suggestive of a seizure, TIA, etc.

Physiotherapy assessment:

- Balance
- Transfers
- Gait

Emotional issues

It can be particularly challenging in the elderly to differentiate between dementia, depression and delirium. The distinction is crucial, as adequate management of both delirium and depression may significantly improve the patient's quality of life.

Dementia

'A syndrome consisting of progressive impairment in two or more areas of cognition sufficient to interfere with work, social function or relationships in the absence of delirium or major non-organic psychiatric disorders.'

Some 5–8% of all people over the age of 65 suffer from moderate to severe dementia, with the prevalence doubling every 5 years reaching over 20% in 80 year olds.

Agitation in the chronically confused

- Up to 70% of patients with dementia may suffer from insomnia or 'sun-downing', a syndrome of increasing confusion during the evening
  - daytime exercises, a consistent bedtime routine and minimizing daytime napping can help improve sleep patterns
  - encouraging patients to participate in their own grooming and bathing may decrease agitation
  - sponge baths and adjusting water temperature may make bathing less threatening
  - familiar music and frequent social activities may also exert a calming influence
- Low doses of neuroleptics can ameliorate confusion, hallucinations and delusions
- Where medication is required then haloperidol 0.5mg p.o. can be given two-hourly up to a maximum dosage of 5mg in 24 hours. (British Geriatric Guidelines, Jan 2006) While second-generation antipsychotic drugs (risperidone and olanzapine) cause less extrapyramidal toxicity than first-generation antipsychotics, concern about cardiac side-effects limit their use in this situation. All patients still need to be monitored for parkinsonism, and doses should always be started as low as possible to minimize side-effects
- Successful management of agitation can prevent hospital admissions and nursing home placement

Anxiety

Being elderly and ill can often provoke considerable anxiety. Such anxiety may relate to:
- Concern about the process of dying: they may have had bad experiences of illness and death which lead them to anticipate that their end of life will inevitably be painful, undignified and difficult
- Concerns about leaving dependent relatives
- Concerns about unresolved conflicts or issues within the family
- Concerns about financial or housing matters

Anxiety may be helped by open discussion and isolation of the particular points of concern. General, non-specific, 'don't worry' advice tends to increase rather than decrease anxiety levels, as patients need a plan as to what they can do to address their concerns.

Prescribing in the elderly

This is a huge issue, and each year many patients (particularly the elderly) are admitted to hospital due to the effects of injudicious prescribing.
    Particular concerns include the following:

- Decreased renal function and liver metabolism places elderly patients at higher risk of drugs accumulating to toxic levels
- Multiple complex physical and psychological conditions can lead to a wide range of medication being prescribed for different complaints, with increasing likelihood of drug interactions causing dangerous side-effects
- Complex prescribing schedules and lack of support networks can lead to irregular medicine ingestion, with higher risks in a population where memory, eyesight and dexterity may not be as good
- It is easier to increase medication than it is to reduce or stop drugs which have been started by another specialist team
- Elderly patients may be particularly sensitive to the confusional side-effects of medication; therefore, it is important to exclude iatrogenic cause(s) in situations where patients suddenly exhibit confusion
- Medication which a patient has taken faithfully for many years to help with a symptom due to, for example, high blood pressure may no longer be strictly necessary, but the patient or family may have a belief in that particular tablet, which makes stopping it even in the last days of life very difficult
- Routes of administration can become an important issue in prescribing if an elderly patient loses the ability to swallow

General rules

- Give as few medications as possible
- Start medication at low doses and slowly increase
- Regularly review medication and reduce any unnecessary tablets
- Use pre-filled drug administration boxes or other devices that may help with concordance
- Remember that age should not exclude patients from either effective, expensive or innovative drug therapy where it is appropriate, and prescribe with care and consultation

Ethical issues

Artificial nutrition and hydration (📖 See Chapter 1)

General issues

- Patients suffering from end-stage dementia as well as other chronic neurological illnesses may develop dysphagia, which predisposes them to aspiration pneumonia
- In the late stages of dementia, patients frequently refuse food, clamp their mouths shut, or hold food without swallowing
- Feeding may become a frustrating battle between the patient and caregiver, who may feel that the patient is deliberately being difficult.

Carers will need support and information to understand that this may be involuntary and due to the dementia

Possible management options
- Changing the texture of the diet to a purée, or liquids thickened with cornstarch or potato starch, may support safe swallowing
- Improving the taste of food may provide increased enjoyment of the process of eating
- Training caregivers to feed the patient in an upright position, with the head forward, using small spoonfuls

---

Artificial nutrition and hydration is an emotionally charged issue for many caregivers. They may believe that their loved one would suffer hunger without artificial nutrition and hydration.

Family members should understand that loss of appetite is an integral part of the dying process.

Full assessment is necessary to exclude a reversible cause.

Decisions regarding the appropriateness of commencing artificial feeding need to be taken with great care and sensitivity and involve the full multidisciplinary team as well as the patient's formal and informal carers.

The process of decision formation at this critical time needs to be conducted thoroughly so that where possible a consensus can be reached.

Very little is known about the degree to which patients with severe dementia experience hunger or thirst, but great comfort can be given to caring families if they can continue to provide their loved one with small amounts of comfort food

---

For a fuller discussion of these issues 📖 see Chapter 1.

Common sources of suffering and discomfort in the elderly

- Patients may suffer even when they are free of pain or other symptoms
- Healthcare professionals need to ask about suffering as well as pain
- Questions should be open-ended in order to help make the patient feel comfortable with discussing fear, anxiety and other non-physical symptoms: 'How are you feeling inside yourself?'
- A sample question to family members is, 'Are you concerned that your family member may be suffering or uncomfortable?'

As in younger patients, relief of pain goes hand in hand with treatment of the emotional and spiritual components that contribute to it.

Care of the carer

Carers of elderly patients in the end-stage of chronic disease often need as much or more attention from the medical team as the patient. While family carers may take enormous satisfaction from their ability to provide safe and loving care for their loved one, most also feel varying degrees of exhaustion, guilt and frustration.

- By listening to and trying to help address the concerns of carers, the medical team conveys the fact that the carer is not alone and that their concerns are legitimate and important
- Carer stress does not end after placing the patient in a nursing home
- Carers continue to worry about the patient as well as suffering guilt over the necessity of nursing home placement
- Carers universally have to face difficult medical (and goals of care) decisions when the questions arise of tube feeding, hospitalization for predictable infection and use of antibiotics

Hospice care and the elderly population

Concern exists within the palliative services of being overwhelmed by elderly patients with chronic long-term care needs:

- Although hospice care may be appropriate for certain patients with end-stage dementia and other chronic illnesses, a hospice is accessed less frequently for these patients than for those with cancer. This may be because it is more difficult to accurately identify a limited prognosis among such patients
- The needs of elderly patents suffering from long-term illnesses in the last year of life may far exceed the needs of patients with malignancy, yet the services available to meet those needs are often much fewer
- Quality palliative care does not require admission to a hospice, but does require access to a healthcare team committed to providing holistic, individualized, planned and communicated care in whatever setting is appropriate for the particular patient

Conclusions

Growing old is a natural process which often changes our bodies, minds and what we regard as being important. A life which has been well lived can provide an elderly person with great comfort and satisfaction as they contemplate their pending death.

Having the opportunity to 'sort things out' and to 'tidy up loose ends' can provide ease of mind to someone who is coming to the end of their life, and is a process that should be facilitated and not regarded as 'morbid'.

The essence of palliative care is providing holistic care tailored to the particular needs of the individual patient. The same can be said of care of the elderly.

Remaining open to all the possibilities of old age and the dying journey will prevent our care of the elderly in this very important part of their lives becoming stereotyped or sentimental and will help carers face the realities of their own mortality.

Further reading

Books

Hughes J. (2006) *Palliative Care in Severe Dementia*. London: Quay Books.

Meier D., Monias A. (2004) Palliative Medicine in care of the elderly. In *Oxford Textbook of Palliative Medicine* (3rd edn) (ed. D. Doyle, *et al*), pp. 935–944. Oxford: Oxford University Press.

Articles

Aminoff B., Adunsky A. (2005) Dying dementia patients: too much suffering, too little palliation. *American Journal of Hospice and Palliative Medicine*, **22**(5): 344–8.

Aminoff B., Adunsky A. (2006) Their last 6 months: suffering and survival of end-stage dementia patients. *Age and Ageing*, **35**(6): 597–601.

Bernabei R., *et al.* (1998) Management of pain in elderly patients with cancer. SAGE Study Group: Systematic assessment of geriatric drug use via epidemiology. *Journal of the American Medical Association*, **279**(23): 1877–82.

Convey V. (2008) How are the carers being cared for? A review of the literature. *European Journal of Palliative Care*. **15**(4): 182–185

Feldt, K. S., Gunderson J. (2002) Treatment of pain for older hip fracture patients across settings. *Orthopedic Nursing*, **21**(5): 63–4; 66–71.

Krulewitch H., *et al.* (2000) Assessment of pain in cognitively impaired older adults: a comparison of pain assessment tools and their use by nonprofessional caregivers. *Journal of the American Geriatrics Society*, **48**(12): 1607–11.

Lawlor P. G., *et al.* (2000) Delirium at the end of life: critical issues in clinical practice and research. *Journal of the American Medical Association*, **284**(19): 2427–9.

Oldred E., Bryant C. (2008) Dementia Care, Part 3: end-of-life care for people with advanced dementia. *British Journal of Nursing*. **17**(5): 308–314.

Toye C., *et al.* (2006) Fatigue in frail elderly people. *International Journal of Palliative Nursing* **12**(5): 202–8.

Spiritual care

Spirituality is a construct, a way of thinking about human experience that can be helpful, but only up to the point at which one begins to believe it exists.

The word 'spirit' is widely used in our culture. Politicians speak about the 'spirit' of their party, veterans talk about the war-time 'spirit'; religious people discuss the 'spirit' as that part of human being that survives death, whereas humanists might regard the human 'spirit' as an individual's essential, but non-religious, life force. Related words are equally common and diverse: footballers describe their team as a spiritual home; there are spiritual healers, spiritual life coaches, spiritual directors, spiritual music, spiritual art, and spiritually revitalizing beauty care products.

Increasingly, the terms 'spirit', 'spiritual' and 'spirituality' are used by healthcare professionals. But these complex words need to be used with care and understanding. Their origins are essentially theological and/or philosophical and as such their primary meanings denote technical theological and philosophical ideas. However, they have also developed more commonly used secondary or derived meanings, and it is these that connote some of the more popular understandings.

Beneficial effects of religion and spirituality

A number of studies report reduced mortality rates among religious and spiritual people. One US study found those attending religious services weekly were:

- 53% less likely to die from coronary disease than those who did not
- 53% less likely to die from suicide;
- 74% less likely to die from cirrhosis[1]

The religious community seems to be protected from the effects of social isolation. Religion provides and strengthens family and social networks, gives a sense of belonging and self-esteem and offers spiritual support in times of adversity. A study by Bernardi et al.[2] showed that rosary prayer and yoga mantra had an effect on autonomic cardiovascular rhythms. Recitation of the rosary, and also of yoga mantras, slowed respiration to 6/minute and enhanced heart rate variability and baroreflex sensitivity. Reduced heart rate variability and baroreflex sensitivity are powerful and independent predictors of poor prognosis in heart disease. Spirituality helps to induce calm, improve concentration and create a sense of well being by reducing adrenaline and cortisone levels and increasing endorphins.[2]

1 Pandya L (2005) Spirituality, religion and health. *Geriatric Medicine*, May.

2 Bernardi L, et al. (2001) Effect of rosary prayer and yoga mantras on autonomic cardiovascular rhythms: comparative study. *British Medical Journal*, **323**; 1446–1449.

Definitions

The root of 'spirit' is breath (Latin: *spiritus*) and it is easy to imagine how it became associated with the idea of life essence: when an ancient died their breath (*spiritus*) departed them.

Western theological/philosophical traditions

In the West, spirit is the third component of human being, alongside body and soul. (With Descartes 'soul' becomes 'mind'.)

> May God himself, the God of peace, sanctify you through and through. May your whole spirit [*pneuma*], soul [*psyché*] and body [*sōma*] be kept blameless at the coming of our Lord Jesus Christ.
>
> The New Testament, 1 Thessalonians 5:23

- 'Spirit', or breath, is that which gives life to the body
- Soul—or mind (psyche)—is conceived in terms of 'the essential imma-terial part of a human, temporarily united with its body'.[3]
- The Western tradition has been more interested in soul than spirit.

Eastern theological/philosophical traditions

Eastern spiritual teachers shared similar interests, although their emphasis on consciousness led to their tendency to speak about 'the self', atman.

- Early Vedic texts links the *atman* with the life breath (*prana*)
- In the later Upanishads, *atman* becomes consciousness, the essence of human being that transcends the body and its experiences
- Buddhist 'non-self' highlights the inter-being of all states of awareness

Separation of spirituality and secular medicine

The separation of spirituality from the practices of modern, secular medi-cine is rooted in eighteenth century Enlightenment debates about the nature of science and religion. The success and subsequent dominance of scientific method has left little place for the non-material soul.

Freud's hostility towards religion and mystical experience is taken as further support for rejecting language of the soul as anachronistic. However, in coining the name 'psychoanalysis', Freud made conscious ref-erence to the myth of Eros and Psyche (the soul).

> It was Freud's emphasis on the soul that made his analysis different from others. What we think and feel about man's soul—our own soul—is all important in Freud's view.
>
> Bruno Bettelheim[4]

Healthcare professionals need to be clear about the concepts they are using. And an effective definition is needed that can, for a contemporary context, make sense of the theological–philosophical roots of these ideas.

---

3 Swinbourne R. G. (1995) Soul. In: *The Oxford Companion to Philosophy* (ed. T. Honderich), p. 823. Oxford: Oxford University Press.

4 Bettelheim B. (1983) *Freud and Man's Soul*. New York Alfred A. Knopf.

A humanistic–phenomenological definition

The humanistic-phenomenological definition of spirituality proposed by Elkins et al.[5] is helpful insofar as it regards spirituality in very broad terms as 'a way of being':

> Spirituality...is a way of being and experiencing that comes through awareness of a transcendent dimension and that is characterized by certain identifiable values in regard to self, others, nature, life, and whatever one considers to be the Ultimate.[5]

In these terms, spirituality, as a way of being, is characterized by how one relates to:
- one's self
- others
- nature
- life
- that which one considers to be Ultimate:
  - God
  - Spirit
  - The transcendent Self
  - Nature/the Universe

Such a humanistic–phenomenological definition makes possible a much closer association of areas of thought and practice that have too long been kept separate and discrete. For this reason, psychotherapists and spiritual carers are beginning to speak of 'psychospiritual care'—a care for the spirit that unites traditional pastoral care, the 'cure of souls', with psychotherapy, which 'attends to the soul'.[6]

> If I were to choose a phrase that encapsulates the way I currently see myself working, it would be soul attender which...is a literal translation of the word psychotherapist.[7]

Most importantly, a humanistic–phenomenological definition of spirituality allows healthcare professionals, who may not be in any way religious, to be much clearer about spiritual care and their involvement in it.

5 Elkins D. N., et al. (1988) Towards a humanistic–phenomenological spirituality. *Journal of Humanistic Psychology*, **28**(4): 10.

6 Nolan S. (2006) Psychospiritual care: a paradigm (shift) of care for the spirit in a non-religious context. *The Journal of Health Care Chaplaincy*, **7**(1): 12–22.

7 West W. (2004) *Spiritual Issues in Therapy: Relating Experience to Practice*, p. 128. Basingstoke: Palgrave Macmillan.

Spirituality and religion

In contemporary speech, 'spirituality' is increasingly used as a contrast to 'religion'—usually in its institutional forms and often with the inference that that which is spiritual is more authentic than that which is religious.

The two orders are intimately related, but while it is possible to be authentically spiritual without being religious, it is difficult to be authentically religious without being spiritual. For this reason, religion can be viewed as one way in which people express their spirituality; but it is by no means the only way.

The effect of culture on individual spirituality

An individual's spirituality is shaped by the culture in which they live. So, where the language, foods, dress, social structures and customs are shaped by religious beliefs and practices, say in Roman Catholic, Hindu or Muslim countries, spirituality will be expressed through those cultural forms; and effective spiritual care will aim to support the expression of those cultural/religious forms.

When Rajendra was admitted to the Hospice it was clear that his prognosis was very limited. His district nurse had asked that he be admitted to a side room because his family, who were devoutly Hindu, wanted to be able to fulfil their familial and spiritual responsibilities to him without upsetting other patients. The family were extremely attentive to his personal physical care and also to his religious requests.

Through the reading of the Hindu scriptures and the burning of incense Rajendra seemed to derive great comfort.

The Hospice was a Christian foundation, with strong links to the local churches and an active chaplaincy department, which visited Rajendra regularly at his request.

Several members of staff found the overt Hindu practices very distressing as they were concerned about demonic influences. A decision was taken that such members of staff would be assigned to different patients.

Several weeks after his death the family returned to say how much they had valued their last days together with Rajendra in the Hospice. They had been nervous when admission had been suggested because they had been aware of the Christian ethos of the Hospice.

They also shared how Rajendra's greatest spiritual comfort and solace in his last days had come from the sense of love, care and acceptance he had received from hospice staff, particularly because in his business life as a shop owner, he had had to put up with a great deal of racial and religious harassment.

In secular Western cultures, where beliefs and values are transmitted in the home and/or the faith community, spirituality finds expression in a variety of forms, not necessarily religious. Again, effective spiritual care will understand that spiritual needs are none the less pressing for being non-religious.

The effect of personal journey on individual spirituality

Spirituality is also shaped by the individual's life journey, the experiences they have and their encounters with others. In particular, being faced with one's own mortality has a profound spiritual impact, which can fundamentally disturb long–held beliefs and values. This may not in itself be a bad thing, and patients may come to value the kind of freedom a changed perspective brings. However, the distress provoked by re-evaluating beliefs can be upsetting for carers, professionals and family alike, and a person experiencing the doubt, conflict and confusion that goes with the disintegration of existing belief, may need sensitive support in order to find a place of reintegration.

Equally, a life-threatening illness may reawaken dormant beliefs in those who have no particular affiliations with any faith group. But this reawakening may be sustaining or threatening depending on how the individual perceives it.

Research on belief and the 'good death'

The assumption underpinning much literature on spirituality, i.e. that a terminal illness intensifies patients' search for meaning, lacks empirical support. However, there is some research supporting anecdotal evidence that, in a terminal illness, what matters is not so much *what* a patient believes, but the *strength* of their beliefs.

- McClain-Jacobson *et al.* found that belief in an afterlife was associated with lower levels of end-of-life despair (desire for death, hopelessness, suicidal ideation), but was not associated with levels of depression or anxiety, and concluded that spirituality has a much more powerful effect on psychological functioning than afterlife beliefs.[8]
- Smith *et al.* noticed a significant curvilinear relationship between a patient's perspective about death and their actual fear of death, 'suggesting that [actual] beliefs are a less critical determinant of death fear than is the certainty with which these beliefs are held'.[9]

The findings indicate the majority did not seek religious comfort or conversion as a response to the challenge of terminal illness, even when this was seen as desirable. Although participants were not actively inspired to be religious as a result of their illness, they did hold a number of spiritual perspectives that were actively at play.[10]

8 McClain-Jacobson C., *et al.* (2004) Belief in an afterlife, spiritual well-being and end-of-life despair in patients with advanced cancer. *General Hospital Psychiatry*, **26**(6): 484–6.

9 Smith D. K., Nehemkis A. M., Charter R. A. (1983) Fear of death, death attitudes, and religious conviction in the terminally ill. *International Journal of Psychiatry in Medicine*, **13**(3): 221–32.

10 McGrath P. (2003) Religiosity and the challenge of terminal illness. *Death Studies*, **27**(10): 881–99.

Faith practices

It is **always unhelpful** to make assumptions about how a patient may value their faith and its practices.

It is important to remember that, in most cultures of the world, spirituality has a practical, social and material impact on people's daily lives—it is the experience of Western culture that is exceptional.

Spirituality plays a vital role in the well-being of large numbers of British residents, and in a pluralistic culture many will value being able to express their spirituality through their religious and cultural traditions.

The complexion of British multicultural society is increasingly diverse, and it is very difficult for non-specialists to understand the nuances of faith traditions. Chaplains or Spiritual Care specialists are an important resource for addressing patients' religious and cultural requirements, but the real experts will be the patients themselves and/or their faith community leaders/spiritual advisors.

Healthcare professionals should always consult the patient directly, or if this is impossible, the patient's family, about their religious and cultural requirements. However, caution will be needed as, while some patients may identify belonging to a particular faith group, they may wish to deviate from what their family consider 'orthodox' practices.

A woman born Roman Catholic and who later converted to Islam, married a Muslim man with whom she raised an Islamic family. Against the wishes of her son and now divorced husband, she wanted to have a Roman Catholic funeral and be cremated. Her nurse referred her to the chaplain!

Spiritual care team

It is normal for members of the spiritual care team to be able to meet the religious and cultural requirements (sacraments, etc.) of the majority of patients, and to act as a resource to the multidisciplinary team for advice on dietary and ethical issues.[11]

- Where patients come from minority faith traditions, as far as possible the spiritual care team will liaise with spiritual advisors/faith community leaders
- The spiritual care team will also be skilled in conducting, arranging or even creating 'bespoke' services that address the pastoral needs of individual patients:
  - informal bedside prayers or meditations
  - *ad hoc* prayers for impromptu family gatherings
  - reaffirmation of marriage vows
  - *in extremis* wedding services
  - baby memorials
  - spiritual healing services, etc.

---

11 For further help, see www.faithandfood.com

- The spiritual care team is likely to have religious artefacts (prayer mats, beads, icons, etc.) and texts that patients will want to use to aid their spiritual practices.

Supporting patients' religious practice

It is important to remember that a patient's frustrations with low energy levels during illness are likely to impact on their ability to follow the routine practices of their faith, which may in turn impact on their spiritual well-being. Religious disciplines are normally relaxed during ill health, for example, the fast during the Muslim holy month of Ramadan.

Faith practices can be particularly helpful in times of stress and change. In the context of illness and the inevitable medicalization inherent in modern treatment pathways, faith practices can help to maintain a person's sense of identity distinct from that of 'patient'.

Around the period of death, faith practices can have particular value, underscoring the transition from life to death. These practices may help patients and relatives:
- Make sense of their loss
- Be supported through the pain of transition and loss
- Provide a framework for dealing with the process of letting go

Spiritual pain

> The realization that life is likely to end soon may well…give rise to feelings of…the unfairness of what is happening, and at much of what has gone before, and above all a desolate feeling of meaninglessness. Here lies, I believe, the essence of spiritual pain.[12]

Saunders' closely identified spirituality with the human search for meaning. Her approach to 'spiritual pain' has been influential:

> Spiritual relates to a concern with ultimate issues and is often seen as a search for meaning.
>
> Peter Speck[13]

> The diagnosis of life-threatening disease has a profound effect on people who are ill and…questions relate to identity and self-worth as patients seek to find an ultimate meaning to their lives.
>
> NICE Guidance on Cancer Services[14]

> [A] number of themes echo through most discussions about spirituality. The link between human spirituality and existential questions about meaning and purpose seems to be at the heart of these themes.
>
> Gillian White[15]

> It is the health care professionals' role to assist individuals to make sense and find meaning in times of crisis such as the acceptance of a terminal diagnosis.
>
> Wilfred McSherry[16], 2006

These assertions seem to be based on Saunders' own conviction, which she draws from the existential psychotherapy of Viktor Frankl. This implies that terminal patients engage (at some level) in a conscious/intellectual process of meaning making. If so, this distorts how Frankl understood 'spiritual'.

Frankl[12] saw the 'spiritual' as the defining mark of what it means to be human: 'human existence is spiritual existence'. He regarded being human as being 'existentially responsible, responsible for one's own existence', and argued that the search for meaning is the making of a response.

12 Saunders C. (1988) Spiritual pain. *Journal of Palliative Care*, **4**(3): 29–32.

13 Speck P. (1988) *Being There: Pastoral Issues in Time of Illness*. London: SPCK.

14 NICE (2004) *Guidance on Cancer Services: Improving Supportive and Palliative Care for Adults with Cancer*. London: NICE.

15 White G. (2006) *Talking about Spirituality in Health Care Practice: A Resource for the Multi-professional Health Care Team*. London & Philadelphia: Jessica Kingsley Publishers.

16 McSherry W. (2006) *Making Sense of Spirituality in Nursing and Health Care Practice: An Interactive Approach* (2nd edn). London: Jessica Kingsley Publishers.

What is the meaning of life?...man is not he who poses the question, What is the meaning of life? but he who is asked this question, for it is life itself that poses it to him. And man has to answer to life by answering for life; he has to respond by being responsible; in other words, the response is necessarily a response-in-action.[17]

Spirituality, then, can be understood as an often unconscious response to the question posed by particular life crises: 'How shall I live?'; 'How will I *be* in this situation?'; 'How will I face *my* dying?'

Because spiritual pain causes patients to suffer, and because palliative care is about the relief of suffering, spiritual pain is often taken as something that healthcare professionals must strive to relieve.

McSherry[18] borrows an expression from St John of the Cross, a sixteenth century Spanish mystic, to describe spiritual pain as 'the dark night of the soul'. But McSherry misrepresents the idea in terms of spiritual search and confusion. Yet the sense of crisis that often accompanies 'the dark night' is not necessarily pathological. Spiritual pain can be the pain associated with spiritual growth, and may:

- Draw out compassion, or even rekindle love between estranged friends/relatives/partners
- Prompt in the patient a reappraisal or re-evaluation of their life
- Lead to the recovery of values, beliefs, talents, ways of being long since lost or forgotten
- Be a transition point along the patient's journey towards greater self-understanding

I was angry, very angry—angry at the world—and that's not me. I'm not like that. I'm usually very calm. That's not the way I want to be. I think that's a quite natural reaction; but I don't want to be angry, I don't want to die angry. But actually, I feel as if I'm moving on from that now. I feel as if I'm moving into trying to making sense of what is ahead.

This is not the old theological idea that humans are sinful and that, there-fore, suffering is necessary and good; rather, it develops Saunders' idea that: 'The last part of life may have an importance out of all proportion to its length.'

- The patient may have important things yet to do, which in the short term may cause distress, but which may ultimately be healing
- The desire always to relieve spiritual pain, even when it is a feature of spiritual growth, may conflict with the patient's need to do 'life-work'
- In which case, the desire to intervene prematurely in spiritual pain may say more about how healthcare professionals deal with pain in others and about how Western culture currently views death and dying

17 Frankl V. E. (2000) *Man's Search for Ultimate Meaning*, p. 29. New York: Basic Books.

18 McSherry W. (2006) *Making Sense of Spirituality in Nursing and Health Care Practice: An Interactive Approach* (2nd edn). London: Jessica Kingsley Publishers.

Spiritual pain can be thought of as the pain of growth associated with the patient's struggle to respond to the question: How shall I *be*—with my self, with others, in the world, nature, and towards the Ultimate—when I am facing my own death?

> However many dying people I've known, this person is dying for the first time and I don't know what they need: everyone has different needs. You must hold your previous experience of dying patterns very lightly... Death reveals that life's about change, so how can we hold to our fixed ideas?
>
> Buddhist staff member of a US hospice

If this is the case, the spiritual pain of a patient poses a profound question to the healthcare professional: 'How will I respond to the patient in front of me?' 'Will I be their...':

- Consultant?
- Social worker?
- Nurse?
- Physiotherapist?
- Chaplain?

'Or will I simply be with them as another human being who has a particular set of knowledge and skills that might be of some help?'

> I couldn't bring rule books about how to be with dying people. When I walked into a room with a person who was dying, there was just the person and me and here we are. And if I'm full of hiding in roles and identities I cut myself off from them and they're left alone, which is the hardest way to die.
>
> Ram Dass[19]

Anticipatory grief

Those who care for a dying person also experience spiritual pain. When circumstances force a carer to live incongruously the experience can be profoundly disturbing.

- Awareness of their own needs—repressed or suppressed by the demands of constant care—may cause them to feel they are betraying or abandoning their partner, parent or friend
- They themselves may feel betrayed or abandoned by their loved one, and they may be shocked by the strength of their anger towards the one for whom they care
- Anticipating what life will be like after the death, or even planning for the funeral, may seem premature and again shocking, and may arouse strong feelings of guilt

19 Dass R. (1992) *Death is not an outrage.* A talk given by Ram Dass to the National Hospice Organisation. Available from www.ramdasstapes.org

For some time Maureen had been planning a foreign holiday. Caring non-stop for six months, she was feeling in real need of her break. However, her first husband had died while she was away and she feared the same would happen again. Nonetheless, she was determined that she had to go.

When her husband had been admitted to the hospice and was expected not to have long to live, Maureen's immediate question had been, 'Will I still be able to get away?' She felt guilty and embarrassed that her first thoughts had been of herself.

In her carers group she talked about guilt and responsibility, and about what long-term caring for a dying person does to the carer. Maureen spoke about wanting the best for her husband, but felt she needed an end to her stress. The seemingly endless experience created emotions within her that made her think and feel in ways that were incongruent with how she would normally have expected to have thought and felt.

Maureen was being squeezed into a spiritually detrimental situation: living inauthentically against herself over an extended period.

Spiritual assessment

It cannot be assumed that all patients have spiritual needs at all times, and when they do, that they always want or need to share them with health professionals.[20]

Assessment has been defined as 'the process of gathering, analyzing, and synthesizing salient data into a multidimensional formulation that provides the basis for action decisions'.[21] There are two contrasting approaches to spiritual assessment:
• The use of a formalized 'spiritual assessment tool'
• The intuitive use of interpersonal skills

Formalized spiritual assessment

Formalized assessment tools include sets of both quantitative and qualitative questions aimed at understanding the patient's current spiritual needs. These may be based around the taking of a spiritual history.

HOPE[22]
• What sources of **H**ope, strength, comfort, meaning, peace, love and connection does the patient have?
• What role does **O**rganized religion play in the patient's life?
• What is the patient's **P**ersonal spirituality and practices?
• What will be the **E**ffects of these factors on the patient's medical care and end-of-life decisions?

• *Advantages of formalized assessment tools:*
  • provide a frame within which healthcare professionals can open conversations about spiritual issues with a patient
  • promise a means by which any healthcare professional can make a spiritual assessment
• *Limitations of formalized assessment tools*:
  • patients may experience such assessment as intrusive and insensitive to their need to be met at the level of their subjectivity
  • inept use of an assessment tool may dehumanize the patient and hinder the formation of a compassionate therapeutic relationship

20 Farvis R. A. (2005) Ethical considerations in spiritual care. *International Journal of Palliative Nursing*, **11**(4): 189.

21 Hodge D. R. (2001) Spiritual assessment; a review of major qualitative methods and a new framework for assessing spirituality. *Social Work*, **46**(3): 203–15.

22 Anandarajah G., Hight E. (2001) Spirituality and medical practice: Using the HOPE questions as a practical tool for spiritual assessment. *American Family Physician*, **63**(1): 81–8.

Intuitive spiritual assessment

A more intuitive approach to spiritual assessment is the use of interpersonal skills developed through reflective practice on 'being with' patients. This depends entirely on the particular experience, skill and personality of the spiritual assessor, and is rooted in the quality of the relationship between healthcare professional and patient.

- *Challenge of intuitive assessment:*
  - demands high levels of self-awareness and empathy on the part of the healthcare professional
  - requires the healthcare professional to demonstrate 'a personal awareness of the "spiritual" dimension, [be] themselves searching for meaning, have experienced a life crisis, recognize "spiritual" care as part of their role and [be] particularly sensitive and perceptive people'.[23]

The intuitive approach to spiritual assessment relies on careful listening to the stories patients tell about themselves and the particularities of the language they use.

The language of spiritual pain

Loss: As a child, I had a place in my mind where I would go until things became safe again. I need it now, but *I've lost it...I can't find it.*

Helplessness: Ah well, nothing to be done, nothing to be done...nothing to be done.

Isolation: There's no way really to know that what you're going through is normal.

Fear (of losing control): If I could only get control of my emotions then everything would be fine.

Pointlessness: This shouldn't be happening...We used to do this differently. Years ago, they would've just up'd the morphine.

While it is the case that all members of the multidisciplinary team contribute to spiritual care, it is debatable whether all are qualified to undertake spiritual assessment. Farvis questions whether it is even 'reasonable to expect nurses who are unfamiliar with the concept of their own spirituality to engage in spiritual care at all?' [20]

Possible questions for initiating a conversation about spiritual assessment

- What is important to you at the moment?
- How is all this affecting you?
- How's it going?

23 Johnson C. P. (2001) Assessment tools: are they an effective approach to implementing spiritual health care within the NHS? *Accident and Emergency Nursing*, **9**: 177–86.

Skills needed in spiritual care

Spiritual care is less about imparting specialist knowledge, be that of theology, philosophy or ritual practice, than it is about the ability to *be* genuinely present to another person during an episode of spiritual pain. Consequently, spiritual care is not the sole prerogative of paid specialists; any multidisciplinary team member *can* offer spiritual care. However, only those capable of what Walter calls 'watch-with-me vulnerability'[24] actually *do* provide real spiritual care.

The 'cure of souls' ('traditional' spiritual care) and 'soul attending' (psychotherapy) are closely associated, and the skills of psychospiritual care are similar to those of counselling and psychotherapy:

• Self-awareness—understanding how one is affected by others; understanding one's limits and triggers
• Unconditional positive regard—'prizing' the other; love
• Empathy—intuitively sensing the patient's world 'as if' it were one's own, but without ever losing the 'as if' quality
• Active listening
• Sense of humour[25]
• Spiritual integrity—balancing one's personal spirituality with what at times can be the challenging beliefs of others

> When the client's world is this clear to the therapist, and he moves about in it freely, then he can both communicate his understanding of what is clearly known to the client and can also voice meanings in the client's experience of which the client is scarcely aware
>
> Carl R. Rogers[26]

Spiritual companion: *Anam Cara*

Spiritual care, particularly of those facing their own death, demands the response of a wise and compassionate 'spiritual friend' (Celtic: *Anam Cara*). Not every member of the multidisciplinary team will be equipped to offer this level of spiritual care. But each one contributes to enabling patients to find a 'way of being' that will enable them to go through the experience of dying in the way appropriate to them.

24 Walter T. (1997) The ideology and organization of spiritual care: three approaches. *Palliative Medicine,***11**: 21–30.

25 Taylor E. J., Mamier I. (2005) Spiritual care nursing: What cancer patients and family caregivers want. *Journal of Advanced Nursing,* **49**(3): 260–7.

26 Rogers C. (1957) The necessary and sufficient conditions of therapeutic personality change. *Journal of Consulting Psychology* **21**: 95–103.

The spirituality of those who care for the dying must be the spirituality of the companion, of the friend who walks alongside, helping, sharing and sometimes just sitting, empty handed, when one would rather run away. It is a spirituality of *presence*, of being alongside, watchful, available, of being *there*.

Sheila Cassidy

Further reading

Books

Cassidy S. (1988) *Sharing the Darkness*. London: Darton, Longman & Todd.

Doyle D., *et al.* (eds). (2004) *Oxford Textbook of Palliative Medicine* (3rd edn). Oxford: Oxford University Press.

Frankl V. E. (2000) *Man's Search for Ultimate Meaning*. New York: Basic Books.

McSherry W. (2006) *Making Sense of Spirituality in Nursing and Health Care Practice: An Interactive Approach* (2nd edn). London: Jessica Kingsley Publishers.

NICE (2004) *Guidance on Cancer Services: Improving Supportive and Palliative Care for Adults with Cancer*. London: NICE.

O'Donohue J. (1999) Anam Cara: *Spiritual Wisdom from the Celtic World*. London: Bantam Books.

Ram-Prasad C. (2005) *Eastern Philosophy*. London: Weidenfeld & Nicolson.

Speck P. (1988) *Being There: Pastoral Issues in Time of Illness*. London: SPCK.

Stanworth R. (2004) *Recognizing Spiritual Needs in People who are Dying*. Oxford: Oxford University Press.

Wilcock P. (1996) *Spiritual Care of Dying and Bereaved People*. London: SPCK.

White G. (2006) *Talking about Spirituality in Health Care Practice: A Resource for the Multi-professional Health Care Team*. London & Philadelphia: Jessica Kingsley Publishers.

Articles

Marie Curie Cancer Care. *Spiritual & Religious Care Competencies for Specialist Palliative Care*. Available at http://www.mariecurie.org.uk/forhealthcareprofessionals/spiritualandreligiouscare/

The contribution to palliative care of allied health professions

Introduction

Palliative care has been very successful at taking ideas, values and techniques from other disciplines in healthcare. Such borrowing of ideas has nearly always included considerable adaptation from the parent discipline. However, the notion of cross-boundary, interdisciplinary working is now highly developed in palliative care. Some disciplines such as medicine and nursing have become core parts of the specialist team, whereas others have been accessed on an as-required basis. Increasingly, individual allied health professions have seen the need to evolve the palliative care specialism within the generic discipline. Allied health professionals (AHPs) include occupational therapists, physiotherapists, nutritional experts, speech and language therapists, clinical psychologists, social workers and chaplains, pharmacists, art and music therapists.

Rehabilitation

Palliative rehabilitation aims to improve the quality of survival. The emphasis of palliative rehabilitation is to attempt to restore quality of life by a maintenance and compensatory approach even if a 'normal' functional level is not possible.

The length of survival for most patients with cancer and other chronic progressive cardiac, respiratory and neurological illnesses has increased over the past 25 years. In some patients this is associated with prolonged disability due to the disease itself and/or the side-effects of treatment.

In general medicine, rehabilitative techniques are generally associated with chronic benign disease and disability with an aim of restoring functional independence. In palliative care, rehabilitation shares the same principles of maximizing a person's potential regardless of life expectancy.

Most patients are fearful of being dependent on others, however they can be helped to be as independent as possible and to live a fulfilled life within the constraints of their illness. This not only helps patients but also relieves the stress of caregivers. Patients within palliative care settings are deteriorating and techniques need to be individually tailored to the rate of clinical deterioration. Techniques include setting realistic and achievable goals which are determined in conjunction with the multidisciplinary team. These goals must be reassessed continually in parallel with the exacerbations and remissions of disease and symptoms. In the later stages of the disease trajectory the goals may have to be reassessed on a day-to-day or even hour-to-hour basis. At different stages of the illness the purpose of goals may vary. It may be appropriate for a patient with a prognosis of weeks/months to set goals for mobilizing with comfort in order to get away for a holiday or to attend an important family event. For patients with a prognosis of days/weeks, goals may include providing physical, emotional, social and spiritual support to both patient and carers to enable them to manage a home death with confidence.

Palliative rehabilitation

- Helps patients gain opportunity, control, independence and dignity
- Responds quickly to help patients adapt constantly to their illness
- Takes a realistic approach to goal setting
- Takes the pace from the individual
- Looks at restoration of quality of life
- Adds life to patient's days not days to their lives[1]
- Is an attitude as well as a process
- Adopts a compensatory approach with a focus on problem solving and the promotion of coping strategies

Assessment of potential for successful palliative rehabilitation

Biological/medical status

A careful medical assessment of the underlying disease, and other disease pathologies which may be contributing to morbidity, needs to be undertaken in order to direct treatment to optimize the control of symptoms (e.g. correction of anaemia or congestive heart failure, treatment of spinal cord compression). In the absence of reversible pathology the empirical control of symptoms is paramount. Consideration should also be given to prognosis. In this way, patients will be in the best position to be able to achieve their own realistic goals.

Psychological status

Patients experience many losses as their illness progresses. These include loss of mobility, self-esteem, position or role in the family as well as expectations for the future. These factors, together with loss of control over their lives, may intensify their feelings of anger, apathy, depression and hopelessness, which will have a negative impact on rehabilitation.

A lack of motivation may need to be explored, to ensure that there are no reversible factors such as clinical depression which may impede their ability to think in any positive way about the future. A competent unwillingness to participate in rehabilitation, on the other hand, should be respected. Palliative rehabilitation offers positive psychological support to overcome lack of confidence, poor motivation and to adjust to losses.

- **Decreased cognition:** patients must be able to follow instructions and retain information in order to benefit maximally from palliative rehabilitation. However, limited functional goals can still be met despite limited cognition
- **Social and environmental factors:** such factors as family and social support, emotional (and sometimes financial), impact on a patient's confidence in goal-setting and achievement

---

1 Twycross (2003). *Introducing Palliative Care*, p. 3 (4th edn) Abingdon: Radcliffe Medical Press.

Successful palliative rehabilitation depends on:

- Speed of team response
- Setting of realistic goals
- Adapting constantly to changing circumstances
- Supporting patients and carers through change

Rehabilitation team

- The patient, family and carers
- Medical staff
- Nursing staff—ward- and community-based
- Occupational therapist
- Physiotherapist
- Speech and language therapist
- Social worker
- Chaplain
- Psychologist
- Complementary therapists
- Dietician
- Other specialists, according to need

Members of the rehabilitation team will have specific expertise and skills to optimize the benefit of rehabilitation, but it is important to understand that there will be some overlap of treatments and roles.

The palliative rehabilitation approach is holistic, taking place at any stage of a person's disease process and in the environments of the ward, home or day hospice.

Further reading

Book

Crompton S. (2000) *Fulfilling Lives: Rehabilitation in Palliative care*. London: National Council for Hospice and Specialist Palliative Care Services.

NICE (2004) *Improving supportive and palliative care for adults with cancer*. London: NICE.

Articles

Eva G., Lord S. (2003) Rehabilitation in malignant spinal cord compression. *European Journal of Palliative Care*, **10**(4): 148–50.

Fialka-Moser V., et al. (2003) Cancer rehabilitation: particularly with aspects on physical impairments. *Journal of Rehabilitation Medicine*, **35**(4): 153–62.

Hopkins K. F., Tookman A. J. (2000) Rehabilitation and specialist palliative care. *International Journal of Palliative Nursing*, **6**(3): 123–30.

Montagnini M., Lodhi M., Born W. (2003) The utilization of physical therapy in a palliative care unit. *Journal of Palliative Medicine*, **6**(1): 11–17.

Schleinlich M.A. (2008) Palliative care rehabilitation survey: a pilot study of patients' Priorities for rehabilitation goals. *Palliative Medicine*, **22**(7): 822–831.

Young I. (2004) The importance of cancer rehabilitation. *Cancer Nursing Practice*, **4**(3): 31–4.

Occupational therapy

Occupational therapy enables people to achieve health, well-being and life satisfaction through participation in occupation (College of Occupational Therapy).[1] In working with people who are terminally ill, occupational therapists value an individual's remaining life, help a client live in the present, recognize an individual's right to self-determination and acknowledge and prepare for the approaching death. The occupational therapist (OT) uses an activity-based, symptom-led rather than a disease- or diagnosis-led approach to treatment. The OT assesses various factors prior to advising on an appropriate intervention strategy.

Occupational history

A profile of the patient is built up based on family history, past self-care abilities, work experience, leisure and recreational patterns. A functional assessment is then made which includes:

- **Self-maintenance:** looking after oneself
- **Productivity:** productive to life, either in the form of domestic activities or earning a living
- Leisure

Self-esteem

A degree of social equilibrium and homeostasis is needed for a peaceful life, in harmony with all that life brings. When patients are diagnosed with a life-threatening illness and are changing from being totally independent to fluctuating or increasing levels of dependency, chaotic feelings can emerge. The natural protective reactions to this assault on self-esteem include anger, loss, resentment, bitterness and hostility.

These feelings are energy wasting, serve no useful purpose and can lead to withdrawal, apathy and depression: behaviours that can significantly impact on an individual's quality of life. Furthermore, carers are inevitably entrenched in this vicious circle of trying to cope not only with their own feelings but those of the patient, who may be continuing to verbalize that their present life is unacceptable. This extra burden and stress can trigger feelings of helplessness, hopelessness and uselessness in both patients and carers.

People are only able to feel self-worth if they are in a position to contribute, as a result of which they can engender respect in others. The role of the OT is to help identify and analyse the cause of these feelings and reactions and to provide the patient with coping strategies to facilitate empowerment and a sense of control. This may be through the interview process or through the selective use of a more specific psychological approach such as cognitive behavioural therapy (CBT).

1 *Occupational Therapy Standard Terminology Project* (2005) London: College of Occupational Therapists: Appendix B.

Physical systems

An analysis of the patient's physical capabilities will depend on the diagnosis and the course of the illness. The OT will need to have an understanding of the likely symptoms and prognosis in order to advise realistically, sensitively and appropriately while recognizing palliative patients' dual states of both living and dying.

The OT assesses physical dysfunction as it relates to muscle strength and endurance, assessing the degree to which disuse may have affected this and to what extent some rehabilitative potential might exist. The OT will need to be aware of muscle spasms and other pain and what factors trigger them. They will also assess ambulation and balance. The impact of cognitive and perceptual abilities will also be relevant and techniques will be found to compensate for these.

Quality of life

Quality of life is defined by the individual. As professionals, we can see potential and give advice that we believe might improve satisfaction (subjectively) in the patient and carer, and from which achievement can be measured (objectively). However, it is ultimately the choice of the individual, which must be valued and respected, to take or reject advice. A patient may, for example, feel that they gain more by not fighting physically or mentally to retain any vestige of their independence.

Goals

With the patient's full cooperation, the OT can help to set realistic goals. The goals must be feasible and structured. If a patient has always been very independent and is 'internally motivated', it may be very difficult for them to accept having to adapt to different methods of performance and what they perceive as unacceptably low goals yet still maintain their pride and dignity.

Carers may find pursuing goals a burden. For instance, they may worry about hurting the patient or themselves. They should not be asked or be required to do more than they are physically or emotionally capable of doing. Carers are often reassured by being told that they will be taught what to do. They need support from health professionals and other support groups, and advice for the often unspoken, unrecognized and unrewarded burden of care. Occupational therapy also has a role in educating both patient and carers about energy conservation, lifestyle changes, leisure activities and alternative means of carrying out activities of daily living.

Treatment planning

Patients and families are vulnerable and often fearful of the uncertain future. They may vacillate chaotically between objective, logical thought and subjective, emotional despair. The aim is to work alongside these feelings and to raise the level of functioning by helping independence. A problem-solving compensatory approach is usually required to achieve this. Both patients and carers can regain a semblance of order, structure, purpose and control. Sometimes, however, change or deterioration can happen quickly or unexpectedly and OTs will need to be able to react to that. Continuous review is essential to ensure that the therapist is still working towards the priorities of the individual and that priorities are still realistic and achievable.

Examples of occupational therapy interventions

- Carrying out home assessments and modifications to enable independence
- Retraining in personal activities, including toileting, feeding, bathing and dressing
- Retraining in domestic activities with the use of appropriate equipment, e.g. kitchen activities
- Ensuring a safe environment, for example devising and implementing complex manual handling plans using adaptive equipment
- Liaising with appropriate organizations in the community for packages of care
- Encouraging increasing engagement in purposeful activity. Teaching time management and the usefulness of daily routines. Redeveloping a sense of purpose and accomplishment to increase self-esteem
- Facilitating lifestyle management with continued engagement in hobbies and leisure pursuits. Promoting therapeutic activity programmes, such as involvement in creative activities and socialization, while encouraging the achievement of individual treatment goals
- Providing relaxation training and stress management. Training in energy conservation and work simplification techniques to cope with fatigue either as individual sessions or group work
- Supporting and educating carers
- Facilitating psychological adjustment to loss of function, e.g. through the use of CBT. Retraining in cognitive and perceptual dysfunction, e.g. learning compensatory techniques to improve procedural memory during domestic tasks
- Assessing for and prescribing wheelchairs, pressure-relief posture management and seating. Assessing muscle flexibility and positioning. Where necessary, having splints made and aiding transfers as well as incorporating both indoor and outdoor needs

Occupational therapists define a clear, structured, graded plan of action with the patient and carers to provide strength of purpose and dignity. Life is a delicate balance: a matter of coping and adapting to a situation in which being productive and feeling valued are paramount. The OT is critical to facilitating a person's sense of mastery and competence and for re-instilling substance and control into the quality of living.

Further reading

Book

Cooper J. (ed.) (2006) *Occupational Therapy in Oncology and Palliative Care* (2nd edn). Chichester: Wiley.

Articles

Armitage K., Crowther L. (1999) The rôle of the occupational therapist in palliative care. *European Journal of Palliative Care*, **6**(5): 154–7.

Bye R. (1998) When clients are dying: occupational therapists' perspectives. *Occupational Therapy Journal of Research*, **18**(1): 3–24.

Ewer-Smith C., Patterson S. (2002) The use of an occupational therapy programme within a palliative care setting. *European Journal of Palliative Care*, **9**: 30–3.

Graff M., *et al.* (2006) Community based occupational therapy for patients and their caregivers: randomized controlled trials. *British Medical Journal*, **333**(7580): 1196–9.

Pearson E., *et al.* (2007) How can occupational therapists measure outcomes in palliative care? *Palliative Medicine*, **21**(6): 477–85.

Dietetics and nutrition

> Laughter is brightest where food is best.

Nutrition is not solely concerned with refuelling the body, but has profound emotional and cultural significance. Food preparation symbolizes tangible care and affection and, as far as possible, should continue to be part of daily social interaction. For carers, a good intake by the patient is often thought of as a hopeful sign, whereas a decreasing intake, particularly as the patient deteriorates, often causes much conflict and distress. The patient may feel guilty for not eating and often forces him/herself to eat in order to please the family.

> You must eat up if you want to get better.

A good assessment of factors affecting nutritional status is important. Nutritional intervention focuses on ensuring that symptoms of disease or side-effects of treatment are managed well and on initiating appropriate dietary advice and strategies to prevent further morbidity. The aims of nutritional support in palliative care will change as the disease progresses.
Aggressive nutritional intervention is needed during the earlier stages of illness, allowing the patient to cope with:
- Metabolic demands of illness and treatment
- Repair of tissue and prevention of infection
- Maintenance of well-being and quality of life

Palliative nutritional care, on the other hand, concentrates on symptom control and targeted nutritional intervention later in the disease process, in order to enhance quality of life.
   The incidence of malnutrition in patients with cancer is high and nutritional screening is required for all patients.

Anorexia (📖 see Chapter 6c)
Anorexia is the absence or loss of appetite despite obvious nutritional needs. Reversible causes of anorexia must be addressed.

Cachexia
Cachexia is the metabolic inability to use nutrients effectively, resulting in weight loss, lipolysis, loss of muscle and visceral protein, anorexia, chronic nausea and weakness.

Role of the dietitian in palliative care

State registered dietitians are experts in nutrition and are, therefore, able to translate scientific theory into practical advice for patients, carers and other health professionals depending on the patient's needs. They can be accessed within the hospital or the community setting and work closely with other members of the multidisciplinary team. Their role is to enhance quality of life.

Tasks for the professional advising on nutrition:
- Assess a patient's nutritional status
- Elicit the patient's goals regarding nutrition
- Provide specialized nutritional advice at diagnosis, during treatment and in the palliative phase
- Advise on food preparation/fortification/supplementation as appropriate
- Relax dietary restrictions if possible, i.e. for patients with diabetes and hypercholesterol states
- Recommend and calculate feeding regimens to suit an individual patient's requirements, using enteral or parenteral access
- Provide psychological and emotional support
- Listen to patients' fears

Dietitians don't just give out nice little boxes of milky supplements!

Dietary management of common symptoms affecting nutritional status

The common symptoms experienced require a multidisciplinary team approach.

Loss of appetite
- Eat small frequent meals or snacks
- Eat slowly and relax after meals
- Use nutritious snacks if unable to manage full meals, e.g. baked beans, scrambled egg, cheese on toast, or tinned, frozen or convenience meals, i.e. macaroni, ravioli, cottage pie
- Consider 'take-aways' and pre-cooked, delivered meals: these do not need to be prepared so can be useful for stimulating appetite
- Take simple exercise or a glass of alcohol, if permitted: these can be useful stimulants
- Consider avoiding soups pre-meals: the volume may prevent further appetite for more nutritious foods

Sore mouth
- Choose foods with plenty of sauce or gravy, e.g. casseroles, fish in parsley sauce
- Moisten food with milk, butter, cream
- Choose soft foods, e.g. pasta dishes with sauces, creamy soups, egg dishes, milk puddings and mousses
- Avoid irritants such as citrus fruits (or juice), spicy or salty foods and rough, coarse, dry foods such as raw vegetables, toast, crackers
- Cook foods until they are soft and tender and cut into small pieces
- Use a blender or food processor to puree foods
- Sip fluids rather than gulping: sipping is more refreshing than gulping
- Keep the mouth clean—brush teeth, gums and tongue at least three times a day with a soft toothbrush
- Use mouthwashes regularly
- Suck ice before being treated with 5-fluouracil, other than in head and neck cancer as it helps to prevent mucositis

Nausea and vomiting

- Cold foods may be more acceptable than hot
- Eat small amounts slowly
- For sickness in the morning, eat prior to getting out of bed, e.g. plain biscuits, dry toast, or cracker
- Keep meals dry, do not add gravy or sauces
- Sip fluids after meals
- Keep upright whilst eating and for 2h afterwards
- Drink fizzy drinks—especially ginger ale and soda water which can help with nausea
- Use a fan to direct away odours, especially in hospital
- Grill foods: fatty foods may make nausea worse
- Check for other reversible causes, such as opioid medication, constipation, patient anxiety

Taste changes

- Try chicken, fish, milk, cheese, beans or nuts if the patient finds red meat tastes unpleasant. These foods are bland in taste and may be more acceptable
- Marinate meat in lemon juice or vinegar to improve flavour
- Use herbs and spices to mask the taste of meat
- Freshen the mouth with oranges, grapefruit, pineapple and lemon fruits or juices
- Consider cold food: these may taste better than hot food. It may suit the patient to have frequent cold snacks throughout the day rather than a more traditional three-meal pattern
- Avoid food and drink which contains saccharin or other artificial sweeteners since they may give food a bitter taste
- It is important to keep the mouth clean, brush teeth three times a day and use a recommended mouthwash
- Use plastic utensils if the patient experiences a metallic taste

Diarrhoea

- Discourage a high-fibre intake, i.e. reduce bran, fruit, vegetable, pulses
- Avoid strong tea and coffee which are gut stimulants
- Avoid spicy foods
- Reduce greasy, fatty foods: certain fats may make diarrhoea worse
- Check inappropriate laxative use
- Consider malabsorption

The above includes only some of the advice available and is a guideline only to the merits of a formal dietetic assessment.

Nutritional supplements

In the UK see the *British National Formulary* for a full range and the nutritional composition of prescribable products.

Oral supplementation is available to assist rather than replace food, but it will not increase weight or prolong the life of patients with cancer. Their benefits include increasing calorie and nitrogen intake and stimulating the appetite.

Many products are available on the market which range in nutritional support and can be expensive. Ideally, they should be recommended after the patient has been assessed by a state-registered dietitian who will then select the most appropriate product for that individual, according to their preferred taste and perceived need.

The challenge for dietitians working with patients in the palliative care setting is to use their expertise to cater for the particular needs of the individual patient whose requirements and goals may change rapidly.

Oral nutritional supplements can be divided into the following categories:

Oral sip feeds
- Some are nutritionally complete and provide a full range of vitamins and minerals
- Milk, juice or yoghurt options are available
- A good source of protein and energy

Fortified puddings
- Provide protein and calories in small volumes
- Are useful for dysphagic patients

Modular supplements
- Are a concentrated source of carbohydrate/protein fat
- Beneficial only if used in conjunction with a diet plan to ensure that a range of nutrients is provided
- Carbohydrate drinks are unsuitable for diabetics without supervision
- In powder form they can be incorporated into foods without increasing volumes
- Need to be calculated to patient requirements to maximize use and reduce risk of volume overload

Tube feeding
Tube feeding is generally nasogastric, or gastric through a percutaneous endoscopic gastrostomy (PEG) or radiologically inserted gastrostomy (RIG) but rarely may be duodenal or jejunal. The aim of feeding may be to replace normal food intake or to supplement it.

There is some evidence that artificial feeding prior to definitive oncological treatment, including surgery, may assist in stabilizing weight, improving quality of life and contribute to better treatment results. However, there is no evidence that artificial feeding prolongs life in those patients with advanced cancer.

The decision to feed artificially requires clinical judgement within the multidisciplinary team and good understanding of the patient's needs and feelings. If used appropriately (e.g. for some patients with neurological conditions when proper counselling and discussion have taken place, and occasionally in patients with head and neck cancer), it can be useful and take the pressure off patients and carers when eating has become a burden and food can no longer be tolerated or enjoyed.

Future developments
There has been a lot of interest in using eicosapentaenoic acid (EPA; an omega-3 fatty acid present in oily fish) as a treatment for patients with cancer for a variety of reasons, including modulation of aspects of the inflammatory response implicated in cancer cachexia, halting and reversing weight loss and prolongation of survival in some patients. The therapeutic potential in the management of end-of-life malnutrition includes its efficacy

in reducing weight loss and improving quality of life. EPA is given either as a capsule or enriched oral nutritional supplement. However, further research is required before a consensus is reached on its value.

Ethical issues

Healthcare professionals working within the palliative care setting are faced with ethical dilemmas daily. Decisions should be made with the support of the team and consideration of the patient and carers. In order to make a justifiable, considered decision, the following questions should be considered prior to commencing artificial feeding:

• What are the patient's wishes?
• What benefit will it bring to the patient?
• How much discomfort is caused by eating and drinking normally?
• How keen or able is the patient to continue eating and drinking?
• What are the risks and discomforts associated with artificial feeding?

Documents are available to offer guidance on nutrition and hydration to health professionals and some are listed below.

Further reading

Books

British Medical Association (2007) *Withholding and Withdrawing Life-Prolonging Medical Treatment: Guidance for Decision making* (3rd edn). London: BMA.

Lennard-Jones, J. E. (ed.) (1998) *Ethical and Legal Aspects of Clinical Hydration and Nutritional Support*. Redditch: The British Association for Parenteral and Enteral Nutrition.

National Council for Palliative Care (2007) *Artificial Nutrition and Hydration—Guidance in End of Life Care for Adults*. London: NCPC and APM.

Article

Elia M., *et al.* (2006). Enteral (oral or tube administration) nutritional support and eicosapentaenoic acid in patients with cancer: A systematic review. *International Journal of Oncology*, **28**: 5–23.

Physiotherapy

A physiotherapist is a healthcare professional concerned with human function and movement and maximizing potential'. A physiotherapist will use physical approaches in the promotion, maintenance and restoration of an individual's physical, psychological and social well-being, taking account of variations in health states.

In palliative care, the role of the physiotherapist is to reduce the degree to which disabilities, caused by the disease or the treatment, interfere with everyday life. This is particularly pertinent for those patients whose disease trajectory may be short and are deteriorating rapidly.

Physiotherapists are important members of the multidisciplinary palliative care team. They may be involved in all healthcare settings in the treatment of patients with any progressive deteriorating condition, which most commonly includes cancer, chronic end-stage respiratory, neurological and cardiac disease.

As part of the rehabilitation team, the specialist physiotherapist is in a good position to identify the needs and coordinate the responses of colleagues working in a wide variety of complementary fields.

The physiotherapist, with a knowledge of the underlying pathological condition, adopts a problem-solving approach in which goals of treatment are planned jointly with the patient. This gives the patient, who may feel helpless because of a loss of independence, a measure of control. These goals must be realistic and achievable for the phase of the disease and must be continually reassessed. Goals may be simple (to be able to sit comfortably in bed) or more complex (to attend and enjoy a wedding). This is known as 'active readaptation'.

A physiotherapist has a detailed knowledge of functional anatomy and ergonomics, and is able to analyse movement and posture in its relationship to the environment. For instance, weakness and immobility may lead to poor posture, which places a strain on muscles and ligaments and can cause pain, particularly around joints. These stresses may be relieved by strategic physical positioning.

The physiotherapist may be the first professional to be alerted to the signs and symptoms of spinal cord compression due to malignant disease. Alongside immediate medical treatment, the initial aim will be an attempt to minimize loss of function. Should a more complete picture of motor, sensory and autonomic impairment develop, the physiotherapist will be instrumental in helping the patient cope with adapting to a drastic reduction in functional ability by helping the patient to develop a strategy for the future. This may involve balance training, development of upper body strength, instruction in transfers and the use of a wheelchair. Relatives and other carers will also require instruction in passive movements, the positioning of paralysed limbs, the use of wheelchairs and in moving and handling techniques.

Physiotherapy interventions

Optimizing mobility

As diseases progress, mobility becomes more challenging. Initially, a stick or crutches may be necessary to support independence, but later the provision of a walking frame or working towards independent mobility in a wheelchair may be more appropriate. Facilitating independence of transfers by strategically positioned furniture or the use of a sliding board may allow patients to remain independent within a smaller environment.

Pain management

Bone pain and neuropathic pain due to cancer are notoriously difficult to manage. Relief may be obtained by the use of transcutaneous electrical nerve stimulation (TENS). Local applications of heat, in the form of heat pads or wheat bags, are also used for pain relief. Progressive disease often leads to immobility and pain may be experienced due to stiffness of joints and poor posture.

Maintenance of joint range and muscle power

Massage and exercise therapy are the core skills of all physiotherapists. Maintenance of joint range by the use of active or passive exercises along with therapeutic massage will be beneficial. Therapeutic massage using stroking and gentle kneading may be used to reduce muscle spasm, to relieve pain and aid relaxation.

Maintenance of joint range is also important in the management of neurodegenerative diseases, and passive movements and active assisted exercises need to be implemented and taught to relatives and other carers.

Physiotherapists also provide and fit neck collars, splints and various other supports for weakened muscles. These will help to correct posture or reduce deformities and facilitate improved function.

Breathlessness management

Breathlessness is very frightening and distressing for patients and carers, making them feel out of control. All physiotherapists are trained in giving respiratory care and can teach patients and their carers techniques to reduce the work of breathing, to encourage relaxation, to aid in the expectoration of secretions and to advise on coping strategies in order to improve breathing control. The physiotherapist is a key member of the multidisciplinary team involved in running breathlessness groups.

Some physiotherapists are trained in various complementary therapies that can be used to help the control of breathlessness, e.g. acupuncture, reflexology and aromatherapy.

Physiotherapists often help in the management of patients, using non-invasive ventilation for respiratory failure e.g. secondary to neuromuscular disability such as in Motor Neurone Disease.

Lymphoedema management (📖 see Chapter 6F Skin problems in palliative care)

Chronic oedema may develop in an arm following treatment for breast cancer or as a manifestation of recurrent axillary lymph node disease, or in the legs secondary to impedance of lymphatic drainage from disease in the pelvis. A swollen limb is heavy and affects posture and mobility, placing stresses on weakened muscles and joints.

Lymphoedema management includes using exercise as well as correct positioning, compression hosiery, multilayer lymphoedema bandaging, manual lymph drainage techniques and skin care.

In palliative care, oedema of mixed aetiology is common, resulting in immobile, dependent limbs and oedema of the trunk. The physiotherapist may need to be adaptive in the management of these patients.

Psychological support

The physiotherapist often works on a one-to-one basis with patients. Patients may discuss their hopes and fears with a sensitive listener. They feel safe to ask searching questions in these situations and, therefore, the physiotherapist needs to be adequately prepared and informed to deal with these issues and to communicate relevant issues to the team, within the bounds of confidentiality.

Further reading

Book

Doyle D., *et al.* (2004) *Oxford Textbook of Palliative Medicine* (3rd edn). Oxford: Oxford University Press.

Articles

Chartered Society of Physiotherapy (2003) *The Role of Physiotherapy for People with Cancer— Chartered Society of Physiotherapy Position Statement.* Available at: www.csp.org.uk/uploads/documents/csp_pos_state_cancer1.htm

Oldervoll L., *et al.* (2006) The effect of a physical exercise program in palliative care: a phase II study. *Journal of Pain and Symptom Management*, **31**(5): 421–30.

Robinson D. (2000) The contribution of physiotherapy to palliative care. *European Journal of Palliative Care*, **7**(3): 95–8.

Speech and language therapy

Speech and language therapy (SLT) is necessary in palliative care since patients often have difficulties with communication and swallowing. Some palliative care teams have their own SLT service, others access SLT from local hospital or community services. The abilities to both communicate effectively and swallow safely are integral to being autonomous social creatures and maintaining life, in sickness as well as in health. Therefore, any problem with communication is an adverse symptom and reduces the patient's independence, quality of life and informed decision-making. Similarly, swallowing problems reduce quality of life and give rise to risks of reduced intake, choking and aspiration. The SLT plays an important role in the multidisciplinary team at all stages of disease management, at diagnosis and in symptom control, palliative rehabilitation and terminal care.

Aims and principles of SLT intervention

SLT assessment contributes to diagnosis, monitoring of disease progression and prognosis, and provides accurate identification of the type, severity and causes of the communication or swallowing problem. This allows appropriate and relevant intervention. The aim of SLT input in this context is the maintenance and facilitation of remaining function within the limits of the disease and compensation for deficits, rather than the restoration of original abilities. SLT is helpful in contributing to an assessment of competence and also at times when the patient needs to communicate their wishes or symptoms or to discuss prognosis but communication is difficult, e.g. due to fear, fatigue, pain or to a specific problem with speech.

SLT helps patients make informed, realistic and timely choices, and to set appropriate personal goals for communication and swallowing by:

- Early involvement: to build understanding and trust, monitor progression and anticipate future problems
- Patient-led, whole-person approach: to enable relevant, appropriate and timely management for the individual
- Accurate identification of problems and causes: e.g. differentiating dysphasia from dysarthria, due to cortical vs bilateral brain lesions or brainstem disease
- Immediate strategy formation to maximize function, manage symptoms and reduce risk: e.g. swallow techniques to reduce choking and the risk of aspiration
- Patient, relative, carer and team support, information and education: to increase understanding and improve appropriateness and effectiveness of management
- Anticipation of future problems, preparation and planning

Communication difficulties

The ability to communicate is always important, but particularly so when an individual has to understand unfamiliar or frightening information, ask difficult questions and express emotionally complex ideas, as happens in palliative care. Even apparently mild problems with communication give rise to heavy physical, cognitive, emotional, psychological as well as time burdens on the patient and also on their relatives, friends and healthcare staff. It can result in the patient withdrawing and others avoiding contact. A significant number of palliative care patients have been shown to have previously unidentified communication problems and have also reported concern about their communication, feeling it is impaired.

Dysphasia

Dysphasia is a difficulty with verbal language and the processing of words. It includes problems with word-finding, syntax, writing and spelling (i.e. **expressive dysphasia**) and with understanding spoken words and reading (i.e. **receptive dysphasia**). The type and severity of the expressive and receptive problems vary between patients, but there is almost always an element of comprehension deficit even though this may not be obvious. For a variety of reasons, patients, relatives and even healthcare staff tend to underestimate the degree of comprehension, but it is also important not to underestimate the underlying competence of the patient. Usually, dysphasia is caused by damage to the cortex of the dominant left hemisphere of the brain. It is frequently present in palliative care as a result of stroke or primary or metastatic cerebral disease.

Examples of strategies that may help patients with dysphasia include:
- Allow additional time, not being rushed, and ensure a reduction in background noise and distractions
- Establish a reliable yes/no response
- Word-finding—encourage to talk around the target word or describe the object (circumlocution), substitute another word or focus on the initial sound, or use pointing or gestures
- Auditory comprehension—speaker slows own speech down, simplifies what is being said, shortens sentences and 'chunks' information, uses pauses, repeats and reiterations
- Use of a picture-based communication chart or aid

Dysarthria

This is a motor (movement) problem of speech. There is a reduction in the range, speed or coordination of facial and oral movements, affecting articulation and resulting in slow or slurred speech and reduced intelligibility. The specific type of dysarthria depends on which motor pathway has been affected and where. Dysarthria can be caused by stroke and cerebral tumours, and occurs in almost all the progressive neurological conditions such as motor neurone disease (MND), Parkinson's disease (PD), progressive supranuclear palsy (PSP), cerebellar atrophy, multiple system atrophy (MSA) and multiple sclerosis (MS), dependent on the disease progression. Sometimes cognitive problems complicate diagnosis and management. Ill health, general weakness and breathing difficulties may also give rise to dysarthria.

In addition, articulation difficulties are almost always a problem for those patients with head and neck cancers, due to structural changes as a result of the disease, surgery or oncological treatment (📖 See Chapter 6h—Head and neck cancer.)

Examples of strategies that may help patients with dysarthria:

- Allow additional time and ensure a reduction in background noise and distractions
- Encourage them to sit up straight and breath slowly and deeply
- Encourage them to slow their speech down, shorten phrases, breath between phrases and over-articulate
- Use of an alphabet or text-based chart or aid

Dysphonia

This is a problem with the voice: it may be quiet or hoarse or it may disappear intermittently or completely. The causes in palliative care are numerous. There may be reduced breath support to make the vocal cords vibrate, due to lung disease or general weakness. There may be a vocal cord palsy due to a lesion of the recurrent laryngeal nerve, as can happen in the spread of lung tumours and disease in the neck. Dysphonia can also be caused by cerebrovascular disease and occurs in progressive neurological diseases such as MND, PD and MS.

Patients with head and neck cancers frequently have voice problems caused by structural changes due to the tumour or treatments. In those patients with laryngeal cancer treated by radiotherapy with or without chemotherapy, there are long-term structural changes to the vocal cords which affect how they vibrate and, therefore, the sound they produce. When laryngeal cancer is treated by laryngectomy the larynx, including the vocal cords, is removed and the patient no longer has the anatomy to make normal voice sounds (📖 see Chapter 6h—Head and neck cancer).

Examples of strategies that may help patients with dysphonia:

- Reduce background noise
- Ensure good vocal hygiene—see explanation below
- Encourage adequate breath support, frequent top-ups of breath and not speaking on residual air
- Encourage patients to open their mouths wide to let the sound out and project the voice but not strain it
- Use an amplifier

Vocal hygiene

'Hygiene' is used in the sense of 'good care' or 'cleanliness'. So vocal hygiene means doing things that are good for the voice/vocal cords/larynx and not doing things that are harmful. Speech and language therapists and ear, nose and throat specialists give standard vocal hygiene advice to almost everyone they see with a voice problem, with good explanation and support. Bearing in mind that patients with palliative care needs may have a short time to live and that the emphasis is on quality of life, advice will need adapting to the individual patient's circumstances.

Vocal hygiene includes:

- Increasing fluid intake
- Avoiding carbonated, caffeine-containing or diet drinks
- Managing reflux (with medication as necessary)
- Humidifying the environment if possible

- Avoiding smoky environments and other known irritants, such as car fumes and some cleaning fluids
- Trying not to talk against background noise
- Not shouting
- Stopping habitual throat-clearing and coughing
- Stopping throat lozenges, pastilles and sweets
- Trying steam inhalations
- Trying to build voice 'rest periods' into the patient's timetable
- Stopping smoking
- Avoiding alcohol, especially spirits

Swallowing difficulties

Dysphagia or swallowing difficulties occur when there are structural, malignant or neurological changes to the lips, tongue, cheeks, upper and lower jaw, teeth, palate, pharynx, larynx and oesophagus. It can also occur when the level of responsiveness is reduced, there are cognitive problems or as a secondary effect of disease elsewhere. Dysphagia leads to reduced intake and may result in choking and putting the patient at risk of aspiration. Dysphagia is caused by head and neck, brain and other cancers and their treatments. It is also caused by stroke and is seen in almost all progressive neurological diseases, such as MND, PD and MS. Dysphagia and reduced eating and drinking are also part of the terminal stage of disease and the dying process.

The type and severity of dysphagia depends on which structures are affected, how and why they are affected and how severely. Therefore, an SLT assessment establishes the type and severity of dysphagia, including symptoms requiring palliation, risks and prognosis. The SLT can then suggest strategies to make swallowing easier, more efficient and safer. The SLT works closely with all members of the multidisciplinary team in the management of dysphagia, including the dietitian, physiotherapist and occupational therapist. In circumstances where there is a long-term high risk of repeated choking and aspiration and inadequate intake (such as in MND and some head and neck cancers) it is appropriate to consider stopping or supplementing oral intake using tube feeding via a PEG or RIG.

Examples of strategies that may help patients with dysphagia:

- Ensuring thorough frequent mouth care
- Advising on an upright sitting posture with head in the mid-line
- Limiting the amount eaten and drunk at one time—little and often
- Modifying the consistency of foods and drinks may help to overcome a delayed swallow and make swallowing safer, e.g. soft, wet, mashable foods rather than hard foods, and syrup-thick drinks (pre-thickened, or hand-thickened, e.g. with Nutilis) rather than thin fluids
- Modifying head position and using various swallow manoeuvres may compensate for a weak or ineffective swallow and poor airway protection, e.g. head turn to the affected side, supraglottic swallow

The SLT should be consulted whenever a patient is having difficulties, as described above, in order to explain which strategies are appropriate.

Further reading

Book

Logemann J. (1998) *Evaluation and Treatment of Swallowing Disorders* (2nd edn). Austin, Texas: PRO-ED.

Articles

Barret R., Roe J. (2004) A team approach to the management of dysphagia in advanced cancer. *Complete Nutrition*, **4**(6): 9–11.

Glasgow Allied Health Professions Palliative Care Project 2004. Available at: www.palliativecareglasgow.info/

Patterson J. (2005) Head and neck cancer dysphagia. *Speech & Language Therapy in Practice*, Autumn: 12–14.

Roe J. (2005) Oropharyngeal dysphagia in advanced non-head and neck malignancy. *European Journal of Palliative Care*, **12**(6): 229–32.

Salt N., Davies S., Wilkinson S. (1999) The contribution of speech and language therapy to palliative care. *European Journal of Palliative Care*, **6**(4): 126–9.

Salt N., Robertson S. (1998) A hidden client group? Communication impairment in hospice patients. *International Journal of Language & Communication Disorders*, **33**: 96–101.

Clinical and other applied psychology in palliative care

Psychologists do not necessarily draw a sharp distinction between work in palliative care and oncology. Job descriptions may require that they work across this range and the evidence-base indicates similar roles and activities are required in both fields. Even so, the workforce is tiny and, although in recent years numbers have been growing, demand has outstripped the supply of suitably qualified and experienced practitioners to take on the responsibilities asked of them.

The alternative is to access existing services within community mental health teams and primary care. If considering referring to these services it is necessary to bear in mind:

- Access to these services is often restricted to those with significant mental health pathology
- Mental healthcare professionals have little training in the special issues of patients with palliative care needs and may struggle to adapt their skills accordingly
- Patients may have difficulty with the perceived stigma of being referred to services for the mentally ill, and may see this as a sign that they are not believed and may refuse this help

Much of the work of psychologists in palliative care is directed towards supporting or working in collaboration with other staff: this can only be achieved by becoming an integral member of the palliative care team.

Mindful of the fact that those turning to this section of the Handbook are likely to be considering contacting or employing a psychologist there is a need to clarify:

- The roles a psychologist may perform, together with some of the terminology used in job titles and treatments
- Who can claim, with justification, to be suitably trained to develop and lead palliative care psychology services

Roles for the applied psychologist in palliative care

Professional training incorporating psychology modules has changed clinical practice, and many healthcare professionals can identify ways in which their psychological knowledge benefits the care of patients, from communication skills to symptom management. One consequence is that any description of the role of the psychologist in palliative care is likely to meet a chorus of 'but I do that' from other members of the team. The palliative care psychologists usually spend a substantial amount of their time working with patients, but a major role for them is multidisciplinary teamwork, supporting and reinforcing the psychological work of other team members, adding new perspectives and updating knowledge as research-led developments occur.

The activities of applied psychologists can be considered under five main headings: treatment; assessment; teaching and training; consultancy; research and audit.

1. Treatment
Often the primary reason for including a psychologist in the palliative care team is to provide additional treatment. Because of a broadening of the definition of 'palliative care' and improvements in treatments, more people receiving palliative care have a lifespan that enables psychological interventions to be effective. Changed circumstances lead to changed perspectives, priorities and duties for the palliative care patient. Psychological intervention can facilitate adjustment, resilience and restitution of an essentially normal life. Commonly occurring problems include:

• Difficulties adjusting to change
• Loss of hope
• Lack of purpose and direction
• Passivity and dependency induced by being cared for
• Fear of the future
• Poor anger control
• Communication difficulties in the family and with health professionals
• The need for better coping strategies

The body of psychological research in cancer and chronic pain has been especially productive in devising intervention strategies to facilitate:

• Constructive acceptance and adjustment to disability and shortened lifespan
• Beneficial emotional expression and regulation, including anger control
• Skilful coping and personal control despite disease progression
• Purposeful living and improved motivation
• Effective communication with carers
• Enhancement of self-esteem despite appearance changes and loss of roles

Mental ill-health problems of anxiety, depression and anger are often reasons for referral, whilst pain management referrals are also appropriate where prolonged experience of chronic pain is experienced.

Cognitive behavioural therapy (CBT) encourages people to modify their unhelpful thoughts and behaviours, thereby constructively changing situational outcomes (e.g. resolving a dilemma), emotional responses (e.g. raising low mood) and physical reactions (e.g. reducing muscle tension). The attraction of this therapeutic approach is partly because of its brief pragmatic interventions focused on current problems, and partly because of the substantial research evidence-base on which this approach is developing. However, a characteristic that often distinguishes psychologists from counsellors is a reluctance to be closely allied to any one particular treatment model. Evidence-based techniques often determine psychologist interventions rather than therapeutic models. Thus psychologists, may, for example, use a mix of CBT methods with others selected from the psychodynamic ways of working (exploring the effects of early life experiences) and a systemic approach (examining interactions and roles, particularly within the family).

2. Assessment

The psychologist's basic history and information gathering is identical to any good in-depth initial interviewing conducted by other healthcare professionals, but it may also include some less common features such as the use of questionnaires and between-session record-keeping.

Tools measuring psychological adjustment and psychopathology are used to assess distress and changes in a patient's mental state, and to screen the need for psychological interventions. The psychologist's role is to make professional interpretation and comparison of results with these assessment instruments, especially those that have been less rigorously evaluated. Other psychometric tools—including measures of cognitive functioning, intellectual ability, attainments, personality and aptitudes—rarely form part of the palliative care psychologist's role.

Since devising new rating scales and questionnaires is a skill for which psychologists receive training, they can, therefore, also assist others who are developing assessment tools.

3. Teaching and training

Many psychological skills are transferable to other professionals.[1] Applied psychologists expect to keep updating their fellow team members in relevant psychological knowledge and skill developments.[2] The NICE guidance[3] places particular emphasis on this role and that of supervision for staff working at lower levels in their model of psychological assessment and support.

Psychologists frequently use an educational approach ('psycho-education') to groups of patients in preference to a therapy group as an effective means of enhancing insight and coping skills.

4. Consultancy

Giving advice and support to fellow team members is often more appropriate than seeing the patient personally. This is particularly true towards the patient's end of life when time may be of the essence and meeting new professionals should be minimized. The psychologist can offer advice (and sometimes techniques) to staff that enables them to proceed in providing skilful assistance with more self-assurance; team meetings and case reviews can be strengthened by this means as well.

5. Research and audit

Some psychologists are involved in aspects of healthcare primarily from a research perspective. A culture of undertaking research is integral to psychologist training, so most psychologists seek to develop or support local research and audit projects.

1 Mannix K., *et al.* (2006) Effectiveness of brief training in cognitive behaviour therapy techniques for palliative care practitioners. *Palliative Medicine*, **20:** 579–84.

2 Sage, N., *et al. CBT for Chronic Illness and Palliative Care:
A Workbook and Toolkit.* Chichester: John Wiley & Sons. (In press).

3 NICE (2004). *Improving Supportive and Palliative Care for Adults with Cancer.* London: NICE.

Types of applied psychologist employed in healthcare

- **Assistant psychologists** are psychology graduates without additional training. They carry out research and clinical support tasks under the supervision of a vocationally trained psychologist and are not normally employed in other roles.
- **Research psychologists** who have an academic background and no vocational training similarly limit their role to supervised or non-clinical activities as agreed within local clinical governance arrangements. (Role 5 above.)
- **Health psychologists** have postgraduate training focused around the psychological aspects of illness, healthy and unhealthy behaviours, health-related attitudes, health promotion and communication, as well as research into psychological aspects of healthcare delivery. Although health psychologists are few in number and are a very new group of qualified and experienced applied psychologists, their skills are relevant in palliative care, particularly with reference to communication skills, information needs and service provision research. (Roles 2–5 above.)
- **Counselling psychologists** are also a relatively new breed of applied psychologist, but numbers have increased substantially in the past few years and they are now present in many psychology services. Training tends to be focused around a thorough knowledge of therapeutic models; therefore they are especially well equipped to provide specific therapy services for patients and carers. (Roles 1–5 above.)
- **Clinical psychologists** remain the most common of all the applied psychologists offering clinical care. They have been part of the healthcare system for over fifty years and their training aims to provide a wide experience of different aspects of that system and its clientele. Breadth of psychological knowledge is often greater than that of the health or counselling psychologist, but is perhaps achieved by limiting depth during training. The all-rounder quality of training makes the clinical psychologist a good choice in the development of palliative care psychological services. (Roles 1–5 above.)

All applied psychologists need to receive supervision of their work from more experienced applied psychologists. In the first instance, new or small palliative care services should employ psychologists with at least five years practice or arrange contracts with larger local psychology services.

Further reading

Books

Moorey S., Greer S. (2002). *Cognitive Behaviour Therapy for People with Cancer.* New York: Oxford University Press.

Sage N., et al. (2008). *CBT for Chronic Illness and Palliative Care: A Workbook and Toolkit.* Chichester: John Wiley & Sons.

Articles

Mannix K., et al. (2006) Effectiveness of brief training in cognitive behaviour therapy techniques for palliative care practitioners. *Palliative Medicine*, **20**: 579–84.

Payne S., Haines R. (2002) The contribution of psychologists to specialist palliative care. *International Journal of Palliative Nursing*, **8**(8): 401–6.

Social work

Social workers are an integral component of the palliative care team, and address many non-physical issues crucial to the holistic care of patients and their families. It is relatively easy to recognize physical problems such as shortness of breath, but healthcare professionals often assume that health concerns are the most important issues in the patient's mind, whereas family relationships and problems of everyday living may be just as, or more, important. When someone suffers from a life-threatening illness it affects all family members and changes the dynamics, roles and relationships within the family. The social worker's focus is on the effects of the illness on the family, and other social and community networks important to the patient. He or she is, therefore, often in the best position to enable patients to express and deal with emotional, psychological and social issues in their lives, helping them to reduce fear and anguish and enabling them to feel reconnected with friends, family and community.

Social work has three main roles:

1 To strengthen people in managing and dealing with emotional, psychological and social consequences of what is happening to them
2 To enable people to make the best possible use of welfare services and family, social network and community resources that will help them
3 To develop community organizations and groups to provide mutual help and support for people in dealing with the problems in their lives

It is not always possible to treat physical symptoms until the patient's emotional, psychological, social and spiritual distress is understood and addressed, and until difficulties in accessing and using practical help and welfare services are resolved. All members of the multidisciplinary team attend to some of these needs, but patients may not want to talk about their emotions to the professionals who are giving them physical care. Also, they may be inhibited from raising family and welfare issues with team members whose focus is mainly healthcare. Social workers usually approach clinical problems from a different angle, being guided first and foremost by the patient and their family, empowering them to identify and express what they feel are their most important needs.

Families come in many different shapes and sizes; they are the set of relationships within which a patient experiences kinship, child–parent and caring and support relationships (e.g. a gay or lesbian relationship may be more important for caring and support than the patient's parents, siblings or children). Friends, family members and partners need help to cope with their fear and anger at the situation as well as the patient. They need to feel involved in care and decision-making, which is essential in order to avoid additional grief in their bereavement. Patients, families, partners and friends can be helped to say their goodbyes, to be given the opportunity to heal rifts and to complete unfinished business. Working together to enable a person to die at peace with him/herself is a fundamental goal for all members of the multidisciplinary team, but the social worker's skills specifically equip them to empower patients and those close to them to say, 'I love you', 'Thank you', 'Sorry' and 'Goodbye'—perhaps the most important messages people need to give to each other at the end of life.

Families and individuals who are particularly vulnerable and at risk will be identified following a full social work assessment and offered appropriate interventions and support. A full assessment is often aided by constructing the family genogram (📖 see Figure 19e.1), finding out who is important to the patient and highlighting relationship issues.

Among the issues to think about when preparing and talking about a genogram to a patient or family member are:
- The stage of life that each family member is at
- Their special responsibilities in the family (e.g. caring for a family member with learning disabilities)
- Important memories (e.g. previous deaths) and expectations (e.g. to be cared for in old age)
- Strengths and resources of each member
- The availability of support or likely demands from the extended family, the patient's social networks or community connections
- Moving into 'gaps' (e.g. children 'replacing' a dead person)
- Who cares for whom? Who cares for carers?
- What changes, separations, illnesses, losses, have children and others experienced
- Who was involved in or absent from family crises, deaths, funerals?
- Who confides in whom?
- Who is in conflict with whom? Who gets left out?

The social network may include ethnic and cultural issues that need to be understood to facilitate family communication. A genogram may be adapted to show wider social networks. Alternatively, a network diagram may be a useful addition. This shows links between the patient and others with whom they have regular contact, remembering that the way in which contact is made (e.g. weekly phone call, visits from the contact by car, visits to the contact by bus) will affect its value as the patient's disability increases, and it is helpful to be aware of the importance of the contact to the patient (often weighted from 1–3). Strong, unfamiliar and often conflicting feelings can be a barrier to open communication. Rifts within families and social networks may emerge and will, therefore, need managing sensitively, often allowing the reconciliation and rebonding of relationships. However, barriers to communication can also occur when families want to protect each other from the pain of bad news and the limited future.

Families may need help so that they feel more confident about knowing how to tell and involve their children. They may try to protect children (and other dependants, such as family members with learning disabilities) by trying to keep up an unrealistic front about the illness or prognosis. Telling children and young people about someone in the family suffering from a serious illness early is helpful because it prevents problems arising and reduces difficulties later. Children are helped by feeling included and valued, and they need to be prepared for possible eventualities in much the same way as adults. Children affected by the illness of a close relative include daughters and sons, grandchildren, nephews and nieces. It is natural for adults to want to soften the pain and shock of bad news, but it is important for children to be told when something is wrong. Sometimes adults want to delay telling children bad news because they hope the next test results or treatment will enable the telling to be less painful. However, there is probably never a 'right' time and putting things off usually makes the difficulties greater. A 'good' time may never arrive and it may become increasingly difficult to explain why such important information was not given earlier.

Sometimes adults think that by not saying anything about someone's illness their children will somehow not be affected. However, the reality is that, even if adults try to hide from their children what is happening, children notice when something is wrong and may blame themselves (e.g. 'I made my mum's illness worse because I behaved badly') unless things are properly explained to them. Children who are not included in being helped to understand such profound changes in their family situation may later feel angry at having been excluded.

Social workers can help parents and other close family members think about making memory boxes or writing letters for their children. A memory box is a collection of significant items, including writings, drawings, recordings of favourite music and pictures that will remind a bereaved child or adult of important shared experiences. Usually, a memory box will contain photographs, details of special family events, information about the person who is dying as well as particular items that help a person to understand more about the dying family member later on. A memory box helps a person to understand their own life story by giving information about the past and so helps the person to feel more confident about themselves, their identity and roots.

Social work may also help to address spiritual pain, by helping to relieve isolation and giving comfort, knowing that concerns, even if unanswered, are taken seriously and recognized as being important and valid. Difficulties such as body image, sexuality and intimacy may need discussion with a social worker. Patients rarely volunteer these problems and may need prompting to see if they want to talk about them. Appropriate guidance is needed to help patients and families cope with the changing circumstances.

Practical help involves enabling patients to make decisions and exercise choice, both for practical reasons and also to promote a sense of worth and dignity. They may need basic assistance in obtaining grants to help with the extra costs incurred as a result of their changed circumstances, paying bills, or to execute more complicated tasks such as preparing a will and thinking about the future of dependants. It is important to ensure that patients receive benefits to which they are entitled, for instance Attendance Allowance and Disability Living Allowance. The patient and family may want to know about the law and other social institutions, family and mental health legislation and community services according to their particular situation. Social workers, along with other palliative care professional workers have a duty to ensure that vulnerable people who are unable to make their own decisions are empowered and protected by the statutory framework set out in the Mental Capacity Act 2005.

Ensuring that patients receive packages of care to enable them to stay in their own home is also part of the social work role. Some people may need support making decisions about an alternative placement, such as a nursing home. Funding private nursing care is often a source of real anxiety and the social worker can advise and arrange NHS-funded care if the eligibility criteria are met. Continuing care is a complex and sensitive area of health-care provision and can affect people at a very vulnerable stage in their lives. Social workers can advise people about the different types of NHS funding, including the principles of eligibility and the assessment process, which in England are set out in the National Framework (2007) on NHS continuing healthcare and NHS-funded nursing care.[1]

Carers may be entitled to a Carers' Allowance. Carers themselves are legally entitled under the Carers (Recognition and Services) Act 1995 and the Carers (Equal Opportunities) Act 2004 to an assessment of their own needs while caring for someone, which can be arranged by the pal-liative care social worker. Carers' rights were strengthened by subsequent government policy, including the Carers' Strategy 1999 and the Carers and Disabled Children Act 2000. Carers may need support at such a distressing time and by having their own needs assessed they can receive appropriate help and relief. Caring for someone who is terminally ill can place huge personal, financial, emotional and practical demands on family members and close friends. Carers' groups are often established and facilitated by social workers to give support to people in similar circumstances.

Social workers seek to enable patients and families retain or regain control and promote empowerment and choice, to help people find inner strength and confidence. Families and other carers can feel so powerless in these situations, but social workers can help them to set realistic goals and make plans to enable them to enjoy the important time that is left.

After death, bereavement support is fundamental to the role of palliative care social workers, who commonly work with bereavement support workers and counsellors within the team. Families may be offered individual, family or group counselling. Social workers may also organize and run special bereavement sessions for children and teenagers.

Financial and practical help in the UK

Attendance allowance

This is a non-means tested benefit for people 65 and over who have difficulty looking after themselves (for example, with washing or dressing). It is paid at variable rates according to dependency. People with a terminal illness (prognosis of six months or less) can receive the benefit quicker and the formalities are simpler.

Disability living allowance

This is a non-means tested benefit for people under 65 who have difficulty walking or looking after themselves (or both). Similar rules apply for dependency and terminal illness (see above).

1 Department of Health (2007) *National Framework for NHS Continuing Healthcare and NHS-funded Nursing Care*. London: Department of Health.

Other possible benefits
- Council tax benefit
- Housing benefit
- Statutory sick pay
- Disability working allowance
- Funeral payments (social fund)
- Bereavement payment
- Bereavement allowance
- Widowed parents allowance
- Severe disablement allowance
- Income support
- Invalid care allowance
- Incapacity benefit
- Working tax credit

Social Services may be able to provide:
- Home care for personal care
- Help with housework
- Occupational therapy aids
- 'Meals on wheels' or frozen meals
- Residential/nursing care
- Disabled parking badge (usually blue)
- 'Dial a ride' access to community transport
- Relief for carers
- Respite care

Further reading

Books

Beresford P., Adshead L., Croft S. (2007) *Palliative Care, Social Work and Service Users: Making Life Possible*. London: Jessica Kingsley.

Department of Health (2007) National Framework for NHS Continuing Healthcare and NHS-funded Nursing Care. London: Department of Health.

Monroe B. (2004) Social work in palliative medicine. In *Oxford Textbook of Palliative Medicine* (3rd edn) (ed. D. Doyle, *et al.*), pp. 1007–17. Oxford: Oxford University Press.

Sheldon F. (1997) *Psychosocial Palliative Care: Good Practice in the Care of the Dying and Bereaved*. Cheltenham: Stanley Thornes.

Articles

Murtagh F., *et al.* (2007) The value of cognitive interviewing techniques in palliative care research. *Palliative Medicine*, **21**(2): 87–93.

Payne M. (2007) Know your colleagues: role of social work in end-of-life care. *End of Life Care*, **1**(1): 69–73.

Reith M. (2007) Care of families during and after the death of a loved one. *End of Life Care*, **1**(2): 22–6.

Chaplaincy

Chaplaincy addresses the spiritual, religious, pastoral and cultural needs of patients, relatives and staff in a healthcare context that is increasingly dynamic and pluralistic.

- Cultural needs include the need to be in an environment that reinforces the familiar—this takes in language, food, dress, family and social structures, customs, etc.
- Religious needs include the need for support to practise sacred rituals and hold certain beliefs, and will require provision for prayers, sacraments, Holy books, religious artefacts (e.g. prayer mats, rosary beads)
- Pastoral needs include the need for support at life's critical moments—relationship formation, illness, death, etc.—typically addressed with reference to particular beliefs or values, religious or otherwise
- Spiritual needs include the need for a sense of 'well-being', which is often nurtured by being well related to one's self, others, and one's source of ultimate meaning; some chaplains refer to this as 'psychospiritual need'
  (📖 See A humanistic–phenomenological definition, p. 741.)

All members of the multidisciplinary team contribute to spiritual care, but because chaplains set high value on their own spiritual development, usually formed within the spiritual disciplines of a faith tradition, they are uniquely qualified as specialists in this area. Although most chaplains have a religious affiliation, it is against their codes of professional practice to proselytize—chaplains only address spiritual needs; they never seek to create them.

Religious needs

The appointment of chaplains will often reflect the proportionality of religious affiliation among the patient group.

Networking with local faith communities

Chaplains routinely network among those religious groups not represented on the chaplaincy staff, and so are able to provide local information to address the usual needs of religious minorities. Respect for the religious beliefs and practices of patients, relatives and staff is fundamental to the ethos of Chaplaincy.

Dedicated sacred space/chapel/quiet-room

As far as possible, provision must be made for a dedicated space for quiet reflection and prayer. Respecting the sensibilities and needs of all, this sanctuary/chapel/prayer-room will be available for religious services.

Pastoral needs

Marriage

The sanctuary/chapel/prayer-room may be used for marriages. *In extremis*, registrars normally attend a patient at very short notice; however, divorced people must ensure they present all necessary documents to the registrar. Religious restrictions may put limits on the involvement of some ministers/priests, for example the marriage of divorcees by Church of England clergy. Advice must be sought in advance of any proposed ceremony.

Funerals

Chaplains are an important resource to families with technical questions about funerals, access to services and beliefs.

Many chaplains receive requests to take funerals, either because they have developed a special relationship with a patient or because they were particularly helpful to the patient's relatives. However, the practice of individual chaplains varies:

- Some want to continue an established pastoral relationship, in order to personalize the funeral, or to encourage a more open attitude to the funeral liturgy;
- Others prefer to encourage the community-based provision of bereavement and pastoral aftercare.

Bereavement and remembrance services

Where chaplains are not centrally involved in providing bereavement support they are likely to work closely with the Bereavement Service to organize remembrance events. Most hospices hold regular remembrance services, and many have an annual event, usually around Christmas-time.

Spiritual needs

Chaplains offer themselves to patients and their carers as 'soul friends' and, according to their training, they provide a broad range of support:

- Listening/counsel
- Prayer/sacrament
- Life-review/reminiscence

Sharing the patient's journey—to the extent to which they are invited—chaplains will contain anxiety, absorb hostility (directed at their representative role), challenge and stand by patients and families. Chaplains will be non-judgemental.

Healing (📖 See Spiritual healing, p. 826.)

Healing can be understood as physical cure, medical or miraculous. But it is also applied to a range of therapeutic activities. Most religious traditions include prayers and rituals for healing, and many chaplains have experience or training in healing prayer.

- A ministry of healing is normative in many Christian churches, and ranges from informal prayers to short, formalized liturgical services; either may include 'the laying on of hands'.

- Trained spiritual healers, with no particular allegiance to an established faith tradition, are an emerging feature within spiritual care. Independent, i.e. healers who are not themselves chaplains or not part of the chaplaincy team, should belong to a healing organization regulated by UK Healers,[1] e.g. the National Federation of Spiritual Healers.

---

1 UK Healers: PO BOX 207, Leeds LS16 5WX. www.ukhealers.info.

Chaplains as professional colleagues

Multidisciplinary working

Chaplains bring a particular perspective to the multidisciplinary team, and expect to participate fully in team meetings. Because chaplains work with the highest regard for confidentiality, there should be an easy flow of communication between chaplains and multidisciplinary colleagues.

Training levels

Currently, there is no universally required qualification for palliative care chaplains. Traditionally, chaplains have been recruited from within the faith traditions, and will normally have a religious formation. However, the professionalization of healthcare chaplaincy is beginning to demand graduate entry, and several Masters level programmes are available. Professional bodies (Association of Hospice & Palliative Care Chaplains, College of Health Care Chaplains, Scottish Association of Healthcare Chaplains) now expect ongoing, in-service training as well as continuing professional development.

Assessment (☐ See Spiritual assessment, p. 750.)

A number of assessment models are available, but it is often inappropriate to attempt a formal assessment of spiritual need.

Chaplains will consider a patient's spiritual, religious, pastoral as well as their cultural needs, and will welcome insights from colleagues on the multidisciplinary team. Chaplains will continually assess patients' spiritual needs, which they will document in patient notes as appropriate.

Availability

Chaplaincy provision is a requirement of specialist palliative care, but staffing levels depend upon the resources of the individual unit. The chaplaincy time with patients will vary. Most units have 24-hour cover from chaplains, sometimes with support (voluntary or paid) from local clergy; some units have teams of chaplains.

Staff support

Chaplains invariably have a role in staff support within the organization. This may be in one-to-one counselling/support, in clinical supervision of individuals or groups, or it may be in the spiritual support of the organization by creating memorials and/or ceremonies to mark important moments in the life of the institution.

Education and research

Many chaplains are involved in teaching staff, and some also undertake research. Subjects depend on individual interests, experience and expertise, and are often published in peer-reviewed journals, including *The Journal of Health Care Chaplaincy* and the *Scottish Journal of Health Care Chaplaincy*.

Awareness of religious diversity

All religions contain a wide range of variation, from orthodox practitioners, for whom correct procedures are vitally important, to liberal groups, who are less likely to take offence if treated with sensitivity, respect and openness. Religious obligations frequently relate to:

- Alcohol
- Cross-gender care
- Food
- Religious objects
- Privacy
- Washing
- Touching/preparing the body after death

All religions have a concern with death and provide rituals and customs associated with the processes of dying. Some religious ministers may be required to carry out particular rituals, while some faiths allow suitably experienced lay people to officiate.

Avoiding assumptions in caring for religious needs

Even when patients identify with a religious group it should be kept clearly in mind that people are individuals and that their belonging will always be particular to them. It is not unusual for the beliefs and the behaviours of a healthy individual to change, sometimes dramatically, when they become terminally ill: a religious label noted on a hospital form is a poor indicator of an individual patient's past or current beliefs or practices.

If a dying patient is to be sensitively and efficiently cared for it will be necessary to understand their philosophy of life, religious beliefs and their expectations about what might happen after death. Chaplains are skilled in gaining this kind of information by a sensitive mix of observation, careful listening and tactful questioning of the patient and family.

The following guidelines indicate only very general points around 'Care for the dying' and 'Procedure at death' for patients from faiths most commonly encountered in the UK.

Two helpful principles:

- **Always check** with the patient (and/or family) concerning beliefs and practices, even if these are many years past.
- **When in doubt**, follow the more orthodox procedures.

Buddhists

Care of the dying

- A basic Buddhist belief is that a person's state of mind at the moment of death influences the character of their rebirth
- Some patients may want help to find quiet for meditation, and they may welcome Buddhist chanting to influence their state of mind
- Some may wish to avoid palliative treatments that lessen conscious capacity or awareness as they approach the moment of death
- Buddhists may require vegetarian food

Procedure at death

- It may be necessary to contact a Buddhist priest after a death
- Buddhists normally prefer cremation to burial

Christians

Care of the dying

- Most Christians will want access to a Bible. Some may welcome a prayer book or hymn book
- Even where the chaplain shares their faith, practising Christians may want their own religious minister to pray with/for them
- Pentecostal Christians may want to pray for physical healing, even if the patient is close to death. The patient may welcome this, but staff should be clear about the patient's desires and respond appropriately
- Roman Catholic/Orthodox Christians will want a priest to hear their confession, bring Holy Communion and offer the Sacrament of the Sick

Procedure at death

- There are no special requirements

Hindus

Care of the dying

- For Hindus, there is religious significance in dying at home, and Hindu patients may welcome support to die in their home setting
- In-patients may welcome the priest (*pandit*) to read holy texts and perform holy rites

Procedure at death

- Non-Hindus should not touch or wash the dead body, and family members will want to wash and prepare their dead relative
- In the absence of family members, healthcare staff should:
  - use disposable gloves to straighten the limbs and close the eyes
  - leave jewellery, sacred threads and religious objects on the body
  - wrap the body in a plain sheet
- Hindus normally request cremation

Jews

Care of the dying

- Orthodox Jews will want Jewish (*kosher*) food, which their relatives may want to provide; the family or a rabbi should be consulted for advice and they may need help to meet this requirement
- There are no 'last rites', although a Jewish patient may want a rabbi to visit; staff should try to find the appropriate rabbi for the patient, i.e. orthodox for orthodox, liberal for liberal
- The Jewish emphasis on the present life may mean that patients or families question treatments that could be seen to weaken the fight for life

Procedure at death

- If possible, the body should not be touched by non-Jews. However, if this causes difficulties, even the strictest Jews will permit healthcare staff to do the following:
  - bind the lower jaw
  - straighten the arms and lay the hands at the side of the body
  - wrap the body in a plain sheet
- Ideally, the dead body should not be left alone, and some Jews have watchers to stay and recite Psalms

- The family, or in their absence a Jewish undertaker, should be informed immediately and (except during the Sabbath [Friday dusk to Saturday dusk] or festivals) a funeral held as soon as practicable, preferably within 24 hours
- Post-mortem examinations are forbidden unless ordered by the coroner, in which case they must be carried out as soon as possible

Muslims

Care of the dying

- Fasting during the Holy month of Ramadan is a requirement of all Muslims, however, sick patients are exempt
- The majority of Muslims will want Islamic (*halal*) food; some will not accept medicines if they contain alcohol
- Muslims will need facilities for washing as an essential prerequisite to performing their daily prayers

Procedure at death

- People of the opposite sex should only touch the body if absolutely necessary and should wear disposable gloves; family members will want to prepare their dead relative for burial
- In the absence of family members, healthcare staff should:
  - turn the head towards the right shoulder so that the body can be buried facing *Makkah* (Mecca)
  - avoid washing the body
  - wrap the body in a plain sheet
- Because Islam teaches the resurrection of the body, normally Muslims will request burial, which should be arranged as soon as possible
- Post-mortem examinations are forbidden unless ordered by the coroner, in which case they should be carried out as soon as possible.

Sikhs

Care of the dying

- As an act of faith, Sikhs wear five symbols (known as the Five Ks): uncut hair (*Kesh*); small comb in the hair (*Kangha*); steel wrist band (*Kara*); dagger (*Kirpan*); white shorts (*Kaccha*)—these symbols must be respected at all times
- Sikhs may get strength from reciting hymns from their holy book, the *Guru Granth Sahab*; any practising Sikh may help with this

Procedure at death

- Family members will want to wash and prepare the body, but there are no restrictions on non-Sikhs attending a dead Sikh
- In the absence of family members, healthcare staff should:
  - pay special regard to the Five Ks
  - refrain from cutting or trimming the hair or beard
  - straighten the limbs and wrap the body in a plain sheet
- Sikhs normally request cremation

Further reading

Books

Gatrad R., Brown E., Sheikh A. (2006) *Palliative Care for South Asians: Muslims, Hindus and Sikhs*. London: Quay Books.

Neuburger J. (2004) *Caring for Dying People of Different Faiths* (3rd edn). Oxford: Radcliffe Medical Press.

Rinpoche S. (2002) *The Tibetan Book of Living and Dying*. London: Rider.

Speck P. (1988) *Being There: Pastoral Issues in Time of Illness*. London: SPCK.

Weller P. (ed.) (2001) *Religions in the UK: A multi-faith Directory*. Multi-Faith Centre at the University of Derby in association with the Inter Faith Network for the United Kingdom.

Articles

AHPCC (2006) *Guideline for Hospice and Palliative Care Chaplaincy.* (rev. edn). Association of Hospice & Palliative Care Chaplains.

AHPCC (2006) *Standards for Hospice & Palliative Care Chaplaincy*. (2nd edn). Association of Hospice & Palliative Care Chaplains.

AHPCC, CHCC & SACH (2005) Association of Hospice and Palliative Care Chaplains *et al. Health Care Chaplains Code of Conduct* (2nd edn).

Nolan S. (2006) Psychospiritual care: a paradigm (shift) of care for the spirit in a non-religious context. *The Journal of Health Care Chaplaincy*, **7**(1): 12–22.

Useful websites

Chaplaincy websites

www.ahpcc.org.uk—Association of Hospice and Palliative Care Chaplains

www.healthcarechaplains.org—College of Health Care Chaplains

www.sach.org.uk—Scottish Association of Healthcare Chaplains

www.mfghc.com—Multifaith Group for Healthcare Chaplaincy

Religion/culture websites

www.bbc.co.uk/religion—BBC Religion & Ethics

www.faithandfood.com—Food & Faith

www.derby.ac.uk/multifaith/religions—MultiFaithNet

www.shap.org—The Shap Working Party on World Religions in Education

Pharmacy

Within the last ten years recognition of the knowledge and skills that a pharmacist can contribute within palliative care has led to an increasing number of hospitals and hospices appointing a specialist palliative care pharmacist to work as an integral member of the multiprofessional palliative care team.

They carry responsibility for specialist medicine and pharmaceutical-related issues in the care of palliative patients. Palliative care patients are often prescribed several medicines to manage the symptoms or side-effects created by their treatment or medication, and the specialist palliative care pharmacist can assist the patient to achieve concordance with the optimal treatment for their particular problems.

The role of the specialist palliative care pharmacist will vary according to local practice but should include most of the following aspects.

Provision of a clinical service to palliative patients

Specialist palliative care pharmacists working within a hospital or hospice will have a clinical responsibility to the inpatients in their respective establishments, and their duties may include some or all of the following:

- Responsibility for specialist advice on the use of medicines in palliative care, especially as many medicines are used off-licence
- Providing assistance in rationalizing patients' medication on admission to the hospital or hospice
- Monitoring inpatient prescribing for appropriate dose, formulation, interactions and compliance with guidelines and policies
- Liaison with other healthcare professionals to resolve any medication-related issues
- Participation in consultant-led ward rounds and multiprofessional team meetings to provide highly specialized advice
- Practice as a supplementary or independent non-medical prescriber to assist in timely alterations to the inpatient prescription in response to change in a patient's symptoms

Helping patients to accept and understand their medication

As patients' symptoms change, their medication regimens will change and the pharmacist will be in a position to counsel and reassure patients and/or their carers by:

- Explaining to patients and/or their carers why their medicines have been prescribed or changed, and how the medicines work to alleviate their symptoms
- Ensuring that medication is in an acceptable form for the patient, whether as solid dose, liquid, buccal, rectal, transdermal or parenteral preparations and advising on alternatives as the patient's condition or symptoms progress
- Ensuring that the patient knows when and how to take their medicines to achieve optimum relief of their symptoms with minimal side-effects,

for example use of a modified-release opioid for regular analgesia and immediate-release opioid to manage breakthrough pain, incident pain or dyspnoea.

Liaison with community pharmacy services and nursing homes on discharge from hospital or hospice

Palliative patients are frequently weak and debilitated, anxious about their medication and they should have access to a prompt and efficient community pharmacy service. The specialist palliative care pharmacist is ideally situated to:

- Communicate with the community pharmacist to ensure consistent standards of care with a continued supply of specialist medication on the patient's discharge from hospital or hospice
- Provide individualized advice to nursing homes on the use of medicines to manage a patient's symptoms
- Provide written information on the specialist use of medicines for the patient and carer, community pharmacist, GP and other healthcare professionals when necessary
- Provide aids to assist the patient and/or their carer in coping with medication at home

Teaching and training other healthcare professionals in palliative care pharmacy-related issues

The principles of palliative care enshrine the principles of good practice for all healthcare professions and a specialist palliative care pharmacist may be expected to:

- Contribute to the provision of training on medicine use in symptom control for pharmacy students, medical students, nurses and other healthcare professionals
- Assist nurse specialists in the provision of syringe driver training for nursing staff
- Assist in training on prescribing for syringe drivers to medical and pharmacy staff

Participation in service development, research and audit

Palliative care is a relatively new specialty within pharmacy and there is an expanding knowledge base on the use of medicines and their accepted side-effects to manage symptoms in palliative care. A specialist palliative care pharmacist is in a position to:

- Contribute to the development of local, regional or national guidelines and protocols in the light of a growing evidence-base
- Audit local prescribing practice for compliance with guidelines and protocols to ensure safe, maximal patient care
- Develop the service within their own locality to provide safe, legal, timely and convenient access to medicines for the optimum benefit of patients and their carers

Art therapy

Art therapy is a form of psychotherapy that uses art media to produce images as its primary mode of communication. Images may be 2D or 3D. Patients need no previous experience or skill in art. The overall aim is to enable a patient to effect change and growth on a personal level through the use of art materials in a safe and facilitating environment.

The relationship between the therapist and the patient is of central importance. Art therapy differs from other psychological therapies in that it is a three-way process between the patient, the therapist and the image. It offers the opportunity for expression and communication and can be particularly helpful when people find it hard to express their thoughts and feelings. Issues may emerge very quickly when working on an image, enabling the patient to explore and resolve them within a limited time frame or even one session.

Art therapists have considerable understanding of art processes which are underpinned by a sound knowledge of therapeutic practice, and work with both individuals and groups in a variety of palliative care settings. The process—what happens in a session—is confidential between the patient and therapist and a degree of privacy is essential. Art therapists have become adept at securing this privacy even when working at the bedside in a busy ward or in the client's home as part of the community team.

Many facilities now have a designated art therapy space with good lighting, an accessible work area and secure storage for images. The art therapist is a key professional in the provision of psychosocial support, working within the interdisciplinary team, attending team meetings and providing assessments and feedback. Art therapists can also provide staff support and team reflection where there has been a particularly difficult or complex death. Bereavement programmes for children and families, partners or parents often have a significant art therapy component.

Art therapists work psychodynamically with complex and challenging issues, which call for skill and sensitivity in working with this particularly vulnerable client group. The training, which combines theoretical and experiential work, is a Postgraduate Diploma to be completed over two years full-time or three years part-time. Art therapists are consequently qualified and experienced to work at levels 3 and 4 in the recommended model of psychological support in NICE guidance.[1]

Art therapists maintain high standards of professional care and must be registered with the Health Professions Council and subscribe to the British Association of Art Therapists (BAAT) Code of Ethics. To protect both the patient and therapist, professional clinical supervision is required (usually on a monthly basis) with an ongoing programme of continuing professional development.

Creative Response (CR) is the special interest group of BAAT whose members work in palliative care, AIDS, cancer and bereavement with

---

1 NICE (2004) *Improving Supportive & Palliative Care for Adults with Cancer*, p. 76. London: NICE.

clients of all ages. CR is a member of the Help the Hospices Network of Professional Associations.

Further reading

Pratt M., Thomas G. (2007) *Guidelines for Arts Therapies and the Arts in Palliative Care Settings*. London: Help the Hospices.

Pratt M., Wood M. J. M. (eds) (1998) *Art Therapy in Palliative Care—The Creative Response*. London: Routledge.

Music therapy

And lull'd with sound of sweetest melody?
William Shakespeare, *2 Henry IV*, III. i. 7–16

References to the therapeutic use of music across many cultures date back to ancient Egypt. In the twentieth century, a growth in interest in the therapeutic properties of music from musicians, psychologists and doctors culminated in the formation of professional groups such as the UKs Association of Professional Music Therapists, and more recently State Registration with the Health Professions Council, alongside other arts therapies and allied health professions. Early work in special needs education laid the foundations for music therapy in a wide range of fields including mental health, neurology, care of the elderly and palliative care. Postgraduate training courses, leading to qualifications at diploma and masters level, equip therapists with an understanding of child development, of psychology, psychodynamic theory and the physical and emotional effects of music. As with art therapy, clinicians are experienced to work at levels 3 and 4 in the recommended model of psychological support in NICE guidance.[1]

Music therapists may use techniques which involve the use of pre-recorded music to meet specific clinical goals such as relaxation or pain control. However, more often they will create music with patients in joint musical improvisation or song writing, where the nature and scope of the work is multidimensional. Such interactive techniques may provide the vehicles for individuals to express their inner feelings relating to suffering and loss, or help them gain a sense of meaning and control over their lives. Whilst no musical skill is required to participate in therapy, the experience of co-producing improvised music and songs with therapists may open up new avenues of creativity as well as providing a sense of accomplishment for patients. Music therapy may take place in designated therapy rooms (ideally sound-proofed), hospital wards, day hospices or the patients' homes.

Palliative care providers are increasingly incorporating music therapy posts as part of their psychosocial provisions for patients, the bereaved and carers, with the discipline's holistic approach providing a natural 'fit' with palliative care philosophy.

1 Pratt M., Thomas G. (2007) *Guidelines for Arts Therapies and the Arts in Palliative Care Settings.* London: Help the Hospices.

This expansion has provided the impetus for a wide range of studies, ranging from those exploring patient and staff experiences of music therapy,[2,3] to the more empirical investigations providing evidence for pain reduction, improved mood, decreased fatigue and increased spirituality.[4]

Music has been described as the most social of all art forms. This is well illustrated by the ability of music therapists to collaborate with a wide variety other disciplines—for example, joint physiotherapy/music and movement work, music reminiscence projects and with spiritual care professionals in planning remembrance services. Sensitively performed live music may also enhance healthcare environments, i.e. providing a humanizing influence on clinical settings such as hospital wards. However, professionals untrained in music therapy wishing to utilize the benefits of music should seek guidance from registered clinicians, as patients may be defenceless against the emotional impact of this powerful medium.

Further reading

Books

Aldridge D. (1999) *Music Therapy in Palliative Care: New Voices*. London: Jessica Kingsley.

O'Callaghan C. (2004) The Contribution of music therpy to palliative medicine. In *Oxford Textbook of Palliative Medicine* (3rd edn) (ed. D. Doyle, *et al.*, p. 1041–6. Oxford: Oxford University Press.

Website address

Association of Professional Music Therapists and British society for music therapy: http://www.apmt.org/

Towersey Foundation (music therapy in palliative care): http://www.towerseyfoundation.org.uk/

2 O'Kelly J., Koffman J. (2007) Multi-disciplinary perspectives of music therapy in adult palliative care. *Palliative Medicine*, **21**(3): 235–43.

3 O'Callaghan C. (2001) Bringing music to life: a study of music therapy and palliative care experiences in a cancer hospital. *Journal of Palliative Care*, **17**(3): 155–60.

4 Hilliard, E. (2005) Music therapy in hospice and palliative care: a review of the empirical data *Evidence-based Complementary and Alternative Medicine*, **2**: 173–8.

Complementary and alternative medicine in palliative care

Introduction

Complementary and alternative medicines (CAM) comprise a diverse array of treatment modalities that are not presently considered part of conventional/mainstream medicine. CAM emphasize a holistic approach towards healthcare, i.e. they are based on the belief that mind, body and spirit are interconnected and that health depends on wholeness and balance between them.

Definitions

- **Alternative** treatments aim to replace conventional treatments.
- **Complementary** treatments are used alongside the conventional treatments
- **Integrated** (or American: integrative) treatments aim to combine best conventional treatments with best complementary treatments: a superfluous term with largely the same meaning as that of evidence-based medicine

Types of therapy

In palliative and supportive care, CAM is primarily used to increase the client's well-being, e.g. by alleviating pain and other symptoms of the disease, improving sleep, reducing stress and anxiety, or by reducing the adverse effects of conventional treatments. They are often used as an addition to conventional treatments. Some CAM modalities claim a direct effect in the prevention or treatment of cancer. Widely practised treatments are acupuncture, aromatherapy, herbalism, homeopathy, hypnotherapy, reflexology, relaxation and spiritual healing.

The individual therapies described in this chapter will be considered under four headings: alternative medical concepts; mind–body interventions, biologically based therapies and manipulative therapies.

Principles of CAM

A central tenet of CAM is the strong belief in the uniqueness and wholeness of the individual and the power of the body to heal itself.

Often, patients who consult complementary practitioners have chronic conditions that are difficult to manage, such as HIV infection, multiple sclerosis, rheumatological conditions and cancer. The interest in CAM in the palliative care setting is perhaps not surprising given the inherent need for the terminally ill to feel supported with regard to physical, psychosocial and emotional domains, in achieving an acceptable quality of life.

Prevalence

Precisely what constitutes complementary medicine differs considerably between countries. Different historical developments and traditions have meant that therapies such as herbal medicine and massage are firmly established in mainstream medicine in many European countries, while they are often classified as complementary outside Europe. Regardless of these national differences and inconsistencies in many surveys, there is evidence that CAM is used by a sizeable proportion of both adult and paediatric populations (see Table 11.1).

Table 11.1 One-year prevalence of CAM in general population samples

Country	Year	Sample (*n*)	Prevalence (%)
UK	2001	669*	28
USA	2004	31 044*	36 (excl. prayer)
Germany	2004	1750*	62.3
Japan	2002	1000**	76

*Representative; **random.

Prevalence studies in patients with life-threatening or chronic illnesses from Europe and the US report an average CAM use in cancer patients of 35–40%. Another survey reports CAM use in cancer patients to be between 7% and 54%. Small surveys in the UK have reported similar results.

An increasing number of departments of oncology in Britain employ at least one type of CAM practitioner in the palliative care setting, with most hospices now offering a range of complementary therapies for their patients. Initially, therapists were largely volunteers but units increasingly recognize CAM as part of basic and expected care. Today, there are an estimated 120 000 CAM practitioners in the UK.

Reasons for seeking CAM

One important and consistent finding is that the majority of CAM use does not occur instead of conventional medical care, but in addition to it. A number of explanations for patients seeking CAM have been proposed. Perhaps the most obvious reason for trying CAM is that, persuaded for instance by the media, or by personal past experience, many consumers are convinced that CAM is effective and improves psychosocial functioning. CAM is often also wrongly perceived as the *only* medicine that addresses the cause of an illness rather than the symptoms.

Certain fundamental premises of most forms of CAM contribute to its persuasive appeal. One of these is the perceived association of CAM with nature. It is linked with certain terminology such as 'natural' rather than 'artificial', or 'pure' as opposed to 'organic': 'natural' is also often somewhat naively equated with 'safe'. Another fundamental component of CAM is 'vitalism'. The enhancement or balancing of life forces or psychic energy, which is central to many forms of CAM, has an intuitive appeal to patients because of the non-invasive notion of healing from within. Many therapies have long intellectual traditions and sophisticated philosophies contributing to their credibility and authority. Spirituality, which bridges the gap between the domains of medical science and (religious) belief, is a further element in the appeal of CAM. CAM's approach tends to be more person-centred; the language is one of unity and holism in contrast to the often distant, reductionist terminology of normative science.

The main reasons why people use CAM can be categorized in 'push' and 'pull' factors.

Possible factors contributing to CAM use

Push factors
- Dissatisfaction with orthodox medicine:
  - ineffective
  - adverse effects
  - poor communication with doctor
  - waiting lists
- Rejection of orthodox medicine:
  - anti-science or anti-establishment attitude
- Desperation

Pull factors
- Philosophical congruence:
  - emphasis on holism
  - active role of patient
  - explanation intuitively acceptable
  - natural treatments
- Personal control over treatment
- Good relationship with therapist:
  - on equal terms
  - time for discussion
  - allows for emotional factors
- Accessibility

Evaluation

Negative attitudes towards research in the palliative care setting, which encompass ethical and methodological issues, particularly when patients are reaching their last few weeks of life, are pertinent. In addition, there are those who argue that scientific evaluation of CAM in the palliative care setting is not needed since patients feel better after therapy. But these attitudes, and the relative lack of research evidence, have long been a barrier to collaboration between conventional and complementary practitioners. The provision of CAM in mainstream care can, however, only be based on solid evidence and research efforts have been demonstrably increased over the last decade. The evidence for or against CAM treatments in palliative care that have been tested in controlled clinical trials are discussed in the respective therapies sections below.

Safety

A common reason for using CAM is that it is erroneously considered safe, certainly safer than conventional medicines. Even when a particular therapy's effectiveness is in doubt it is often still taken because of the belief that 'it may not work but it won't do any harm'. Although some CAM treatments are associated with only mild and rare risks, others are harmful in a number of ways. Herbal medicines have been associated with toxicity, herb–drug interactions and contamination. Acupuncture and chiropractic have been associated with serious adverse events such as pneumothorax or stroke, hypnosis may be associated with negative physiological and psychological effects.

There are also more general safety issues associated with CAM as a whole. CAM can be dangerous when it causes the patient either to be misdiagnosed or if it delays access to life-saving treatments. CAM is potentially dangerous when patients self-medicate. Often, patients do not tell their doctors about their CAM use, and doctors usually fail to ask patients about it.

The notion that CAM is safe and harmless can be dangerously misleading. The situation is not helped by a serious level of under-reporting of adverse events. To date, no effective system is in place for recording and analysing the occurrence of adverse events.

Practitioner accountability

There is no legislation that restricts the practice of CAM in the UK. Osteopathy and chiropractic are the only two complementary professions that, so far, have achieved statutory regulation in the UK. Since the House of Lords Report on Complementary and Alternative Medicine in 2000 there has been a move towards regulation, but progress is slow as there is considerable fragmentation within the various therapeutic disciplines. Initiatives for regulating acupuncture and herbal medicine are underway. The Faculty of Homeopathy trains and examines medical doctors, veterinary practitioners and other medical professionals, while the Society of Homeopaths is the regulatory body mainly for non-medically qualified practitioners; membership is, however, not compulsory.

The General Medical Council (GMC) provides guidelines regarding the accountability of doctors considering making a referral or delegating a patient's care.

It is important that patients consult a CAM practitioner who is fully qualified and a member of a recognized body or association and holds professional liability insurance cover, and also that the recognized body has a code of ethics and conduct, as well as a complaints and disciplinary procedure.

Useful resources of how to find a practitioner are:
- http://www.nhsdirectory.org/—NHS health professionals can search for suitable practitioners using the NHS health directory, which is a searchable database of CAM practitioners
- http://www.complementaryalternatives.com/—the online magazine *Complementary Alternatives*, published in association with the NHS Trusts Association, also has a searchable practitioner database

- The various CAM organizations hold lists of registered members and can be approached directly. Website addresses of organizations or councils can be found at the end of the respective therapy sections in this chapter

Conclusions

The use of CAM alongside conventional medicine in palliative care is increasing and is perceived as contributing to improvements in symptom control, well-being and satisfaction. It is seen as an important component of best practice in cancer care and is supported by the National Cancer Strategy, and the NICE Guidance on Support and Palliative Care for Adults with Cancer. It is, however, important to use treatment modalities backed up by research evidence and not to deceive patients.

Useful organizations

- **Prince's Foundation for Integrated Health** is a lobby group set up by the Prince of Wales to facilitate the development and delivery of integrated healthcare. The website contains resources for professionals interested in establishing integrated practices, for example databases of training courses, guidelines and reports
http://www.fihorg.uk/; E-mail: info@fihorg.uk; Tel: 020 3119 3100
- **The British Complementary Medicine Association** is an umbrella organization for over 60 CAM organizations/associations, schools and colleges. The website offers information about different CAM modalities, registered therapists and training courses. http://www.bcma.co.uk; E-mail: office@bcma.co.uk; Tel: 0845 345 5977
- **Penny Brohn Cancer Care** (formerly the Bristol Cancer Help Centre) is the UK's leading charity in complementary cancer care. Its vision is to enable world-wide access to complementary care and support through the Bristol Approach. http://www.pennybrohncancer-care.org; E-mail: helpline@pennybrohn.org; Confidential helpline: 0845 123 23 10
- **The Research Council for Complementary Medicine**'s website provides a variety of resources aimed at providing practitioners and patients with information about CAM efficacy. One of the major resources is the Complementary and Alternative Medicine Evidence Online (CAMEOL) database which displays the systematic reviews available for each entry. http://www.rccm.org.uk/; E-mail: info@rccm.org.uk; Tel: none

Further reading

Books

Ernst E.. et al. (2006) *The Desktop Guide to Complementary and Alternative Medicine* (2nd edn). Edinburgh: Mosby.

Ernst E., et al. (2008) *Oxford Handbook on Complementary Medicine*. Oxford: Oxford University Press. (2005)

Jonas, W. B. (2005) *Mosby's Dictionary of Complementary and Alternative Medicine*. St Louis: Mosby.

Micozzi M. S. (2007) *Complementary and Integrative Medicine in Cancer Care and Prevention: Foundations and Evidence-based Interventions*. New York: Springer.

NICE (2004) *Improving Supportive and Palliative Care for Adults with Cancer*. London: NICE.

Spencer J. W., Jacobs J. (2003) *Complementary and Alternative Medicine: an Evidence-based Approach* (2nd edn). St. Louis: Mosby.

Yuan C. S., et al. (2006) *Textbook of Complementary and Alternative Medicine*. London: Informa Healthcare.

Articles

Barton D. L., et al. (2006) Can complementary and alternative medicine clinical cancer research be successfully accomplished? The Mayo Clinic–North Central Cancer Treatment Group experience. *Journal of the Society for Integrative Oncology*, **4**: 143–52.

Cassileth B. R., Deng G. (2004) Complementary and alternative therapies for cancer. *Oncologist*, **9**(1): 80–9.

Deng G., et al. (2004) Complementary therapies for cancer-related symptoms. *The Journal of Supportive Oncology*, **2**(5): 419-26. (Discussion 427–9.)

Ernst E., et al. (2003) Evidence-based complementary medicine for palliative cancer care: does it make sense? *Palliative Medicine*, **17**: 704–7.

Ernst E., et al. (2007) Complementary/alternative medicine for supportive cancer care: development of the evidence-base. *Supportive Care in Cancer*, **15**: 565–8.

Kronenberg F., et al. (2005) The future of complementary and alternative medicine for cancer. *Cancer Investigation*, **23**: 420–6.

Mansky P. J., Wallerstedt D. B. (2006) Complementary medicine in palliative care and cancer symptom management. *Cancer Journal*, **12**: 425–31.

Mao J. J., et al. (2007) Use of complementary and alternative medicine and prayer among a national sample of cancer survivors compared to other populations without cancer. *Complementary Therapies in Medicine*, **15**: 21–9.

Monti D. A., Yang J. (2005) Complementary medicine in chronic cancer care. *Seminars in Oncology*, **32**: 225–31.

Post-White J. (2006) Complementary and alternative medicine in pediatric oncology. *Journal of Pediatric Oncology Nursing*, **23**: 244–53.

Schmidt K., Ernst E. (2004) Assessing websites on complementary and alternative medicine for cancer. *Annals of Oncology*, **15**: 733–42.

Scott J. A., et al. (2005) Use of complementary and alternative medicine in patients with cancer: a UK survey. *European Journal of Oncology Nursing*, **9**: 131–7.

Yates J. S., et al. (2005) Prevalence of complementary and alternative medicine use in cancer patients during treatment. *Supportive Care in Cancer*, **13**: 806–11.

Website

http://www.gmc-uk.org/guidance/

Group 1: Alternative medical systems

Alternative medical systems are complete systems of theory and practice. Examples of alternative medical systems developed in Western cultures are homeopathy and naturopathy. Others have evolved apart from and earlier than the conventional medical approach used in the West, e.g. such as traditional Chinese medicine and Ayurveda.

Acupuncture

Background and theory

The history of acupuncture dates back 2000 years. It is an integral part of traditional Chinese medicine (TCM) and based on its principles. **Acupuncture** involves the stimulation of certain points on the body by inserting fine needles, whereas **acupressure** involves firm manual pressure on these points.

The workings of the human body are thought to be controlled by a vital force or energy called 'qi' (pronounced *chee*) which circulates between organs along channels called meridians. The twelve main meridians are thought to correspond loosely to twelve major functions or organs of the body. On these meridians, more than 350 acupuncture points have been defined, and it is believed that qi energy must flow through each of the meridians and organs for health to be maintained. The acupuncture points are situated along the meridians and through these the flow of qi can be altered. Traditional acupuncture theory is based on the concept of yin and yang, which should be in balance: any imbalance (particularly blockage or deficiency) in the continuous flow of energy causes illness. Acupuncture point stimulation redresses this balance, allowing the healthy unimpeded flow of qi.

There are many different schools of acupuncture. Western medical acupuncturists relate acupuncture points to various physiological and anatomical features such as peripheral nerve junctions. The concept of 'trigger points', has also been recognized, whereby areas of increased sensitivity within a muscle cause referred pain in relation to a segment of the body.

There is no evidence to confirm the physical existence of qi or the meridians. However, attempts have been made to explain the effects of acupuncture within a conventional physiological framework. It is known that acupuncture stimulates A delta nerve fibres which enter the dorsal horn of the spinal cord and mediate segmental inhibition of pain impulses carried in the slower unmyelinated C fibres. Through their connections with the midbrain, descending inhibition of C fibre pain impulses is also enhanced at other levels of the spinal cord. It is also known that acupuncture stimulates the release of endogenous opioids and other neurotransmitters such as serotonin, which are involved in the modulation of pain.

Uses

Acupuncture is used, for example, in the management of pain, anxiety, fatigue and digestive disorders.

Practical application

Acupuncture may be delivered in a number of different ways. Between four and ten needlepoints are typically selected. These points are often located in areas where they represent the relevant local, regional and distant meridians. Needlepoints may also be centred around the area of pain.

In the UK, the practice is to use sterile disposable needles which are usually inserted to a depth of about 5 millimetres (or more deeply into muscle). Needles are left in situ for approximately 15 minutes. Needle sizes differ, but typically measure up to about 30mm long and 0.25mm in diameter. It is possible that the sensation of 'de qi' (pronounced *dechee*) which causes feelings of soreness or numbness at the point of needling is necessary both to indicate that the anatomically correct site has been needled and that the treatment will work well. However, the treatment is also often considered successful in the absence of de qi or any sensation at the point of skin puncture.

Stimulation of the acupuncture point can be increased by gentle turning/manipulation of the needles, using a small electric current, laser beams or ultrasound. Acupuncture studs remain *in situ* and may be pressed by the patient as necessary to give more sustained stimulation. In moxibustion, the needles are heated by smouldering a substance called moxa over the points.

Acupuncture treatments are often given once a week for 6–8 weeks and thereafter as necessary.

Evidence of effectiveness

Good evidence exists to support acupoint stimulation in treating the nausea and vomiting induced by chemotherapy: adjunct stimulation with needles and electroacupuncture reduced the incidence of acute vomiting but not nausea, while acupressure reduced nausea but not vomiting.

For relieving cancer pain some encouraging short-term results have been reported, but there is not enough evidence available to make any firm conclusions. Similarly, insufficient evidence is available for the relief of cancer-related fatigue, chronic obstructive pulmonary disease, dyspnoea, Alzheimer's disease, Parkinson's disease, multiple sclerosis, pain associated with cystic fibrosis and chronic heart failure. Hence, acupuncture is unlikely to be beneficial for neuropathic pain associated with AIDS/HIV.

Safety

Acupuncture is generally considered to be a relatively safe form of treatment with a low incidence of serious side-effects if practised by a skilled practitioner. Some events, such as nausea and syncope, can be mild and transient. While there is no official mechanism for reporting adverse events, there have, however, been accounts of pneumothorax, septicaemia, spinal injuries and hepatitis B/C transmission. The use of acupuncture studs in the ear may result in perichondritis of the underlying cartilage.

Acupuncture should be used with care in any patient in whom there is a risk of infection or bleeding. It should be avoided in patients with valvular heart disease. Acupuncture to spinal muscles should be safe unless there is an unstable spine, in which case it is contraindicated. Extra care should be exercised in those patients receiving their first acupuncture treatment as they may react strongly, with dizziness and drowsiness. The initial treatment should be given supine and patients should be advised not to drive or to operate machinery for a few hours.

Homeopathy

Background and theory

Homeopathy was founded by the German physician Samuel Hahnemann (1755–1843). This method often uses highly diluted preparations of a variety of different substances. Homeopathy is based on two key principles. The first is that 'like cures like'. Here, patients are given preparations whose effects when administered to healthy subjects correspond to the manifestations of the disorder (symptoms, clinical signs and pathological states) in the unwell patient. For instance, hayfever, which presents with lacrimation, stinging and irritation around the eyes and nose, might be treated with the remedy *Allium cepa*, derived from the common onion. According to the second principle, remedies are prepared by a process of serial dilution and succussion (vigorous shaking). The greater the number of times this process of dilution and succussion is performed, the greater the potency of the remedy. Homeopathic medicines are diluted so much that they are unlikely to contain even a single molecule of the original substance.

Prescribing strategies vary considerably. In 'classical' homeopathy, practitioners aim to identify a single medicine that is needed to treat a patient, taking into account current illness, medical history, personality and behaviour. 'Complex' homeopathy involves the prescription of combinations of medicines.

Common homeopathic medicines include those made from plants (such as belladonna, arnica and chamomile), minerals (e.g. mercury and sulphur), animal products (e.g. sepia (squid ink) and lachesis (snake venom), and more rarely, biochemical substances (such as histamine or human growth factor).

Uses

Many different, often chronic and recurring conditions are treated with homeopathic medication. Self-prescription for various conditions such as the common cold, bruising, hayfever and joint sprains is common.

Practical application

A very detailed history is taken in order to find the optimally matching drug ('similimum'). Information is also gathered about mood and behaviour, likes and dislikes, responses to stress, personality and food reactions. A 'symptom picture' is thus built up and matched to a 'drug picture' described in the homeopathic *Materia Medica*. One or more homeopathic medicines are then prescribed, usually in pill form, either as one or two doses or on a more regular basis.

A patient's initial symptom picture commonly matches more than one drug picture. Follow-up allows the practitioner to define the best medication for a particular patient.

Evidence of effectiveness

Controlled clinical results report encouraging but not fully convincing results for homeopathic treatment of chemotherapy-induced stomatitis and radiodermatitis. No convincing effects of homeopathy have been reported for general radiotherapy-related side-effects, menopausal symptoms in breast cancer survivors and oestrogen withdrawal in breast cancer patients.

The effectiveness of homeopathic remedies for HIV/AIDS has not been established. Overall, there is no convincing evidence of the effectiveness of any homeopathic remedy for any condition.

Safety

Serious adverse effects of homeopathic medicines are rare. However, symptoms may become acutely and transiently worse (aggravation reactions) after starting treatment and patients should be warned of this possibility. The occurrence of an aggravation reaction is interpreted by homeopaths as a sign that the treatment will be beneficial.

The more serious issue is the view of some practitioners who adamantly believe that conventional medication reduces the efficacy of homeopathic remedies. Serious adverse effects have occurred when patients have failed to comply with conventional medication.

Further reading

Books

Aung S. K. H., Chen W. P. D. (2007) *Clinical Introduction to Medical Acupuncture*. New York: Thieme.
Owen D. (2007) *Principles and Practice of Homeopathy*. Edinburgh: Churchill Livingstone/Elsevier.

Articles

Bardia A., *et al.* (2006) Efficacy of complementary and alternative medicine therapies in relieving cancer pain: a systematic review. *Journal of Clinical Oncology*, **24**: 5457–64.

Chung A., *et al.* (2003) Adverse effects of acupuncture. Which are clinically significant? *Canadian Family Physician*, **49**: 985–9.

Ernst E. (2006) Acupuncture—a critical analysis. *Journal of Internal Medicine*, **259**: 125–37.

Ezzo J.M., Richardson M.A. Vickers A, Allen C., Dibble S.I., Issell B.F., Lao L., Pearl M., Ramirez G., Roscoe J.A., Shen J., Shivnan J.C., Streitberger K., Treish I., Zhang G. Acupuncture point stimulatiion for chemotherapy-induced nausea or vomiting. *Cochrane Database of Systematic Reviews* 2006, Issue 2. Art. No.: CD002285. DOI: 10.1002/14651858. CD002285.pub2.
http://www.mrw.interscience.wiley.com/cochrane/clsysrev/articles/CD002285/frame.html

Milazzo S., *et al.* (2006) Efficacy of homeopathic therapy in cancer treatment. *European Journal of Cancer*, **42**(3): 282–9.

Mills E., *et al.* (2005) Complementary therapies for the treatment of HIV: in search of the evidence. *International Journal of STD & AIDS*, **16**(6): 395–403.

Sood A. (2007) A critical review of complementary therapies for cancer-related fatigue. *Integrative Cancer Therapies*, **6**: 8–13.

Walach H., *et al.* (2005) Research on homeopathy: state of the art. *Journal of Alternative and Complementary Medicine*, **11**: 813–29.

Professional organization

British Acupuncture Council: http://www.acupuncture.org.uk/

British Homeopathic Society: http://www.trusthomeopathy.org/

Group 2: Mind–body therapies

Mind–body medicine uses a variety of techniques designed to enhance the mind's capacity to affect bodily function and symptoms.

Relaxation therapy

Background and theory

Relaxation therapy uses a range of techniques for eliciting the 'relaxation response' of the autonomic nervous system. This results in decreases in oxygen consumption, heart rate, respiration and skeletal muscle activity and in the normalizing of blood supply to the muscles. One of the most common techniques is progressive muscle relaxation, which consists of progressive clenching followed by the conscious relaxation of all the muscles in the body in parallel with concentration on breathing control. Other relaxation techniques involve passive muscle relaxation, refocusing or imagery. In imagery-based relaxation, the idea is to visualize oneself in a place or situation associated with relaxation and comfort.

Uses

Relaxation therapies are commonly used for the relief of anxiety, stress disorders, musculoskeletal pain and headaches.

Practical application

Relaxation is usually taught in groups or by listening to tapes. With progressive muscle relaxation, the muscle groups are systematically contracted, then relaxed in a predetermined order while the patients lie on their back. In the early stages, an entire session will be devoted to a single muscle group. With practice, it becomes possible to combine muscle groups and then eventually relax the entire body all at once. Several months of daily practice are needed in order to be able to evoke the relaxation response within seconds.

Evidence of effectiveness

In cancer palliation, relaxation has been shown to be a useful adjunct for preventing nausea and vomiting associated with chemotherapy and other treatment-related symptoms in patients undergoing, for example, radiotherapy, bone marrow transplantation or hyperthermia. It has also proved to have a significant effect on anxiety. Encouraging effects have been reported for the reduction of tension and amelioration of the overall mood, but not enough data are available.

Similarly, data from rigorous trials into the benefits of relaxation therapy are too scarce to make any recommendations for its use in cancer-related fatigue, hot flushes in breast cancer patients, dyspnoea associated with chronic obstructive pulmonary disease and chronic heart failure.

Safety

Relaxation techniques are not associated with any serious safety concerns. They are, however, contraindicated in schizophrenic or actively psychotic patients. Those techniques requiring inward focusing may intensify depressed mood.

Further reading

Book

Payne R. (2004) *Relaxation Techniques: A Practical Handbook for the Health Care Professional.* Edinburgh: Churchill Livingstone.

Articles

Kwekkeboom K. L., Gretarsdottir E. (2006) Systematic review of relaxation interventions for pain. *Journal of Nursing Scholarship*, **38**: 269–77.

Rheingans J. I. (2007) A systematic review of nonpharmacologic adjunctive therapies for symptom management in children with cancer. *Journal of Pediatric Oncology Nursing*, **24**(2): 81–94.

Sood A. (2007) A critical review of complementary therapies for cancer-related fatigue. *Integrative Cancer Therapies*, **6**: 8–13.

Tipton J. M., *et al.* (2007) Putting evidence into practice: evidence-based interventions to prevent, manage, and treat chemotherapy-induced nausea and vomiting. *Clinical Journal of Oncology Nursing*, **11**(1): 69–78.

> You see things; and you say, 'Why?' But I dream things that never were;
> and I say, "why not?"
>   George Bernard Shaw (1921), *Back to Methuselah*, Part 1, Act 1

Hypnotherapy

Background and theory

Hypnotherapy involves the induction of deep physical and mental relaxation, inducing an altered state of consciousness which leads to a greatly increased susceptibility to suggestion. Once patients are guided into a hypnotic trance, they may recall memories not easily accessed by their conscious minds. The dissociation between the conscious and the unconscious mind can be used to give therapeutic suggestions, thereby encouraging changes in behaviour and the relief of symptoms. The goal of hypnotherapy is to gain self-control over behaviour, emotions or physiological processes. A fundamental principle of hypnotic phenomena is that the hypnotized individual is under his own control and not that of the hypnotist.

Uses

Hypnotherapy is more commonly used for anxiety, for disorders with a strong psychological component (such as asthma and irritable bowel syndrome) and for conditions that are modulated by levels of arousal, such as pain.

Practical application

Sessions typically last between 30 and 90 minutes, with an average course comprising 6–12 sessions. The initial visit involves gathering a history and discussion about hypnosis, suggestion and the client's expectations of the therapy; various tests for hypnotic suggestibility may also be conducted. The hypnotic state is achieved by first relaxing the body, then shifting attention away from the external environment towards a narrow range of objects or ideas suggested by the therapist. Sometimes hypnotherapy is carried out in group settings.

Evidence of effectiveness

In children with cancer, hypnosis has potential as a clinically valuable intervention for procedure-related pain and distress. It has also been shown to be helpful for anticipatory and post-chemotherapy nausea, again particularly in children. More data are required for its usefulness in the relief of pain, anxiety, fatigue and of hot flushes in patients with breast cancer.

Safety

Hypnosis is generally safe when it is practised by a clinically trained professional. It can, however, sometimes exacerbate psychological problems and is contraindicated in psychosis and personality disorders.

Further reading

Book

James U. (2005) *Clinical Hypnosis Textbook: A Guide for Practical Intervention.* Oxford: Radcliffe Publishing.

Articles

Anbar R. D. (2006) Hypnosis: an important multifaceted therapy. *Journal of Pediatrics*, **149:** 438–9.

Bardia A., *et al.* (2006) Efficacy of complementary and alternative medicine therapies in relieving cancer pain: a systematic review. *Journal of Clinical Oncology*, **24:** 5457–64.

Richardson J., *et al.* (2006) Hypnosis for procedure-related pain and distress in pediatric cancer patients: a systematic review of effectiveness and methodology related to hypnosis interventions. *Journal of Pain and Symptom Management*, **31:** 70–84.

Richardson J., *et al.* (2007) Hypnosis for nausea and vomiting in cancer chemotherapy: a systematic review of the research evidence. *European Journal of Cancer Care* **16:** 402–12.

Professional organization

The British Association of Medical Hypnosis. http://www.bamh.org.uk/

Guided imagery and visualization

Background and theory

Guided imagery is a visualization technique based on the notion that the mind can affect the body. It uses imagination and mental images to encourage physical healing, promote relaxation and bring about a change in attitude or behaviour. Stimulating the brain through visualization may have direct effects on the endocrine and nervous systems and may lead to changes in immune and other functions.

Uses

Imagery is commonly used by those patients undergoing conventional cancer treatment or surgery, for stress and anxiety as well as chronic pain conditions.

Practical application

Imagery is generally taught in small classes. Sessions usually last for 20–30 minutes, or longer if needed, once or twice weekly for several weeks. Patients will either sit in a chair or lie on a treatment table or a floor mat. Sessions usually begin with general relaxation exercises and then move on to more specific visualization techniques, introduced by the practitioner. Patients will be led to build a detailed image in their mind. Patients with cancer, for example, may be asked by their practitioner to picture their cancer being attacked by their immune system, their tumours shrinking or their body freeing itself of cancer.

Evidence of effectiveness

In cancer patients, guided imagery seems to be psychosupportive, decreasing anxiety and depression and increasing comfort. Although some encouraging effects on cancer-related pain have been reported, the available data are insufficient to make any firm recommendations. Guided imagery may increase oxygen saturation in patients with chronic obstructive pulmonary disease, but further data are required to make any firm recommendations. Not enough data are available for its usefulness in patients with AIDS and multiple sclerosis; it is unlikely to be beneficial for chemotherapy-associated nausea and vomiting.

Safety

Although guided imagery and visualization are generally safe, they are contraindicated in those with severe mental illness, latent psychosis and personality disorders.

Further reading

Books

Hall E., et al. (2006) *Guided Imagery: Creative Interventions in Counseling and Psychotherapy.* Thousand Oaks, CA: Sage Publications.

Articles

Bardia A., et al. (2006) Efficacy of complementary and alternative medicine therapies in relieving cancer pain: a systematic review. *Journal of Clinical Oncology,* **24**(34): 5457–64.

Roffe L., et al. (2005) A systematic review of guided imagery as an adjuvant cancer therapy. *Psychooncology,* **14**: 607–17.

Professional organization

National Federation of Spiritual Healers: http://www.nfsh.org.uk

Meditation

Background and theory
Meditation refers to a range of practices aimed at focusing and controlling attention to suspend the strategies of thoughts and relax body and mind. It is believed to result in a state of greater physical relaxation, mental calmness and psychological balance. Meditation comprises a very diverse array of practices, most of which are rooted in Eastern religious or spiritual traditions (e.g. transcendental meditation, Sahaja yoga/meditation, mindfulness meditation as well as meditative prayer). They are based on listening to breathing, repeating a mantra, detaching from the thought process or self-directed mental practices. Meditation is aimed at inducing physiological changes, e.g. altering the fight or flight response. It is believed to reduce activity in the sympathetic nervous system and increase activity in the parasympathetic nervous system. The specific mechanisms remain, however, unknown.

Uses
Meditation is often used for the relief of anxiety, asthma, stress, drug and alcohol addiction, epilepsy, heart disease, hypertension.

Practical application
Two common approches to meditation are mindfulness meditation and transcendental mediation. In mindfulness meditation the meditator learns to concentrate on the sensation of the flow of the breath in and out of the body and focus on what is being experienced, without reacting to or judging that experience. Eventually the meditator should learn to experience thoughts and emotions in normal daily life with greater balance and acceptance. Transcendental meditation uses a mantra or e.g. a word, sound, or phrase repeated silently, in order to prevent distracting thoughts from entering the mind. Eventually this should allow the mind to come to a quieter state and the body into a state of deep rest.

Meditators are initially instructed by a teacher in several sessions and should then practise regularly twice daily for 15–20 minutes. Continuous regular practice is expected to increase the effects.

Evidence of effectiveness
Positive results in patients at the end of life have been reported for mood disturbance, anxiety, depression, anger/hostility, emotional suppression, psychological distress, stress, intrusive images, confusion and coping mechanisms. For other symptoms and signs there are not enough data available for and including nausea and vomiting, quality of life, sleep disturbance and fatigue.

Meditation may improve the quality of life in patients with chronic heart failure, but not enough data are available. For stress, anxiety or anger in AIDS patients, there are too few data available to make any recommendations.

Safety
Although meditation is generally safe, patients suffering from psychiatric problems who wish to take up meditation should be supervised by a qualified psychiatrist or psychotherapist experienced in the use of such techniques in a therapeutic context. People with epilepsy or those at risk of developing epilepsy should consider the theoretical risk of precipitating attacks before proceeding.

Further reading

Articles

Canter P. H. (2003) The therapeutic effects of meditation. *British Medical Journal*, **326**: 1049–50.

Krisanaprakonkit T., Krisnaprakornkit W., Piyavhatkul N., Lagopaiboon M. Meditation therapy for anxiety disorders. *Cochrane Database of Systematic Reviews* 2006, Issue 1. Art. No.: CD004998. DOI: 10.1002/14651858.CD004998.pub2.
http://www.mrw.interscience.wiley.com/cochrane/articles/CD004998/frame.html

Lafferty W. E., *et al.* (2006) Evaluating CAM treatment at the end of life: a review of clinical trials for massage and meditation. *Complementary Therapies in Medicine*, **14**: 100–12.

Ott M. J., *et al.* (2006) Mindfulness meditation for oncology patients: a discussion and critical review. *Integrative Cancer Therapies*, **5**: 98–108.

Spiritual healing

Background

Spiritual healing uses spiritual means in treating disease. A healer and a patient interact with the intention of generating improvements or a cure of the illness. Healers believe they channel 'energy' (for example, of cosmic or divine origin) into patients which helps the body heal itself. The concept is not supported by scientific plausibility.

Uses

Healing is used to alleviate symptoms and recovery in a variety of clinical situations including anxiety, pain and general well-being.

Practical application

Spiritual healing is generally given in two ways, *laying-on of hands* or *distant healing*. In the former, healers hold their hands near to but not touching (or only lightly touching) the body, detecting areas of concern and transmitting 'energy' into the patient's body, which allegedly enhances self-healing. In the latter, healers send signals mentally as meditation, prayer or healing wishes from a location that can be many miles away from the patient.

A session may last 30–60 minutes. Typically, weekly sessions are pre-scribed. A series of treatments may consist of 6–10 sessions, which may be repeated regularly.

Many varieties of healing are available. While therapeutic touch is the most familiar, there is also: *Reiki*, derived from Japanese traditions; *Shamanism* which may include chanting and dancing; intercessory prayer; *Johrei*; faith healing; psychic healing; and paranormal healing

Evidence of effectiveness

There is not enough evidence available to support spiritual healing as a treatment for any condition. Although encouraging results for healing touch on cancer-related pain are available, the data are not sufficient to make any firm recommendations. Spiritual healing has shown encouraging results in reducing anxiety levels and increasing well-being, but studies are methodologically weak. Not enough data are available for its efficacy in reducing anxiety in AIDS patients.

Safety

Healing is generally a safe treatment and has no known serious side-effects, although it is contraindicated in those patients with psychiatric illnesses.

Further reading

Books

Jonas W. B., Crawford C. (eds) (2003) *Healing, Intention, and Energy Medicine*. Edinburgh: Churchill Livingstone.

Articles

Bardia A., *et al.* (2006) Efficacy of complementary and alternative medicine therapies in relieving cancer pain: a systematic review. *Journal of Clinical Oncology*, **24**(34): 5457–64.

Professional organization

National Federation of Spiritual Healers: http://www.nfsh.org.uk/

Creative therapies (📖 See Art and Music therapies pages 803–6)

Background and theory

In creative therapies art, music, prose and poetry are used as alternative forms of expression and communication. Therapy may release suppressed deep fears and feelings and evoke memories that, with careful and sensitive guiding by the therapist, may be used in trying to help the patient work through them constructively and positively. Receptive music therapy uses the analgesic and anxiolytic properties of music, which are mainly due to the lowering of stress levels and stress hormone production similar to the relaxation response.

Uses

Art and music therapies are popular in palliative care, helping with the patients' feelings of loss, fear, anger, guilt, anxiety and depression.

Practical application

Both art and music therapists work in a wide range of settings using art or music to achieve therapeutic goals. Art therapy combines traditional psychotherapeutic theories and techniques with an understanding of the psychological aspects of the creative process, especially the affective properties of the different art materials. In music therapy, the most basic distinction is between receptive music therapy (listening to music played by the therapist or recorded music) for relaxation and pain relief and active music therapy (the patient is involved in music-making) as a form of expression.

Evidence of effectiveness

Only preliminary data exist for the evaluation of art therapy. They relate to improving coping resources in women with primary breast cancer undergoing radiotherapy and increasing positive and collaborative behaviour in children during painful procedures.

Music therapy has been shown to be beneficial for procedure-related anxiety. In a range of conditions, music therapy has shown encouraging effects but there are not enough data available to draw any firm conclusions. Clinical music therapy might improve quality of life in patients with terminal cancer; preliminary data are positive for psychological problems in cancer palliation; and it may have some effect in relieving nausea and vomiting associated with chemotherapy. Similar encouraging, yet only preliminary, results have been reported for recorded music as an adjunct during routine chest physiotherapy for cystic fibrosis, for reducing agitation and aggressive behaviour in Alzheimer patients, strengthening of respiratory muscles through the coordination of breath and speech in multiple sclerosis, and for motor, affective and behavioural functions in Parkinson's patients. The data are methodologically too limited in patients with dementia.

Safety

There are no known safety concerns associated with art or music therapy.

Further reading

Books

Gilroy A. (2006) *Art Therapy, Research and Evidence-based Practice*. London: Sage Publications.

Karkou V. (2006) *Arts Therapies*. Edinburgh: Elsevier Churchill Livingstone.

Articles

Hilliard R. E. (2005) Music therapy in hospice and palliative care: a review of the empirical data. *Evidence-based Complementary and Alternative Medicine*, **2**: 173–8.

Oster I., *et al.* (2006) Art therapy improves coping resources: a randomized, controlled study among women with breast cancer. *Palliative & Supportive Care*, **4**: 57–64.

Scott JT, Harmsen M, Prictor MJ, Sowden AJ, Watt I. Interventions for improving communication with children and adolescents about their cancer. *Cochrane Database of systematic Reviews* 2003, Issue 3. Art. No.: CD002969. DOI: 10.1002/14651858.CD002969.
http://www.mrw.interscience. wiley.com/cohrane/clsysrev/articles/CD002969/frame.

Professional organization

The British Association of Art Therapists: http://www.baat.org/

The British Society for Music Therapy: http://www.bsmt.org/

Group 3: Biologically-based practices

Herbal medicine

Background and theory

Plants have been used for medicinal purposes since the dawn of humanity. They form the origin of many modern medicines, e.g. digoxin from *Digitalis purpurea* (foxglove) or salicin from *Salix* spp. (willow). Herbal extracts contain plant material with pharmacologically active constituents. The active principle(s) of the extract, which is in many cases unknown, may exert its effects at the molecular level and may have, for instance, enzyme-inhibiting effects (e.g. escin). A single main constituent may be active, or a complex mixture of compounds produces a combined effect. Known active constituents or marker substances may be used to standardize preparations.

Modern Western herbalism or phytomedicine as practised in many European countries such as Germany is integrated into conventional medicine with compulsory education and training for physicians and pharmacists. It follows the diagnostic and therapeutic principles of conventional medicine.

Other more traditional systems include Chinese herbal medicine, which is based on the concepts of yin and yang and qi energy. In China, ill health is seen as a pattern of disharmony or imbalance and Chinese herbal medicines are believed to harmonize these energies and ultimately restore health. In Japan, this system of traditional herbal medicine has evolved into *kampo*. Ayurveda, the traditional Indian medical system, frequently uses herbal mixtures. Characteristic of these systems is a high degree of individualization of treatments. In contrast to modern phytomedicine, all traditional herbal medicine systems predominantly use complex mixtures of different herbs.

Uses

Herbal medicine is generally used for a wide range of conditions. In palliative care it is used for anxiety, depression, pain, radiation-induced dermatitis, chemotherapy-induced nausea and vomiting, hot flushes and quality of life, as well as for the prevention and treatment of cancer.

Practical application

During an initial treatment session the practitioner will usually take the patient's medical history. Information may also be sought on the patient's personality and background, which may influence the selection of herbs. Individualized combinations of herbs may be prescribed. Follow-up appointments may be arranged and the herbal preparations and regimen reviewed. The regimen depends largely on the nature and severity of the condition, but consists generally of either one or two appointments per week for a treatment period ranging from one to several weeks. Medication is usually administered orally in the form of tablets, capsules, tinctures or teas. Topical applications, e.g. ointments and compresses, are also used.

Evidence of effectiveness

No convincing evidence exists for any herbal medicine in the treatment of **cancer**. The effectiveness of a range of herbal medicines in cancer palliation is unclear due to insufficient data being available: cannabinoids for pain-control, appetite or quality of life; ginkgo (*Ginkgo biloba*) for lymphoedema; ginseng (*Panax ginseng*) for fatigue and quality of life; marigold (*Calendula officinalis*) for radiation-induced dermatitis in breast cancer; the Chinese herbal remedy huangqi for nausea and vomiting induced by chemotherapy. *Aloe vera* showed no convincing effects on radiation-induced skin irritation or oral mucositis. The results regarding black cohosh (*Actaea racemosa*) on hot flushes are contradictory and it has been associated with liver damage. Cranberry (*Vaccinium macrocarpon*) and phytoestrogens showed no efficacy in the treatment of prostate cancer symptoms or for hot flushes, respectively.

In patients with **AIDS** the effectiveness of boxwood (*Buxus sempervirens*) as well as tea tree oil (*Melaleuca alternifolia*) for oral candidiasis are unknown. Many different preparations of Chinese herbal mixture exist but the data are not encouraging for their use in patients with AIDS. No evidence of effectiveness is available for St John's Wort (*Hypericum perforatum*) on antiviral activity or for topical application of capsaicin to reduce pain.

Ginkgo (*Ginkgo biloba*) improves cognition and function in **Alzheimer's disease**. The Kampo medicine choto-san might lead to a general improvement. Not enough data are available for *Huperzia serrata*, lemon balm (*Melissa officinalis*) and sage (*Salvia officinalis*). Ginseng (*Panax ginseng*) is likely to be ineffective for improving somatic symptoms, depression and anxiety.

In **chronic obstructive pulmonary disease** the effects of Chinese herbal mixtures, ginseng (*Panax ginseng*) on lung function and ivy (*Hedera helix*) leaf extract for dyspnoea are not clear. Studies of pomegranate (*Punica granatum*) juice were negative.

In **chronic heart failure**, extracts from the leaf and flower of the hawthorn (*Crataegus* spp.) improve maximal workload, while milk vetch (*Astragalus* spp.) has been shown to improve left ventricular ejection fraction. The evidence for shengmai, a combination product including *Panax ginseng, Ophiopogon japonicus* and *Schisandra chinensis,* is inconclusive due to the low quality of the studies. Not enough data are available to make any firm recommendations for Ayurvedic medicines, Chinese medicines, Ginseng (*Panax ginseng*) and Kanlijian.

St John's Wort (*Hypericum perforatum*) has been shown to be effective in the treatment of mild to moderate **depression**.

The results so far from studies of cannabis (*Cannabis sativa*) for **multiple sclerosis** are somewhat contradictory, but some data suggest there is an improvement in mobility, pain and sleep. It might also reduce the number of incontinence episodes but not enough data are yet available. It is unlikely to be beneficial in reducing tremor. Some preliminary data for Ginkgo (*Ginkgo biloba*) suggest it may improve fatigue, symptom severity and functionality but not cognitive function.

In **Parkinson's disease**, preliminary data are encouraging for the use of *Mucuna pruriens*, a traditional Ayurvedic herbal medicine, which is a natural source of L-dopa. Cannabis (*Cannabis sativa*) is unlikely to reduce tremor.

Safety

Because plant extracts have pharmacological effects, their potential for adverse effects and interactions needs to be considered. They vary for each individual herb and should be evaluated individually. St John's Wort (*Hypericum perforatum*), for example, interacts with warfarin and the contraceptive pill, while kava kava (*Piper methysticum*) has been associated with liver damage. In general, those patients taking herbal medication on a regular basis should receive regular follow-up and appropriate biochemical monitoring. Patients should always be asked about self-prescription use of herbal medicine. There is currently no reporting system for adverse events and interactions of herbal medicines.

Other safety issues associated with herbal medicines are toxicity, contamination (in particular traditional Chinese medicines), adulteration, misidentification or quality issues.

Further reading

Books

Basch E. M., Ulbricht C. E. (eds) (2005) *Herb and Supplement Handbook: The Clinical Bottom Line*. St Louis, MO: Elsevier Mosby.

Braun L., Cohen M. (2005) *Herbs and Natural Supplements: An Evidence-based Guide*. Sydney: Elsevier Mosby.

Capasso F., *et al.* (2003). *Phytotherapy: A Quick Reference to Herbal Medicine*. Berlin: Springer.

Articles

Birks J, Grimley Evans J. Ginkgo biloba for cognitive impairment and dementia. *Cochrane Database of Systematic Reviews* 2007, Issue 2. Art. No.: CD003120. DOI:10.1002/14651858.CD003120.pub2. http://www.mrw.interscience.wiley.com/cochrane/clsysrev/articles/CD003120/frame.html

Linde K., *et al.* (2005) St John's Wort for depression. *Cochrane Database of Systematic Reviews*, **2**: CD000448.

Liu JP, Manheimer E., Yang M. Herbal medicines for treating HIV infection and AIDS. *Cochrane Database of Systematic Reviews* 2005, Issue 3. Art. No.:CD003937. DOI: 10.1002/14651858. CD03937.pub2. http://www.mrw.interscience.wiley.com/cochrane/clsysrev/articles/CD003937/frame.html

Pittler M. H., *et al.* (2003) Hawthorn extract for treating chronic heart failure: Meta-analysis of randomized trials. *American Journal of Medicine*, **114**: 665–74.

Zajicek J., *et al.* (2003) Cannabinoids for treatment of spasticity and other symptoms related to multiple sclerosis (CAMS study): multicentre randomised placebo-controlled trial. *Lancet*, **362**: 1517–26.

Databases

Natural Standard: http://www.naturalstandard.com/

The Natural Medicines Comprehensive Database: http://www.naturaldatabase.com/

Professional organization

The British Herbal Medicine Association: http://www.bhma.info/

Aromatherapy

Background and theory

Aromatic plants, and the infusions prepared from them, have been employed in medicines and cosmetics for thousands of years. Aromatherapy uses oils extracted from plants, which are usually referred to as 'essential oils'. These are the pure, concentrated hydrophobic liquids containing the volatile essences of plants: flowers (e.g. rose), leaves (e.g. peppermint), barks (e.g. cinnamon), fruits (e.g. lemon), seeds (e.g. fennel), grasses (e.g. lemongrass), bulbs (e.g. garlic) and other plant substances. Fresh plant material usually yields 1–2% by weight of essential oil on distillation. A typical essential oil contains a complex mixture of over 100 different chemical compounds which give the oil its smell, therapeutic properties and, in some cases, its toxicity. Essential oils are highly toxic if ingested undiluted.

Essential oils are considered to act not only on the body, by stimulating physiological processes, but also on the emotions and the mind. Odour stimulates the olfactory senses and these relay to the limbic system, which is central to the emotions and memory. In turn, the limbic system is associated with the hypophyseal–pituitary axis which regulates the endocrine system, affecting a person's reactions to fear, anger, metabolism and sexual stimulus.

Practical application

Usually, diluted essential oils are applied to the skin through gentle massage. The individual choice of oil is determined by the experience of the therapist. Occasionally, essential oils are also used in baths or diffusers. One session typically lasts around 1 hour. A full series may include about ten sessions.

Evidence of effectiveness

Aromatherapy in combination with massage has positive short-term effects on psychological well-being in cancer patients, with the effect on anxiety supported by limited evidence. However, the effects on physical symptoms such as nausea are not supported by sufficient evidence. Evidence is mixed as to whether aromatherapy enhances the effects of massage.

Encouraging results have been reported for reducing agitation and neuropsychiatric symptoms in dementia patients and symptom control and well-being in patients with Alzheimer's disease, but there are insufficient data to make any firm recommendations. Aromatherapy failed to show benefits in terms of symptom control in cancer patients, pain control, anxiety or quality of life in hospice patients, as well as on psychological outcomes during radiation therapy.

Safety

Essential oils should not be taken orally or used undiluted on the skin. Some oils cause photosensitivity. Allergic reactions are possible with all oils. Some oils have carcinogenic potential and certain oils should be avoided in cancer patients.

Patients with cancer are often highly sensitive to the sense of smell, which may have altered due to chemotherapy. Certain smells can be very nauseating, and this should be assessed with the patient before therapy.

Further reading

Books

Lis-Balchin M. (2006) *Aromatherapy Science: a Guide for Healthcare Professionals*. London: Pharmaceutical Press.

Articles

Fellowes D., Barnes K., Wilkinson S. Aromatherapy and massage for symptom relief in patients with cancer. *Cochrane Database of Systematic Reviews* 2004, Issue 3. Art No.: CD002287. DOI: 10.1002/14651858.CD002287.pub2
http://www.mrw.interscience.wiley.com/cochrane/clsysrev/articles/FD002287/frame.html

Graham P. H., *et al.* (2003)Inhalation aromatherapy during radiotherapy: results of a placebo-controlled double-blind randomized trial. *Journal of Clinical Oncology*, **21**: 2372–6.

Soden K. (2004) A randomised controlled trial of aromatherapy massage in a hospice setting. *Palliative Medicine*, **18**: 87–92.

Thorgrimsen L., *et al.* (2003) Aroma therapy for dementia. *Cochrane Database of Systematic Reviews*, Issue 3.

Wilcock A., *et al.* (2004) Does aromatherapy massage benefit patients with cancer attending a specialist palliative care day centre? *Palliative Medicine*, **18**: 287–90.

Wilkinson S. M., *et al.* (2007) Effectiveness of aromatherapy massage in the management of anxiety and depression in patients with cancer: a multicenter randomized controlled trial. *Journal of Clinical Oncology*, **25**: 532–9.

Professional organization

The Aromatherapy Council: http://www.aromatherapycouncil.co.uk/

Group 4: Manipulative and body-based therapies

These therapies in CAM are based on manipulation and/or movement of one or more parts of the body. Some examples include chiropractic or osteopathic manipulation, and massage.

Massage

Background and theory

Massage is one of the oldest healthcare practices in existence. It was documented in Chinese texts more than 4000 years ago and has been used in Western healthcare since Hippocrates in the fourth century BC. Massage therapy is the manipulation of the soft tissues of the body for therapeutic purposes. It consists of manual techniques that include applying pressure and traction. The friction of the hands as well as the mechanical pressure exerted on cutaneous and subcutaneous structures affect all body systems, in particular the musculoskeletal, circulatory, lymphatic and nervous systems.

Uses

Massage is widely used in the treatment of a variety of conditions including lymphoedema, stress, anxiety, back and other pain, and insomnia. Through the relaxation of muscle tension and the relief of anxiety, massage therapy may reduce blood pressure and heart rate. Massage may also enhance the immune system. Abdominal massage may be useful for constipation.

Practical application

Either the whole body or relevant specific parts may be treated. The practitioner may play background music depending on the patient's preference. Patients may be encouraged to breathe steadily and to communicate with the therapist. Oils, including aromatherapy oils, may also be used, depending on the individual patient and the aims of treatment. Massage usually lasts one hour, and one or two sessions per week for a treatment period of 4–8 weeks are recommended initially.

Evidence of effectiveness

Both massage and/or aromatherapy have been shown to have positive effects on the well-being of cancer patients in general, and on anxiety in particular. The question whether essential oils are important remains unanswered. It has also been shown to be beneficial for the relief of anxiety of various causes.

Encouraging results exist for the effect of massage in chemotherapy-related nausea as well as anxiety and depression in multiple sclerosis, but further data are required. Although massage may improve quality of life, anxiety and low mood in HIV patients, its effects on immune function are not clear. For Alzheimer's disease there is only a limited amount of reliable data available which prevents any firm conclusions.

The relaxing effects of massage may have some, albeit non-specific, influence on the well-being of most patients.

Safety

Massage is comparatively safe and adverse effects are extremely rare. There is no evidence that it encourages the spread of cancer, although it is contraindicated where it might damage tumour or frail normal tissue, particularly in treatment-related areas.

It is generally contraindicated in patients who have advanced heart disease, phlebitis, thrombosis and embolism, kidney failure, infectious diseases, contagious skin conditions, acute inflammation, infected injuries, unhealed fractures, conditions prone to haemorrhage and psychosis. It is also contraindicated in the acute flare-up of rheumatoid arthritis, eczema, goitre and open skin lesions.

(📖 For aromatherapy massage, see the Aromatherapy section, p. 833.)

Further reading

Books

Rich G. J. (2002) *Massage Therapy: the Evidence for Practice*. Edinburgh: Mosby.

Articles

Corbin L. (2005) Safety and efficacy of massage therapy for patients with cancer. *Cancer Control*, **12**: 158–64.

Fellowes D., Barness K., Wilkinson S. Aromatherapy and massage for symptom relief in patients with cancer. *Cochrane Database of Systematic Reviews* 2004, Issue 3. Art. No.: CD002287. DOI: 10.1002/14651858.CD002287.pub2
http:\\www.mrw.interscience.wiley.com/cochrane/clsysrev/articles/CD002287/frame.html

Professional organization

Massage Therapy UK: http://www.massagetherapy.co.uk

Reflexology

Background and theory

The therapeutic use of hand and foot pressure for the treatment of pain and various illnesses existed in China and India over 5000 years ago.

It is suggested that there are ten longitudinal, bilateral reflexes or zones running along the body which terminate in the hands and feet. All systems and organs are reflected onto the skin surface, particularly that of the palms and soles. By applying gentle pressure to these areas it is possible to relieve blockages or imbalances of energy along the zone. It is believed that specific organs as well as the interrelationship between organs and bodily systems can be influenced to regain and maintain emotional, physical and spiritual homeostasis resulting in the relief of symptoms and facilitating the prevention of illness and the promotion of healing.

Malfunction of any organ or part of the body is thought to cause the deposition of tiny calcium and uric acid crystals in the nerve endings, particularly in the feet. These deposits are then broken down and eliminated by gentle pressure. This is referred to as 'detoxification', which may lead to a 'healing crisis' including 'flu-like symptoms, a feeling of being light headed and lethargic, feeling cold 3–4 days' post-treatment, a reduction in blood pressure, an increase in excretory functions and an alteration in sleep pattern.

Uses

Reflexology is used for a variety of clinical problems. Of particular relevance to palliative care are control of pain and anxiety, induction of deep relaxation and improvement in sleep.

Practical application

Although there are different schools of teaching in the application of reflexology, the underlying principles are consistent. The foot is treated by applying gentle pressure along each zone systematically until the dorsum, sides and sole have been covered. The practitioner then repeats the treatment on the other foot. Initially, gentle massage and stroking movements are used, followed by deep thumb and finger pressure. The reflex areas on the foot may feel tender or painful if 'blocked', but is relieved as the treatment works and the 'blockage' is removed. Treatment may take up to an hour and be repeated weekly as necessary.

Evidence of effectiveness

There is no convincing evidence of the effectiveness of reflexology from controlled clinical trials to support its use for any indication, including symptom control in chronic obstructive pulmonary disease, agitation in dementia, motor sensory and urinary symptoms in multiple sclerosis. It is unlikely to be beneficial in improving quality of life in patients with cancer.

Safety

Contraindications to reflexology include its use in the first trimester of pregnancy. Care should be taken in patients with depressive and manic states, epilepsy and acute conditions.

Patients receiving reflexology may notice an increase in urination and body discharges, leading to fears that medicinal drugs such as chemotherapy agents might be eliminated more quickly from the body and thus be less effective. However, there is no evidence for this.

Further reading

Books

Barraclough J. (ed.) (2007) *Enhancing Cancer Care: Complementary Therapy and Support*. Oxford: Oxford University Press.

Ernst E. (2007) *Complementary Therapies for Pain Management: An Evidence Based Approach*. St Louis: Mosby.

Mackareth P., Tiran D. (ed.). (2002) *Clinical Reflexology: A Guide for Health Professionals*. Edinburgh: Churchill Livingstone,

Articles

Devlin B. (2006) The art of healing and knowing in cancer and palliative care. *International Journal of Palliative Nursing*, **12**(1): 16–19.

Stephenson N. L. N., *et al.* (2000) The effects of foot reflexology on anxiety and pain in patients with breast and lung cancer. *Oncology Nursing Forum*, **27**(1): 67–72.

Professional organization

The Reflexology Forum: http://www.reflexologyforum.org/

Palliative care in the home

Palliative care at home embraces what is most noble in medicine: sometimes curing, always relieving, supporting right to the end.[1]

The major part of continuing care for palliative patients is provided by the primary healthcare team, whether with malignant or non-malignant diagnoses: such continuing care cannot realistically be the responsibility of specialist palliative care. The reality is that primary care and the generic hospital services currently provide, and will continue to provide, the great majority of palliative care.[2]

Palliative care in the community is important. Primary care contributes a vital role, which is greatly appreciated by patients and carers, and has a significant impact on other services. Many general practitioners (GPs) and district nurses feel that palliative care represents the best of all medical care, bringing together the clinical, holistic and human dimensions of primary care. They know their patients well, and are in a key position to provide the best support for them and their families at this most crucial stage, with the backing of specialist palliative care and hospice expertise, advice and resources. GPs and district nurses often prioritize care of the dying, some claiming that it reconnects them with their reasons for entering healthcare and also affects their standing in a community. However, care at home can break down or become suboptimal for a variety of reasons such as lack of planning, poor communication, limited round-the-clock coordination, difficulties in symptom control, inadequate support for carers, misunderstanding of the specialists' role and availability out of hours, etc.

Good palliative care is appreciated by our patients and their families, and is at the core of good primary care, and in many ways is probably the best thing we do.

(A Northern Ireland GP)

---

1 Gomas J.-M. (1993) Palliative care at home: a reality or 'mission impossible'? *Palliative Medicine*, **7**(Suppl. 1): 45–59.

2 Barclay S. (2001) Palliative care for non-cancer patients: a UK perspective from primary care. In *Palliative Care for Non-cancer Patients* (ed. J. Addington-Hall, I. Higginson), pp. 156–172. Oxford: Oxford University Press.

First paradox of community palliative care[3]

Most dying people would prefer to remain at home, but most of them die in institutions.

Second paradox of community palliative care

Most of the final year of life is spent at home, but most people are admitted to hospital to die.

Despite most patients expressing a preference to remain at home and to die there if adequately supported, most patients die in institutions. Disturbingly, most are not even formally consulted as to their wishes.

Home is the place that reminds us of living as well as dying and is where we feel more fully ourselves.

The community provision of palliative care services is a vital part of integrated palliative care, and affects hospital and hospice admission rates and capacity, particularly for non-cancer patients.

Many more patients with non-malignant disease, and as many cancer patients, die in care homes as in hospices, so good palliative care in this setting, where a fifth of all people die, is also essential.

The goal is that quality palliative care should be available to patients who need it irrespective of their diagnosis or the setting.

Many hospice-based, hospice-at-home services successfully supplement and support generic services.

The original palliative care principles are being mainstreamed into standard healthcare across the world. From the early days of the movement the proliferation of hospices was discouraged in favour of broad dissemination of 'terminal care' principles throughout the health service, including acute hospital and community services.

Ideally, there should be a means to optimize generalist palliative care at home so that, regardless of the setting, the diagnosis and the possible disease timescale, patients should receive the highest standard of palliative care at all times, i.e. the '...care of the dying should be raised to the level of the best' (NHS Cancer Plan England 2000).

I think that terminal care is probably if not the most important then certainly one of the most important things that GPs can become involved in. I feel it's that personal involvement that is often the most important thing.[4]

3 Thorpe G. (1993) Enabling more dying people to remain at home. *British Medical Journal*, **307**: 915–18.

4 Jeffrey D. (2000) *Cancer from Cure to Care: Palliative Care Dilemmas in General Practice* Manchester Hochland and Hochland.

Community palliative care key facts

- 90% of the final year of life for most patients is spent at home
- People are now living longer with serious illnesses, and mainly in the community
- GPs have always been, and will continue to be, the main providers of palliative care for the majority of patients
- Patients especially appreciate:
  - continuity of relationship
  - being listened to
  - an opportunity to ventilate feelings
  - being accessible
  - effective symptom control
- GPs' palliative care role can be optimized by specialist support, especially if there is some formalized engagement.[5] 'It is better to help a colleague with a difficult case than to tell him he is wrong, and that he should make way for the expert'[6]
- On average, each GP will look after 30–40 patients with cancer at any one time, or about 200 patients per practice team of 10,000 patients, or 3500 for every Primary Care Trust (PCT)
- On average, 8 patients will be newly diagnosed with cancer/GP per year, 50 per practice and 750 per PCT
- The 'average' UK GP will have about 20 patient deaths/year, of which about 5 will be from cancer, 5 from organ failure (e.g. heart failure or COPD), 7 or 8 as a result of multiple pathology, dementia and decline, and 2 or 3 sudden deaths, e.g. myocardial infarction, road traffic accident, etc.
- Palliative care occupies a greater proportion of a district nurse's time, including out-of-hours care, than patient numbers would indicate
- There is less support available for patients and carers with non-malignant end-stage illness, and limited support for GPs managing such patients
- There is a steady shift in the place of care for many patients with palliative care needs, away from the hospital setting into the community, for the majority of their last year of life
- Hospital death is more likely if patients are poor, elderly, have no carers, are far from other services or have a long illness trajectory
- The home death rate in England is low (23% for cancer patients and 19% for all deaths)
- The hospital death rate in England is high (55 % for cancer patients and 66 % for all deaths)
- There is a clear preference from most patients and carers for a home death and an increasing choice of hospice death

5 Mitchell G. (2002) How well do general practitioners deliver palliative care? A systematic review. *Palliative Medicine*, **16**: 457–64.

6 Pugsley R., Pardoe J. (1986) The specialist contribution to the care of the terminally ill patient. *Journal of Royal College of General Practitioners*, **36**: 347–8.

- For hospitals, improving community palliative care services will help: reduce the numbers of patients with palliative care needs from occupying acute beds; improve capacity and waiting lists; and reduce the standard hospital mortality ratio
- According to the National Audit Office, it is estimated that 4000 patients a day could be discharged from hospital if there were adequate community places for them
- Gaps are apparent in community care, e.g. for symptom control management, 24h nursing care, night sitters, access to equipment, out-of-hours support—and there are concerns that this picture may worsen in future with changes in out-of-hours provision
- Specialist palliative care has raised standards of care and symptom control
- Hospice care is changing: with the average length of stay now reduced to two weeks
- 50% of patients admitted to hospices will be discharged back to the community
- Improved palliative care services can have a very positive effect on a family's bereavement journey
- GPs and district nurses repeatedly demonstrate they are keen to improve the quality of the palliative service they provide, and they regard palliative care as important and intrinsic to primary care
- In England, national directives emphasize the vital role of community palliative care*

The care of the dying is a test of a successful NHS
NHS Chief Executive Sir Nigel Crisp, March 2003

* www.goldstandardsframework.nhs.uk
www.mcpcil.org.uk/liverpool-care-pathway
www.endoflifecareforadults.nhs.uk.

Patients' needs

The user viewpoint

You matter because you are you. You matter to the last moment of your life and we will do all we can not only to help you die peacefully but to live until you die.

Dame Cicely Saunders

John had wanted to stay at home as he became weaker. But suddenly one weekend it all went badly wrong and he went into hospital in the middle of the night. He never came home. I will never forgive myself for this. I will have to live with this feeling of guilt all my life, wishing I could have done more.

Mary, wife of John, a cancer patient

Listening to patients

The care provided both in the provision of day-to-day clinical care at the bedside and, strategically, in the planning of services must be based on the needs of patients. Listening to the 'user view' is obvious, increasingly important in both scenarios, yet sometimes still avoided. The importance of the views of the patient and their carers is becoming recognized more formally with the emergence of user groups in cancer networks and elsewhere.

How much do we listen to patients' needs and respond accordingly? Unfortunately, workload pressure and the daunting task of facing sensitive situations that require good communication skills can easily deflect from taking time to acquire the patient's view. Some assessment tools have been developed to help facilitate this important task, such as the Problems and Concerns Assessment Tools or Patient/Carer Feedback sheets.

I think that the most important thing is that we must listen to what the question is and try to hear what is behind the actual words used.

Cicely Saunders[7]

Truth telling, communication skills and retaining control

Patients and carers cannot be full participants in decision-making without having clear information; if they are left uninformed, they will have less sense of retaining autonomy and control. There is a common, well-intentioned but misguided assumption, present at all stages of cancer care, that what people do not know does not harm them.

'Truth may hurt but deceit hurts more.'[8] Healthcare professionals often censor the information they give to patients in an attempt to protect them from potentially hurtful, sad or bad news. However, less than honest

---

7 Clark D. (2002) *Cicely Saunders, Founder of the Hospice Movement—selected letters 1959–1999.* Oxford: Oxford University Press.

8 Fallowfield L. J., Jenkins V. A., Beveridge H. A. (2002) Truth may hurt but deceit hurts more: communication in palliative care. *Palliative Medicine*, **16**: 297–303.

disclosure and the desire to shield patients from the reality of the situation often create even greater difficulties for patients, carers and other members of the healthcare team. Although it may be well meant, such a conspiracy of silence often results in a heightened state of fear, anxiety and confusion for patients who may even feel betrayed by such a process, which actually does little to promote patient calm and equanimity. Ambiguous or deliberately misleading information may afford short-term benefits, but denies individuals as well as their families opportunities to reorganize and adapt their lives towards the attainment of achievable goals, realistic hopes and previously planned-for aspirations. Having said this, breaking bad news is always difficult. Skills in discussing sensitive information can be learned and practised, and most areas run communication skills' learning, now an integral part of the Supportive and Palliative Care Guidance in England.

As the Age Concern's 12 Principles of a Good Death confirms (Table 12.1), in 8 out of 12 assertions, retaining control is a vital element for patients, and our role should be more to enable than to instruct, ever respectful of the boundaries set by our patients.

Table 12.1 Age Concern's 12 principles of a good death[9]

1	To be able to retain **control** of what happens
2	To have **control** over pain relief and other symptom control
3	To have **choice and control** over where death occurs (at home or elsewhere)
4	To have **access** to hospice care in any location, not only in hospital
5	To have **control** over who is present and who shares the end
6	To be able to issue **Advance Directives** which ensure wishes are respected
7	To know when death is coming, and to understand what can be expected
8	To be afforded dignity and privacy
9	To have **access** to information and expertise of whatever kind is necessary
10	To have **access** to any spiritual or emotional support required
11	To have time to say goodbye, and **control** over other aspects of timing
12	To be able to leave when it is time to go, and not to have life prolonged pointlessly

9 Henwood M. (1999) *The Future of Health and Care of Older People*. London: Age Concern.

Preferred place of death

Asking and noting where patients would like to be cared for in their dying phase is a very significant step towards tailoring services to meet patients' preferences and needs. This is a key issue in developing a real sense of choice, maintaining some control and self-determination in a world seemingly turned upside down for patients and their carers. The literature confirms that where someone has been asked about preference for place of care it is more likely to be attained, and choice of place of death is increasingly seen now as a patient's right. However, many may express a preference for home or hospice care, but are currently unable to achieve this. Carers are our patients in primary care and also have their own needs, as the toll of caring for the dying patient may be considerable.[10]

Table 12.2 Place of death

Higginson I (2003) Priorities for End of Life Care in England Wales and Scotland National Council				
Place:	Home	Hospital	Hospice	Care Home
Preference	56%	11%	24%	4%
Cancer	25%	47%	17%	12%
All causes	20%	56%	4%	20%

Patient needs

We all have needs, whether acknowledged or not. In 1943, Maslow proposed that we are all motivated by our wish continually to satisfy our needs. He commented that there were at least five sets of goals which he called 'Basic needs'. Briefly, these are:

• Physiological (food, sleep, warmth, health)
• Safety (security, protection from threats)
• Social (belonging, association, acceptance, friendship, love)
• Esteem (self-respect, reputation, status, recognition)
• Self-actualization (personal growth, accomplishment, creativity, achievement of potential).
• Spiritual, involving non-clinicians

Maslow described a hierarchy of needs to show that at any moment we concentrate almost exclusively on one of our unmet needs. We do not bother much about our social status if we are starving. Once the most immediate need is fairly well satisfied we are impelled to move on to the next most pressing need. Patients recently diagnosed with cancer find themselves returned starkly to the bottom of Maslow's hierarchy, to the level of the need to survive.

Dying is not just a physical or medical journey, for it is essentially a human one, common to us all: something of metaphysical or spiritual significance that is set within a cultural context. If we, as healthcare professionals, can fully support our patients in the first two stages of the hierarchy above,

10 Simon C. (2001) Informal carers and the primary care team. *British Journal of General Practice*, **51**: 920–3.

i.e. as far as possible maintain comfort, freedom from symptoms and provide a sense of security and support, then our patients are more likely to be able to proceed with other stages of their journey towards greater depths of relationships, self-acceptance and spiritual peace. By alleviating symptoms and reducing fear we create the space for people to travel. Our prime business is to play our role within the medical context; hence, maintaining patients symptom-free, secure, supported and enabled to die in their place of choice. These are three of the goals of the Gold Standards Framework.[11]

The essential concept is that the doctor, or at least the practice, will stay firmly with the patient and relative at their time of need and not desert them…When a patient is dying at home, it makes a big difference if the doctor continues to call regularly…otherwise patient and family are likely to feel abandoned and deserted when they least expect it…The promise of a regular visit gives a special kind of support unlike any other.[12]

What do patients and carers want from the services?

- *Being treated as a human being.* People want to be treated as individuals, and with dignity and respect
- *Empowerment.* The ability to have their voice heard, to be valued for their knowledge and skills, and to exercise real choice about treatments and services
- *Information.* Patients and carers should receive all the information they want about their condition and possible treatment. It should be given in an honest, timely and sensitive manner. Always document and do not forget updating with new data as available
- *Having choice.* Patients and carers want to know what options are available to them from the NHS, voluntary and private sectors, including access to self-help and support groups and complementary therapy services
- *Continuity of care.* Good communication and coordination of services between health and social care professionals working across the NHS and social sectors is essential
- *Equal access.* People want access to services of similar quality wherever they are delivered
- *Meeting physical needs.* Physical symptoms must be managed to a degree acceptable to patients
- *Meeting psychological needs.* Patients and carers need emotional support from professionals who are prepared to listen to them and are capable of understanding their concerns
- *Meeting social needs.* Support for the family, advice on financial and employment issues and provision of transport are necessary
- *Meeting spiritual needs.* Patients and carers should have support to help them explore the spiritual issues important to them.

From *Cancerlink* survey, Cancer Supportive
Care Services Strategy, User's Priorities and
Perspectives 2000

11 www. goldstandardsframework.nhs.uk
12 Brewin T. (2001) Personal view: deserted. *British Medical Journal*, **322**: 117.

Examples of needs-based predicting and fulfilling needs

Two examples of refocusing and structuring care around patients' needs are:

- **The Seven Promises**, produced in the USA by Joanne Lynn, President of ABCD (Americans for Better Care of the Dying) and co-director of the Institute of Healthcare Improvements Breakthrough Series[13]
- **Summary of suggested needs-based care**, which was the basis of the development of the Gold Standards Framework in the UK (Table 12.2)

Lynn, writing about the current position of end-of-life care in the USA, asks why we feel 'lucky' if things go well in the final stages of life, in an age when we are surrounded by highly complex and sophisticated innovations that we take for granted at any other stage.

Ask any American about the death of a family member or friend and you will usually hear a sad tale of pain, fear, confusion, along with a mismatch of services offered and services needed. Less often, you will hear about a decent close of life, one that included appropriate and respectful health-care, time with family and friends and support from the community. Even so, that good story will have a strange conclusion: 'Weren't we lucky!' How odd! We don't attribute good conclusions from other important events to luck—we know that airplanes land safely and patients wake up after surgery because lots of people do their jobs well, in systems designed to help people do their jobs well. Yet, we accept almost without question that the last few months or years of life—when we are most often chronically ill, dependent and frail—will be miserable. Should our final days be comfortable only with good luck?

How did we come to do so poorly on care at the end-of-life? A fundamental reason is we have simply never been here before. We face problems our grand-parents would envy—the problems that come from growing quite old and dying rather slowly...So what will we need when we have to live with eventually fatal chronic disease? More than anything else we need reliability. We need a care system we can count on. To make excellent care routine we must learn to do routinely what we already know must be done...All it takes is innovation, learning, reorganisation and commitment. People should not expect end-of-life care to be miserable and meaningless...we should get good care for our expense without having to hope for good luck.[14]

13 Lynn, J (2000) *Improving Care for the End of life: a sourcebook for Health Care Managers and Clinicians.*

14 Accelerating Change Today (2000) *Promises to keep: Changing the Way we Provide Care at the End of Life.* Boston, USA: The National Coalition on Health Care and the Institute for Healthcare Improvement

The Seven Promises—a vision of a better system

For patients in the advanced stages of serious illnesses, it is impossible to promise cure or restoration of health. However, here are seven promises that really seem to make a difference to such patients. In each case, we define the promise, its core statement and list a few examples of what it might mean to put practices in place to deliver on that promise.

1 Good medical treatment:
   - You will have the best of medical treatment, aiming to prevent exacerbation, improve function and survival, and ensure comfort
   - Patients will be offered proven diagnosis and treatment strategies to prevent exacerbations and enhance quality of life, as well as to delay disease progression and death
   - Medical intervention will be in accord with best available standards of medical practice and evidence-based when possible

2 Will never be overwhelmed by symptoms:
   - You will never have to endure overwhelming pain, shortness of breath or other symptoms
   - Symptoms will be anticipated and prevented when possible, evaluated and addressed promptly and controlled effectively
   - Severe symptoms, such as shortness of breath, will be treated as emergencies
   - Sedation will be used when necessary to relieve intractable symptoms near the end-of-life

3 Continuity, coordination and comprehensiveness:
   - Your care will be continuous, comprehensive and coordinated
   - Patients and families can count on having certain professionals to rely upon at all times and reassured that professionals talk to each other
   - Patients and families can count on an appropriate and timely response to their needs
   - Transitions between services, settings and personnel will be minimized in number and made to work smoothly

4 Well-prepared—no surprises/crisis:
   - You and your family will be prepared for everything that is likely to happen in the course of your illness
   - Patients and families come to know what to expect as the illness worsens, and what is expected of them
   - Patients and families receive supplies and training needed to handle predictable events

5 Customized care, reflecting your preference:
   - Your wishes will be sought and respected, and followed wherever possible
   - Patients and families come to know the alternatives for services and expect to make choices that matter
   - Patients never receive treatments they refuse
   - Patients who want to live out the end of their life at home, usually can

6 Use of patient and family resources—financial, emotional and practical:
   - We will help you and your family to consider your personal and financial resources, and we will respect your choices about the use of your resources

- Patients and families will be aware of services available in their community and the costs of those services
- Family caregivers' concerns will be discussed and addressed
- Respite, volunteer and home aid care will be part of the care plan when appropriate
7 Make the best of every day:
  - We will do all we can to see that you and your family will have the opportunity to make the best of every day
  - The patient is treated as a person, not a disease, and what is important to the patient is important to the care team
  - The care team responds to the physical, psychological, social and spiritual needs of the patient and family. Families are supported before, during and after the patient's death

Barriers to community palliative care

The care of all dying patients must improve to the level of the best.
DoH, The NHS Cancer Plan, September 2000

Palliative care is a barometer for all our other care...and we only have one chance to get it right.
A district nurse, Liverpool

Several studies confirm that GPs, district nurses and other community professionals prioritize the care of the dying. Yet, despite this high priority, service provision can be less than optimal. This may be due to lack of pre-planning and communication, poor team working, out-of-hours factors, limited carer support or difficulties with symptom control. However, commonly, the major problem is that the different instruments in the orchestra are not playing together.

> The challenge is to orchestrate the service so that the patient and carers feel enveloped in professional, seamless, supportive care allowing them 'a good death' in the place of their choice.

Current gaps in community palliative care provision include (key factors in bold):
- Clinical competence:
  - assessment of symptoms and diagnostic skills
  - **symptom control** and drug usage. Ability to predict evolution of symptoms depending on diagnosis
  - when to refer or seek help
- Organizational:
  - communication and information transfer
  - access to other support—social care and **carer support**
  - continuity, including **out-of-hours**
  - primary care issues—workforce, time and workload
  - **teamwork** and co-working with specialists. Clarification of specialists' role, and cross-boundary working
- Human dimension:
  - individual's **control**, autonomy and choice
  - **supportive care**
  - listening to deeper underlying needs and spiritual reflections

Specific issues
- **Role of the primary healthcare teams**. Primary care teams play a pivotal role in the delivery and coordination of care. The use of a framework to increase consistency of standards and formalize good practice ensures fewer patients 'slip through the net'. Community or district nurses play a crucial role in needs' assessment, the development of a therapeutic relationship and are well placed to liaise across the boundaries of care between community and inpatient services

- **The main barriers to effective community palliative care** however, are the lack of an organized system or plan of care
- **Out-of-hours palliative care and 24h district nurses**. The out-of-hours gap in provision can cause significant breakdown in home care and inappropriate crisis admissions to hospitals. Anticipatory planning, along with better access to information (e.g. via a handover form), drugs left in the home or carried by the on-call provider (as in palliative care bags held by out of hours providers) and better access to support at home and specialist advice, can prevent many crises. Lack of out-of-hours district nursing is an important issue and is a first step to improving community palliative care. More terminally ill patients are kept at home where 24h district nursing is available
- **The social care of patients and carers at home** is seen consistently as one of the key factors that will prevent institutionalized care, as confirmed in the literature and the experience of professionals. So the availability and coordination of night sitters, Marie Curie nurses, social services input, rapid response teams, etc. play a vital role in maintaining home care. This is sometimes overlooked in strategic planning of services. Well functioning cooperation between healthcare and social services is crucial, with continuing care funds or their equivalent, carer assessments, non-medical support, respite care, carer support groups, grants and financial advice being of vital importance
- **Preferred place of care.** Care customized to patient need is another crucial factor, and one vital element of this is choice over where a person wishes to be in their final days. Most people would choose to remain at home to die, but this is less likely to occur with some groups of patients, particularly the poor, the elderly, women, etc. *Asking and recording the patient's preferred place of death/care has been shown to make this more likely to be fulfilled. This requires time, good communication skills and a trusting relationship with the patient and carers.* Good use should be made of: assessment tools, discussions with the patient and family of their management plans (Advance Care Planning), Advance Directives, discussion of 'do not resuscitate' (DNR) decisions (and informing ambulance staff) and 'route-maps' of likely options. These all help to involve patients and families in decisions, enabling some retention of control and self-determination. In addition, better planning and communication may also prevent some disasters, e.g. emergency calls, failed attempted resuscitations in the ambulance or inappropriate coroners' cases (📕 see chapter 19a and b)
- **Specialist palliative care and effective symptom control**. There is a need for specialists to work effectively with generalists and there are many good examples of this working well in the UK. Clear referral criteria and regular formalized contact at primary care team meetings, plus the availability of telephone advice, can enable more effective working relationships. Symptom control in the community can be difficult, so supportive relationships with specialists helps, along with targeted education programmes, better assessment tools, and agreed guidelines
- **Communication and transfer of information.** Poor organization in this area can create an unbridgeable chasm for all involved, reducing

patients' confidence in their professional carers and adding stress to staff. Several factors have been shown to improve information transfer:
- using practice registers
- handover forms for out-of-hours providers
- patient-held records or medication cards, electronic transfer of information
- ensuring patients and carers have written information at home to consult when problems arise
- home packs (potentially needed medication and equipment)

- **Non-cancer patients.** There is less access to specialist palliative care for patients with non-malignant disease than for cancer patients. GPs will have more patients dying from organ failure, e.g. heart failure or COPD, than cancer, yet the disease trajectory is less predictable and the end-stages harder to recognize. Crisis hospital admissions are more frequent,
  but there is less specialist involvement or access to supportive cancer-related services such as Marie Curie or Macmillan nurses. Those dying from chronic 'multiple pathology' illnesses causing general decline or dementia may be disadvantaged further. The learning gained from cancer patients may be transferred to the care of other patients with end-stage illnesses (as in the Gold Standards Framework (🔲 see Table 12.2)), and it is well recognized that patients with other end-stage illnesses should be able to benefit from palliative care symptom control, advice and services.

- **Other care settings.** Some patients dying in other settings may be significantly disadvantaged, as they currently do not fully benefit from specialist palliative care services or even from generalists within the primary care teams. Provision for good palliative care in other settings therefore needs to be included in the area-wide strategic plan, e.g. in care homes, community and private hospitals, and prisons

Improving community palliative care—the Gold Standards Framework (📖 see also Table 12.2)

Increasingly within primary care there are agreed protocols of care, just as in the management of patients with other conditions such as diabetes or hypertension. Often, however, there are no such systems for the effective organization of care for the most seriously ill patients nearing their end of life. Not every patient has diabetes or hypertension, yet every one of our patients eventually dies. There is a need to formalize a model of good care to ensure that every dying patient receives top quality care. Hospices and palliative care specialists have largely led the way in this, but this needs also to be mainstreamed into generalist care, to encompass all dying patients. In primary care, use of a framework, such as the Gold Standards Framework in community palliative care, can bridge this gap; it can also enable local ownership and release the creativity of staff to respond to the needs of patients relevant to their area of care.

> GSF is the bedrock of community palliative care. In our team, we didn't have a system of care before for dying patients so sometimes patients would slip through the net—now we do, and we all feel better for it, patients and their families, as well as doctors and nurses.

Developing a system-best care for every patient every time

It is said that care should be:
- Knowledge-based—best science, best practice, best evidence
- Systems minded—*cooperation across boundaries, working at systems delivery*
- Patient centred—*put patients in control of their care, ACTIVELY customize care to patients' needs*[15, 16]

In other words:
- **Clinical competence**—*knowledge-based*, e.g. assessment and diagnostic skills, knowledge of what to do, which treatments to use, when to refer, symptom control, etc., the *'what to do'—the head*.
  Response: Education and training, audit, etc.
- **Good organization**—*systems-minded* protocols/processes /systems, e.g. communication and information transfer, accessing other support, coordination and continuity, out-of-hours provision, workload issues and managed systems of care—the *'how to do it'—the hands*
  Response: improve the system—e.g. Gold Standards Framework

15 Berwick D. (2002) A users manual for the IOM's Quality Chasm Report. *Health Affairs*, **21**(30): 80.

16 Berwick D., Nolan T. (1998) Understanding medical systems. *Annals of Internal Medicine*, **128**: 293–8.

- **Affirmation of the human dimension of care**—this includes the commitment to improve the patient's experience of care, compassion, preserving patient dignity, patient and carer autonomy/choice, 'loving medicine'—the *'why' we do it*—the heart
  Response: e.g. patient/carer involvement, needs focused, preference of place of care, etc.

We know what we'd like to do—but it doesn't always seem to happen.

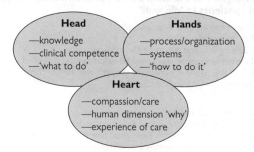

Fig. 12.1 The head, hands and heart of palliative care.

We need all three elements—focusing purely on education will miss the importance of developing practical systems or protocols that will lead to continuous quality improvements.

It is most often the systems organization or 'hands' that let us down.

The Gold Standards Framework (GSF)[17]
The aim of the Gold Standards Framework is to develop a practice-based system to improve and optimize the organization and quality of supportive/palliative care for patients in their last 6–12 months of life.

GSF is recommended as an example of a generalist community framework in the Improving Supportive and Palliative Care for Adults with Cancer guidance[18] and is currently being used extensively across the UK to improve the delivery of primary palliative care.

17 Thomas K. (2003) *Caring for the Dying at Home: Companions on the Journey.* Oxford: Radcliffe Medical Press. (Or contact gsf@macmillan.org.uk)

18 NICE (2004) *Improving Supportive and Palliative Care for Adults with Cancer.* London: NICE.

There are three central processes of the GSF, all of which involve improved communication.
- **Identify** the key group of patients, i.e. using a register
- **Assess** their main needs, both physical and psychosocial, and that of the carers
- **Plan** ahead for problems, including out-of-hours—move from *reactive* to *proactive* care by anticipation and prevention

> **The five goals of the Gold Standards Framework are to enable patients to 'die well'**
>
> - **G1** Symptom-free as far as possible
> - **G2** In their preferred place of choice
> - **G3** Feeling safe and supported with fewer crises
> - **G4** Carers feeling supported, involved, empowered and satisfied with care
> - **G5** Staff feeling more confident, satisfied, with better communication and teamworking with specialists

Essentially, the GSF is a simple, common-sense approach to formalizing best practice, so that good care becomes standard for *all* patients *every* time. GSF users find it affirms their good practice, regularizes quality palliative care activities and improves consistency of care.

> We are doing much of it 'piecemeal' already, but it formalizes and coordinates what we do, so under pressure it's more likely to happen.
>
> A GP, Halifax

> The GSF is the one thing in palliative care over recent years that has really made a difference.
>
> A district nurse, Glasgow

> It is in the attention to such details, in the context of an overall management plan, that transforms the quality of palliative care provision in the community.

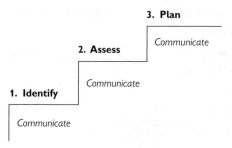

Fig. 12.2 The three central processes of the Gold Standards Framework.

Key elements of the Gold Standards Framework[19]

The seven 'gold standards' of community palliative care—The Seven Cs

- **C1** Communication
- **C2** Coordination
- **C3** Control of symptoms
- **C4** Continuity, including out-of-hours
- **C5** Continued learning
- **C6** Carer support
- **C7** Care in the dying phase

The seven C's

C1: Communication

Practices maintain a supportive care register (paper or electronic) to record, plan and monitor patient care, and act as a focus for regular monthly PHCT meetings. The aims of these meetings are:
- To improve the flow of information
- Advanced care planning/proactive care
- Measurement and audit, to clarify areas for future improvement at patient, practice, PCT and network level

C2: Coordination

Each PHCT has a nominated coordinator for palliative care (e.g. a district nurse) to ensure good organization and coordination of care in a practice by overseeing the process, i.e.:
- Maintaining the register of problems/concerns, summary care plans, symptom sheets, handover forms, audit data, etc.
- Organizing PHCT meetings for discussion, planning, case analysis, education, etc.
- Using tools such as a checklist of potential symptoms that need to be assessed

Coordinators meet regularly together with the local facilitator to share experience and discuss ways to overcome local barriers to good care.

C3: Control of symptoms

Each patient has their symptoms, problems and concerns (physical, psychological, social, practical and spiritual) assessed, recorded, discussed and acted upon, according to an agreed process. The focus is on actively assessing and responding to the patient's agenda.

---

19 Thomas K. (2003) *Caring for the Dying at Home: Companions on the Journey.* Oxford: Radcliffe Medical Press.

C4: Continuity

Transfer of information to the out-of-hours service for palliative care patients, for example, using a handover form, ensuring appropriate drugs are available in the home and use of an out-of-hours protocol.

This builds in anticipatory care to reduce crises and inappropriate admissions. Information should also be passed on to the other relevant services, such as hospice/oncology departments. Record and minimize the number of professionals involved, i.e. note lead GP, lead district nurse, etc.

C5: Continued learning

The PHCT will be committed to the continued learning of skills and information relevant to patients seen: 'learn as you go'.

- Practice-based or external teaching, lectures/videos
- Use of Significant Event Analysis (SEA)
- Practice and personal development plans
- Audits/appraisal
- A practice reference resource
- Learning involves clinical, organizational/strategic and attitude domains
- Involvement and co-working of specialists is crucial
- Protected time for a review meeting, e.g. after six months, allows audit, assessment of current practice, planning for improvement and development of a practice protocol

C6: Carer support

Carers are supported, listened to, kept fully informed, encouraged and educated to play as full a role in the patient's care as they wish. They are regarded as an integral part of the team.

- Practical support:
  - practical hands-on support is supplied where possible, e.g. night sitter, respite, commode
- Bereavement:
  - practices plan support, target 'high risk bereavement', organize visits, tag notes, keep others informed, etc.
- Staff support:
  - inbuilt, leading to better teamwork and job satisfaction
  - a shift to no-blame culture (e.g. SEA) enables 'systems thinking' and improving care
  - debriefing sessions for complex situations

C7: Care of the dying (see Table 12.3)

Patients who are in their last days of life (terminal phase) are cared for appropriately, for example by following the Liverpool Integrated Care Pathway. (See Chapter 13.)

This includes:

- Stopping non-essential interventions and drugs
- Considering comfort measures
- Psychological and religious/spiritual support
- Bereavement planning
- Communication and care after death being assessed, recorded and acted upon

Table 12.3 Minimum protocol for the dying—C7 of GSF

1	Diagnosis of dying—awareness of signs of the terminal phase
2	Current medication assessed, non-essentials discontinued, essential treatment converted to subcutaneous route via syringe driver
3	As-required drugs written up as per protocol, including pain, agitation, respiratory secretions and nausea and vomiting
4	Ensure the carers know the patient is dying
5	Spiritual, religious needs assessed and met regarding patient and carers
6	There is an agreed plan of ongoing assessment and care, including symptom control (pain, agitation, respiratory tract secretions, mouth care, pressure areas, psychosocial support)
7	Relatives are aware of what to do when the patient dies at home
8	Communication with others—handover form for out-of-hours providers updated, secondary/specialist services informed and hospital appointments cancelled after a death, etc.

Adapted from the Liverpool Care Pathway[20]. (See also Chapter 13)

Once the above minimum protocol is established, consider developing this further as an area/PCT, by adopting an integrated care pathway for the dying (e.g. the Liverpool Care Pathway, used in the last few days of life) to ensure standardizing and benchmarking best care. Contact lcp@marie-curie.org.uk, or see Ellershaw and Wilkinson.[19]

Doing both?

Suggested plan for the introduction of the GSF and Liverpool Care Pathway (LCP)
- In the community—GSF first then add LCP
- In care homes—LCP then add GSF
- In hospitals and hospices—LCP then link with GSF practices

The Gold Standards Framework has transformed our practice's approach to the care of the dying. The whole team no longer perceives palliative care as all doom and gloom and is more confident that we can make a positive contribution. The teamworking, care coordination and anticipation of problems mean that our patients experience fewer crises and have a much better outcome. We are so pleased that we have decided to start applying the principles of the Gold Standards Framework to all of our cancer patients from the point of referral onwards.

A GP, Runcorn, GSF Phase 2

20 Ellershaw J., Wilkinson S. (2003) *Care of the Dying: A Pathway to Excellence.* Oxford: Oxford University Press.

How to do it

Gold Standards Framework—how to implement it in your primary healthcare team

- **Identify** palliative care patients within the practice population who are approaching the end of their lives—using a register to centralize information. Discuss these patients as a team regularly—encouraging better proactive planning, communication. Give someone in the practice the task of coordinating the care, e.g. handover form sent, drugs left in home, patient's choice of place of death noted, etc. (C1 and C2)
- Use tools to **assess** patient and carer choices, needs, symptoms and problems and **respond or refer**, as appropriate (C3):
  - reflect on your practice, linking in learning with palliative care specialists, e.g. local hospice community nurse
  - audit your care to target changes and commission better local resources
  - link with practice clinical governance and set your own standards
  - measure improvement and celebrate teamwork and success (C5)
- **Proactive planning** and **improved communication**:
  - send the handover form to the out-of-hours' team and leave the appropriate drugs and equipment in the home (C4)
  - link with social services. Consider carers' needs and provide information and contact details, especially for a crisis (C6)
  - build in bereavement care and be aware of other local services for the bereaved
  - plan for good care in the last days of life (C7 checklist)
  - review and reflect on achievements and learning after six months
  - agree a practice protocol for all dying patients, so that the best of care becomes normal practice—'this is what we do for our palliative care patients'

Gold Standards Framework—a 6–12 month plan of how to implement it in an area (such as a UK Primary Care Trust)

For more details and resources see the websites—www.gsf.org.uk and www.macmillan.org.uk

- Each area funds a **GSF facilitator**, e.g. one day a week with administrative back-up
- Facilitator **introduces GSF** to a few interested practices, e.g. 4–10 at a time
- Each practice team agrees to use GSF for at least 6–12 months, nominates a practice **GSF coordinator** (DN or manager) (C2) backed up by a supportive GP and DN, and undertakes a baseline questionnaire
- GSF facilitator **links** with a larger group, e.g. Cancer Network, Macmillan, project team, etc. and receives training in GSF and ongoing support plus resources, to be distributed to each practice team via a coordinator

- GSF facilitator organizes regular **GP pratice coordinators' meetings** (e.g. monthly) to teach GSF principles, share experiences, audit, develop local commissioning, develop new ideas, etc. This group is an important backbone of the work as it nurtures relevant local ownership and momentum, commissions local changes and also develops sustainability. It raises awareness of palliative/supportive care and builds better relationships between teams and with specialists. Specific teaching can be tailored to learning needs
- Practice coordinator sets up supportive care **registers** using the suggested templates provided (amended if needed) (C1). Criteria for inclusion outlined in Prognostic Indicator Guidance in GSF. 📖 see p. 871
- This can be prioritized into those with most need, moderate need and future need, e.g. colour-coded, star-rated, 'poorlies and pending', etc.:
  - pre-printed forms for identification, planning and handover are available
- Practice coordinator **organizes** a regular primary healthcare team meeting to discuss relevant patients on the register, patient and carer needs, management plan, preferences for place of care and patients anticipated requirements—this builds in better communication and proactive care. Palliative care specialists can be invited and teaching integrated
- Practice coordinator develops a **system of tasks,** i.e. sends and ensures delivery of information/handover form to the out-of-hours provider (C4), agrees assessment tools in line with local arrangements (C3), provides information to carers, e.g. home pack (C6), uses a minimal protocol for the last days of life or a care pathway (C7), etc.
- Practice coordinator plans a team **review meeting**, e.g. six monthly, to review and audit care, reflect on positive and negative issues (e.g. use of significant event analysis), to develop and refine an agreed practice protocol which then embeds changes into mainstream care.
- **Extend** application of GSF to patients with other end-stage illnesses, to other settings (e.g. in care homes or community hospitals) and to supportive care at an earlier stage (e.g. from diagnosis). Improve carer support and patient information and empowerment. Introduce, e.g. Liverpool Care Pathway for the Dying if agreed locally, and continually improve generalist palliative care in the community with education and strategic planning of services

The results in practice

One of the big shifts in practice using such a framework is the move from reactive to proactive care. Here are two examples of typical patient journeys, as described by two district nurses, Rosie Norbury and Anne Fearnley of West Yorkshire. NB The first may not be considered to be a 'bad death' by many, but one that may be suboptimal but not untypical, especially after team reflection or discussion with the carer.

Reactive patient journey before GSF

Mr B. in the last months of his life

GPs and district nurse *ad hoc* visiting arrangements—no agreed care plan and no preferred place of death discussed or communicated among the team

Problems with symptom control—high anxiety—carer uninformed

Crisis call out-of-hours, e.g. no information, plan or drugs available

Admitted to hospital (inappropriate use of an 'acute' bed)

Dies in hospital—(over-intervention/medicalization of natural process)

Carer given minimal support in grief

No reflection or improvements by primary care team

Proactive patient journey using GSF

Mrs W. in the last months of her life

On Supportive Care Register—needs and care plan discussed at team meeting

Social benefits administration such as the UK DS1500 form and information given to patient + carer (e.g. home pack)

Regular support, visits, phone calls—anticipatory not reactive visits

Assessment of symptoms—referral to specialist palliative care services—customized care to patient and carer needs

Carer assessed, including psychosocial needs—information given for crises

Preferred place of care noted and provision organized

Handover form sent to out-of-hours service—drugs issued for home

Minimal protocol for terminal care/Liverpool Care Pathway used

Patient dies in preferred place—bereavement support

Staff reflect—significant event analysis, audit gaps, learn, improve care

Twenty measurable outcomes in GSF Seven Cs goal
(see pp. 862)

 1 Identification of palliative care patient using a register* C1 G2
 2 Team meeting to discuss advanced care planning* C1 G2
 3 Co-working with specialists C1 G1, G3
 4 Team coordinator named—cross-boundary communication C2 G2
 5 Management plans including advanced care planning noted C2 G2
 6 Preference for place of care/death noted* C2 G2
 7 Preferred place of death attained* C2 G2
 8 Staff teamwork satisfaction and confidence* C5 G5
 9 Symptom control better—assessment tools used C3 G1
10 Confidence in assessment of symptoms and management* C3 G1
11 Out-of-hours information/handover form sent* C4 G3
12 Required drugs left in home* C4 G3
13 Crises reduced, e.g. fewer acute admissions in last days* C4 G3
14 Review meeting (e.g. six monthly), audit and reflection C5 G5
15 Targeted learning, use of SEA and protocol developed C5 G5
16 Information given specifically to carer* C6 G4
17 Carer separately assessed and supported* C6 G4
18 Staff support, communication and teamwork improved* C6 G5
19 Use of protocol for last days of life* C7 G1
20 Application to non-cancer patients, other settings, etc.
   * = most important

Four levels of GSF Adoption

It is easiest to take GSF in stages, or four gears, but once the basics are
established at Level 1, to move on beyond this to include all areas for
maximum effect. The first stage may take about 2-3 months to establish
but all can be achieved within 6-12 months. A few teams remain at Level 1,
with just a register and meeting, but most benefit is gained when teams
develop and integrate GSF more deeply into level 2, 3 and 4

Level 1 - First Gear

Set up Register, Meeting and Coordinator

Level 2 - Second Gear

Assessment Tools, out of Hours Handover, Education, Audit and
Reflective Practice

Level 3 - Third Gear

Carer/ family support, bereavement plan and care in the final days

Level 4 - Fourth Gear (sustain embed extent)

Sustain and build on all developments as standard practice
Embed - develop a practice protocol
Extend - to other settings e.g. care homes, non Cancer, Advanced Care
Planning, pathway for the last days (LCP) and other areas

Prognostic Indicator Guidance - three triggers suggesting inclusion on the supportive/palliative care registers

1 **Surprise question** - would you be surprised if the patient was to die within 1 year
2 **Patient preference** for comfort care/need
3 **Clinical indicators** for each specific disease eg co-morbidity, metastatic cancer, NY Stage, FEV1, functioning score, etc*

Benefits of GSF

1 **Attitude awareness and approach**
   - **Better quality** of care perceived
   - Greater confidence and job satisfaction
   - Immeasurable benefits-communication, teamwork, roles respected especially that of nurses
   - Focus and proactive approach
2 **Patterns of working, structure/processes**
   - **Better organisation + consistency** of standard, even under stress
   - Fewer slipping through the net-raising the baseline
   - Better communication within and between teams, co-working with specialists
   - Better recording, tracking of patients and organisation of care
3 **Patient outcomes**
   - **Reduced crises/hospital admissions**/length of stay
   - More patients dying in preferred place
   - More recorded advanced care planning discussions

*www.goldstandardsframework.nhs.uk

Specific issues in community palliative care

Out-of-hours palliative care

> It was awful, I—just panicked! My husband was in agony. It was three o'clock in the morning. We were at home all alone. It was dark and frightening and we didn't know what to do or who to turn to. Things all came together to make his pain seem much worse than it really was.

Reducing the burden of symptoms suffered by patients and their carers at home remains a challenging round-the-clock priority. For this to be addressed we need to plan for out-of-hours palliative care services in the community, dovetailing generalist palliative care from GPs, district nurses and their out-of-hours providers with the available specialist palliative care skills and resources.[21] Several protocols have been developed[22]—one such four-point plan has been shown to improve care as judged by practitioners' experience.[23]

21 Thomas K. (2000) Out-of-hours palliative care—bridging the gap. *European Journal of Palliative Care*, **7**: 22–5.

22 Munday D. (2002) Out-of-hours and emergency palliative care. In *Primary Palliative Care* (ed. R. Charlton), pp. 97–111. Oxford: Radcliffe Medical Press.

23 King N., Bell D., Thomas K. (2003) An out-of-hours protocol for community palliative care. *International Journal of Palliative Nursing*, **9**(7): 277–82.

Suggestions to improve out-of-hours palliative care in the UK

- Develop a local protocol—coordinate a meeting of all out-of-hours health professionals involved in the care of the seriously or terminally ill. This would include the GP cooperative, the deputizing service, PCT or health authority, district nurses and specialist doctors. Improve anticipatory care and proactive planning by the PHCT
- Look at communication and the efficient transfer of information between those working in-hours and out-of-hours. Use a paper or electronic handover form which is kept by the patient/the district nurse and out-of-hours service. Make sure the patient and the carer know what to do in an emergency
- Ensure 24h carer support, including 24h access to nursing care. Night sitters and respite care should also be easily available, thereby preventing a breakdown in the carer system, which is key to avoiding inappropriate crisis admissions
- Make best use of the specialist advice out-of-hours and expertise available through the local hospice/SPC service.
- Keep in the patient's home an adequate supply of drugs (including a range for increases in doses) and p.r.n. drugs for predictable symptoms, e.g. hyoscine, midazolam, diamorphine and cyclizine or haloperidol. Coordinate equipment access. On-call cars or out-of-hours centres could hold special palliative care bags.

See the five recommendations of the Macmillan Out of hours Palliative Care report at: www.macmillan.org.uk or info@goldstandardsframework.nhs.uk

Improving access to palliative care drugs

- Suggested list of drugs to be left in the home of every palliative care patient: morphine, cyclizine, midazolam, hyoscine butylbromide
- Suggested drug list in palliative care bags carried by out-of-hours provider to be locally agreed:
  - midazolam, haloperidol, cyclizine, hyoscine butylbromide, levomepromazine, rectal diazepam, dexamethasone, metoclopramide, glycopyrronium, diclofenac controlled drugs used with special CD measures—morphine, oral morphine solution

Summary of four point plan for out-of-hours palliative care

From Calderdale and Kirklees Health Authority West Yorkshire

1 Communication:
   • use handover form—GP/DN to write and fax to on-call service, keep in DN notes
   • inform others e.g. hospice
   • does the carer know what to do in a crisis?
2 Carer support:
   • coordinate pre-emptive care e.g. nightsitters, 24h district
   • nursing service
   • give written information to carers
   • emergency support e.g. Rapid Response Team
3 Medical support:
   • anticipated management in handover form
   • crisis pack, guidelines etc and ongoing teaching
   • 24h specialist advice available from hospice
4 Drugs/equipment:
   • leave anticipated drugs in home
   • Special palliative care bag with drugs and information available on-call
   • on-call stocked pharmacists

Communication—handover form

The handover form has two important functions:
• To improve information transfer
• To build in anticipatory care

The process of completing such a form is part of the benefit—if you think that a patient might become agitated or develop a 'rattly chest' over a weekend, leave some midazolam or hyoscine in the home for administration either by the on-call doctor or district nurse. If the on-call doctor presented with the handover form notes that the patient has stated a preference to remain at home, there is more chance that they will be enabled to do so. Many of the handover forms are developed electronically and are being used by central coordinating agencies, e.g. NHS Direct. Once discussed with the family (as well as the patient, if possible), some have added 'not for CPR' or 'Do Not Resuscitate' statements, to inform emergency staff and prevent the tragic indignity of inappropriate resuscitation. Confirming written details with the carers of what to do in an emergency and informing other agencies such as hospice staff is also important.

Carer support

Round-the-clock access to nursing care is a basic prerequisite for good palliative care in the community. Some areas have 'Rapid Response Teams', a crisis-only service for patients who would otherwise be admitted to hospital. There are examples of good coordination of care with a centralized number for all services (NHS Direct may increasingly be involved in this in England).

Medical support

Handover forms inform the visiting on-call doctor of the GP's care plan and the patient's current medication. When faced with a difficult medical symptom, crisis symptom sheets (often kept in the palliative care bags in the on-call cars) or local guidelines are invaluable, backed by teaching. Most specialist palliative care services provide some on-call advice.

Drugs and equipment

For drug access, there are three suggestions:
- Leaving anticipated drugs in the home, prompted by the handover form
- Keeping a stock of drugs with the out-of-hours service
- Stocking the on-call pharmacist with an approved list of drugs

Carer support

It is worth reminding ourselves that the principal providers of care are actually the relatives. We are still not doing nearly enough to empower, strengthen, educate and support carers and to use imaginative means to help and support them through this difficult time.[24]

> When my wife, Joy, was diagnosed with cancer of the liver, our excellent GP said three things: first, we can do a great deal to control pain these days; second, we must see that the quality of life will be as good as it can be; third, we must see that she dies at home. With the help of our Macmillan nurse all these points were met. At every stage of the next 14 months our GP, district nurse and Macmillan nurse were on hand to suggest, reassure and predict, helping not only Joy but me and our children. Their assistance in dark days was priceless.
>
> M. C., widower and carer

If the needs of carers cannot be addressed, an almost inevitable result will be the breakdown of home care, with the majority of patients dying in institutions.

Carer support is one of the most important aspects of the care provided by primary healthcare teams. The experience of most healthcare professionals, reflected clearly in the literature, is that carer breakdown is often **the** key factor in prompting institutionalized care for dying patients. Some suggest that the impact of cancer (or other serious illness) on the carer can be even greater than that on the patient. Certainly, there is resounding evidence that without the support from family and friends it would be impossible for many patients to remain at home. Those without carers are less likely to be able to remain at home to die—they present particular difficulties for primary care.

Carers' anxiety is rated alongside patients' symptoms as the most severe problems by both patients and families.[25]

24 Doyle D. (1998) The way forward. In National Council for Hospice and Specialist Palliative Care Services: Promoting Partnership: Planning and Managing Community Palliative Care, pp. 44–50. London: NCHSPCS.

25 Ramirez A., Addington-Hall J., Richards M. (1998) ABC of palliative care; the carers. British Medical Journal, **316**: 208–11.

> The reason my husband had to go into a nursing home in the end was quite simply that I couldn't lift him to the commode. It all came to a head after a fall and I felt I couldn't cope on my own any more. We were both heartbroken.
>
> Elderly carer of a cancer patient

For the carer, despite their natural feelings of trepidation beforehand, there can be a great sense of consolation in bereavement if they have been able to fulfil the patient's wishes to remain at home during their final days. However, this places a great strain on carers, both emotionally and physically.

The NHS Executive White Paper *Caring about Carers: A National Strategy for Carers*[26] describes the difficulties that carers face, and emphasizes that carers should be treated as partners in the team but with specific and sometimes unmet needs of their own.

> We intend to make progress so that more carers—and eventually all carers feel adequately prepared and equipped to care if that is what they choose to do, feel cared for themselves, and feel their needs are understood.

---

26 Department of Health (1999) *Caring about Carers.* London: DoH.

A primary care team response to carer needs[27,28]

- Acknowledge carers, what they do and the problems they have
- Flag the notes of informal carers so that in any consultation you are aware of their circumstances
- Treat carers as you would other team members and listen to their opinions
- Include them in discussions about the person they care for
- Give carers a choice about which tasks they are prepared to take upon themselves
- Ask after the health and welfare of the carer as well as the patient
- Provide information about the condition the person the carer is looking after suffers from
- Provide information about being a carer and support available
- Provide information about benefits available
- Provide information about local services available for both the person being cared for and the carer
- Be an advocate for the carer to ensure services and equipment appropriate to the circumstances are provided
- Liaise with other services
- Ensure staff are informed about the needs and problems of informal carers
- Respond quickly and sympathetically to crisis situations
- Provide training, e.g. in lifting, giving medication, etc.
- Allow carer time to confide in and be listened to, express their needs and feel supported, often outside the home
- Discuss coping strategies, both internal (faith, positive attitude, etc.) and external (social networks)
- Develop a bereavement protocol and raise awareness of bereaved patients in practice teams. Assemble a list of local contacts for bereavement support

I was terrified at first when they said they would discharge him home—I didn't think I could cope. But in looking after Peter dying at home, I felt I was fulfilling his wishes and we were a real family—this really helps me now. Our GPs and district nurses were really caring and professional and kept pace with us at every stage—we felt very grateful to them. Although it was so sad, it was also in some ways a very good and satisfying experience, etched forever on our minds. The children and I are glad that we were able to look after him at home, where he wanted to be, with the help of our marvellous team.

Maureen, wife of Peter, a cancer patient

27 Piercy J. (2002) The plight of the informal carer. In *Primary Palliative Care* (ed. R. Charlton), pp. 143–153. Oxford: Radcliffe Medical Press.

28 Simon C. (2001) Informal carers and the primary care team. *British Journal of General Practice*, **51**: 920–3.

The vast majority of care in the last year of life is not provided by professionals, but by relatives and friends of the patient, especially wives and daughters. The support provided by a family caregiver may make all the difference to the dying person in their place of death: some have reported that up to 90% of terminal admissions to hospice are due to the stress of caring on the relatives, or a lack of resources available to support the patient at home. The relationship between carers and professionals is often an ambiguous one. For over half of the carers, the only supportive service they are in touch with is their GP.[29]

Bereavement (📖 see Chapter 17)

The loss of a loved person is one of the most intensely painful experiences any human being can suffer, not only is it painful to experience, but it is also painful to witness.[30]

There is a significant increase in morbidity and mortality in grief, making dying of a broken heart a reality for some. The main causes of bereavement-associated death are heart disease, alcohol-induced cirrhosis, suicide, road accidents or other violent death. Bereavement is the greatest psychological trauma people can go through, and yet in some cases the carers are not given the 'preventive care' that could ameliorate future problems. The immediate bereavement visit straight after a death is much appreciated, but will not in itself constitute the kind of help that heals. Initiating regular support and contact, actively listening, planning even brief follow-up care, tagging notes, awareness of risk factors, etc. as well as referral to specialist groups are all proactive means of caring for carers and preventing the feeling of desertion at this most vulnerable time. Recognizing the sense of loss that staff may feel is also important, and this is where the development of a team approach through shared meetings can be of benefit, especially when there is a sense of guilt regarding less than perfect care. Care of dying patients, though very rewarding, is also an area of care that many professionals find stressful and challenging, so support for staff is essential.

Other providers of community palliative care include

Specialist palliative care services

Clinical nurse specialists, Macmillan and Marie Curie nurses, hospice general staff and home care teams as well as the Hospice at Home initiatives have long been involved in bringing quality palliative care services into patients' homes.

However, this can only be successfully achieved in *partnership* with generalists from the patient's usual primary care team.

---

29 Barclay S. (2001) Palliative care for non-cancer patients: a UK perspective from primary care. In *Palliative Care for Non-cancer Patients* (ed. J. Addington-Hall, I. Higginson), p. 172–188. Oxford: Oxford University Press.

30 Bowlby J. (1969) *Attachment and Loss, Vol. 1*. Harmondsworth: Penguin.

• Specialist palliative care services eg CNS, Macmillan/Marie Curie nurses/ Hospice home care teams	• Allied Health professionals
• Hospice at home as rapid response teams	• GPs with a special interest (GPwSI)
• Community hospitals	• Social Services specialist support;
• 'Key workers' community matrons etc.	
• 'Night sitters' and support for other care assistants	

Developments of GSF

1. **Prognostic Indicator Guidance** - Better identification of patients approaching the end of their lives – guidance on which patients to include on the register
2. **EOLC Strategic planning**- as part of life care supportive care strategy SC Framework
3. **GSF adapted for use in other settings**
   • GSF Care Homes Programme
   • Community Hospitals
   • GSF used in prisons
   • GSF in-reach to hospitals
4. **Advance Care Planning**
   • Use of ACP and DNAR
   • Communication
5. **Education**
   • Resource Packs
   • Links with The Princess Alice Certificate in Essential Palliative Care
6. **Childrens GSF**
7. **OOHs 'Just in Case Boxes'**
8. **Patient Informatiion**
9. **Measures and evaluation**
   After Death Analysis tool – comparative and benchmarking
10. **Needs/Support Matrices** - describing the right support required at key times
11. **Admission avoidance**
12. **Examples of good practice + Resource packs**
    are a new initiative, especially useful in areas short of palliative medicine specialists.

DH End of Life Care Strategy July 2008

http://www.dh.gov.uk/en/Publicationsandstatistics/Publications/Publications
PolicyAndGuidance/DH_086277
EOLC website - http://www.endoflifecareforadults.nhs.uk/eolc/
ADRT website - http://www.mcpcil.org.uk/liverpool_care_pathway
PPC wevsute - http://www.cancerlancashire.org.uk/ppc.html
GSF website to PIB - http://www.goldstandasframework.nhs.uk/gp_contract.
php
GSF website to ACP - http://www.goldstandardsframework.nhs.uk/advanced_
care.php

Working partnerships with palliative care specialists

Good effective partnerships with palliative care specialists will ensure the best care for patients and their families. Involvement of specialists in primary palliative care can be very fruitful, e.g. in local education and training programmes, targeted teaching on individual patient case histories, invitations to team meetings, agreed use of assessment tools and templates, out-of-hours protocols and advice, the strategic planning of services and hospice outreach, etc. With good relationships and lines of communication, and with roles and responsibilities clarified, there can be excellent dovetailing of generalist and specialist skills, for the benefit of all.

Referral to specialist palliative care services

Eligibility criteria for specialist palliative care help clarify what is expected of both generalist and specialist palliative care providers.[31] By attempting to crystallize and improve 'generalist' palliative care, and better integration with the 'specialist' services available then a more comprehensive and equitable service for those in the last stages of life could be provided.

Eligibility criteria for referrals to specialist palliative care services[32]

Eligible patients have:
- Any active progressive and potentially *life-threatening* disease
- *Anticipated or actual unresolved*, complex needs that cannot be met by the caring team, i.e. physical, psychological, social and spiritual needs, for example complicated symptoms, specialist nursing needs, difficult family situations, ethical issues regarding treatment decisions
- Been recently *assessed* by a member of one of the specialist palliative care teams

---

31 Ellershaw J. E., Boyes L.M., Peat S. (1995) Assessing the effectiveness of a hospital palliative care team. *Palliative Medicine*, **9**: 145–52.

32 Bennett M., et al. (2000) Leeds Eligibility Criteria for specialist palliative care services. *Palliative Medicine*, **14**(2): 157–8.

Further reading

Books

Addington-Hall J., Higginson I. (eds) (2001) *Palliative Care for Non-cancer Patients*. Oxford: Oxford University Press.

Charlton R. (ed.) (2003) *Primary Palliative Care*. Oxford: Radcliffe Medical Press.

Cooper J. (ed.) (2000) *Stepping into Palliative Care: a Handbook for Community Professionals*. Oxford: Radcliffe Medical Press.

Doyle D., Jeffrey D. (2000) *Palliative Care in the Home*. Oxford: Oxford University Press.

Ellershaw J., Wilkinson S. (2003) *Care of the Dying: A Pathway to Excellence*. Oxford: Oxford University Press.

Lee E. (2002) *In Your Own Time: A Guide for Patients and their Carers Facing a Last Illness At Home*. Oxford: Oxford University Press.

Lynn J. (2000) *Improving Care for End of Life: A Sourcebook for Health Managers and Clinicians*. New York: Oxford University Press.

Thomas K. (2003) *Caring for the Dying at Home: Companions on the Journey*. Oxford: Radcliffe Medical Press.

Useful websites

www.goldstandardsframework.nhs.uk/gsf

www.ncpc.org.uk

www.macmillan.org.uk

www.palliativedrugs.com

www.palliative-medicine.org

Respite care

Evidence suggests that 90% of terminally ill patients spend the majority of their last year of life at home.[33] It is widely accepted that keeping patients at home weighs heavily on those family members who will provide care and support. Caring for someone on a daily basis can be very tiring, both physically and emotionally, leading some carers to feel unable to manage, which may result in unplanned admissions to hospital.[34] One strategy to help carers in this situation is for hospices to offer planned respite care, either as an in-patient or on a day basis within a day hospice, to enable carers to have a rest from caring. This may be sufficient to enable them to 'recharge their batteries' and continue the care they provide, thus allowing their family member to stay at home.

Respite care can be for as short as a few days or as long as two weeks. The exact length is often negotiated at the time of referral and varies from organization to organization. One of the benefits of having allocated beds is that respite can be booked in advance, so providing carers with the comfort of knowing that a rest is planned and enabling families to book a holiday for the future.

Hospices may need to review their respite provision, with specialist palliative care being offered to patients who have life-limiting illnesses other than cancer. Many patients with non-malignant diseases will have long-term conditions with complex treatment regimes and routines. Carers may have been looking after their family member for many years and developed strategies and routines to manage. It is often difficult and stressful to relinquish this role. Hospices need to consider how to develop strategies to enable a smooth transition for the patient from home to hospice and then to return home which causes least amount of stress to the patient and their carer.

What should be the key factors for respite care?
- To provide a place of care within fixed dates which have been agreed prior to admission
- To continue the patient's normal routine as closely as possible, with changes only being made if clinically indicated.

If respite care is about providing a place of care whilst a carer has a break, the main focus of care should be nursing care that enables the patient to maintain their normal routine and return home after an agreed time. Medical intervention should be kept to a minimum. That is not to say that the patient's condition may not change or deteriorate during their admission, in which case the focus of care would, therefore, need to be reviewed.

---

33 Hinton J. (1994) Which patients with terminal cancer are admitted from home care? *Palliative Medicine*, **8**: 197–210.

34 Skilbeck J., et al. (2005) An exploration of family carers' experience of respite services in one specialist palliative care unit. *Palliative Medicine*, **19**(8): 610–18.

One example of respite care is the nurse-led approach. The respite nurse would carry out a home visit prior to the patient's admission to discuss their care needs during admission, write a care plan that includes the patient's routine and answer any questions. The same nurse would liaise with in-patient staff prior to admission about any specific requirements, e.g. nutritional needs, mattresses, equipment, etc. This respite nurse would then admit the patient to the hospice, review them during the admission and assist in organizing their discharge. Only if there was a clinical need would doctors or allied health professionals become involved.

Palliative care in the community: A perspective from a resource-poor country

The number of people living on less than $US1 per day has exceeded 1.3 billion and is steadily rising. The income of the 500 richest people in the world exceeds that of the poorest 416 million. This, coupled with the increasing commercialization of healthcare, with decreasing public spending on healthcare and the introduction of high-technology interventions means good healthcare is becoming less accessible to people with chronic and incurable diseases living in resource-poor countries. To add further burden to this already difficult situation, 80% of deaths from chronic diseases occur in resource-poor settings.

Of the 56 million people dying annually, 44 million reside in developing countries, and it is estimated that 33 million would benefit from palliative care services (80% only present at a late stage).[1] The cruel reality is that palliative care services are an unattainable luxury for the majority of people in resource-poor countries, with isolated services providing care for few. It is precisely those in greatest need of health care who are least able to afford and obtain it.[35]

Palliative care should be readily accessible and provided in a manner appropriate to the patient's needs and culture. Putting this into practice using an institutionalized model is very difficult. Institutions provide high-quality care for the few, for specified periods. Numerous studies have highlighted the fact that patients consistently wish to be cared for in their own home by their relatives and trained professionals wherever possible.

When this argument is transferred to the global realm of palliative care needs, the idea of an institutional model for delivery of palliative care becomes untenable. Therefore, there is a need for a culturally appropriate system of palliative care, accessible to those who need it and provided in the communities in which they reside, at a cost they can afford.

A 'public health' or 'primary care' approach to palliative care has been discussed for some time as the only realistic option for reaching the millions in need, supported by specialist services. The idea of creating community-based primary healthcare systems involving local people and resources from the locality is not new. In 1979, the WHO issued the Alma Ata Declaration, urging healthcare providers at all levels to provide appropriate and sustainable healthcare with meaningful coverage at the community level. Analysis of this almost 30 years on is a depressing read, but it remains the only realistic option to get good care to many.

The financial implications of end-of-life care can be prohibitive. An exception to this, which has caught the attention of the WHO, is a pioneering initiative in Kerala, south India, called the 'Neighbourhood Network in Palliative Care' (NNPC).

35 Stjernsward J., Clark D. (2004) Palliative medicine and a global perspective. In: *Oxford Textbook of Palliative Medicine* (3rd edn) (ed. D. Doyle et al.) p. 1199.

The 'Neighbourhood Network in Palliative Care' is an initiative started in 2001, in an attempt to provide comprehensive, long-term supportive and palliative care to those in need in northern Kerala. It empowers the community to provide high-quality emotional, psychological, financial and spiritual support, working with professionals who provide the medical and nursing care, thus realizing the concept of 'total care' in its truest sense.

The NNPC programme:

- A public awareness session is conducted, to tell people about palliative care, what it is, why it is important and how they can help
- Those interested and who can spare 2 hours per week take part in a structured training programme, with 16 hours of interactive theory sessions and 4 supervised clinical days, followed by an evaluation
- On completion, the volunteers either join existing clinics, or start a new one in an area of need
- The umbrella organization, NNPC, helps with guidance about how to set up a clinic and also provides doctors and nurses trained in palliative care and initial funding
- The volunteers organize the running of the clinic and fundraising, the majority of clinics becoming financially independent within 6 months
- The initiative does not aim to replace healthcare professionals with volunteers. Instead, it aims to augment the service provided by both doctors and nurses
- With the limited time they have to see the large number of patients, physical symptoms are, understandably, the priority
- Continuity of care and out-of-hours care is difficult as the large number of patients means it is simply not practical for doctors and nurses to see each patient each week
- The type of emotional, psychological and spiritual problems faced by the patients may be new to the healthcare professionals and they may be unable to empathize as fully as someone from the patient's own neighbourhood
- The volunteers receive extensive training in communication skills, counselling and basic psychological interventions, how to handle collusion and other difficult issues and bereavement support. In this way they are actually more qualified than medical or nursing graduates, as these areas, along with palliative care, are largely missing from their undergraduate curricula

Thus the Kerala initiative aims to empower the local community to look after the chronically ill and dying people in their community with the support of trained professionals. The belief underlying the NNPC programme is that chronic illnesses are social problems with medical aspects, rather than the commonly held converse view. In this way, different people in the community must be mobilized to take care of financial, spiritual and emotional problems and to find the means of dealing with them. Trained doctors and nurses support the process.

Quotes from community volunteers:

Many of these people were socially active in the past. They are now bedridden and brooding over their fate. These people can have a lot of problems, they can feel social isolation. Similarly in the spiritual domain, there can be a lot of problems. A doctor can address only a small fraction of these. Most of the others can be addressed by laypeople in the community. They can address social isolation by visiting the patient regularly, listening to him, his worries and fears. When the family do not have food, the patient's main worry will be about the children starving; in June, when the school opens, many parents worry more about the expenses in sending the child to school than about his pain. A doctor cannot do anything about these. A doctor who sees a patient once a week or once a month is incapable of intervening in most of these issues. But a supportive neighbourhood that knows the patient can do a lot in all these areas...It was the realization that the problems of the patient can be addressed only by the community that made us take this work to the community.

This helps the togetherness of the community. People are often not aware of other's problems. Getting them together and linking them to those in difficulty can enhance the attitude in the community to help the needy. Such collectives in a community are positive on their own.

In many, gramasbhas in the area have recently started hearing raised voices about the problems of incurable patients alongside demands for roads and electricity

I believe this can be successfully established in any place once we find a group and pass on the message. It doesn't involve a particular belief system or anything magical. Anyone should be able to find a team like this. Begin with it...initiate and plan to involve everyone in the region, people with a similar attitude will be there in any place, any time.

He said he didn't believe in God but his conviction was that he would participate in this work if it meant the relief of pain in one person. That's it. Those in the movement with religious convictions and those without such faith, means this thing, that with their work they can relieve a brother's discomfort, that is the common factor.

It grew beyond Malappuram to the rest of northern Kerala because there was the attitude to help each other. The potential exists not just here, but everywhere. Such projects can, in all places where people form collectives, address issues.

Hospital liaison palliative care

Introduction

The hospital, probably more than any other healthcare setting, is a challenging environment in which to support the human dimension in patient care. The focus is on investigation, treatment and cure; priorities, such as quality-of-life issues, can get overshadowed. Developments, such as the National Cancer Plan[1] and the recent emphasis on End of Life Care[2] initiatives from the Department of Health, including the widespread introduction of the Liverpool Care Pathway[3] for the dying patient, have helped raise the profile of palliative care and have engaged clinicians but there are still many challenges.

Most hospitals in the UK currently have some form of hospital liaison support, varying from a single nurse to consultant-led multidisciplinary teams. Models exist for in-patient hospital beds where the palliative care specialist provides clinical leadership, but the majority of teams work in an advisory capacity and are known as Hospital Specialist Palliative Care Teams (HSPCTs). Many teams have direct relationships with the local specialist palliative care providers, through joint working contracts.

---

1 Department of Health (2000) The NHS Cancer Plan: a plan for investment, a plan for reform. London: DoH. www.dh.gov.uk/publications

2 www.endoflifecareproducts.nhs.uk/eolc.

3 www.mcpciL.org.uk/liverpool_care_pathway.

The need for a hospital palliative care liaison service

- Up to 90% of patients receive some form of hospital care in their last year of life.[4] Approximately 22% of hospital bed days are taken up by people in their last year of life[5]
- Some 5–23% of hospital in-patients have been estimated to have palliative care needs at any one time[6]
- The large majority of patients die in hospitals, despite the research clearly showing that the majority of people would want to die at home[7]
- Just under 50% of cancer deaths in the UK occur in hospital, and this percentage is much higher for those with a non-cancer diagnosis. Although some of the factors involved in preventing this need to be addressed within the community, there are also many challenges for hospital services.
- Studies show that the experience of dying in hospitals is often poor: high prevalence of symptoms which are poorly assessed and managed; poor communication and patient involvement in decision-making; poor recognition of dying; lack of privacy; and lack of emotional support[8,9]
- These unmet needs are even greater in those patients with a non-cancer diagnosis,[10] who, until recently, have not had ready access to specialist palliative care (SPC) support. Although this is changing, the large majority of patients under SPC teams still have a cancer diagnosis. Given the high proportion of patients with non-cancer diagnoses dying in acute hospitals, this is a particular challenge for hospital teams
- The ready availability of intensive treatments can skew the balance of patient-centred care and lead to the over-treatment of some patients. Many elderly patients at the end of life prefer a treatment plan focused on comfort[11]

4 Fallon M., Hanks G. (2006) *ABC of Palliative Care* (2nd edn). Oxford: Blackwell Press.

5 Skilbeck J., Small N., Ahmedzai S. (1999) Nurses' perceptions of specialist palliative care in an acute hospital. *International Journal of Palliative Nursing*, **5**(3): 110–15.

6 Gott C., Ahmedzai S., Wood C. (2001). How many in-patients at an acute hospital have palliative care needs? Comparing the perspectives of medical and nursing staff. *Palliative Medicine*, **15**: 451–60.

7 Higginson I., Sen-Gupta G. (2000) Place of care in advanced cancer: a qualitative systematic literature review of patient preferences. *Journal of Palliative Medicine*, **3**: 287–300.

8 Dunne K., Sullivan K. (2000) Family experiences of palliative care in the acute hospital setting. *International Journal of Palliative Nursing*, **6**(4): 170–8.

9 Willard C., Luker K. (2006) Challenges to end of life care in the acute hospital setting. *Palliative Medicine*, **20**: 611–15.

10 The SUPPORT Principal Investigators (1995) A controlled trial to improve care for seriously ill hospitalized patients: the study to understand prognosis and preferences for outcomes and risks of treatments. *Journal of the American Medical Association*, **274**: 1591–8.

11 Lynn J., et al. (1997) Perceptions by family members of the dying experience of older and seriously ill patients. *Annals of Internal Medicine*, **126**(2): 97–106.

- The majority of complaints received by hospital trusts involve communication problems. The highly emotive situation of end-of-life care, compounds this
- Despite these identified needs, HSPCTs have been shown to be under-utilized[12]

Challenges to enable more patients to be discharged to die at home

- Early recognition of dying, in order to stop investigations and treatments that are not going to impact on outcome and to allow the change in focus which can enable a safe and timely discharge
- Recognition of the potential for dying, in order to facilitate discussions around future care preferences
- Improving communication skills to support discussions around end-of-life care
- Good multidisciplinary team (MDT) structures to support timely assessments and planning for discharge to die at home
- Recognition by the MDT that dying at home is possible

12 Lagman R. et al. (2007) The underutilization of palliative medicine services in the acute care setting. *Journal of Palliative Medicine.* **10**(4): 837–8. (Letter)

The challenges in an acute hospital setting

- **Busy, stretched staff**: in one study, ward nurses had an average of 3 minutes per patient per shift for psychological care[13]
- **Lack of consistency in treating teams**: e.g. shift working, multiple ward moves, weekly team change-over of junior medical staff, changing consultant team of the week and frequent staff turnover
- **Variability in models of communication amongst the MDT**: there are some good models of MDT working but this is not consistent
- **Difficulty accessing clinical information**: this is particularly important on admission to hospital and when a patient comes to A&E. Good communication between community/hospital teams and hospital/hospital teams is invaluable. The use of electronic records, where available, should facilitate communication. In the absence of this there is no substitute for consulting widely. Inadequate information leads to inadequate care!
- **Environment**: there is frequently lack of privacy; lack of quiet rooms in which to talk; lack of attention of dignity; difficulty accessing outside green spaces; difficulty for loved ones to stay overnight; lack of free and/or convenient parking for visitors
- **Attitudes and skills**: there is variability in knowledge and acceptance of a palliative care approach; generalists may see palliative care professionals as 'giving up' on patients; there is fear in prescribing drugs used for symptom control eg. morphine
- **Bureaucracy as a limit**: to creativity and empowering patient-centred choices: strict visiting times; lack of flexibility in food choices
- **Hospital-acquired infections**: with the vulnerable being most at risk
- **Providing support out of hours**: given the small size of many hospital teams and lack of funding, out of hours provision is often inadequate

13 McDonnell M., et al. (2002) Palliative care in district general hospitals: the nurse's perspective. *International Journal of Palliative Nursing*, **8**(4): 169–75.

Aims and evaluation of a hospital specialist palliative care team

Aims

- Integrate hospice values and practice into the acute care setting
- Be a visible and practical support and resource within the hospital
- By working in an advisory capacity, support the needs of both patients and their families
- Be dedicated specialists, with the time and focus to truly influence the patient experience
- Develop models of MDT working and communication; foster trusted relationships with consultant colleagues and other specialists involved in caring for those patients with advanced progressive illnesses, e.g. clinical nurse specialists working with neurodisabilities, such as Parkinson's disease, Motor Neurone Disease
- Help identify and be present at junctures in the patient's experience, to ensure review and resetting of treatment plans in the light of (changing) patient preferences, e.g. close working with oncology colleagues by attendance at cancer site-specific MDTs and outpatient clinics; presence at ward rounds or outpatient clinics for e.g. heart failure/end-stage renal disease
- Optimize collaborative working with the local community and hospice services. Different models exist which range from joint appointments of staff working across multiple settings, community team attendance at hospital MDT meetings or outpatient clinics, to fully integrated community/hospital palliative care teams
- Develop MDT education programmes to raise standards throughout the hospital, covering all aspects of holistic care, e.g. physical, emotional, social, spiritual and ethical elements. Provide informal and formal teaching covering a wide variety of staff, including those at the periphery of patient care who may still be affected and interact with patients, e.g. porters and ward clerks
- Provide and/or develop patient information in an accessible form
- Promote clear ethical decision-making through joint working with clinicians and education/participation in hospital clinical ethical committees
- Promote audit and research to evaluate service and ensure best care
- Influence policy development and raise the profile of palliative care within the hospital, through involvement at all levels. It is crucial to engage with management in order to change culture
- Represent and participate in hospital and regional groups, e.g. cancer locality groups, cancer or other disease networks
- Be a role model and mentor; empower and enthuse professional colleagues and encourage the next generation of palliative care specialists

Evaluation

There are inherent difficulties in evaluating hospital palliative care teams. The evidence-base showing a benefit for HSPCTs is limited,[14] reasons for which include the difficulty in evaluating advisory teams, attrition rate of patients and bias, and the clinical complexity of patients with whom palliative care teams are involved e.g. those who have intractable pain or difficult psychosocial problems. However, there are a few established tools, such as the Palliative Care Assessment Tool (PACA) and Palliative care Outcome Score (POS) which have shown benefit from HSPCT involvement in a variety of areas, such as pain, symptom control and patient and carer insight.

14 Higginson I. J., et al. (2002) Do hospital-based palliative teams improve care for patients or families at the end of life? *Journal of Pain and Symptom Management*, **23**(2): 96–106.

Things to think about when considering a referral to the hospital palliative care team

- What are your team's plans for ongoing care?
- What treatment options are available?
- What are the patient's wishes for care or place of care?
- If there are symptoms, what do you think is the underlying cause and what steps have already been taken to address them?
- If the referral is for terminal care, has your team reached a consensus that this is the aim of care? Is this reflected in the care which is being provided?
- Have you thought through and identified the specialist palliative care needs of your patient, e.g. difficulties with pain and symptom management, psychological and social needs and dying?
- Have you made sure the patient is aware of and in agreement with any referral? This will usually imply a level of understanding of their illness and prognosis
- Do you want to refer to the HSPCT or the community SPCT? There may be a separate referral route for the latter

Of course, difficulties in the above areas may be the exact reason why you want to refer to the HSPCT. By thinking these issues through before contacting the HSPCT you will pre-empt their questions!

Urgent discharge of a dying patient who wants to die at home

Sometimes, following sudden realization of a rapid decline, a patient may decide that he/she wants to go home to die. In these changing circumstances, time can be short and clinicians need to be flexible for this to be possible. Steps are outlined below to aid clinicians facilitate safe discharge. There is a new Department of Health Fast Track Pathway process for NHS Continuing Healthcare, which allows speedy access to continuing care support for such patients.

Steps

(Adapted from the resource pack for healthcare professionals from the South West and South East London Cancer Networks, Supportive and Palliative Care Subgroups.)

Communication

Remember to enhance understanding through consideration of first language, learning disability and literacy skills. Use of interpreters or advocates may be needed.

Patient
- Ensure it is the patient's wish to die at home
- Explain the level of care available and ensure he/she is aware of limitations in support and the impact of the discharge on carers
- Re-check that the patient still wants to go home to die

Family/carer, where possible with patient
- Is the family/carer in agreement with the patient's wishes?
- Are they aware of the aims of care and the short prognosis?
- Does the family understand the medications?
- Ensure the family knows which community agencies will be involved and what their roles and level of commitment are
- Give the family contact numbers for 'in-hours' and 'out-of-hours' GP, district nursing, community palliative care and other involved agencies
- Advise the family that when a patient dies at home, they must inform the GP

Ward nurse
- Verbal referral supported by fax to district nurse
- Nursing letter should include details of the patient's diagnosis, their nursing needs, medication, poor prognosis, understanding and wishes. Indicate other referrals made
- Consider local supports that may be available, including Marie Curie night nursing, hospice-at-home schemes, etc. (Liaise with the HSPCT.)
- Provide a letter/form to go with the patient, for the in-hours/out-of-hours district nursing service
- Verbal referral supported by faxed referral/update to the Community Specialist Palliative Care Team (CSPCT)
- If patient is oxygen-dependent, check adequate oxygen availability at home. If not, ensure arrangements are made for home oxygen through local policies. There is the facility for urgent provision, where time is short

- Ensure urgent referral for Continuing Care Category 1 utilizing the Fast Track Tool, to optimize the level of care available. The more detailed form can follow on after discharge
- Ensure regular liaison with MDT members involved in the patient's discharge from hospital discharge, e.g. coordinators, occupational therapists, etc.
- Book ambulance: ensure the ambulance service is aware that the patient is not for resuscitation, and that a written DNAR order is with the patient (e.g. in the form of a letter, or a copy of the hospital DNAR order; local policies will apply)
- Liaise with the HSPCT for advice and support

Doctor
- Verbal update supported by fax to the GP ± out-of-hours GP service. Emphasize the patient's wish to die at home. List the medications. Ensure an early review by the GP who will also need to undertake death certification
- Complete and fax out-of-hours handover forms, where available, to local GP out-of-hours service and, where agreements exist, the local ambulance service
- Ensure DNAR form is both signed and current

Medication
Doctor
- Prescribe at least 1 week of **oral medication**. Include p.r.n. analgesia and antiemetics
- Even if the patient can swallow on discharge, they are likely to become unable to swallow in the near future, so **subcutaneous medication must** also be prescribed
- Prescribe regular medication needs for delivery via syringe driver, plus p.r.n. medication needs for possible distressing symptoms. (📖 see Chapter 16, The terminal phase). Remember also to prescribe water for injection
- Doctors must write a prescription chart for the syringe driver and p.r.n. sc medications to go home with the patient, so that district nurses can administer medications. This can be in the form of a letter or utilization of local charts, as available

Nurse
- Provide a written medication chart to go home with the patient. Include information about the reason for the medication, dosage and frequency
- Explain to the patient and family and ensure understanding

Equipment
Ward nurse's responsibility for equipment needed for discharge:
- For patients with a syringe driver, **either**:
  - supply a clearly labelled syringe driver for early return by district nurse, or other explicit arrangement; **or**:
  - give stat medications prior to transfer to cover the known symptoms and arrange for the district nurse to set up the syringe driver shortly after the patient's arrival at home

- When sending the patient home with a hospital syringe driver, Remember to include:
  - a spare battery
  - a range of Luer-lock syringes: 2mL, 10mL, 20mL, 30mL (× 4)
  - needles: orange, blue and green (× 4)
  - syringe driver lines (× 4)
  - Tegaderm (× 4)
  - labels for barrel of syringe
  - water for injection
  - sharps box (× 1)
- For patients with additional needs discuss with the district nurses the need for:
  - dressings (× 4)
  - incontinence pads
  - catheter bags for patients who are catheterized
  - colostomy/ileostomy/ileal conduit bags
  - vomit bowls
  - urine bottles, bed-pan, commode
  - hospital bed/mattress
  - gloves, apron
  - mouth sponges

  It may not be possible to provide all the equipment, but don't let this stop you from fulfilling the patient's wishes. Where items are not available, discuss possible solutions with district nurse/patient/family.
  Communication is key to a successful discharge
  - At any stage, liaise with the HSPCT for advice and support

Case

A 95-yr-old widower was admitted to hospital with pneumonia. He had had previous strokes, which significantly affected his mobility. He lived alone and had no children or close family. Early in the admission he said that he didn't want any more treatment and wanted to be allowed to die.

His infection caused intermittent confusion and the treating team were concerned that he did not have capacity to refuse treatment. They felt he could benefit from treatment and so continued to offer antibiotics. He then became increasingly distressed and mistrustful of staff and started to refuse all treatment, including symptomatic measures such as pain control. He was referred to the HPCT for symptom control, support and in the knowledge that, despite their efforts, he was probably dying.

On meeting him, the HPCT were able to talk through his understanding of his condition and his wishes for care. He had nursed his wife through a long illness and saw her death as a blessing. He had also lost close friends recently. He felt he had a poor quality of life due to his strokes and did not want to prolong his life any more. He had agreed to come in to the hospital so he could die in a place of safety, but he had not anticipated the battle to keep him alive. He understood there would be friends who would be upset by his dying, but said he had spoken to them and said his goodbyes. He was, at that moment, competent in his refusal of life-sustaining treatment. He also had many other symptoms that had either not been addressed (nausea, shortness of breath associated with his anxiety, constipation), or had been inadequately managed (regular analgesia had been prescribed, but he had refused). The HPCT were able to talk through his drug chart, rationalize medication for comfort only and spoke with staff so they would explain clearly what was being given.

By meeting with the treating team, the team were able to clarify aims of care and to ensure consistency of care. This reassured him. He did not want a single room, as he liked the activity of the open ward. He deteriorated steadily and within 24 hours was started on the Liverpool Care Pathway for the dying patient. A syringe driver and p.r.n. medications were advised and he died comfortably a few hours later.

Dying in the intensive care unit (ICU)

A large number of patients who die in hospital spend some time on the ICU during their last admission.[15] But the experience of dying on an ICU is reported as variable, with a high prevalence of symptoms and poor communication around the end-of-life preferences. In such an aggressive treatment environment focused on saving life, ensuring a peaceful death may get lost as a central goal of clinical care.

In the US SUPPORT (the Study to Understand Prognosis and Preferences or Outcomes and Risks of Treatments) study[7], from the perspective of patients who died, 60% of patients would have preferred comfort care. Poor communication around end-of-life issues may, therefore, influence admissions to ICU and lead to invasive treatment which does not always follow patients' wishes.

A study that looked at the quality of dying in an ICU, from the perspective of bereaved relatives, showed that 24% of patients were never aware of dying and that 34% were only aware in their last week of life.

The most important aspects of the perceived quality of dying were good pain control, being prepared for death, having control over events, feeling at peace, maintaining dignity and self-respect.

More than 70% of deaths on an ICU can be predicted, e.g. by withdrawal of treatment that has failed. Withdrawal of treatment can precipitate, in some circumstances, a very rapid death within minutes to hours. Some patients will be stable enough to be transferred to other areas.

HSPCTs clearly have a role in supporting end-of-life care in an ICU and the challenge is to develop relationships with ICU colleagues to allow this. Opportunities include: developing joint education programmes to raise the profile of a palliative care approach, for it to be seen as a core goal of care, not a failure of care; ensuring clear criteria for referral to HSPCTs; looking at models of MDT working; adapting approaches to the dying phase in the light of the often fast clinical deterioration and by highlighting variations in routes and types of medications needed.

The National Liverpool Care Pathway Centre has developed an ICU version of the LCP which is currently being evaluated. The HSPCT can actively support the transition of dying patients who are transferred from ICU to other settings. Throughout the hospital, the team has a role in promoting the need for early communication around end-of-life preferences with patients, enhancing their control over events and supporting the staff in the communication skills needed in these difficult situations.

15 Rady M., Johnson D. (2004) Admission to intensive care unit at the end of life: is it an informed decision? *Palliative Medicine*, **18**: 705–11.

Using the Liverpool Care Pathway for the dying patient (LCP) in the hospital setting

The LCP was originally developed to bring the hospice model of care of the dying to the acute hospital setting. It has since been disseminated to other settings and is one of the three End of Life Care initiatives promoted by the Department of Health.

Experience with the LCP in the acute hospital setting shows that more than 50% of dying patients have a non-cancer diagnosis, so it is successfully reaching patients who have not previously accessed hospice care.

There is widespread enthusiasm amongst staff who feel they are empowered by the LCP (📖 see box, p. 942). Senior doctors are given flexibility within the Variance to allow individualized care and clinical judgement. Within an acute hospital setting, it is essential to ensure senior medical involvement in the decision to start the LCP, and this is ensured by the paperwork requiring the consultant or their agreed deputy (usually the specialist registrar) to agree.

The structure of the tool is welcomed by busy ward staff. It provides an effective audit and educational tool, which also reinforces other palliative care education programmes. Analysis of Variances can help reflection and support learning. However, it is essential to monitor quality beyond the purely paper assessment, and sustaining the LCP in a busy hospital with large staff turnover has its challenges. Although a tool for generalists, its implementation has been largely led by the HSPCTs.

One of the challenges, especially in the treatment-focused hospital, is the recognition of dying and patient involvement in decision-making. There is a need to raise skills in communication at the end of life as well as using ethical frameworks for reflection and decision-making.

Quotes on the use of the LCP by healthcare professionals

…'a very good tool to explain to the family care of the dying patient and reassure them about the existence of such a protocol'

Pre-registration house officer in care of the elderly

'I find it simple and easy to understand. I don't miss any care or comfort measures for the patient and family, as everything is there to remind me'

Sister, Medical Unit

'The thing I like about the LCP is that a firm decision is made by the team and you don't get a half-hearted approach to terminal care'

Medical Pre-registration house officer

'Having a specific plan of nursing care for the patient facilitates open communication with the family'

Staff nurse, Medical Unit

'I have noted that it has improved the confidence of ward nurses in dealing with dying patients and their families'

Staff nurse, Medical Unit
Kingston Hospital Pride of Nursing Prize 2007

Further reading

Articles

Cunningham C., Archibald C. (2006) Supporting people with acute dementia in acute hospital settings. *Nursing Standard*, **20**(43): 51–5.

Formiga F., et al. (2007) Dying in hospital of terminal heart failure or severe dementia: the circumstances associated with death and the opinions of care givers. *Palliative Medicine*, **21**(1): 35–40.

Willard C., Luker K. (2006) Challenges to end of life care in the acute hospital setting. *Palliative Medicine*, **20**(6): 611–15.

Palliative care for people with learning disabilities

People with learning disabilities are a part of us rather than being apart *from* us

Todd, 2006

Learning disability has been described as a significantly reduced ability to understand new or complex information and to learn new skills, and a reduced ability to cope independently, which started before adulthood, with a lasting effect on development. Around 2.5% of the population in the UK has a learning disability, with figures higher in deprived and urban areas. It has been suggested that the number of people with learning disabilities may increase by around 1% each year over the next fifteen years; and, due to their increased longevity and age-related disease, people with learning disabilities are more likely to require palliative care services in the future. About one-third of people with Down syndrome over 35 years of age may be expected to show clinical evidence of dementia. In the presence of Down syndrome and dementia, the person's health can often deteriorate quite quickly. The highest cause of death in people with a learning disability is respiratory disease.

People with learning disabilities tend to have:
- Higher healthcare needs, but less access to healthcare services
- A late diagnosis of cancer, due in part to lack of access to screening, and a subsequent poor prognosis
- A higher incidence of gastrointestinal cancer
- An increased incidence of dementia (and significantly earlier onset in people with Down syndrome)

The diagnosis of an advanced progressive disease is equally one of the most distressing and traumatic life experiences for the person with a learning disability as it is for anyone else. Yet people with a learning disability are a disadvantaged and devalued group, who, for a variety of reasons, are often excluded from discussions about death, dying and bereavement, which makes it particularly difficult for these people to be actively involved in necessary decision-making. It seems that the more complex the disability, the less likelihood there is of the person being actively involved in these discussions.

Key points
- People with a learning disability have the same needs as any other patient group at the end of life, and may also have additional needs as a result of their disability
- Meeting the needs of someone with a learning disability at the end of life may present a challenge to professionals' working practices

- Partnership and collaboration between palliative care and learning disability services is essential to ensure the exchange and fusion of knowledge and skills in meeting the needs of this vulnerable population
- Palliative and end-of-life care for people with learning disabilities should be patient-centred and family-oriented
- People with learning disabilities have more similarities to people without learning disabilities than differences, particularly at the end of life

Communication

It is a truism that people 'cannot not communicate'. It is important to remember that all people with learning disabilities have communication abilities, even when these do not appear immediately apparent. For many people with learning disabilities the spoken word may not be their 'first language'.

- Take time to establish a relationship with the person with learning disabilities and their carers
- Undertake any assessment over a length of time, possibly in a range of settings and with the support of people who know the person
- A clear positive, focused assessment that provides an indication of receptive and expressive communication abilities and needs should be undertaken in collaboration with family members, carers and the speech and language therapist, if necessary
- In seeking to establish effective communication, it may be necessary for staff to refine their skills in observation and listening, as well as in explaining new information

General Breaking Bad News' models require adapting for someone with a learning disability who may not understand the 'warning shot' or the need to ask questions in order to get information. The language used should be straightforward, non-euphemistic, consistent and be supplemented or supported in a variety of different ways, such as using books, photographs, pictures or picture boards (Table 14.1).

Whenever possible, a familiar person, of the patient's choice, should be actively involved. Allow time for the patient to inspect and digest new information, either verbally or visually. People with learning disabilities should be given the opportunity to be involved as much as possible (and as much as they are able to be) in communication about his or her illness, subsequent treatment options and eventual death.

Table 14.1 A model to promote communication when breaking difficult news

Prepare ↓	The environment should not be too noisy, busy, over-stimulating or intimidating
	Liaise with family/carers to determine what the person's levels of understanding and communication are, and what resources are already present (e.g. a person-centred plan or communication passport)
	Establish the patient's previous experience of serious illness and any fears or phobias, e.g. 'needle phobia'
Ask ↓	Always use the person's name. Find out what he or she already knows. Use straightforward questions and non-euphemistic language to elicit information. Find out what the person wants to know. Remember that some people with learning disability take longer to process questions or new information, so allow extra time between questions or statements. Be aware of the danger that the person is acquiescing to what they perceive is wanted rather than really understanding or expressing their own opinion.
Repeat and clarify ↓	Be prepared to go over information time and time again, and make use of a variety of media (e.g. books, photographs, etc.). Simplify language using concrete statements. Actively listen. Be guided by the individual. Remember that people with learning disability sometimes have difficulty in sequencing information and, therefore, they will require such explanations which facilitate this.
Check level of understanding ↓	Explore what the person understands (cognitively); and what they have 'taken in'. Explore the potential impact. Go back to a previous stage, if necessary. Be guided by the individual.
Help the person to express their feelings ↓	Encourage expression; acknowledge feelings and give constructive feedback; where appropriate, help the person to describe their feelings; explore what they feel they might need next. Explore the future support options. Follow up where necessary.
Follow-up ↓	It is unlikely that the information will be completely understood or retained after only one visit and, therefore, a follow-up appointment will need to be offered. This should be with the lead physician or another member of the team who can take a lead role in ongoing communication and liaison.

The pressure from family, or other carers, to maintain a 'conspiracy of silence' rather than truth telling may be immense. In a client group who often already lack control and choice this can result in a greater loss of autonomy, and skill and sensitivity and time are, therefore, required in dealing with this situation.

Consent

All people with learning disabilities can make some decisions; a key question is determining which decisions they can make. All adults, including people with learning disabilities, are considered capable of providing consent unless demonstrated otherwise. Furthermore, all people with learning disabilities have the right to give, withdraw and withhold consent to examination, treatment and care; withholding/ withdrawing consent is not equal to non-compliance.

- It is not permissible to say that a person with learning disabilities can make no decisions
- The person's ability to make each decision must be considered.
- The only way to establish that a person cannot give valid consent is to seek to obtain it
- Remember that in doing so it is necessary to make all 'reasonable adjustment' in providing information and to do this throughout the decision-making process
- Staff should seek advice in relation to any Disability Discrimination and Capacity/Incapacity legislation, which must be followed

If an adult cannot give consent, including a person who has learning disabilities, no one can consent on their behalf and a consent form must **not** be signed. Instead, a careful and clearly documented process of 'best interests' decision-making should be followed. Central to this is being able to clearly show that any decision taken was primarily in the best interests of the person with learning disabilities.

Pain and symptom assessment

- Adults with a mild learning disability are often able to locate pain in the same way as those who do not have a learning disability
- A body map, photographs and the involvement of a carer (with support for their needs as carers) who knows the person well may be helpful
- In people with more severe disabilities the presence of pain may be expressed in atypical ways, such as a behavioural change (both positive and negative), or vocalization such as the use of a specific word, phrase, mannerism or laugh
- In palliative and end-of-life care the concept of 'total pain', which reflects the multidimensional suffering (physical, emotional, spiritual and social) that can occur, influences holistic pain assessment and its multidisciplinary management.

There is a recognized need for effective symptom assessment tools for people with learning disabilities. The DisDAT (Disability Distress Assessment Tool) is one tool which has been developed in the UK to assist in the identification of distress. Identifying the source of distress, whether physical pain or another cause, is pivotal.

People with learning disability may tolerate symptoms or express them through irritability, inactivity, loss of appetite or sleep disturbance. Carers need information that will assist them to recognize signs of potential ill-health, such as weight loss, clothes being to loose or too tight, loss of appetite or changes in toilet habits. Careful assessment is required in patients with learning disabilities who have gastrointestinal cancer, i.e. due to the risk of intestinal obstruction which may not be readily diagnosed.

Loss, grief and bereavement

People with learning disabilities do experience grief, but may express it in idiosyncratic or different ways, and it may take time for the reality of the loss to be realized.

They may experience multiple and successive losses too, as their main carers die and alternative accommodation is urgently organized. Therefore, accurate record keeping is crucial to long-term effective support. Carers may be anxious about involving people with learning disabilities in bereavement, perhaps because they remain unsure as to how that person may react, or they feel uncomfortable in this area of support. The most important point to remember is to be human, kind and understanding. People deliberately excluded from participating in bereavement are likely to experience disenfranchised grief, which may lead to complicated grief.

- Be prepared to repeat information often
- Keep language clear and consistent and avoid using euphemisms about death that may only confuse the person over time
- Use everyday opportunities (such as stories on the TV or news items) to encourage individuals to talk about loss and death and to minimize the taboos around the topic with this population

Some people with a learning disability may feel uncomfortable when carers rely on spoken language only. It, therefore, remains important to be creative when acknowledging and facilitating feelings, giving accurate information and creating time and a confidential space. There are easy to read, pictorial books to help in this process. Memory books and life-story books, in accessible formats, are constructive and helpful ways of helping the person to remember their loved ones, and serve to create continuing links with loved ones who have died.

Richard's story

I live in my own flat supported by an outreach team. This is about what I went through when my dad died. My dad died in hospital. He had been sick for about ten months and had been having treatment in hospital. My sister wrote to me because I am not able to use telephones because I am also deaf. She wrote to tell me that our dad was in hospital. I was able to visit him before he died. I used to visit him on my own.

This was very hard because I didn't know about cancer and what it does to people. No-one in the hospital told me what was happening to him. I didn't know that he was going to die. I thought he was going to get better. I only knew he was going to die just before he died because I could see that he was very weak. He wasn't eating or drinking. No-one in my family told me that he was going to die either.

The last time I went to the hospital to visit him, he wasn't there. I didn't know where he was. I asked a nurse what was happening to him. She took me to a private room and told me that he had died. She didn't tell me anything else and I was too upset to ask her any questions. My dad had died the same day.

The nurse didn't tell me that I could have seen my dad after he had died. I didn't get to say goodbye to my dad. The nurse didn't tell me where they had taken his body. She didn't tell me that there was a chaplain that I could talk to. She didn't tell me that there was a quiet place that I could go to…She didn't tell me about these people that you can talk to when a person dies. It would have been better if she had told me about these things. It would have been better if everything was written down in an easy way so that I could have looked at it later.

I think that it would have been better if the health people had talked to me about cancer and radiotherapy and chemotherapy. I think it would have been easier for me to understand what was happening to my dad.

I want to end with these messages:

People with learning disabilities should be given the same information about death and dying that other people are given

Information needs to be accessible, using pictures, photographs, easy words and/or video

This information should be given to us by everyone who works with people with learning disabilities, for example health, social services, voluntary people, family, etc.

It would be good to plan and work with people with learning disabilities who have cancer and talk about how services can make their needs better

People with learning disabilities need support when going through something like this (where they have lost someone who has died)—support can come from family and friends as well as people who work with us

Richard highlights how people with a learning disability are often excluded in the name of protecting them and are treated as children, shielded away from the painful and raw realities of life. Sometimes, individuals are left having to make sense of things that are happening around them because they are not kept fully informed about what is happening and what to expect. They subsequently lack the knowledge and information to make informed decisions regarding coping with the loss of those close to them. They may also become unnecessarily anxious about the health of their remaining carers and their own health.

• Collaboration is the key to effective support, this requires the development of mutual trust between people with learning disabilities, carers and people delivering palliative care, in both learning disability and generalist/specialist palliative care services
• Carers, be they family members or other carers, supporting people with learning disabilities at such sensitive times need support too

Useful contacts

National Network for Palliative Care of People with Learning Disabilities (NNPCPLD); website: http:www.helpthehospices.org.uk/NPA/uk

website: www.bereavementanddisability.org.uk

Further reading

Books

Blackman N. (2003) *Loss and Learning Disability*. London: Worth Publishing.

Blackman N., Todd S. (2005) *Caring for People with Learning Disabilities who are Dying*. London: Worth Publishing.

Doka K. J. (ed.) (2002). *Disenfranchised Grief: New Directions, Challenges and Strategies for Practice.* Illinois: Research Press.

McEnhill L. (2004) Disability. In *Death, Dying and Social Differences* (ed. D. Oliviere, B. Monroe), pp. 97–118. Oxford: Oxford University Press.

McEnhill L. (2006) The role of hospices. In *Palliative Care for People with Learning Disabilities* (ed. S. Read), pp. 13–25. London: MA Healthcare.

Read S. (2006) *Palliative Care for People with Learning Disabilities*. London: Quay Books.

Read S. (2006) Communication in the dying context. In *Palliative Care for People with Learning Disabilities* (ed. S. Read), pp. 91–104. London: MA Healthcare.

Read S. (2007). *Bereavement Counselling and Support: A Manual to Develop Practice*. London: Quay Books.

Royal College of Nursing (2006) *Meeting the Health Needs of People with Learning Disabilities*. London: RCN.

Todd S. (2006) A troubled past and present—a history of death and disability. In *Palliative Care for People with Learning Disabilities* (ed. S. Read), pp. 13–25. London: MA Healthcare

Articles

Department of Health (2001) *Valuing People: A New Strategy for Learning Disability for the 21st Century.* London: DoH.

Deudney C. (2006) *Patients with Autistic Spectrum Disorders: Information for Health Professionals.* London: NAS Information Centre.

Read S., Elliot D. (2003) Death and learning disability: A vulnerability perspective. *Journal of Adult Protection*, **5**(1): 5–14.

Regnard C.,*et al* (2003) Difficulties in identifying distress and its causes in people with severe communication problems. *International Journal of Palliative Nursing*, **9**(3): 173–6.

Ryan K. R., McQuillan R. (2005) Palliative care for disadvantaged groups: people with intellectual disabilities. *Progress in Palliative Care*, **13**(2): 70–4.

Tuffrey-Wijne I. (2003) The palliative care needs of people with intellectual disabilities: a literature review. *Palliative Medicine*, **17**: 55–62.

Tuffrey-Wijne I., Davies J. (2006) This is my story: I've got cancer. *British Journal of Learning Disabilities*, **35**: 7–11.

http://www.intellectualdisability.info/mental_phys-health/DadDied_west.html

Emergencies in palliative care

While this chapter focuses on the common oncological emergencies in palliative practice, other emergencies include a wider range of issues such as:

- An emergency discharge so a patient's wish to die at home can be met
- Emotional emergencies, with high levels of expressed anxiety
- Spiritual/existential/social emergencies with pressure to 'sort things out' before it is too late

It is important to have a clear understanding of the management of emergencies in palliative care as clear thinking is crucial in handling such situations. Providing transparent decisiveness to the patient, their family and staff can transform a crisis situation filled with anxiety.

Faced with an emergent, acute problem in the palliative care setting, clinicians would do well to establish quickly the answer to three simple questions:

- Where is the patient on their disease trajectory?
- What is causing this particular problem at this particular time?
- What ideas, concerns and expectations does the patient/family have?

The time frame for normal hospice and palliative care interventions are modulated by the need for calmness and patient comfort. There are, however, several emergency situations which can occur for hospice patients requiring urgent and prompt diagnosis and management. This may create some dissonance among staff and other patients. It is vital that all staff appreciate the nature of these emergencies and the appropriateness of an urgent response.

Sepsis in the neutropenic patient

All clinical staff should be acutely aware of the serious risk and precarious condition of patients who have become neutropenic and febrile following oncological treatments. If not managed rapidly and effectively, these patients will die from overwhelming infection.

An absolute neutrophil count of less than 0.5×10^9/L is defined as severe neutropenia, although the risk of infection increases as the count falls below 1.0×10^9/L

Initially, patients may develop general influenza-type symptoms, highlighting the need for vigilance and a high index of suspicion in patients who have recently received either cytotoxic chemotherapy or immunosuppressant therapy.

Patients should be admitted to a unit where essential investigations can be carried out rapidly and where intravenous antibiotics can be given and suitable monitoring maintained. Appropriate facilities are not usually available within a hospice unit. Occasionally, patients may develop neutropenic sepsis while in a palliative care setting, which can create a dilemma. After full discussion, emphasizing the gravity of the situation and the high chance of a good response to optimal management in an acute unit, patients may still refuse transfer, preferring to stay in the hospice and receive suboptimal care. This should be discussed with their oncologist if possible.

Empirical treatment of a febrile neutropenic patient should be instigated and an appropriate antibiotic regime started, *with advice from the local bacteriologist since antibiotic regimes vary across the country.*

A regime currently being advocated at The Royal Marsden Hospital is outlined below as an example

- Tazocin 4.5g q.d.s. + gentamicin 5mg/kg IV o.d.

  or, if allergic to penicillin:
- Ceftazidime 2g IV t.d.s. + gentamicin 5mg/kg IV o.d.

  If still febrile after 48h:
- Add vancomycin 1g IV b.d.

  If still febrile after 96–120h:
- Stop tazocin + gentamicin
- Start ciprofloxacin 400mg IV b.d.
- Add amphotericin 0.75mg/kg per day IV (or 1mg/kg per day for haemato-oncology patients)
- Treat for a minimum of seven days and continue until neutrophil count >0.5×10^9/L[1].

---

1 Antibiotic Guidelines for the Royal Marsden Foundation Trust (2008)

Spinal cord compression

Signs of spinal cord compression

- Back pain (present in 90% of cases)
- Weak legs
- Increased reflexes
- Sensory level
- Urinary hesitancy (late feature)

Spinal cord compression occurs in 3–5% of patients with cancer, and 10% of patients with spinal metastases develop cord compression,[2] the frequency being highest in multiple myeloma and cancers of the prostate, breast and bronchus.

- Malignant causes:
  - intramedullary metastases
  - intradural metastases
  - extradural compression (80%)
    —vertebral body metastasis
    —vertebral collapse
    —tumour spread
    —interruption of vascular supply

It is important to have a high index of suspicion for possible cord compression, because of the consequences of paraplegia and urinary and faecal incontinence with a delay in diagnosis.

Symptoms and signs

- Spinal cord compression must be considered in all cancer patients with back pain. Pain often pre-dates neurological changes by some considerable time
- A sensation of weakness in the legs and often vague sensory symptoms in the legs may be early manifestations. Patients may complain of a band-like pain, particularly on coughing or sneezing
- For those presenting with profound weakness, a sensory 'level' and sphincter disturbance, which are relatively late features, the outcome is poor and the compression is much less likely to be reversible
- Tenderness along the bony spine may be present

The site of compression is:

- thoracic in 70%
- lumbosacral 20%
- cervical 10%

Lesions above L1 (lower end of spinal cord) will produce upper motor neurone signs and often a sensory level, whereas lesions below L1 will produce lower motor neurone signs and perianal numbness (cauda equina syndrome). Multiple sites of compression may produce different and confusing neurological signs (Table 15.1).

Table 15.1 Neurological signs of upper and lower motor neurone lesions

	Upper motor neurone lesion	Lower motor neurone lesion
Power	Reduced/absent	Reduced/absent
Tone	Increased	Reduced
Sensation	Sensory loss	Sensory loss
Reflexes (plantars)	Increased (upgoing)	Absent/reduced (downgoing)

Management

High dose corticosteroids (dexamethasone 16mg/day) to relieve peritumoural oedema (with proton pump inhibitor cover); urgent referral to oncology centre.

Spinal cord compression is an **emergency** and two questions need to be answered urgently:

- Does this patient have a reasonable likelihood of having spinal cord compression?
- Would this patient benefit from instituting emergency investigation and treatment?

Does this patient have a reasonable likelihood of having spinal cord compression?

Even the most skilled clinician is unable to diagnose spinal cord compression with absolute certainty. Often by the time clinical signs are 'classic', it is too late for patients to benefit from treatment, as it has a limited role in reversing symptoms which are already established. Thus if intervention to prevent paraplegia is to be successful, potential compression needs to be diagnosed early.

The keys to diagnosing spinal cord compression include:

- Having a high index of suspicion in patients with spinal metastases, particularly in patients with breast, lung and prostate cancer and with pain and tenderness on palpation or percussion of the vertebra at the level of the suspected lesion
- Taking patients' complaints about back pain, odd sensations in the legs and difficulties in passing urine seriously

Would this patient benefit from instituting emergency investigation and treatment?

The patient will need to be transferred to a specialized unit where an MRI scan can be carried out and treatment given. In the context of metastatic cancer, radiotherapy is often the most appropriate treatment, but surgery may need to be considered in specific circumstances.

Deciding whether the particular course of treatment is appropriate for a particular patient involves an overall assessment.

Key questions in deciding on emergency investigations and management

- Does the patient want emergency management?
- Is the patient still walking?
- Is the patient suffering from severe back pain?
- Does the patient already have established cord compression?
- Does the patient have a short prognosis (e.g. week by week deterioration)?

Where suspicion of spinal cord compression is high, it is quickest to telephone the oncological team in the cancer centre where the patient has been managed, who can then coordinate the necessary scan and appropriate emergency treatment (Table 15.2).

Table 15.2 Definitive treatment of spinal cord compression

Indications for surgical decompression	Indications for radiotherapy
- Uncertain cause—to obtain histology - Radiotherapy has not been effective or symptoms persist despite maximum radiotherapy - Radioresistant tumour, e.g. melanoma, sarcoma - Unstable spine - Major structural compression - Cervical cord lesion - Solitary vertebral metastasis	- Radiosensitive tumour - Multiple levels of compression - Unfit for major surgery - Patient choice

Patients with spinal cord compression provide great challenges to the multidisciplinary team. These challenges include:
- Mobility management (risk of venous thrombosis)
- Skin management in a patient confined to bed (risk of pressure sores)
- Bowel management
- Urinary system management
- Psychological management.

There is no consensus on the optimum time to start mobilizing patients diagnosed with cord compression. In general, if the spine is stable and the pain is relatively well controlled it would seem wise to introduce physiotherapy as soon as possible to maintain muscle tone and motor function.

The occupational therapist will be crucial in helping with goal-setting and rehabilitative techniques.

Steroids are usually continued at high dose to start with, and then tailed off gradually and completely discontinued after some time (4–6 weeks), or to the lowest dose that maintains stability. Radiation-induced oedema may exacerbate symptoms and the dose of steroids may need to increase temporarily during treatment.

Prognosis

Overall, 30% of patients may survive for one year. A patient who is ambulant after treatment may survive for 8–9 months, but the life expectancy for a patient who remains paraplegic is a few weeks only. Function will be retained in 70% of patients who were ambulant prior to treatment, but will return in only 5% of those who were paraplegic at the outset. Return of motor function is better in those with incomplete spinal compression and particularly so with partial lesions of the cauda equina. Loss of sphincter function is a bad prognostic sign.

In practice, most patients with an established diagnosis are relatively unwell and have multiple metastases, and will be referred for radiotherapy, achieving similar results to those of surgery.

Superior vena cava obstruction

Superior vena cava obstruction (SVCO) may be due to external compression, thrombus formation inside the SVC, or direct invasion of the vessel by malignancy. It is caused most commonly by carcinoma of the bronchus (75%)—particularly small or squamous cell—and lymphomas (15%). Cancers of the breast, colon, oesophagus and testis account for the remaining 10%.

Symptoms and signs

Symptoms are those of venous hypertension, including breathlessness (laryngeal oedema, tracheal or bronchial obstruction/compression), headache or fullness particularly on bending or lying down (cerebral oedema), visual changes, dizziness and swelling of the face, neck and arms.

Signs include engorged conjunctivae, periorbital oedema, non-pulsatile dilated neck veins and dilated collateral veins (anterior chest, forehead and arms). If the latter sign evolves, the symptoms of SVCO may stabilize. Papilloedema is a late feature.

Management

In the palliative care setting, the diagnosis (usually of carcinoma of the bronchus) is already established. SVCO can present acutely, resulting in very distressing symptoms. The patient should be referred to the oncology centre for urgent management.

- Dexamethasone 8–16mg p.o. or IV (with proton pump inhibitor cover). There is no good evidence for the efficacy of steroids, but they may be helpful in reducing oedema (if there is associated stridor), or as an anti-tumour agent for lymphoma
- Furosemide 40mg p.o. or IV
- Consider a prophylactic anticonvulsant as these patients are at risk of seizures
- Appropriate analgesia may be necessary for the relief of headache
- Supplemental oxygen may be indicated where breathlessness is associated with hypoxia
- Treatment is the standard oncology treatment for the particular underlying cancer, e.g.: chemotherapy for small-cell lung cancer (SCLC) and lymphoma; radiotherapy for non-small cell carcinoma of the bronchus
- An intraluminal stent can be inserted via the femoral vein and is the treatment of choice for patients with severe symptoms
- Thrombolysis may be considered prior to stenting

Prognosis

Without treatment, SVCO can progress over several days leading to death. Prognosis is poor in a patient presenting with advanced SVCO unless the primary cancer is responsive to radiotherapy or chemotherapy. Generally, the prognosis is that of the underlying tumour.

Haemorrhage

Haemorrhage may be directly related to the underlying tumour, or caused by treatments, e.g. steroids or non-steroidal anti-inflammatory drugs (NSAIDs) resulting in gastric/duodenal erosion. A generalized clotting deficiency, seen in thrombocytopenia, hepatic insufficiency or anti-coagulation therapy are also contributory factors in patients with cancer.

Non-acute haemorrhage

Treatments for non-acute haemorrhage include oncological, systemic and local measures. Palliative radiotherapy is very useful for treating superficial tumours and those of the bronchus and genitourinary tract. If radiotherapy is not appropriate, coagulation should be enhanced with oral tranexamic acid 1g t.d.s., but caution is necessary with haematuria since clots may form resulting in further problems such as urinary retention. Local measures for superficial tumours, such as topical tranexamic acid or adrenaline (1:1000) soaks, may be useful. Sucralfate may act as a local astringent to stop stomach mucosal bleeding in addition to a proton pump inhibitor such as lansoprazole.

Acute haemorrhage

Erosion of a major artery can cause acute haemorrhage, which may be a rapidly terminal event. However, it may be possible to anticipate such an occurrence, and appropriate medication and a red blanket to reduce the visual impact should be readily available. Relatives or others who witness such an event will need a great deal of support. If the haemorrhage is not immediately fatal, such as with a haematemesis or bleeding from the rectum, vagina or superficially ulcerated wound, the aim of treatment is local control (if possible) and sedation of a shocked, frightened patient. Rectal or sublingual diazepam (Stesolid)10mg or midazolam 10mg SC or buccally act quickly.

Members of the palliative care team need to balance the anxiety of alerting and preparing the family for such an event against the likelihood of it occurring. If the patient chooses to be looked after at home, the issues of managing acute haemorrhage need to be discussed with the family and the home care team and a clear plan worked out.

It may be appropriate to have emergency medication in the home to sedate the acutely bleeding patient. Such a strategy needs lengthy discussion with the family, carers and the patient's GP, along with clearly documented plans.

Convulsions (see Chapter 6J)

Hypercalcaemia (📖 see Chapter 6i Endocrine and metabolic complications of advanced cancer)

Hypercalcaemia occurs in 10% of patients with cancer. The pathogenesis of hypercalcaemia in malignancy may be related to lytic bone lesions, the production of parathyroid hormone-related peptide (PTHrP) or uncontrolled vitamin D conversion. Calcium is released from bone, and there may also be a decrease in the excretion of urinary calcium. Malignancies most commonly associated with hypercalcaemia include squamous cell carcinoma of the bronchus (and other squamous cell tumours), carcinoma of the breast, prostate and renal tract, multiple myeloma and lymphoma.

A corrected plasma calcium concentration above 2.6mmol/L defines hypercalcaemia. It is often mild and asymptomatic and significant symptoms usually only develop with levels above 3.0mmol/L, but the rate of rise of blood calcium dictates the symptoms and signs. Levels of 4.0mmol/L and above will cause death in a few days if left untreated.

Symptoms include drowsiness, confusion, nausea, vomiting, thirst, polyuria, weakness and constipation.

Management

Treatment is only necessary if there are symptoms of hypercalcaemia and may be unnecessary if the patient is very near to death. Patients should be encouraged to mobilize if appropriate. The absorption of calcium from the gut is generally reduced, so patients may eat what they wish regardless of the calcium content of food.

Hypercalcaemia usually responds to specific antitumour therapy if appropriate.

Fluid replacement

Patients are usually dehydrated and need adequate fluid replacement. A high oral intake of fluid should be encouraged as appropriate for the individual clinical situation. Alternatively, extra fluid should be given intravenously. Fluid replacement alone improves symptoms but rarely achieves total control.

Bisphosphonates

Bisphosphonates inhibit osteoclast activity and thereby inhibit bone resorption. Because of poor alimentary absorption, they are usually given intravenously initially. Both disodium pamidronate or sodium clodronate are effective in 70–80% of patients for an average of two to three weeks. Zoledronic acid can be given over a shorter period and the effect lasts for longer. However, patients receiving bisphosphonates may develop transient fever and bone pains; they may also become hypocalcaemic and need to be monitored.

- e.g. zoledronic acid 4mg in 50mL sodium chloride 0.9% over 15 minutes
- e.g. disodium pamidronate 60–90mg in sodium chloride 0.9%, 500mL over 2–4h
- e.g. sodium clodronate 1.5g in sodium chloride 0.9%, 500mL over 4h

Plasma calcium levels start to decline after 48h and fall progressively for the next six days. Oral bisphosphonates have been reported to delay the recurrence of hypercalcaemia and may be important for maintenance.

The introduction of once- or twice-daily oral bisphosphonates have made compliance easier.

Prognosis

Some 80% of cancer patients with hypercalcaemia survive less than one year.

Further reading

Books

Currow D., Clark K. (2006) *Emergencies in Palliative and Supportive Care*. Oxford: Oxford University Press

Doyle D., *et al (eds)* (2004) *Oxford Textbook of Palliative Medicine* (3rd edn). Oxford: Oxford University Press.

Falk S., Reid C. (2006) Emergencies in Fallon M., Hanks G. *ABC Palliative Care* (2nd edn.) 40–43.

Kaye P. (1999). *Decision-Making in Palliative Care*, pp. 162–163. Northampton: EPL Publications.

The Royal Marsden Hospital (2008) *Prescribing Guidelines, including Symptom and Control Guidelines*, London: Royal Marsden NHS Trust.

Twycross R., Wilcock A. (2001) *Symptom Management in Advanced Cancer* (3rd edn). Oxford: Radcliffe Medical Press.

Articles

Chaichana K I. (2008) Predictors of ambulatory function after decompressive surgery for metastatic epidural spinal cord compression. *Neurosurgery* **62**(3): 683–692.

Cole J. S. (2008) Metastatic epidural spinal cord compression. *Lancet Neurology* **7**(5): 459–466.

Drudge-Coates J. (2008) Diagnosis and management of spinal cord compression Part 1. *International Journal of Palliative Nursing* **14**(3): 110–115.

Drudge-Coates J. (2008) Diagnosis and management of spinal cord compression Part 2. *International Journal of Palliative Nursing* **14**(4): 175–180.

Eva G., Lord S. (2003) Rehabilitation in malignant spinal cord compression. *European Journal of Palliative Care*, **10**(4): 148–50.

Falk S., Fallon M. (1997) ABC of Palliative Care. Emergencies. *British Medical Journal*, **315**(7121): 1525–8.

George R., Jeba J., Ramkumar G., Chacko A. G., Leng M., Tharyan P. Interventions for the treatment of metastatic extradural spinal cord compression in adults. Cochrane Database of Systematic Reviews 2008, Issue 4.

Heatley S. (2004) Metastatic bone disease and tumour-induced hypercalcaemia: treatment options. *International Journal of Palliative Nursing*, **10**(1): 41–6.

Hillier R., Wee B. (1997) Palliative management of spinal cord compression. *European Journal of Palliative Care*, **4**: 189–92.

Kramer J. A. (1992). Spinal cord compression in malignancy. *Palliative Medicine*, **6**: 202–11.

Penas-Prado M. (2008) Spinal cord compression in cancer patients: review of diagnosis and treatment. *Current Oncology Reports* **10**(1): 78–85.

Rowell N. P., Gleeson F. V. (2005) Steroids, radiotherapy, chemotherapy and stents for superior vena cava obstruction in carcinoma of the bronchus. *Cochrane Database of Systematic Reviews* (2): CD001316.

Saunders Y., et al. (2004) Systematic review of bisphosphonates for hypercalcaemia of malignancy. *Palliative medicine*, **18**(5): 418–31.

Smith A. M. (1994) Emergencies in palliative care. *Annals of Medicine*, **23**(2): 186–90.

Walji N. (2008) Common acute oncological emergencies: diagnosis, investigation and management. *Postgraduate Medical Journal* **84**: 418–427.

Watkinson A. F. (2008) Endovascular stenting to treat obstruction of the superior vena cava. *British Medical Journal* **336**: 1434–7.

Weissman D. E. (2004) Decision making at a time of crisis near the end of life. *Journal of the American Medical Association*, **292**(14): 1738–43.

The terminal phase

Death is not extinguishing the light; it is putting out the lamp because the dawn has come.

Rabindranath Tagore

Prognosis

Patients frequently ask, 'How long have I got?' It is notoriously difficult to predict when death will occur, and it is wise to avoid the trap of making a prediction or an incorrect guess. If pushed to do so, it should be made clear that any predictions are only a guide. It is best to talk in terms of 'days', or 'weeks' or 'months', as appropriate.

For example:

"When we see someone deteriorating from week to week we are often talking in terms of weeks,; when that deterioration is from day to day then we are usually talking in terms of days, but everyone is different."

Patients may have expressed wishes regarding the manner and place of their death. A key factor to facilitating these wishes is for the health professional to know when the patient is dying. However, predicting when someone is going to die is infrequently simple and often complex, particularly when caring for a patient with a long-term chronic illness.

Signs and symptoms of death approaching[1]

The clearest signs of approaching death are picked up by the day-by-day assessment of deterioration (Table 16.1).

Table 16.1 Signs and symptoms of approaching death

Profound tiredness and weakness	Reduced interest in getting out of bed
	Needing assistance with all care
	Less interest in things happening around them
Diminished intake of food and fluids	
Drowsy or reduced cognition	May be disorientated in time and place
	Difficulty concentrating
	Scarcely able to cooperate and converse with carers
Gaunt appearance	
Difficulty swallowing medicine	

1 National Council for Hospice and Specialist Palliative Care Services (2006) *Changing Gear—Guidelines for Managing the Last Days of Life in Adults* (Revised ed). London: NCPC.

Should such symptoms develop suddenly over a matter of days instead of the usual weeks, it is important to exclude a reversible cause of the deterioration such as infection, hypercalcaemia or adverse effects of medication changes.

Goals for the last 24h

- Ensure the patient's comfort physically, emotionally and spiritually
- Make the end-of-life peaceful and dignified
- By care and support given to the dying patient and their carers, make the memory of the dying process as positive as possible

It is very important to continually seek the patient's views on the treatment, and their feelings about it, while they remain conscious, even when the weakening state makes communication difficult. Relatives also need to be given time to have their questions, concerns and requests for information listened to and answered as clearly as possible. As the patient deteriorates, the family's advocate role becomes more important, though their wishes need to be balanced with the palliative care team's understanding of the patient's best interest.

Where possible, families and carers should be offered the opportunity to participate in the physical care of patients. Carers should be invited to stay, if they want to, while nursing and medical procedures are carried out. Very occasionally, relatives would like to participate in carrying out the last offices after death, and this can be a very important part of their last 'duty' on behalf of their dead loved one.

The events and the atmosphere which are present at the time of a patient's death can greatly influence the grieving process of those left behind.

Different cultures

Different religious and cultural groupings have divergent approaches to the dying process. It is important to be sensitive to their possible beliefs. If in doubt, ask a family member. Offence is more likely to be caused by not asking than by asking. (💻 see Chapter 1Oh Chaplaincy).

The patient's wishes

The process of dying is a very individual event. Helping to explore patients' wishes about death and dying should, if possible, take place before final days of life are reached. Important discussions can still, however, take place even at this late phase and professionals should encourage this dialogue. The family gain great comfort in knowing that they have made the most of precious moments and that they have the answers to issues that are important to them. Some of these questions can include preferred place of death or burial/cremation and financial or 'unfinished' business issues. Time to say the last goodbyes to close family members, children and dependants and time to forgive and bury guilt can be crucial to enable a normal bereavement.

Collaborative multidisciplinary approach

Effective terminal care needs a team approach. No single member of the palliative care team, no matter how committed or gifted, can meet all the palliative care needs of a patient and his/her family.

Effective multidisciplinary working depends on:

- Recognizing the centrality of patient and family needs
- Good communication
- Clear understanding and respect for the value, importance and role of other professionals
- Early referral to specialist palliative services if needed

Referral to specialist palliative care services is appropriate when:

- One or more distressing symptoms prove difficult to control
- There is severe emotional distress associated with the patient's condition
- There are dependant children and/or elderly vulnerable relatives

Assessment of patients' needs

The focus of assessment in the last few days of life is to discover what, apart from dying itself, the patient is most concerned about and which concerns need to be addressed. Patients may under-report their symptoms which distress families. Although families may be very helpful in understanding non-verbal cues, in their own distress, they may also misinterpret and exaggerate the patient's symptoms, which needs careful handling.

Physical needs

Common problems that need to be addressed are nausea, pain, oral problems, sleep disturbance, weakness, feeling confused (and sometimes hallucinating), pressure sores as well as the burden of having to take medication. Skilled nursing care can be crucial to ensuring that the patient's comfort is maintained, e.g. using a pressure-relieving mattress to reduce the risk of pressure sores and the need for frequent turning; offering the patient a urinary catheter if they are too weak to get out of bed; and ensuring the mouth is kept clean and moist when nutrition and fluid input is reduced. Patients rarely worry about nutritional and fluid intake, but this may be a major concern for the family.

Psychological needs

The key to psychological assessment is finding out what the patient wants to know in a sensitive and unhurried manner. Gently assessing how the patient feels about their disease and situation can shed light on their needs and distress (Table 16.2). How the patient interprets their disease and its symptoms may be a cause of suffering itself. However, deep probing at this stage is inappropriate as the goal is psychological comfort and peace, **now**.

Anxiety and agitation may need to be managed with medication. Patients are more often concerned about their family at this stage than about themselves.

Table 16.2 Patients' fears

Fears associated with symptoms	e.g. 'the pain will escalate to agony', 'breathing will stop if I fall asleep'
Other emotional distress	e.g. dependence on family ('I am a burden and it would be better if I was out of the way')
Past experience	e.g. past contact with patients who died in unpleasant circumstances and with unresolved issues
Preferences about treatment or withholding treatment	e.g. 'What if nobody listens to me or takes my wishes seriously?'
Fears about morphine	e.g. 'If I use morphine now, it will not work when I really need it'
Death and dying	e.g. Patients frequently adapt to the fact that they will die, but are fearful of the process leading up to death

Dignity (see p. xxxiv)
The palliative care team needs to have as a goal the maintenance of the patient's dignity in a manner which is appropriate to that particular patient. What is dignified for one patient may not be for another, which is one of the reasons why many hospices have both single rooms and small wards.

Spiritual needs
Particular religious tasks may need to be accomplished, for instance absolution, confession or other forms of religious preparation. Spiritual disquiet or pain may be relieved by allowing the expression of feelings and thoughts, particularly of fear and loss of control. Patients are more often concerned about the family at this stage than about themselves and may need to address issues of unresolved conflict or guilt.

Families often want to know that the patient is comfortable and not suffering. If appropriate, it may be helpful for them to be aware of the experiences of people who have had near-death experiences, which are described as tranquil and peaceful. Many mechanisms have been used to explain this phenomenon, including the release of endorphins (natural analgesics), retinal hypoxia with resultant neuronal discharge (particularly in the fovea where there are many neurones) so that a bright spot looks like the end of an inviting tunnel. Temporal lobe seizures may also provide an explanation. Whatever the mechanism, nature seems to have a way of allowing dying people to feel comforted and at peace at the end.

Talking about death and dying

As a taboo subject, few people feel comfortable about discussing death and dying, even though it is natural, certain and is happening all around us all the time.

Opening up discussion can be very liberating to patients who can feel they have not been given permission to talk about dying before as this would be admitting defeat.

Sometimes the direct question 'Are you worried about dying?' is most appropriate.

Often a patient's biggest fears are groundless and reassurances can be given. Where reassurance cannot be given, it is helpful to break the fear down into constituent parts and try to deal with the aspects of the fear that can be dealt with (☐ see Chapter 2 Communication).

Physical examination

Examination at this stage is kept to the minimum to avoid unnecessary distress. Examine:
- Any site of potential pain. Patients may be comfortable at rest but in pain on being turned, which they may not readily admit
- Any relevant area of the body that might be causing discomfort as suggested by the patient's history or non-verbal signs
- Mouth

Investigations

Any investigation at the end of life should have a clear and justifiable purpose, such as excluding reversible conditions where treatment would make the patient more comfortable. There is little need for investigations in the terminal stages.

Review of medication

At this stage comfort is the priority. Unnecessary medication should be stopped but analgesics, antiemetics, anxiolytics/antipsychotics as well as anti-convulsants will need to be continued. If the patient is unable to swallow their essential medicines, an alternative route of administration is necessary. These changes needs to be explained to relatives, who may become anxious that tablets which the patient has had to take for years have now suddenly stopped (☐ see Management of diabetes p. 456–460).

Routes for medicine delivery in the terminal phase

- The **intramuscular** route for injections should be avoided as it is too painful
- If **buccal** medicines are given it is important that the mouth is kept moist
- The **rectal** route can be very useful for certain patients, although it is more or less accepted in different cultures
- **Topical** fentanyl or buprenorphine patches should be avoided for pain in the terminal stage unless they have been used before this time, since it takes too long to titrate against a patient's pain
- In many instances a **syringe driver** is used so that finer adjustments can be made in accord with the patient's changing state

Even when patients are dying, it is often possible to communicate with them and to get their consent for certain treatment, such as subcutaneous medication. As the patient becomes less aware, however, it is the family and the nursing staff who become the patient's advocate. At this point a clear plan of goals needs to be agreed between the doctors, nurses, family members and other carers.

- The potentially sedative side-effects of analgesia needs to be explained
- The use of alternative routes of medication need to be discussed, as the oral route may be more difficult
- The treatment plan should define clearly what should be done in the event of a symptom breakthrough

Common problems in the last 48 hours

- Respiratory tract secretions
- Restlessness/anguish
- Pain see p. 215
- Breathlessness see p. 363–371
- Nausea/vomiting see p. 308–313
- Myoclonic twitching see p. 243

Respiratory Tract Secretions

Weakness in the last few days of life can result in an inability to clear respiratory secretions leading to noisy, moist breathing (death rattle). It occurs in 50% of dying patients and is caused by fluid pooling in the hypopharynx. This is often very distressing to family members, and should be treated prophylactically as it is easier to prevent secretions forming than removing those that have gathered in the upper airways or oropharynx.

Management

General measures include re-positioning the patient and reassuring the relatives. Explain to the family that the noise is due to secretions collecting which are no longer being coughed or cleared as normal. They should also know that the secretions are not causing suffocation, choking or distress.

Specific measures

These specific guidelines are for patients who are imminently dying and develop 'rattling' or 'bubbly' breathing (the death rattle). The following guidelines should be used with caution, particularly if the patient is still aware enough to be distressed by the dry mouth that will result from treatment.

(Acute pulmonary oedema should be excluded, and treated with furo-semide.)

- Give hyoscine hydrobromide 200–400mcg stat subcutaneously, and start hyoscine hydrobromide 1.2–1.6mg/24h CSCI
- Wait for 30min and reassess the patient
- If there is still an unacceptable rattle, and there has not been a marked improvement:
  - give a further dose of hyoscine hydrobromide 200-400mcg stat SC
  - wait for half an hour and reassess
- If the noise has been relieved, but recurs later, give repeat doses of hyoscine hydrobromide 400mcg to a maximum of 800mcg in any 4h
- Increase CSCI to 2.4mg/24h

NB Hyoscine hydrobromide can cause sedation and confusion.

If the patient is conscious, and their respiratory secretions are not too distressing, it may be adequate to use a transdermal patch (Scopaderm 1.5mg over three days or sublingual tablets (Kwells).

- Alternatives to hyoscine hydrobromide include:
  - glycopyrronium bromide 0.2mg stat or CSCI 0.6–1.2mg/24h (glycopyrronium does not cause sedation or confusion. It is useful for the patient who is still conscious and wishes to remain as alert as possible)

- hyoscine butylbromide (Buscopan) 20mg SC stat. and 60–90mg CSCI. Buscopan does not cross the blood–brain barrier, so is less sedating than hyoscine hydrobromide
- If the respiratory rate is >20 breaths/min, the noise may be reduced by slowing the respiratory rate: give e.g. morphine 2.5–5mg SC (or one-sixth of the 24h dose if already on CSCI) and repeat after 30min if the respiratory rate still above 20/min
- If the patient is deeply unconscious, try using gentle suction
- Ensure that the patient is not distressed, using sedative drugs such as midazolam if necessary

Restlessness/Anguish

All potentially reversible causes of agitation (see the 'Think list' below) in the terminal phase should be excluded. A diagnosis of terminal agitation can only be made if reversible conditions are excluded or are failing to respond to treatment. If the patient is clearly distressed, some degree of sedation will probably be warranted. This decision should be discussed with the patient, if at all possible, and the family if they are also involved in the discussions.

'Think list' for some common reversible causes of terminal agitation:
- Pain
- Urinary retention
- Full rectum
- Nausea
- Cerebral irritability
- Anxiety and fear
- Side-effects of medication
- Poor positioning

Management

Examination and explanation

Once any treatable causes of agitation have been excluded it is important to inform the family in attendance of your clinical findings, and of the management options, emphasizing clearly that the goals of treatment in this situation are primarily comfort and dignity.

Medication

- Midazolam 5–10mg SC stat. and 30–60mg/24h given by CSCI. If the patient remains distressed, other medication (e.g. levomepromazine) should be added. Clonazepam (1–4mg CSCI/24h) is sometimes used instead of midazolam, particularly if the patient has neuropathic pain and can no longer take effective medication by mouth.
- Levomepromazine 25mg SC stat and 50–100mg/24h by CSCI. It is unusual for patients to require larger doses but, if necessary, up to 200mg/24h can be given.
- Haloperidol 5mg SC stat. and 10–20mg/24h **CSCI** may be used but extrapyramidal symptoms can occur, particularly at higher doses.
- Phenobarbital 100mg SC stat and 300–600mg/24h by CSCI should be effective but higher doses may be needed; a second syringe driver is needed as phenobarbital is incompatible with most other drugs.

If a syringe driver is unavailable, alternative phenothiazines or benzodiazepines may be given sublingually or rectally, e.g. chlorpromazine 25mg per rectum 4–6 hourly with escalation to response (up to 100–200mg 4h) and/or diazepam rectally 10mg p.r.n. or clonazepam sublingually 0.5mg and titrate upwards.

- Propofol, an anaesthetic agent, has been used intravenously to treat intractable cases, although under specialist supervision.

Cerebral oedema

Rising intracranial pressure due to cerebral oedema, in the terminal stages of cerebral tumours, can cause a rapid and severe escalation of headache (which can be made worse by opioids) and terminal agitation. Generous doses of opioids, however, may be effective in addition to an NSAID and midazolam. Avoid drugs that will lower the seizure threshold such as levomepromazine unless given with adequate doses of a benzodiazepine. In a dying unconscious or semiconscious patient, it should not be necessary to replace oral steroids with subcutaneous steroids provided that adequate pain control and sedation is given. Usually by this stage the oedema is not well controlled by steroids and, at best, may only serve to prolong the dying phase.

The Liverpool Care Pathway for the dying patient

Sections detailing the last few days of life, practical issues and bereavement in this Handbook clearly outline good practice for the care of the dying. The Liverpool Integrated Care Pathway for the Dying Patient (LCP) aims to translate such best practice into a template of care to guide health-care professionals with limited or infrequent experience of caring for dying patients. The LCP provides guidance on the different aspects of care required, including comfort measures, anticipatory prescribing of medicines and discontinuation of inappropriate interventions. In the UK the LCP is widely used within hospitals, hospices, care homes and the community setting.

There are three sections of the LCP for the dying patient:
1 Initial assessment
2 Ongoing care
3 Care after death

Initiating the Liverpool Care Pathway for the dying patient (LCP)—diagnosing dying

Before a patient is commenced on the LCP it is important that the MDT has agreed that the patient is in the dying phase. This decision in itself can sometimes lead to conflict within the team, but it is important to make a clear diagnosis if appropriate care and communication is to be achieved.

In cancer patients, if the patient's condition has been deteriorating over a period, i.e. the last weeks/days, and two of the following four criteria apply:
• Bed-bound
• Semi-comatose
• Only able to take sips of fluid
• Unable to take tablets

it is likely that the patient is entering the dying phase. **These criteria may not be appropriate in a non-cancer population**. It is important to highlight that a patient who is clinically in the dying phase may occasionally recover and stabilize for a time. However, this should not prevent the clinical team from using the LCP to provide the appropriate physical, psychological, social and spiritual care.

The three sections of the Liverpool Care Pathway for the dying patient

Section 1—Initial assessment see Fig. 16.1
This section identifies the key goals that should be achieved when a patient enters the dying phase. These goals are directly related to and support the guidance referred to this chapter. A key component of the LCP is the supporting guidelines for the symptoms of pain, nausea/vomiting, agitation and respiratory tract secretions. These guidelines ensure that the appropriate oral medication is converted to a subcutaneous regimen and that patients have p.r.n. (as required) medication available should they require it.

In care settings where the LCP is not in common usage, healthcare professionals can use the goals of care in Fig. 16.1 to guide and inform their practice.

Section 2—Ongoing care
The LCP promotes multidisciplinary working and a joint approach to the care of the patient and their family. In caring for a dying patient, at least four-hourly observations of symptom control should be made, and the appropriate action taken if problems are identified. Particular attention is given to pain, agitation, respiratory tract secretions, nausea and vomiting, mouthcare and micturition problems. In addition, support regarding the psychological, social and spiritual aspects of care for both the family and the patient need to be continued in the dying phase.

Section 3—Care after death
The LCP incorporates the certification of death within the document, identifies any special needs for the patient who has died and support for the family and carers immediately after death. It particularly focuses on the information needs of the family at this distressing time.

How does using the Liverpool Care Pathway benefit patients?
In providing a template of care for the dying phase, the LCP promotes discussion within the clinical team with regard to the diagnosis of dying, and facilitates the initiation of care that is appropriate for the dying phase. The LCP integrates local and national guidelines into clinical practice. This powerful educational tool can be used to facilitate the role of specialist palliative care teams and to empower generic health workers to deliver a model of excellence for the care of the dying. Healthcare professionals also benefit by knowing that they have delivered a good standard of care to the patient. In the words of the National Cancer Plan 'The care of all dying patients must be improved to the level of the best.'

Example of Chart in LCP - Initial Assessment.

COMFORT MEASURES	**Goal 1: Current medication assessed and non essentials discontinued** Yes ☐ No ☐ Appropriate oral drugs converted to subcutaneous route and syringe driver commenced if appropriate Inappropriate medication discontinued
	Goal 2: PRN subcutaneous medication written up for list below as per protocol (see blue sheets at back of ICP for guidance) Pain — Analgesia — **Yes ☐ No ☐** Nausea and vomiting — Antiemetic — **Yes ☐ No ☐** Agitation — Sedative — **Yes ☐ No ☐** Respiratory tract secretions — Anticholinergic — **Yes ☐ No ☐**
	Goal 3: Discontinue inappropriate interventions Blood test — **Yes ☐ No ☐ N/A ☐** Antibiotics — **Yes ☐ No ☐ N/A ☐** i V's (fluids/medications) — **Yes ☐ No ☐ N/A ☐** Not for cardiopulmonary resuscitation — **Yes ☐ No ☐** (Please record below & complete appropriate associated documentation–policy/ procedure)
	Goal 3a: Decisions to discontinue inappropriate nursing interventions taken **Yes ☐ No ☐** Routine turning regime – reposition for comfort only – consider pressure relieving mattress–and appropriate assessments re skin integrity–Taking Vital Signs
	Goal 3b: Syringe driver set up within 4 h of Doctor's order **Yes ☐ No ☐ N/A ☐**
PSYCHOLOGICAL/ INSIGHT	**Goal 4: Ability to communicate in English assessed as adequate** a) Patient — **Yes ☐ No ☐ Comatosed ☐** b) Family/other — **Yes ☐ No ☐**
	Goal 5: Insight into condition assessed Aware of diagnosis a) Patient — **Yes ☐ No ☐ Comatosed ☐** b) Family/other — **Yes ☐ No ☐** Recognition of dying c) Patient — **Yes ☐ No ☐ Comatosed ☐** d) Family/other — **Yes ☐ No ☐**
RELIGIOUS/ *SPIRITUAL SUPPORT*	**Goal 6: a) Religious/spiritual needs assessed with patient** **Yes ☐ No ☐ Comatosed ☐** **b) Religious/spiritual needs assessed with family/other** **Yes ☐ No ☐** Patient/other may be anxious for self/others Consider support of chaplaincy team Religious tradition identified, if yes specify:................ **Yes ☐ No ☐ N/A☐** Support of chaplaincy-team offered **Yes ☐ No ☐** In-house support Tel/Bleep No: .... Name .... Date/Time .... External support Tel/Bleep No: .... Name .... Date/Time .... Special needs now, at time of impending death, at death and after death identified:- ....
COMMUNICATION WITH FAMILY/OTHER	**Goal 7: Identify how family/other are to be informed of patient's impending death** **Yes ☐ No ☐** At any time ☐ Not at night-time ☐ Stay overnight at hospital ☐ Primary contact name .... Relationship to patient .... Tel no: .... Secondary contact .... Tel no:.........
	Goal 8: Family/other given hospital information on:- **Yes ☐ No ☐** Concession car parking; accommodation; dining room facilities; payphones; washrooms and toilet facilities on the ward; visiting times. Any other relevant information
COMMUNICATION WITH PRIMARY HEALTHCARE TEAM	**Goal 9: GP Practice is aware of patient's condition** **Yes ☐ No ☐** GP Practice to be contacted if unaware patient is dying
SUMMARY	**Goal 10: Plan of care explained & discussed with:-** a) Patient — **Yes ☐ No ☐ Comatosed ☐** b) Family/other — **Yes ☐ No ☐**
	Goal 11: Family/other express understanding of plan care. **Yes ☐ No ☐** Family/other aware that LCP commenced and their concerns identified and documented

Fig. 16.1 Initial assessment and care of the dying patient. (Adapted from The Liverpool Care Pathway for the Dying Patient[2])

2 Ellershaw J. E., Wilkinson S. (eds) (2003) *Care of the Dying: A Pathway to Excellence*. Oxford: Oxford University Press.

International perspectives in care pathways

An integrated care pathway for India

The successes of the Liverpool Care Pathway (LCP) in the UK have led to considerations of its use further afield. As an example, this section details the development of an integrated care pathway for end-of-life care in India.

Palliative care in India

There are currently 100 palliative care physicians working in India, a country with a population of over one billion. Despite islands of high-quality palliative care, the national average for coverage of palliative care remains under 1%. With the burden of chronic diseases being increasingly shouldered by resource-poor countries, the development of comprehensive palliative care services is an imperative. Attempts to develop these services should focus on the provision of services in areas of unmet need, to measure and improve the quality of existing centres as well as the capabilities for training health professionals in palliative care.

The role of the LCP in India

- To improve existing services through the process of setting standards of best practice and audit
- To facilitate the spread of skills from established palliative care centres to new, developing services (*specialist–specialist*)
- To facilitate the spread of skills and knowledge from palliative care centres to general healthcare settings (*specialist–generalist*)
- As an educational tool for both specialist palliative care workers and general healthcare workers

The Indian project

One of the fundamental principles of an integrated care pathway is that it reflects locally determined best practice. Ownership is critical for the success of the LCP. Thus, a pathway developed in one setting cannot be exported and used in another, but must be redesigned to incorporate local needs. The process of the multidisciplinary team sitting together to determine their standards of best practice is integral to the success of the LCP.

The pathway was redesigned in an established centre of excellence by multidisciplinary focus groups 'blind' to the goals of the LCP. This produced a generic pathway for use in the Indian setting. The LCP Central Team UK recommend that the goals of care remain the same during the translation process and, therefore, were coded in sequence to enable the future benchmarking of LCP's success across sector, organizations and countries. The LCP India fully complied with this process and was ratified by the LCP Central Team UK.

The pathway is now undergoing piloting in four centres around the country, after being adapted locally at each setting. These pilot centres cover a range of settings, from hospice and hospital to the community.

Results from the first pilot centre

A comparison of the documentation pre- and post-implementation of the pathway shows improvement in almost all parameters, from anticipatory prescribing to the discussion of emotional issues with family members. Analysis of the improvement showed both an increase in documentation of care and in the care actually given.

A series of semi-structured interviews was conducted with the original focus group, six months after the introduction of the pathway. There has been a very positive reception to the project. Comments centred around five main themes:

Improved documentation
'The pathway means we have improved documentation of things like the patient's address which has stopped a lot of confusion at the time of the death certificate. Generally, we can see what care we have given the patient over the past day. This was really needed.'

Addressing emotional issues
'Emotional issues of the patient and family are a higher priority now we are using the pathway'

Communication
'It allows us to tell the family what is happening directly and clearly'

Improved observations
'The regular checking of symptoms is good and improves the interaction and relationship with the patients and relatives.'

Training
'If there is a new member of staff it is easy to teach them how best to care for the dying on the ward'

Difficulties

The concept of 'variance' has proved difficult to explain to staff. This has often led to the pathway being used as a set of guidelines rather than an integrated care pathway. New staff require training before using the pathway, which can take a significant amount of time. Staff members are reluctant to stop recording information in the original case sheet, leading to a duplication of documentation. Variance analysis must be undertaken by staff and this is an added burden for a busy team.

The future

After completion of the four pilot projects in India generic documentation for each of the settings will be produced. A core team of national trainers will then be developed to allow training days to be run for new centres interested in using the pathway. The pathway will then be launched nationally and a formal evaluation will follow.

Further reading

Books

de Luc K. (2000) *Developing Care Pathways*. Oxford: Radcliffe Medical Press.

Department of Health (2000) *The NHS Cancer Plan—A Plan for Investment, A Plan for Reform*. London: DoH.

Ellershaw J. E., Wilkinson S. (eds) (2003) *Care of the Dying: A Pathway to Excellence*. Oxford: Oxford University Press.

Fenwick P., Fenwick E. (2008) *The Art of Dying*. London: Continuum.

Articles

Campbell. *et al.* (1998) Integrated care pathways. *British Medical Journal*, **316**: 133–7.

Ellershaw J. *et al.* (2001) Care of the dying. *Journal of Pain and Symptom Management*, **21**: 12–17.

Elllershaw J. E., Ward C. (2003) Care of the dying patient: the last hours or days of life. *British Medical Journal*, **326**: 30–4.

Wee B.L. (2008) Death battle: its impact on staff and volunteers in palliative care. *Palliative Medicine* **22**(2): 173–176.

Bereavement

> How small and selfish is sorrow. But it bangs one about until one is quite senseless.
>
> Queen Elizabeth the Queen Mother, in a letter to Edith Sitwell shortly after the death of King George VI

Grief is a normal reaction to a bereavement or other major loss. Its manifestations will vary from person to person but will often include physical, cognitive, behavioural and emotional elements. For a close personal bereavement, grief is likely to continue for a long time and may recur in a modified form, stimulated by anniversaries, future losses or other reminders. Although people are likely to be changed by the experience of grieving, most, in time, find they are able to function well and enjoy life again. A compassionate approach surrounding the death can positively impact on bereavement.

Normal manifestations of grief

Physical manifestations

Symptoms experienced by a bereaved person may include a hollow feeling in the stomach, tightness in the chest or throat, oversensitivity to noise, shortness of breath, muscle weakness, lack of energy and dry mouth. People may misinterpret these symptoms as indications of a serious illness and require reassurance.

Emotional manifestations

For many, a sense of shock and numbness is the initial emotional response to bereavement. Feelings of anger (directed at family, friends, medical staff, God, the deceased or no one in particular) and feelings of guilt (relating to real or imagined failings) are common, as is a yearning or desire for the return of the deceased. Anxiety and a sense of helplessness and disorganization are also normal responses. Sadness is the most commonly recognized manifestation of grief, but the greatest depth of sadness, something akin to depression, is often not reached until many months after the death. Feelings of relief and freedom may also be present, although people may then feel guilty for having these feelings.

Cognitive manifestations

Disbelief and a sense of unreality are frequently present early in a bereavement. The bereaved may be preoccupied with thoughts about the deceased and ruminate about the lost person. It is also not uncommon for the bereaved to have a sense (visual, auditory, etc.) of the presence of the deceased. Short-term memory, the ability to concentrate and sense of purpose are frequently detrimentally affected.

Behavioural manifestations

Appetite and sleep may be disturbed, and dreams that involve the deceased, with their attendant emotional impact for the bereaved, are not infrequent. The bereaved person may withdraw socially, avoid reminders of the deceased or act in an absent-minded way. They may also engage in restless overactivity, behaviour which suggests that they are at some level searching for the deceased, or visit places or carry objects that remind them of the deceased. Some people contemplate rapid and radical changes in their lifestyle (e.g. new relationship or move of house), which may represent a way of avoiding the pain of bereavement. Such rapid changes soon after a bereavement are not normally advisable.

Psychological/psychiatric models

He was my North, my South, my East and West,
My working week and my Sunday rest,
My noon, my midnight, my talk, my song;
I thought that love would last forever: I was wrong.
W.H. Auden (1907–73): *Funeral Blues*, 1936

Grief and bereavement have been analysed over many years, and it is generally agreed that there are no single 'correct' or 'true' theories that explain the experience of loss or account for the emotions, experiences and cultural practices which characterize grief and mourning. Within broad cultural constraints, individuals manage bereavement in different ways, reflecting the diverse range of human responses and cultures. In the UK there are a number of accepted ways to behave, but most are characterized by stoicism and emotional restraint, especially in public. In contrast, bereavement support services emphasize the importance of emotional expression, acknowledgement of the reality of the loss and the sharing of thoughts and feelings with others.

Theories of grief

Most cultures provide accounts of what happens after death (such as religious accounts of an after-life) and provide guidance about how the bereaved should feel and behave, but in an increasingly secular society these may now have less influence. The range of beliefs, practices and rituals associated with death is large, particularly in multicultural societies, although many adapt to the customs of the host culture.

Psychological models

These are based on developmental notions of change and growth. It is assumed that bereavement is a process in which there is an outcome: individuals need to progress through phases or stages and tasks need to be accomplished. The theories are based on the assumption that people have some control over their feelings and thoughts and that these can be accessed through talk. Individuals need to accept the reality of the loss so that the emotional energy can be released and redirected.

The effortful, mental process of withdrawing energy from the lost person is referred to as 'grief work'. It is regarded as essential to break relationships with the deceased, and to allow reinvestment of emotional energy in new relationships with others.

The most influential and earliest theories emerged from psychoanalysts such as Freud,[1] who also described normal and pathological grief. Bowlby[2] proposed a complex theory of close human relationships in which separation triggers intense distress and behavioural responses. Parkes[3] proposed that people progress through phases in coming to terms with their loss and that they have to adapt to changes in relationships, social status and economic circumstances. Kubler Ross[4] also proposed a staged model of the emotional expression of loss, described in terms of shock/denial, anger, bargaining, depression and ultimately acceptance.

Worden[5] based his therapeutic model on phases of grief and tasks of mourning. He suggested that grief was a process, not a state, and that people needed to work through their reactions to loss to achieve a complete adjustment. Tasks that need to be accomplished in order to allow recovery from mourning included:

Task 1—To accept the reality of the loss
Task 2—To experience the pain of grief
Task 3—To adjust to an environment in which the deceased is missing
Task 4—To emotionally relocate the deceased and move on with life

Each of these theories have been modified and developed by their authors and, despite subsequent criticisms, they remain very popular ways to explain bereavement and grief and are used by the public and health professionals. Staged or phased models provide guidance that bereaved people are progressing satisfactorily along a path over time, even though this progression may not be linear. However, some people may become 'stuck' and unable to move through grief satisfactorily. Various techniques are used to support and encourage people to move forward and to begin engaging in life again.

Stress and coping model

These ideas are based on an assumption that if certain things, called 'stressors', are present in sufficient amounts, then they trigger a stress response which is both physical and psychological. People are able to adapt to most things, but things that challenge the adaptation process are considered to be stressful. Lazarus and Folkman's transactional model of stress and coping[6] proposed that any event may be seen as threatening, and that cognitive appraisal is undertaken to estimate the degree of threat needed to mobilize the resources to cope with it. Coping may focus on

1 Freud, S. (1961) Mourning and melancholia. In *The Standard Edition of the Complete Psychological Works of Sigmund Freud*, Vol. 14 (ed. and transl. J. Strachey), pp. 243–58. London: Hogarth Press. (Original work published 1917.)

2 Bowlby J. (1969) *Attachment and Loss*, Vol. 1. Harmondsworth: Penguin.

3 Parkes C. M. (1996). *Bereavement* (3rd edn). London: Routledge.

4 Kubler-Ross E. (1969) *On Death and Dying*. London: Tavistock Publications.

5 Worden J. W. (1991) *Grief Counselling and Grief Therapy* (2nd edn). London: Routledge.

6 Lazarus R., Folkman S. (1991) *Stress and Coping* (3rd edn). New York: Columbia University Press.

dealing with the threat directly (problem-focused), or may emphasize the emotional response (emotion-focused). Stroebe and Schut[7] developed this idea, proposing that after death people oscillate between restoration-focused coping (dealing with everyday life) and grief-focused coping (e.g. expressing their distress). People move between these extremes but become more restoration-focused with time. This is known as the 'dual processing model'.

Social and relationship-focused models

This is based on an assumption that people wish to maintain feelings of continuity and that, even though physical relationships may end at the time of death, relationships become transformed but remain important within the memory of the bereaved individual. Walters[8] in the UK and Klass et al.[9] in the US, have suggested that continuing relationships (emotional bonds), emphasize the importance for the living of integrating the memory of the dead into their ongoing lives, recognizing the enduring influence of the deceased.

7 Stroebe M., Schut H. (1999) The dual process model of coping with bereavement. *Death Studies*, **23**: 197–224.

8 Walters T. (1996) A new model of grief. *Mortality*, **1**: 7–25.

9 Klass D., Silverman P., Nickman S. (eds) (1996) *Continuing Bonds*. London: Taylor & Francis.

Bereavement support

Give sorrow words. The grief that does not speak whispers the o'er-fraught heart, and bids it break.

William Shakespeare, *Macbeth*, iv, iii, 209–10

In practice, bereavement support, whether through GPs or professional accredited counsellors, helps clients tell their story. GPs may become involved in grief counselling, but their main role is to screen for people who may be most at risk (📖 see p. 875–6) from a complicated bereavement. Most bereaved people manage well with their own resources and with the help of community and faith groups such as Cruse (a charity offering free bereavement counselling and support groups).

Specialist palliative care and bereavement

The philosophy of the hospice movement encompasses the care of patients and their families after death and into the bereavement period. The provision of bereavement support is regarded as integral to their services. Most services are based on the assumption that bereavement is a major stressful life event but that a minority of people experience substantial disruption to their physical, psychological and social functioning. A multidisciplinary team (MDT), including social workers, nurses, chaplains, counsellors and doctors, is usually involved. But, occasionally, clients present such difficult and complex problems that psychiatrists, clinical psychologists or other specialist healthcare workers may be required. NICE[10] recommends that three levels of support should be available, depending upon the complexity of the needs of the bereaved person.

- **Component 1**: All bereaved people should be offered information about grief and how to access support services
- **Component 2**: About one-third may require additional support to help them deal with the emotional and psychological impact of loss by death
- **Component 3**: Specialist interventions are required by a small proportion (7–10%), which will involve referral to a range of services including mental health services, psychological support services, specialist counselling services, etc.

There is evidence that offering support to people who have adequate internal and external resources can be disempowering and detrimental to their coping. Bereavement support may include a broad range of activities such as social evenings, befriending, one-to-one counselling and support groups, etc. (Table 17.1).

10 NICE (2004) Services for families and carers, including bereavement care. In *Improving Supportive and Palliative Care for Adults with Cancer*. Chapter 12. London: NICE.

Table 17.1 Types of hospice and palliative care bereavement support for adults

Social activities	Supportive activities	Therapeutic activities
Condolence cards	Drop-in centre/coffee mornings	One-to-one counselling with professional or trained volunteer
Anniversary (of death) cards	Self-help groups	Therapeutic support groups
Bereavement information leaflets	Information support groups	Drama, music or art therapy
Bereavement information resources (videos/books)	Volunteer visiting or befriending	Relaxation classes
Staff attending the funeral		Complementary therapies
Social evenings	Psychotherapy	
Memorial service or other rituals		

From M. Lloyd-Williams (ed.) (2003) *Psychosocial Issues in Palliative Care.* Oxford: Oxford University Press.

Complicated grief

Normal and abnormal responses to bereavement cover a continuum in which intensity of reaction, presence of a range of related grief behaviours, and time course betray the presence of an abnormal grief response.

Complicated grief involves the presentation of certain grief-related symptoms at a time beyond that which is considered adaptive. We hypothesize that the presence of these symptoms after approximately 6 months puts the bereaved individual at heightened risk for enduring social, psychological and medical impairment.

Prigerson, *et al.*, 1995

Complicated mourning means that, given the amount of time since the death, there is some compromise, distortion or failure of one or more of the…processes of mourning.

Full realization of the pain of living without the deceased is denied, repressed or avoided The deceased is held on to as though alive. Symptoms do not resolve spontaneously and need active intervention

Rando, 1993

…is more related to the intensity of a reaction or the duration of a reaction rather than the presence or absence of a specific behavior.

Worden, 1982

Risk factors for developing complicated grief

Personal
- Markedly angry, ambivalent or dependent relationship with the deceased
- History of multiple losses and/or concurrent losses
- Mental health problems
- Perceived lack of social support

Circumstantial
- Sudden, unexpected death, especially when violent, mutilating or random
- Death from an overly lengthy illness such as dementia
- Loss of a child
- Mourner's perception of loss as preventable

Historical
- Previous experience with complicated grief
- Insecurity in childhood attachments

Personality
- Inability to tolerate extremes of emotional distress
- Inability to tolerate dependency feelings
- Self-concept, role and value of 'being strong'

Social
- Socially unspeakable loss (e.g. suicide)
- Socially negated loss (e.g. loss of ex-spouse)
- Absence of social support network
- Absence of a body on which to conduct funeral rites (e.g. lost at sea)

Complicated grief includes the following in abnormal intensity or duration (Table 17.2):
• Symptoms of depression
• Symptoms of anxiety
• Grief-specific symptoms of extraordinary intensity and duration that include:
  • preoccupation with thoughts of the deceased
  • disbelief
  • feelings of being stunned
• Lack of acceptance of the death
• Yearning for the deceased
• Searching for the deceased
• Crying

Common psychiatric disorders related to grief include:
• Clinical depression
• Anxiety disorders, alcohol abuse or other substance abuse and dependence
• Psychotic disorders
• Post-traumatic stress disorder (PTSD)

While frank psychiatric disorders following bereavement are reasonably straightforward to diagnose, it is more difficult to pick up complicated grief, in which the pathological nature of the grief response is only distinguishable from normal grief by its character. Recognition of complicated bereavement calls for an experienced clinical judgement that does not 'rationalize' the distress as understandable.

Table 17.2 Clinical presentations of complicated grief

Category	Features
Inhibited or delayed grief	Avoidance postpones expression
Chronic grief	Perpetuation of mourning long-term
Traumatic grief	Unexpected and shocking form of death
Depressive disorders	Both major and minor depressions
Anxiety disorders	Insecurity and relational problems
Alcohol and substance abuse/dependence	Excessive use of substances impairs adaptive coping
Post-traumatic stress disorder	Persistent, intrusive images with cues
Psychotic disorders	Manic, severe depressive states, and schizophrenia

From Doyle D. H., et al. (eds). (2004) *Oxford Textbook of Palliative Medicine* (3rd edn), p. 1140. Oxford: Oxford University Press.

Warning signs of complicated grief

- Long-term functional impairment
- Exaggerated, prolonged and intense grief reactions
- Significant neglect of self-care
- Substance overuse or abuse
- Frequent themes of loss in conversation, activity, behaviour
- Idealization of the deceased
- Impulsive decision-making
- Mental disorders following loss
- PTSD-like symptoms

Ways of helping a bereaved person

- 'Being there' for them
- Non-judgemental listening
- Encouraging them to talk about the deceased
- Giving permission for the expression of feelings
- Offering reassurance about the normality of feelings and experiences
- Promoting coping with everyday life and self-care (e.g. adequate food intake)
- Screening for damaging behaviours (e.g. increased alcohol use, smoking, etc.)
- Providing information, when requested, about the illness and death of their loved ones—also about the range of grief responses
- Educating others (family members and other support networks) about how best to help the bereaved person
- Becoming familiar with your own feelings about loss and grief
- Offering information about local bereavement support services, e.g. hospice services or Cruse

Bereavement involving children

One feature of the grief of most children is that they do not sustain grief over continuing periods of time, but tend rather to dip in and out of grief—jumping in and out of puddles, rather than wading through the river of grief.

Adults should be aware that children will learn what is 'acceptable grief' from the adults around them.

Childhood bereavement services seek to support children with their loss experience and to help parents deal with a bereaved child.

Payne and Rolls (2008)

Children's grief

Children may be bereaved of family members (e.g. siblings, parents or grandparents) and this will precipitate a cascade of changes and loss. They will become a child of bereaved parents who may need help in dealing with their own loss and also help in how to parent a bereaved child. Children will be helped by knowing that the expression of feelings is acceptable. Children may express their emotions and grief in many ways, e.g. through play, artwork, music, drama, etc.

Children's understanding, responses and needs will be affected by many factors, including their previous experiences of loss and how these were handled. It is also important to consider the age and the developmental level of the child, although any attempt to consider responses according to age will require flexibility as there is, of course, considerable crossover between different children.

Children under the age of 2–3 years may have little concept of death, but will be aware of separation and may protest against this by detachment or regressive behaviour. Children of this age need a consistent caregiver, familiar routines and the meeting of their physical and emotional needs.

Children aged between 3 and 5 years do not see death as irreversible. Rather, their concerns will relate to separation, abandonment and the physical aspects of death and dying. Their response may include aggressive and rejecting behaviour. They may also become withdrawn or demonstrate an increase in clinging or demanding behaviour. There may also be regression to infant needs. Routine, comfort, reassurance and a simple answering of their questions will help a child of this age. They should be allowed to participate in family rituals and to keep mementos of the deceased. Adults should be aware of the words they use since they can be misinterpreted (e.g. do not associate death with sleep or a long journey).

Children aged between 6 and 8 years seek causal explanations. A whole range of behaviours may be evidence of their response to grief—withdrawal, sadness, loneliness, depression, acting-out behaviour or becoming a 'perfect' child. Short, honest, concrete explanations will help a child of this age, as will maintaining contact with friends and normal activities. Short-term regression may be allowed and they should be reassured that they will always be cared for. Involvement in the family's grief-related rituals will also help.

Pre-teenage children appear to have a calmer and more accepting attitude to death. They often have a good factual understanding of what has happened. The child should be encouraged to talk about the deceased and be provided with clear and truthful answers to their questions. The feelings of adults do not need to be hidden, allowing the child to provide mutual help and reassurance.

Teenaged-year children are engaged in a search for meaning and purpose in life and for their identity. They feel that they have deep and powerful emotions that no one else has experienced. Teenagers may exhibit withdrawal, sadness, loneliness and depression, or else they may act-out in an angry, hostile and rejecting way. They may seek to cover up fears with joking and sarcasm. Young people of this age need as much comfort as possible, involvement, boundaries, a sense that their feelings are being taken seriously and reassurance that their feelings are normal. Continuing contact with their peers should be encouraged. Young people will often identify for themselves someone with whom they feel comfortable to talk.

Risk factors for complicated grief in bereaved children

These may be divided into three groups:

Features of the loss
- Traumatic
- Unexpected

Features of the child
- History of psychiatric disorder
- Multiple losses
- Child under 5 years old
- Adolescent

Features of the relationship
- Ambivalent/conflicted
- Unsupportive family
- Death of a father (adolescent boys)
- Death of a mother (very young children)
- Mental illness in surviving parent
- Child of a single parent who has died

Bereavement due to death of a child

The death of a child is a devastating loss, particularly in times where most childhood illness can be prevented or cured. It profoundly affects all those involved—parents, siblings, grandparents, extended family, friends and others involved in caring for the child. As a community we rarely experience the death of a child, which makes it all the more difficult when we do. There is a sense that the natural order of things has been upset.

Principles for working with bereaved parents
- Make early contact and assess the bereaved parents
- Provide assurance that they can survive their loss, but acknowledge the uniqueness of their pain
- Allow adequate time for parents to grieve
- Facilitate the identification and expression of feelings, including negative feelings such as anger and guilt
- Encourage recall of memories of the deceased child
- Maintain a professional and realistic perspective—not all pain can be 'fixed'
- Allow for individual differences in response relating to gender, age, culture, personality, religion and the characteristics of the death
- Assist in finding a source of continuing support
- Promote confidence in their parenting of their surviving children
- Identify complicated grief reactions and refer to the appropriate services

Interpret resolution of grief to parents, and that it is not a betrayal of their deceased child. Health professionals need to recognize the significance they may have in a family's life. Many children are treated over long periods and the hospital/hospice may become something of a second home. Health professionals also care for families during the intense highs and lows of serious illness, and may even be present at the time the child dies. The significance of this cannot be overstated. These relationships cannot be abruptly ended and many (but not all) families will want ongoing contact with those people they feel truly understand what they have experienced. A follow-up appointment with the child's paediatrician should always be offered to discuss the child's illness and treatment, the results of any outstanding investigations including post-mortem examinations and how the family is coping.

Sibling grief

Siblings almost universally experience distress, but many feel unable to share this for fear of burdening their already fragile parents. One of the many factors which influence sibling grief is developmental level and the impact this has on the child's understanding of illness and death.

Most children learn to recognize when something is dead before they reach three years of age. However, at this early age, death, separation and sleep are almost synonymous in the child's mind. As children develop and experience life, their concept of death becomes more mature. Table 17.3 shows the six subconcepts acquired during this process (average age of attainment in brackets).

Table 17.3 Six subconcepts of children's understanding of death

Separation (age 5)	Dead people do not coexist with the living
Causality (age 6)	Death is caused by something, be it trauma, disease, or old age
Irreversibility (age 6)	A dead person can not 'come alive' again
Cessation of bodily functions (age 6)	The dead person does not need to eat or breathe
Universality (age 7)	All living things will die
Insensitivity (age 8)	The dead can not feel fear or pain

Supporting bereaved children

- Adjusting to the loss of a loved person does not necessarily require 'letting go' of the relationship. Indeed, bereaved children (and adults) often maintain a connection to the dead person. The relationship is reconstructed over time and maintained by remembering the person, keeping their belongings and sometimes talking to them. Children spend most of their time in the care of their parents. It is therefore important to empower parents to support siblings by equipping them with knowledge and ideas. Staff can encourage the family to:
  - **provide information** in simple, developmentally appropriate language
  - **be alert to misunderstandings** which may arise as a consequence of an incomplete death concept
  - set aside special **time** for the child/young person

- openly **express** emotion
- recruit family, friends and teachers to help
- **allow the child to play** with friends and reassure them that it is OK to have fun
- help the child **create memories**, e.g. stories, photos, drawings, memory books
- **maintain normal routines and discipline** as much as possible
- allow the child/young person opportunities to feel in control
- resist any temptation to 'fix their grief'
- encourage them to do what feels right for them
- be there—to provide love, reassurance and routine
- **allow the child time alone**. Private 'space' is important
- **talk** about the death
- **answer questions**, no matter how explicit
- do not be surprised if children use symbolic play, stories and art to make sense of their experience.

School grief

The following is adapted from *A Practical Guide to Paediatric Oncology Palliative Care*, Royal Children's Hospital, Brisbane, 1999.

After the family, the school community may contain the people most affected by the death of a child—friends, fellow students, teachers, administrative staff. Parents form part of a wider school community. It may well be the first bereavement experience for the child's peers, their parents and teachers. Close attachments are formed between children and their teachers, so that the death of a child may be a personal as well as a professional loss.

In a school, there will be a range of grief responses. It is anticipated that both staff and students will be vulnerable to stress and may express themselves differently. For the student, the closer they were to the child the more profound will be the consequences. Teachers may notice a change in the other student's behaviour, thought processes, concentration and academic performance. A greater level of support, monitoring and care may be warranted, even for those students who may not be expressing their grief in an obvious way.

People who may be at increased risk are:
- Those who have already experienced significant loss in their lives
- Those who have a close relationship with the child who has died or the child's siblings, and those who have similar health problems themselves or in their family

The school is in an ideal position to provide opportunities for students to be supported as well as to identify those who may be experiencing difficulty. The child's parents should always be consulted before any information is released so that their privacy and the best interests of any siblings are considered and respected.

Ways in which the school can help include:
- Informing staff and students of the child's death as a priority. Anxiety and misinformation are fuelled by uncertainty and delay
- Senior staff need to acknowledge the sadness of what has happened, perhaps by way of assemblies, class announcements and letters home

- Staff and children need the opportunity to talk about what has happened, to ask questions and to express their feelings. This is best done in familiar small groups, though it may also be appropriate to set aside a time when people can come and talk together. Students can also be given opportunities to write farewell letters or tributes, and to create artwork as an expression of their thoughts and feelings
- A sense of routine provides reassurance to staff and students who have experienced trauma. It is, therefore, important that the school continues to function as a supportive and stable part of the staff and students' environment
- Staff need their own support. Staff meetings provide an opportunity to provide information, monitor the reactions of the children and discuss feelings. In some cases, it may be helpful to hold a special meeting facilitated by someone with expertise in this area. Senior staff are usually required to manage the immediate crisis and may experience a 'delayed reaction'
- The school can maintain contact with the family in a number of ways. This may be through friends or formal rituals. Some families welcome the participation of the school in the funeral for example, and may wish to be involved in school memorial services. The child may also have expressed wishes regarding the involvement of their school friends

Assessment of bereavement risk

The assessment of bereavement risk presupposes that some individuals will display a grief reaction that does not fit a 'normal' or expected pattern or level of intensity. The factors that influence complicated bereavement are:

- Stage of the life cycle particularly when:
  - the bereaved parent is an adolescent and family support is perceived as inadequate
  - the surviving parent of a deceased child is a single mother/father as a result of divorce or being widowed
- A history of previous losses, particularly if unresolved. Losses may include:
  - loss of a pregnancy
  - loss of a job
  - divorce
- The presence of concurrent or additional stressors such as:
  - family tension
  - compromised financial status
  - dissatisfaction with caregiving
  - reliance on alcohol and psychotropic medications, pre-bereavement
- Physical and mental illness particularly:
  - current/past history of mental health problems that have required psychiatric/psychological support
  - family history of psychiatric disorders
- High pre-death distress
- Inability or restriction in use of coping strategies such as:
  - maintenance of physical self-care
  - identification of prominent themes of grief
  - attributing meaning to the loss

- differentiation between letting go of grief and forgetting the bereaved
- accessing available support
- Isolated, alienated individuals
- Low levels of internal control beliefs, such as:
  - feeling as if he/she has no control over life
- The availability of social support particularly if:
  - people in the immediate environment are, or are perceived to be, unsupportive
  - support from family and friends immediately prior to death was good and following death it subsided
- The bereaved lack a confidant with whom to share their feelings, concerns, doubts, dreams and nightmares
- The bereaved is dissatisfied with the help available during their child's illness

Further reading

Books

Dyregrov A. (2008) *Grief in young children: a handbook for adults.* London: Jessica Kingley.

Dyregrov A. (2008) *Grief in children: a handbook for adults.* 2nd ed. London: Jessica Kingsley.

Payne S., Rolls L. (2008) Support for bereaved family carers. In *Family Carers in Palliative Care* (ed. P. Hudson, S. Payne). Oxford: Oxford University Press.

Rando T. A. (1993) *Treatment of Complicated Mourning.* Champaign: Research Press.

Articles

Becker G., et al. (2007) Do religions or spiritual beliefs influence bereavement? A systematic review. *Palliative Medicine,* **21**(3): 207–17.

Prigerson H. G., et al. (1995) Inventory of complicated grief. *Psychiatry Research,* **59**: 65–79.

Roberts A. (2008) The nature and use of bereavement support services in a hospice setting. *Palliative Medicine* **22**(5): 612–626.

Winston's Wish: www.winstonswish.org.uk.

Zhang B., et al. (2006) Update on bereavement research: evidence-based guidelines for the diagnosis and treatment of complicated bereavement. *Journal of Palliative Medicine,* **9**(5): 1188–203.

A Charter for Bereaved Children

"A child can live through anything provided they are told the truth and allowed to share the natural feelings people have when they are suffering" Eda Le Shan

This Charter has been written following our conversations with over 2,000 bereaved children and their families since Winston's Wish began in 1992. Although supporting a bereaved child can seem a daunting challenge, we have found that there are simple and straightforward ways which can make a positive difference to a grieving child. If we live in a society that genuinely wants to enable children and young people to re-build their lives after the death of a family member, then we need to respect their rights to the following:

1. Adequate Information

Bereaved children are entitled to receive answers to their questions and information that clearly explains **what** has happened, **why** it has happened and **what** will happen **next**.

Daddy died of a tumour, but I don't know what a tumour is.' Alice, age 6, whose father died of stomach cancer.

2. Being Involved

Bereaved children should be asked if they wish to be **involved** in important decisions that have an impact on their lives (such as planning the funeral, remembering anniversaries).

'I helped to choose mum's favourite music which they played at her funeral.' Kim, age 12.

3. Family Involvement

Bereaved children should receive support which **includes their parent(s)** and which also respects each child's confidentiality.

'Meeting other parents in exactly the same situation as me was so helpful.' John whose wife died from a brain haemorrhage.

4. Meeting Others

Bereaved children can benefit from the opportunity of **meeting other children** who have had similar experiences.

'Often I want to break down and cry but I can't do that in front of my school mates... meeting all the other kids who have been through the same thing – I don't feel alone any more.' Colin, age 12, whose mother died.

5. Telling the Story

Bereaved children have the right to **tell their story** in a variety of ways and for those stories to be heard, read or seen by those important to them. For example, through drawing, puppets, letters and words.

'My picture shows the car banged dad on the head, he fell off his bike, hit his head and died later in hospital.' Georgina, age 7, whose father died in a road accident.

6. Expressing Feelings

Bereaved children should feel comfortable expressing **all** feelings associated with grief such as anger, sadness, guilt and anxiety, and to be helped to find appropriate ways to do this.

'It's alright to cry and OK to be happy as well.' James, age 9, whose dad died from a heart attack.

7. Not to Blame

Bereaved children should be helped to understand that they are **not responsible and not to blame** for the death.

'I now understand it wasn't anyone's fault.' Chris, age 12, whose dad died by suicide.

8. Established Routines

Bereaved children should be able to choose to **continue** previously enjoyed activities and interests.

'I went to Brownies after Meg died, I wanted my friends to know.'

9. School Response

Bereaved children can benefit from receiving an appropriate and positive response from their **school or college**.

'My teacher remembers the days which are difficult, like father's Day and dad's birthday.' Alex, age 9.

10. Remembering

Bereaved children have the right to remember the person who has died for the rest of their lives if they wish to do so. This may involve re-living memories (both good and difficult) so that the person becomes a comfortable part of the child's on-going life story.

'I like to show my memory book to people who didn't have the chance to know my dad.' Bethany, age 8, whose father died from cancer.

Fig. 17.1 A charter for bereaved children.© Winston's wish 2002. Charity registration number 1061359.www.winstonswish.org.uk/reproduced with permission.

Self-care for health professionals

It is your responsibility to your patients/clients and your human right for yourself, to nurture and maintain your physical, emotional, intellectual and spiritual being.

Brigid Proctor

Impact of caring for dying people

Background

Sources of stress are multiple, may be accumulative and are linked to all areas of an individual's life. Working with dying people may be stressful, particularly if staff experience personal bereavement and loss, and where such work can put staff in touch with personal anxiety about loss and death.[1,2,3] Palliative care staff also find it very stressful to deal with patients who experience intractable pain, those who have young children and those patients who are afraid to die. Symptoms that leave nurses feeling helpless, useless and impotent are the most stressful to deal with, as is dealing with distressed relatives.[4]

Overall, however, stress and burnout in palliative care has been found to be less than in other specialties. Some research has shown that this is an area where there is very high degree of job satisfaction, and that staff feel they are privileged to be in the position to provide this care.[1,2,3] Working with dying people has also been found to influence the attitude of staff towards death and dying. In death anxiety scoring, people who coped well in this field of work scored higher on inner-directedness, self-actualizing value, existentiality, spontaneity, self-regard, self-acceptance, acceptance of aggression and capacity for intimate contact. They were also more likely to live in the present, rather than the past or future.[1,2,3]

It is suggested that the reason for lower stress and burnout within hospice palliative care units is probably due to the recognition that stress may be inherent to the field of death, dying and bereavement, and consequently more robust support mechanisms have been built into those organizations that provide palliative care.[1,2,3]

1 Vachon M. (1995) Staff stress in hospice/palliative care: a review. *Palliative Medicine*, **9**: 91–122.

2 Vachon M. (1997) Recent research into staff stress in palliative care. *European Journal of Palliative Care*, **4**(3): 99–103.

3 Vachon M. (2005) The stress of professional caregivers. In *Oxford Textbook of Palliative Medicine* (3rd edn) (ed. D. Doyle, *et al.* (eds), pp. 992–1004. Oxford: Oxford University Press.

4 Alexander D.A., Richie E. (1990) 'Stressors' and difficulties in dealing with the terminal patient. *Journal of Palliative Care*, **6**(3): 28–33.

Hospice and hospital palliative care teams differ considerably, and it has been found that palliative care physicians based in hospitals experience more stress than their hospice colleagues. However, a comparison of 401 specialist registrars' experience of occupational stress in palliative medicine, medical oncology and clinical oncology showed there was no significant difference between the specialties.[5] One in four of the specialist registrars (SpRs) experienced stress and more than one in ten showed clinically important levels of depression. The most common suggestions for reducing stress were improved relationships with colleagues and having 'supportive seniors'. The importance of coping strategies received far more emphasis from the group of palliative medicine trainees than those SpRs in clinical or medical oncology.[5]

Supportive environments

The Health and Safety Executive recommend that all organizations have a stress policy that outlines the responsibilities of managers and staff to identify stress in the workplace, and provides strategies that may be used to manage this stress and support the staff within the organization. Of note, they recommend the provision of specialist advice and awareness training. A supportive environment and supportive working relationships are essential ingredients in managing the potential stress of working with dying and bereaved people; in addition, it has been found that satisfaction with support in training is protective against stress. Of importance are: regular team meetings, where time is provided to evaluate and reflect on difficult situations encountered by the team; promoting shared decision-making in the management of patient care as the norm; and respecting each other's expertise.

Organizations also need to provide effective training for their staff who work with dying and bereaved people, such as the development of advanced communication skills and 'professional competence', i.e. knowledge, technical skills, relationship insight and the appropriate attitudes.

One means by which this can be achieved is through education in ethics: specifically, virtue ethics or philosophy of care. This is an important component of education in fields of care that involve intense human interactions, as occurs in palliative care.[6] Another is to the provision of protected time for clinical supervision and/or reflective practice sessions that support clinical learning and development within a supportive framework. Furthermore, there is a need to support staff in developing realistic expectations of clinical interventions in order to minimize any sense of failure and helplessness.[4]

Sources of stress

Personal life

- Personal relationships—spouse/partner, children, carer responsibilities, no close relationships/loneliness

5 Berman R. *et al.* (2007) Occupational stress in palliative medicine, medical oncology and clinical oncology specialist registrars. *Clinical Medicine*, **7**(3): 235–41.

6 Olthuis G., Dekkers W. (2003) Professional competence and palliative care: an ethical perspective. *Journal of Palliative Care*, **19**(3): 192–7.

- Illness—in self or one close to self
- Recent bereavement
- Minority related stress—victim of racism, sexism, ageism, disability prejudice, etc.
- Gender related stress—pressure to do everything/pressure to provide

Patients/clients
- Inability to create relationships
- Negative attitudes—hostility, open dislike, anger
- Potential/actual physical violence
- Emotional pressures
- Problems of emotional involvement
- Guilt feelings—feeling responsible
- Dependent clients

Colleagues
- Inability to create relationships
- Lack of support
- 'Each doing their own thing'—no teamwork
- Open conflict—practice undermined
- Bullying
- Negative/pessimistic attitudes to work
- Bringing problems at home to work
- Own anxieties about work
- Resentful of others' positions—professional jealousy

Managers
- Lack of support—no supervision, etc.
- No attention paid to personal development
- 'Routines' before 'people'
- Little positive feedback
- Discriminatory behaviour
- Bullying
- Given inappropriate client group, caseload, etc.
- Practice skills not recognized
- Overwork, heavy demands
- Faced with crises
- Lack of involvement in decision-making

Organizational issues
- Lack of resources
- 'Routines' before 'people'—bureaucracy
- Impersonal links with 'hierarchy'
- Poor pay/poor conditions of service
- Lack of clarity in roles
- Little professional 'expertise'
- Administrative procedures/paperwork
- Functions limited by resources
- Lack of clarity of work expectations—low status
- Poor Staffing ratios
- Staff shortages/vacancies not filled

Warning signs of prolonged stress

Physical
- Palpitations
- Chest pains
- Recurrent headaches
- Heartburn
- Stomach cramps
- Stomach full of gas

Intellectual
- Memory problems
- Poor concentration
- Anxiety
- Errors in judgement
- Feeling 'woolly' headed
- Inability to make decisions

Emotional
- Frequent feelings of anger, irritation and frustration
- Feeling dull and low
- Feelings of helplessness and insecurity
- Inability to love and care
- Feeling tearful
- Sleep disturbance

Strategies for coping with stress

Organizational
- Developing a supportive culture within the organization
- Opportunities to express work-related feelings and discuss problems in the workplace
- Regular team meetings
- Mandatory clinical supervision
- Provision of a counselling service for staff
- Support in developing competencies for working in palliative care
- Robust education programmes for staff that include: developing insight into individual/personal potential areas of difficulty; avoiding excessive involvement with particular clients; handling emotions; advanced communication skills; etc.

Personal coping strategies
- Having a sense of competence, control and satisfaction in working in palliative care
- Having control over workload
- Taking time off
- Having non-job-related outside activities
- Engaging in physical activities and diversions
- Ensuring adequate sleep and nutrition
- Using relaxation techniques, e.g. physical activity, yoga, meditation, complementary therapies
- Developing a personal philosophy regarding death that may or may not relate to individual religious or spiritual beliefs

Legal and professional standards of care

Doctors like all other healthcare professionals (HCPs) work in an increasingly litigious climate, which is paralleled by increasing legal regulation of healthcare. Sadly, for both patients and doctors, a simple failure by doctors to appreciate the nature and extent of their legal and professional responsibilities is one of the commonest errors leading to significant medicolegal problems. Thus, in addition to familiarity with the high standards set by the GMC within its professional codes of conduct and statements of professional responsibility, it is just as essential that doctors be acquainted with the medicolegal requirements of care. This is particularly true in palliative medicine, where doctors are involved at a highly emotional time in patients' and families' lives when numerous ethical issues are encountered, e.g. deciding best interests or deciding capacity. Recently, the Mental Capacity Act 2005 (MCA 2005), by looking at the legality of interventions for adults who lack the capacity to make their own decisions, has helpfully clarified many key medicolegal aspects of healthcare provision within English statute law, reducing some of the clinical dilemmas created by the previous uncertainty and
legal inconsistency.

Doctors' key legal and professional responsibilities cover:
- Capacity
- Best interests — for children and adults with or without capacity
- Advance decisions (previously advance directives or living wills)
- The right to medical treatment
- Appropriate withholding and/or withdrawing of treatment
- Clinical negligence
- Provision of care for patients with mental health disorders
- Dealing with violent or aggressive patients
- Caring for victims of mental and/or physical abuse
- Informed consent, battery/trespass
- Communication with patients and colleagues
- Medical records: keeping adequate clinical notes and patient access to records — data protection and patient confidentiality
- Witnessing of patients' wills or advance decisions
- Prescribing controlled drugs for patients travelling abroad
- Medical cause of death certification and notification of the coroner
- DVLA notification of patients' fitness to drive

Mental Capacity Act 2005 (MCA)[1]

Before April 2007, doctors in the UK were expected to make decisions on behalf of patients lacking capacity according to common law and accepted best practice. However, it was feared that without clear legislation inconsistencies could follow and that patients' autonomy could be undermined. There were particular concerns around the lack of any formal legal status for a 'next of kin' and the risk of unfair presumptions of incapacity based only on diagnosis. The increasing numbers of people lacking mental capacity, up to 2 million in England and Wales, also added to the pressure for new legislation (e.g. people with dementia, learning difficulties, mental health problems, stroke, brain injuries or intoxication). The Mental Capacity Act 2005 (MCA) was enacted to cement the principles from case law and best practice into UK statute law and to reform the existing relevant statute. It received Royal Assent in April 2005, and came into force in stages between April 2007 and October 2007. The MCA provides England and Wales with a clear legal framework to define and govern the clinical decision-making process for people who lack mental capacity, to protect and promote patients' rights (particularly autonomy), to involve and guide relatives/representatives and to protect and guide professionals (with a binding 'Code of Practice'). Greater clarity, legal backing and the improved options provided within the MCA empower patients' self-determination and improve consistency within decision-making processes after capacity is lost. This has meant that the MCA has been broadly welcomed, despite some inevitable limitations.

The MCA is underpinned by five key principles

- Presumption of capacity:
  - capacity is assumed unless established otherwise
- Supported decision-making:
  - the right to receive all practical support to enhance capacity and hence to be as self-determining as possible
- Acceptability of unwise decisions:
  - the right to make seemingly eccentric or unwise treatment decisions
- The requirement of best interests:
  - any action or decision made for people without capacity must be in their best interests
- Least restrictive interventions:
  - any action or decision made for people without capacity should be the least restrictive of their basic rights and freedoms

1 *Mental Capacity Act 2005.* London: TSO.

The MCA clarifies the legal position when decisions need to made for a person who lacks mental capacity:

- The MCA describes who can act on someone else's behalf; when it is appropriate; and how it should be done
- The MCA specifies the 'test' to assess capacity and the need to support people to enhance their capacity
- The MCA provides a checklist of relevant information and views to consider when deciding best interests. This is broader than the traditional 'medicalized' perspective including:
  - the patient's general welfare
  - multi-professional working
  - the views of family and carers, who gain the legal right to be consulted

The MCA enables people to put plans in place to ensure their health-care wishes are still adequately represented if they later lose capacity

- It specifies the process to make a written statement to refuse treatment (an advance decision)
- It specifies the appointment of substituted decision-makers:
  - 'Lasting Power of Attorney' (LPA)
  - 'Independent Mental Capacity Advocate' (IMCA)
  - 'Court Appointed Deputy'
- It ensures a person's known wishes and feelings are still considered

Realizing the complexity of end-of-life treatment decisions, the uniqueness of each scenario and how a lack of capacity further clouds the picture, it is inevitable that the MCA contains limitations. The MCA's guidance cannot resolve:

- Differing opinions on best interests; where consensus cannot be reached despite all reasonable attempts at resolution, e.g. differing religious beliefs within the same family or conflicts between HCPs and LPAs, when it is questionable who is best representing the patient's views
- Disputes as to the applicability of advance decisions:
  - some doubt will be unavoidable in view of the potential for different interpretations of a patient's actual meaning (particularly if an advance decision uses vague or lay terms or was written by a third party)
  - the inherent difficulty for anyone to reliably predict their wishes for an unfamiliar future event. Patients with capacity can and do change their minds when actually facing situations. And many patients, despite lacking the capacity for complex treatment decisions, may still have an unexpectedly good quality of life
- The required formalities deterring some patients, particularly elderly patients, from making advance decisions
- Legal defensiveness fuelled by an increasing exposure to formal advance decisions that may undermine the value of informal decisions
- Either, the need to re-assess capacity/best interests every time patients lacking capacity move from one setting to another, e.g. on admission to the hospice for terminal care from home, or to opt for a continuity of decisions model, which 'risks' assumptions of persisting validity and applicability of existing non-treatment decisions and adequate

adherence with the legal requirements of the MCA by referring colleagues

MCA 2005 and assessing capacity

Everyone normally has the mental capacity to make everyday decisions for themselves, e.g. what to eat and where to live. This self-determination extends to deciding whether to accept or refuse medical treatments.

The MCA clarifies that anyone from the age of 16 years is assumed to have the capacity to make their own decisions. However, a judgement of capacity must be made if it is felt that a person is unable to make a decision for themselves as a result of a specific brain or mind dysfunction (e.g. dementia, learning difficulties, mental health problems, stroke, brain injuries or intoxication). The MCA specifies the best practice approach (optimistically described as the 'single clear test') to assess whether a person lacks capacity.

Capacity

A person lacks capacity on an issue if, because of their brain or mind dysfunction, they cannot understand, retain and use the relevant information to reach and then communicate their decision on that specific task at that time

The 'burden of proof' lies with confirming that, even after receiving all practical assistance, someone lacks capacity and, crucially, this adjudged lack of capacity is specific only to that decision at that time.

To demonstrate capacity a person must meet all five required domains:
- Brain or mind dysfunction/impairment
- Understand the relevant information:
  - the information must be given in a clear and understandable way; appropriately tailored to a person's needs, e.g. using simple language or visual aids
  - the 'relevant information' includes the nature and need for a decision, in particular the likely consequences, of any accepting/refusing of a treatment, of any alternative options; or of not deciding
- Retain that information:
  - for sufficient time to reach a decision, i.e. not necessarily any longer
- Use or weigh the relevant information:
  - to reach a balanced decision
- Communicate their decision:
  - this can be by any means. Thus 'failure to express wishes' should rarely be given as the sole justification of incapacity, i.e. only where all help to communicate has failed

A lack of capacity cannot be established merely by reference to, or the presumptions around:
- Age, appearance or behaviour
- Any underlying medical conditions
- The likely duration of brain dysfunction

MCA 2005 and deciding best interests

The concept of a patient's 'best interests' is difficult to define precisely. Historically, it has appeared sufficient that any intervention should potentially offer a net benefit to the patient.[2]

A central tenet of the MCA is that any decisions made for people without capacity must be in their best interests. It is down to the person providing the care or treatment to decide what is in the best interests of the person lacking capacity.

Although the MCA does not define 'best interests' directly, it does provide a checklist of factors that any decision-makers must consider when deciding the best interests for a person they reasonably believe lacks capacity. In addition to the relative medical merits, consideration of broader ethical, social and moral components is required. These 'requirements' to determine best interests apply equally to: donee(s) of LPA, court appointed deputies, Independent Mental Capacity Advocates (IMCAs) and professionals within healthcare and social services.

Deciding best interests

- Confirm the person lacks the capacity for that decision at that time
- Weigh the relative medical benefits of the treatment
- Clarify current wishes and feelings of the person who lacks capacity
- Clarify past wishes, feelings, beliefs and values, to deduce what the person would want from:
  - any written statements from the person (formal and informal)
  - views of legally designated decision-makers and all other relevant sources, including carers and family as well as professionals

Deciding best interests is not an individual opinion determining what the person would have wanted (i.e. it is not just a 'substituted judgement'), but an attempt to reach a consensus, as objectively as possible, to decide what would be best for the person after all due consideration. Specifically carers and family members have gained a legal right to be consulted within the process of deciding best interests (previously this was only good practice; a 'next-of-kin' had no legal rights). Also, the MCA formally provides for a person to make an advance decision and/or appoint an LPA.

The presumed wishes of patients who lack capacity should carry the same weight in 'best interests' as a contemporaneous decision from a patient with capacity. This means that doctors are expected to follow a presumed refusal of treatment but they are not obliged to go along with any presumed request for a treatment that goes against their best judgement.

When deciding best interests around life-sustaining treatment, there is a strong presumption in favour of continuing treatment to prolong life:

- Unless the prolonged quality of life would be 'intolerable' for the patient (and so not be in their best interests)
- And any determination to stop treatment must not be motivated by any desire to bring about death

---

2 BMA, (2007). 'Withholding and Withdrawing Life-prolonging Medical Treatment. (3rd Edn.) Oxford: Blackwell.

Ultimately, if there is uncertainty or disagreement after appropriate consultation, it is a judge (not a doctor) who makes the determination of 'best interests' for a patient lacking capacity.

Checklist for determining best interests

When determining a person's best interests it is necessary to consider all the known relevant circumstances (as is reasonable), in particular:

- Confirm that, even after receiving all practical assistance, the person lacks capacity for that decision at that time:
  - if not permanent, can any decisions be put off (without risking irreversible mental or physical harm) until capacity is regained?
- Fully consider the relative medical merits of any healthcare decisions:
  - treatments should offer a realistic chance of a net gain in health, in terms of quality of life and quantity of life, with a reasonable expectation of cost-effectiveness
- Involve the person who lacks capacity to deduce what that person wants:
  - allow, encourage and facilitate the person's ability to participate, as fully as possible, in any decisions
  - include current wishes/feelings
- Include the person's past wishes/feelings to deduce what that person would want:
  - any relevant written statements made before capacity was lost
  - any beliefs and values that would be likely to influence their decision
  - any other specific factors to the decision
- Involve any legally designated decision-makers (as is practicable and appropriate) to deduce what that person would want:
  - a donee of a LPA
  - any deputy appointed by the court
- Consult and take all other relevant views into account (as is practicable and appropriate) to deduce what that person would want:
  - someone named by the person to be consulted
  - anyone caring for the person or interested in their welfare

Conversely, there are factors that are not relevant when determining a person's best interests. Best interests cannot be determined merely on the basis of, or following unjustified assumptions around:

- Age, appearance or behaviour
- Any underlying medical conditions

Background to advance decisions to refuse treatment (previously advance directives or living wills)

Historically, patients with life-threatening illnesses were comparatively content for doctors to make many treatment decisions on their behalf, and doctors would typically presume that most patients would want all available treatments. However, this is no longer the case, with increasing patient-led care and ongoing technological advances within medicine shifting the balance.

Medical developments such as artificial ventilation, artificial hydration/nutrition, renal dialysis and even cardiopulmonary resuscitation, may potentially prolong life, and could theoretically be offered to all dying patients. However, in advanced disease, such interventions may offer relatively little meaningful survival or symptomatic benefit, yet they still come with burdensome toxicities. Thus doctors may be unsure of their true value; many patients may not desire a prolongation of life that is only possible through what they see as 'intolerable' means. Open discussion and agreement with patients prevents the pursuit of inappropriate and undesirable medical interventions.

Respect for patient autonomy is a fundamental aspect of medical professionalism; it is a prerequisite of the doctor–patient relationship and is enshrined in UK law. A patient with capacity can refuse any treatment for any or no reason, rational or not, even if their life may be shortened. In general, a HCP is not even allowed to touch a patient without consent (otherwise it is a battery, even if an intervention has proved helpful). However, there are exceptions; consent has not been needed in common law if there is necessity or in an emergency.

- **Doctrine of Necessity:** acting in the best interests of a patient who is not competent to give valid consent (now reflected in the MCA)
- **Emergency:** to prevent immediate serious harm to a patient or to others or to prevent a crime

Doctors are not as a rule legally obliged to follow any patient's requests for a specific treatment. Patient choice cannot force HCPs to give treatments against their best judgement, i.e. if it appears clinically unnecessary, futile or inappropriate, or lacks any reasonable expectation of cost-effectiveness. However, a demand for artificial nutrition and hydration in order to be kept alive from a patient with capacity must be followed (any failure to comply could leave a doctor at risk of criminal proceedings).

Patients cannot exercise the same autonomy once they lack capacity. The resulting fear is of losing capacity and then being unable to refuse futile treatments; particularly of being kept alive artificially, with no prospect of recovery and no perceived quality of life. This has prompted society to draw up guidance to ensure that patients' right to refuse treatment is not lost when capacity is lost. Similarly, HCPs are keen to be protected when stopping treatments at the end of life, so they do not feel pressured to provide seemingly unbeneficial and burdensome interventions to such patients lacking capacity, merely because those patients are unable to refuse the treatment. Of note, once capacity is lost, patients no longer have the same absolute right to artificial nutrition and hydration to keep them alive.

Advance decisions (or advance directives/living wills) allow a patient with capacity to formally express and register their wishes about future treatment decisions in the event that they may lose capacity (and then be unable to consent or refuse treatment). Following proposals dating from the late 1960s, the first legal decision to validate an advance directive occurred in New Jersey Supreme Court, USA, March 1976. This followed the high profile legal case of Karen Ann Quinlan, which was the first to deal with the dilemma of withdrawing life-sustaining treatment from a patient who lacked capacity but was not terminally ill.

Karen Ann Quinlan

In 1975, 21-year-old Karen Ann Quinlan lapsed into a persistent vegetative state after coming home from a party (as a result of hypoxic brain damage, following two respiratory arrests). Without the legal option for non-treatment (as she was not brain-dead), the hospital refused to stop her artificial ventilation, despite the request of her parents. Subsequently, in 1976, the Supreme Court found that her ventilation could be discontinued, on 'privacy' grounds, if the hospital ethics committee believed her condition was irreversible. The court regretted that it could not discern her supposed choice based on her previous conversations, but had no doubt that Karen would decide to stop the life-support if she could, even if it led to her death. Once off the ventilator, unexpectedly she continued to breathe on her own and remained in a PVS until she died from infection in 1985.

At appeal the judicial principles upheld were:
- When a patient lacks capacity, someone else may exercise their right to make treatment decisions, preferably their families with medical input (rather than the courts)
- End-of-life care decisions should balance any treatment invasiveness against the likelihood of recovery
- Patients can refuse treatment even if this refusal might lead to death

A similar high-profile debate on the role of advance decisions took place in the UK in 1993, following the case of Tony Bland; the first patient to be allowed to die following the decision of an English court to allow the withdrawal of life-prolonging treatment.[3]

---

3 Airedale NHS Trust Bland [1993] I All ER 821.

Tony Bland

Tony Bland was left in a persistent vegetative state aged 18 years, following the crush at the Hillsborough football stadium disaster in 1989. Subsequently, the hospital, with the support of the Bland family, made an application to the court to lawfully withdraw all life-prolonging treatment, because such action at that time would otherwise have amounted to the crime of murder in UK law. On appeal the court decided that:

- Though at no time had Mr Bland actually given 'any indication of his wishes', it was felt that he would not have wished to continue living as a PVS patient
- Artificial nutrition and hydration were to be counted as treatment and not basic care (as previously), so they could be withdrawn legally

A House of Lords Select Committee on Medical Ethics decided that legislation was unnecessary, favouring the development of a 'code of practice'.

Consequently in 1995, the British Medical Association's document *Advance Statements about Medical Treatment* outlined the ethical and legal issues.[4] At that time, the UK Government was satisfied that this BMA document, together with case law, provided sufficient clarity and flexibility to enable the validity and applicability of advance decisions to be decided on a case-by-case basis. However, to improve both clarity and consistency, UK legislation on advance decisions was brought in during 2007 within the MCA.

MCA 2005 and advance decisions to refuse treatment

Advance decision

According to the MCA, an 'advance decision' describes the formal provision of clear instructions to cover any future loss of capacity, so a person can specify which treatment(s) should be then stopped or not started and under which circumstances

By formalizing anticipatory decision-making, the MCA brings statutory rules and clear safeguards to improve the process. Though no set instructions for preparing an advance decision have been formalized (because of their inherently individualized nature), the MCA clarifies the necessary content and ramifications of an advance decision.

In summary, advance decisions;

- Can only be made by informed, adult patients with specific capacity
- Must stipulate the relevant treatments and circumstances
- Only cover refusal of treatment
- Can be oral or written, unless authorizing refusal of life-sustaining treatment, when they must also comply with further formalities, i.e. written, signed, witnessed and clarifying 'even if life is at risk'

---

4 BMA (1995) *Advance Statements about Medical Treatment. Code of Practice with Explanatory Notes.* London: BMJ Publishing Group.

Open discussions with relevant HCPs will help ensure that the patient has the relevant information to complete an advance decision. Advance decisions to refuse treatment are the outcome from, and are not a substitute for, ongoing communication with HCPs and careful deliberation. To make informed choices, patients need to be aware of: the predictable phases of their disease; the diagnosis; prognosis; rehabilitation potential; and all available treatment options. Patients also need to know what will happen if no treatment is carried out.

Advance decisions do not encompass other anticipatory decision-making:

• Advance statements describing a patient's preferences for treatment
• Oral or unwitnessed refusals of life-sustaining treatment
• General commentaries on a patient's fundamental values
• A non-specific desire not to be treated

Though these areas (even if documented) are not legally binding in the same way as specific advance refusals, they remain relevant to deciding 'best interests' and therefore still need to be incorporated into decision-making. That said, nothing in an advance decision (formal or not) can force HCPs to give treatments against their best judgement.

Similarly, an advance decision from a patient under the age of 18 years should be taken into account and accommodated if possible, but a court or a person with parental responsibility can overrule it.

The legal weighting of any undocumented verbal advance decisions may prove uncertain if contested. Where possible, HCPs should record any verbal advance decisions to refuse treatment in the patient's medical notes as fully as is practical.

Healthcare professionals:

• Are liable to follow an advance decision to refuse treatment if it appears valid and applicable to the prevailing circumstances, just as if the person had made a contemporaneous decision with capacity (failure to comply could risk a claim of battery)
• Carry no liability for the consequences of giving or not giving a treatment according to an advance decision that the HCP has sufficient grounds to reasonably believe to be valid and applicable
• Can provide a treatment 'refused' in an advance decision if they are not satisfied that the advance decision is both valid and applicable, and as long as the treatment is in the patient's best interests
• Are protected from any liability if a failure to comply with an advance decision results from their lack of awareness of its existence

If an advance decision is contested, the court can be asked to decide if it exists, if it is valid and if it is applicable to a proposed treatment. Specifically, life-sustaining treatment to prevent a serious deterioration can be provided while awaiting the court's decision. If the validity or applicability of an advance decision remains uncertain, common law suggests the court would be likely to favour continuing with life-sustaining treatments.

Advance decisions to refuse treatment are not valid if...

• Made by someone under 18 years (not binding, but can still carry influence)
• Made by someone who lacked the necessary capacity when the advance decision was completed. If capacity could potentially be open

to subsequent contest, it may be prudent to seek HCP assessment to confirm and document capacity

- The nature or implications of any unwanted treatments were not fully understood when the advance decision was completed. Though not compulsory, it is therefore 'very important' that patients have sufficiently discussed any plans to refuse life-sustaining treatments with HCPs in order to make an informed refusal. Similarly, all other potential stakeholders should be involved in discussions, to limit any later doubts around validity or applicability
- The advance decision has subsequently been altered or withdrawn by the patient when they still had capacity
- A LPA was created after the advance decision that conferred authority over the specific decision. Of note, an advance decision overrules any previously appointed LPA and can still be valid despite the existence of a subsequent LPA if the LPA does not convey the relevant authority
- The patient's subsequent actions are clearly inconsistent with the advance decision remaining fixed, suggesting that the patient might have changed his/her mind before capacity was lost. Regular updates, particularly after any key life events will improve the perceived validity of an advance decision
- Advance decisions to refuse life-sustaining treatment are not valid unless written, signed, witnessed and explicit specifying that the decision stands 'even if life is at risk'. The patient (or someone explicitly directed by the patient) must have signed the document in front of a witness. This witness must then also have signed the document, in the patient's presence, to witness both the signing and that the document was intended to reflect the patient's wishes, but not to witness the presence of capacity (which is presumed). By contrast, if a HCP witnesses an advance decision, satisfactory capacity could be implied, though this alone would not suffice as proof. Thus, it would appear good practice for any HCPs witnessing an advance decision to also perform and document a formal assessment of capacity
- Patients are refusing future basic care. Advance decisions cannot refuse: warmth, comfort, shelter, hygiene or the offer of food and drink
- Made by someone thought to have been coerced, under perceived pressure or clinically depressed when the advance decision was completed, sufficient to undermine the decision
- Applying the advance decision could potentially put others at risk of serious harm

Advance decisions to refuse treatment are not applicable if...

- The patient still has capacity to give or refuse consent, or would regain capacity within an adequate timeframe to allow a delayed capacity-decision with no compromise
- The treatment in question is not specified in the advance decision
- Any circumstances specified in the advance decision are absent
- There are reasonable grounds to believe the existing circumstances had not been anticipated within the advance decision and these would affect any decision

- Refusing treatment that was subject to compulsory treatment under mental health legislation, Part 4 (Consent to Treatment) of the Mental Health Act 1983 which permits treatment without consent

An 'advance decision' to refuse treatment can be...
- Expressed in layman's terms
- Withdrawn or altered at any time by the patient, if capacity is retained
- Withdrawn or altered verbally by the patient, except for the need to be in writing to cover refusing life-sustaining treatments (though a prior refusal of life-sustaining treatments can be revoked orally)

An 'advance decision' cannot be followed if it is not available when needed
- The patient should be encouraged to store the document safely. It is the patient's responsibility to ensure its availability. A copy should be sent to the GP, specialist team and stored in the case notes as well as with carers, family and friends. Patients should consider carrying a specific bracelet or card to flag the existence and whereabouts of an advance decision
- In an emergency situation, HCPs should make all reasonable efforts to acquaint themselves with the contents of the Advance decision if they know or have reason to believe that one is available, but they should not delay treatment in anticipation of finding one

Guidance on a written advance decision

Though there is no set format for written advance decisions, as with any legal document, it should be clear, comprehensive and unambiguous. It must be readily accessible when needed, it should be reviewed regularly (to appear as up-to-date as possible) and all stakeholders should be kept aware of the contents to prevent avoidable distress and disputes when implemented. Meticulous preparation and adherence with the additional requirements is needed for any refusal of life sustaining treatments, to prevent any doubts around validity or applicability, which may otherwise undermine the patient's expressed wishes, if the advance decision were to be contested in court.

Possible format of written advance decisions

- Patient's full name, address and date of birth
- Document name and address of GP, and any other key HCPs stating if they have a copy
- Clarify the extent of HCP advice sought when writing the advance decision; give any additional names and addresses
- Clear statement that the document should apply if the patient lacks capacity to make their own treatment decisions
- If potentially open to question, seek HCP confirmation and documentation of capacity at the time of writing
- Make a clear statement of the patient's decision:
  - clarify the specific treatment(s) to be refused
  - clarify the specific circumstances when the refusal would apply
  - confirm the decision stands 'even if life is at risk' if refusing life-sustaining treatments
- Date of first and any subsequent drafts and the current review
- Clarify if a LPA has been appointed and any other nominated persons who should be consulted:
  - document names, addresses and telephone numbers
  - clarify their awareness of the contents of the document
- Signature of patient or of their nominee (confirming signing for the patient, in the patient's presence)
- Signature of the witness: clarify that it has been signed with the patient present, to witness both the signing and that the signature confirms that the document reflects the patient's wishes
- Witness' full name, address and their relationship to the patient
- Accessibility: details should be given of where all copies of the advance decision are expected to be kept
- Attach a statement to better inform future 'best interests' decisions (not binding but still must be taken into consideration)
  - set out the patient's general wishes, feelings and values
  - make any specific requests for treatment, or a general request to receive all medically reasonable efforts to prolong life
  - state where the patient would like to be cared for

MCA 2005 and designated decision-makers to act for someone who lacks capacity

- A competent person can appoint someone they trust as a 'LPA', who can then have full legal powers to act on their behalf on matters of health, welfare and finances, should they lose capacity (as detailed below)
- Independent Mental Capacity Advocates (IMCAs) are an extra safeguard for particularly vulnerable people in specific situations. An IMCA is appointed to represent and support any person who lacks capacity when there is no one available (as is practicable) to speak on their behalf. An IMCA is required in decisions of 'serious medical treatment' or, as in most cases during the pilot phase, decisions of significant changes of residence (e.g. discharge from hospice to nursing home). The IMCA brings all the factors relevant to a decision to the

attention of the decision-maker, including the person's wishes, feelings, beliefs and values. The IMCA can challenge the decision-maker. The Department of Health website provides a list of IMCA providers (from local authorities or NHS bodies)

- The new Court of Protection will appoint a deputy when facing a series of decisions where the Court cannot resolve the issues with a one-off 'court order'. As specified, deputies can then make decisions on welfare (including health) and/or financial matters, but deputies cannot refuse consent to life-sustaining treatment or override a LPA and they must act in the person's best interests

MCA 2005 and lasting power of attorney (LPA)

A 'power of attorney' is a legal document that enables a person to choose someone else to act on their behalf. The MCA has updated and extended the scope of the previous UK statute on '(Enduring) Power of Attorney' which covered only finances, replacing it with 'Lasting Power of Attorney' (LPA) which can, in addition, cover decisions on health and welfare. The new documents allow a person, the donor, to choose one or more representative(s), the 'donee(s)', to officially act on their behalf. The scope of legal authority passed within a LPA can cover any or all aspects within either or both types of LPA.

Two types of LPA

- **Property and affairs:**
  - replaces the previous Enduring Power of Attorney
  - can be activated either before or after capacity is lost, as specified
- **Personal welfare:**
  - a new option to appoint someone to 'consent' on health and other welfare matters
  - can only be activated once the donor has lost capacity

Thus, a patient can now appoint a trusted representative to cover not only relatively mundane decisions such as access to medical records, diet and daily care routine, but also to accept or decline potentially life sustaining treatment on their behalf should they lose capacity. Such a role carries a 'very heavy burden'; a LPA may have to make potentially life and death decisions for someone they care about, with in practice, limited clear-cut instructions.

Creating a LPA requires:
- The appropriate appointment of a donee(s):
  - donees must be aged 18 years or more (or a trust corporation if only covering property and affairs)
  - donees must not be bankrupt, if the LPA conveys authority over property and affairs
  - two or more persons may act as a LPA jointly (shared role) and severally (independent roles)
  - a replacement donee can only be appointed by the donor

- That the document is drawn up in accordance with the MCA:
  - donor had reached 18 years of age and had the required capacity at the time
  - written and complies with further specific requirements. For an LPA to be able to authorize the giving or refusing of consent to life-sustaining treatment, the document must contain explicit authority
- That the LPA is registered with the Office of the Public Guardian (OPG) (P. 985) before it can be used

The authority conferred by a LPA is subject to:

- Confirmation that, even after receiving all practical assistance, the person lacks capacity for that decision at that time
- The LPA, in the prescribed form, having been registered with the OPG
- The donee being fully informed of the nature, risks and consequences to the donor of accepting or refusing any proposed treatment
- As applicable, consultation with any donee with 'joint' responsibility to reach agreement (by contrast, if multiple donees carry 'several and joint' responsibility, then they can all independently give the needed authority)
- Any specified limitations to the scope of powers, as set by the donor
- Compliance with all the provisions within the Act. In particular, donee(s) must adhere to 'the principles' and so they must make decisions that are in the donor's 'best interests'. Thus, no one person can act as a true patient proxy (i.e. able to give consent); in being obliged to follow best interests, if contested in court the scope of a donee's authority may not prove comparable to that of a patient with capacity or an accepted advance decision
- Consensus with HCPs and other relatives/carers; if conflict cannot be resolved, the case will need referral to the Court of Protection. While discord around 'best interests' decisions should be infrequent, it is not yet clear if LPAs will convey the power of veto, to overrule clinicians. For example, could a LPA refusal prevent the necessary hoisting of a patient lacking capacity, despite the potential health and safety issues for staff (but crucially not the patient), pending any decision by the Court of Protection?

A donee of a LPA cannot authorize restraint unless:

- The LPA reasonably believe the donor lacks the necessary capacity
- The LPA reasonably believe that restraint is necessary to prevent harm to the donor
- The restraint is proportionate to the likelihood and seriousness of harm

MCA 2005 and restraint/deprivation of liberty

The MCA's protection of patients' rights include guidance on the 'restraint' of people lacking capacity.

- Restraint is defined as any restriction to the liberty or movement of an incapacitated person or the use or threat of force should the person resist:
  - restraint is only permitted if the person using it reasonably believes it is necessary to prevent harm to the incapacitated person
  - any restraint must be proportionate to the likelihood and seriousness of potential harm
  - any restraint must represent the least restrictive option

- In 2004, the European Court of Human Rights ruled that a patient had been unlawfully detained, despite being admitted to hospital under the UK Common Law Doctrine of Necessity. This led to an update to the MCA via the Mental Health Act 2007 to fill the 'Bournewood gap'. The 'Bournewood gap' refers to the lack of legal safeguards for patients who lack capacity (but are not covered by the Mental Health Act) when they need to be deprived of their liberty in their best interests. This includes admitting people with significant learning difficulties, dementia or cerebral malignancies for treatment or care (to protect them from harm). To prevent European Convention on Human Rights incompatibilities, there was a need to ensure these patients had recourse to adequate formal legal procedures if admission were needed. Consequently the MCA makes any deprivation of liberty unlawful unless there is 'Bournewood authorisation' or Court of Protection support. In 'an emergency' an institution (e.g. a hospice) can issue urgent authorisation for any patient felt to be at risk of deprivation of liberty while obtaining standard authorization through a local authority.

MCA 2005 and clear parameters for research

The MCA introduces strict safeguards for research involving people lacking capacity. The MCA balances the potential risks of this vulnerable population against the potential benefits of properly conducted research for patients who lack capacity. Specifically, the individual's interests are put ahead of science or society's interests.

Any research involving people lacking capacity must:

- Be sanctioned by an 'appropriate body' of independent experts (e.g. a Research Ethics Committee)
- Be safe and necessary; with a net benefit to the person or to derive new scientific knowledge
- Be intended to help understand or treat the person's condition: and thus not as valuable if as when performed by recruiting people who have mental capacity
- With minimal risk, intrusion or interference with the person's rights (e.g. case-note reviews)
- Have ongoing permission from carers or an independent nominated third party; agreeing that the person lacking capacity would have consented to participate
- Ensure a person is withdrawn if there are any signs of distress, resistance or refusal

MCA 2005 and legal requirements for provision of care

The MCA offers some protection and guidance to clinicians and caregivers. A person can provide care or treatment for a patient who lacks capacity with no additional legal liability, providing reasonable steps are taken to establish that: firstly, the patient lacks capacity; and, secondly, the decisions made appear in the patient's best interests at the time.

Thus the legal liability for any healthcare interventions for patients who appear to lack capacity is exactly the same as that seen for patients with capacity who have consented, providing that:

- Having followed the specified assessment of capacity, HCPs should have a 'reasonable belief' that the patient lacks capacity

- Having followed the specified requirements for deciding best interests, HCPs should have a 'reasonable belief' that any decisions are in the patient's best interests
- The HCP has not acted in conflict with a valid and applicable advance decision or the decision of a LPA or court deputy when acting within their authority and in accordance with the Act

The Code of Practice fleshes out the broad framework set out by the MCA. This Code (running to 302 pages) has legal force and applies to anyone with a prescribed role that impacts on persons lacking capacity including:

- Anyone with formal powers (attorneys, deputies and IMCAs)
- A professional or someone with a paid role, e.g. in health or social care
- Anyone with a research remit covered by the MCA

The Code also serves as a good practice guide for anyone else working with or caring for people who may lack capacity. In addition, the general approach appears transferable to any complex healthcare decision-making process, even in patients with capacity, while consensus is sought.

The MCA has added further legal provisions to protect vulnerable people:

- A legal obligation to comply with the Act is placed on both individuals and employing NHS Trusts
- The MCA introduces a new criminal offence of ill-treatment or wilful neglect of a person who lacks capacity, liable to imprisonment for up to five years. It applies to anyone caring for a person (of any age) who lacks capacity. This includes family carers as well as healthcare and social care staff providing care in any setting (hospital, hospice, care home or home), Court-appointed deputies and LPAs.

The MCA does not cover areas considered too individual or personal to allow someone else to make decisions for a person lacking capacity. These include marriage/civil partnerships, divorce, sexual relationships and voting.

Two new public bodies to support the statutory framework of the MCA 2005

- The Court of Protection is a single specialized Court that combines the previous Court of Protection (property and affairs) and High Court jurisdiction (on welfare including healthcare). The 'Court of Protection', was created to oversee the new legislation, with jurisdiction across the whole Act, and is the final arbiter for complex matters of capacity or best interests. It has trained staff to consider property, affairs and welfare issues, with a regional presence but an informal style. In addition to adjudicating in one-off financial or difficult welfare decisions, if a single court order is insufficient, the Court of Protection can appoint deputies to assist ongoing decision-making
- The 'Office of the Public Guardian' (OPG) has replaced the Public Guardianship Office. The OPG will be the registering and supervising authority for both LPAs and Court-appointed deputies. They will

respond to any concerns raised about the way in which an attorney or deputy is operating and provide guidance to the public and information to the courts. Court-appointed deputies have replaced receivers, and can be appointed to decide on financial or welfare matters or both. The deputy must still allow the person who lacks capacity to make whatever decisions they are able to, and must only make decisions that are in the person's best interests

Clinical negligence

Claims of clinical negligence will result when doctors are deemed to have acted outside of sound medical practice. While clinical opinion may vary, in medical litigation the central question is whether or not a doctor attained the standard of care as required by law. The UK legal standard expected is one of 'reasonable care' as defined by case law. This is judged by taking into account all the circumstances surrounding a particular situation and by balancing the diversity inherent in medical practice against the interests of the patient.

• In determining the required standard of care, the court traditionally uses the Bolam test; a doctor has not been negligent if they can show they acted in line with the accepted practice of responsible peers, even if another body of medical opinion takes a contrary view

• Subsequently, the judgment from the 'Bolitho' case has imposed an additional requirement above the standard of clinical care as was defined by the Bolam test. The courts must now take a more enquiring stance, testing the medical evidence offered by both parties in any litigation, to determine if such opinion is 'reasonable', 'respectable' and 'responsible'. The courts must be satisfied that the medical experts have considered all the risks and benefits to reach a defensible and logical conclusion. Thus, though unlikely, a doctor acting in line with the accepted practice could still be found to be negligent if the court believes the accepted medical practice in question is not sufficiently balanced or logical. That is, just the occurrence of similar medical practices is no longer a sufficient defence in itself; to be defensible, clinical care must also reflect balanced, comprehensive and logical decision-making

The Bolam Test, 1957[5]

In 1954, Mr Bolam underwent electroconvulsive therapy (ECT) for clinical depression. At that time medical opinion differed on how best to minimize the risk of injuries possible from convulsions induced by ECT. In Mr Bolam's case the technique of manual restraint was ineffective and as a result fractured his pelvis. He subsequently argued that the doctor had been in breach of the standard of care in providing treatment and that the hospital had been negligent.

The Judge in his direction to the jury said that a doctor is not guilty of negligence if he has acted in accordance with the practice accepted as proper by a responsible body of medical opinion skilled in that particular art. If, therefore, a medical practice is supported by a body of peers, then the Bolam test is satisfied and the practitioner has met the required standard of care in law. This test has been used on numerous occasions in cases of medical litigation.

5 Bolam v Friern Hospital Management Committee [1957] 1 WLR 582.

Bolitho, 1998[6]

In 1984, a two-year old boy was re-admitted to hospital with breathing difficulties a day after discharge, following a 4-day admission for croup. During this stay a doctor failed to attend when called by nurse colleagues to assess further episodes of breathing difficulties. Subsequently, the child arrested and sustained severe brain damage. By the time of the court case the child had died. A breach of duty from the non-attendance was established, while the doctor's defence that they would not have intubated the child if they had attended was not considered germane.

The question of negligence rested with the need for intubation and if this intubation could have then prevented the arrest. Conflicting medical evidence was given on whether intubation would have been the proper course of action. In line with the Bolam Test, the doctor was initially deemed not negligent since not intubating was supported by one of the two sets of responsible medical opinion.

Though the courts ultimately dismissed the case, it went to appeal and the House of Lords. The Bolam principle was perceived as being excessively reliant upon the medical testimony supporting the defendant. Contrary to the spirit of Bolam the presence of expert medical opinion supporting the defendant was deemed insufficient in itself to avoid a claim of clinical negligence. Rather the court had to be satisfied that any body of medical opinion relied upon by the defence had demonstrated that it had a logical basis, having weighed all the competing risks and benefits. Reassuringly, it was deemed 'very seldom' that a judge would question a competent medical expert opinion.

6 Bolitho v City and Hackney HA [1998] AC 232.

Further reading

Books

BMA, (1995) *Advance Statements about Medical Treatment. Code of Practice with Explanatory Notes'*. London, BMJ Publishing Group.

BMA, (2007). *'Withholding and Withdrawing Life-prolonging Medical Treatment. Guidance for Decision-making'*. (3rd edn.) Oxford: Blackwell.

Articles

Jacoby R, Steer P (2007) How to assess capacity to make a will. *British Medical Journal*, **335**: 7611: 155–157.

Johnston C, (2007) The Mental Capacity Act 2005 and Advance decisions *Clinical Ethics*, **2**: 80–84.

Luttrell S (1996) living wills do have legal effect provided certain criteria are met. *British Medical Journal*, **313**: 1148.

Samanta A., Samanta J., (2006) Advance directives, best interests and clinical judgement; shifting sands at the end of life. *Clinical Medicine*, **6**(3): 274–8.

Sheather J, (2006) The Mental Capacity Act 2005 *Clinical Ethics*, **1**: 33–36.

Travis S., *et al.* (2001) Guidelines in respect of Advance Directives: the position in England. *International Journal of Palliative Nursing*, **7**(10): 493–500.

Department for Constitutional Affairs (2007) 'Code of Practice for. London: The Stationery Office (TSO) The Mental Capacity Act 2005. Available on-line; at: http://www.opsi.gov.uk/acts/en2005/ukpgaen_20050009_en_cop.pdf.

Department of Health (2007) *'Background to the IMCA Service'* from: www.dh.gov.uk/en/socialcare/Deliveringadultsocialcare/mentalcapacity/IMCA/DH_4134876

Mental Capacity Act 2005 London. HMSO.

Re B (Consent to treatment: capacity) [2002] All ER 449.

Death certification and referral to the coroner

Registration of death

Every death occurring in the UK has to be registered in the Register of Deaths local to the place of death. This chapter relates to procedures in England and Wales, although other jurisdictions e.g. Scotland have very similar procedures.

The information recorded in the Register comprises personal details of the deceased person and medical information as to the cause of death. The death must be formally registered (within 5 days) at the Register Office for Births, Deaths and Marriages local to the place of death, although it is now possible to provide the personal details needed to register at any registry.

Personal details

The relevant personal details (including the deceased's full name, home address, dates and places of birth and death, occupation, matrimonial/partner status, etc.) will be provided by the **'informant'** (normally a close relative who has personal knowledge of the deceased) who attends the Register office, and is able to respond to the various questions asked by the registrar.

Medical details and completion of the Medical Certificate of Cause of Death

The medical details will be provided by the registered medical practitioner who has been in attendance on the deceased during his/her last illness. He/she is required to furnish a certificate in the prescribed form ('Medical Certificate of Cause of Death' or MCCD). It should be completed, by the certifying doctor, with the cause of death to the best of the doctor's information, knowledge and belief.

The MCCD should be completed promptly, giving clear statements that set out the sequence of the disease process that led to death. It should not give a 'mode' of death as the only entry nor should abbreviations be used. The doctor is legally responsible for the delivering the MCCD to the registrar, although normally the informant acts as the doctor's agent and hands it to the registrar.

The registrar will copy all the medical details from the MCCD (using the identical words and spelling) into the register.

Reference to the coroner

Deaths that cannot be readily certified as due to natural causes should be referred to the coroner. Once a death has been reported to the coroner, he/she has a duty to investigate the cause of death. This may be done by way of informal inquiry carried out by the coroner or a coroner's officer, by a post-mortem examination made to establish a cause of death or by an inquest. If the family objects to the post-mortem, whether for religious or other reasons, an appeal can be made, but this may delay the funeral.

The registrar (but no one else) has a statutory duty to report any death to the coroner if, on the basis of information coming to the registrar's notice, it may be one that, by law, the coroner is required to investigate (see below). Nevertheless, doctors are encouraged to report voluntarily any death that the registrar may subsequently refer to the coroner. This will save time and reduce uncertainty for the family. **Coroners and their officers are always prepared to discuss individual cases and, in this way, ensure that families are neither inconvenienced nor troubled unnecessarily.**

Coroner's inquiries

The coroner will address the duties of investigating a death by informal inquiry carried out by the coroner or a coroner's officer, by a post-mortem examination made to establish a cause of death or by an inquest.

If the case is one where an inquest is held, the registration in the Register of Deaths is completed by the coroner when the inquest is finally concluded.

A coroner's inquest is a limited public inquiry, convened by the coroner, to find factual answers to who the deceased person was and how, when and where the death occurred. The coroner does not address matters of blame (i.e. liability).

Registrar's duty to report to the coroner

The registrar is required to report the death to the coroner if:
- It appears to the registrar the deceased was not attended during his last illness by a registered medical practitioner
- The registrar has been unable to obtain a duly completed MCCD
- The deceased was not seen by the doctor:
  - either after death, *or*
  - within 14 days before death
- The cause of death appears to be:
  - unknown, *or*
  - unnatural, *or*
  - the death was caused by:
    —violence, *or*
    —neglect, *or*
    —abortion; *or*
  - the death was attended by suspicious circumstances; *or*
  - the death occurred:
    —during an operation, *or*
    —before recovery from the effect of an anaesthetic; *or*

- the death appears to have been due to:
  —industrial disease, or
  —industrial poisoning

24 hours
In addition, it is sometimes argued that if the deceased was only under the care of the doctor for less than 24 hours before death ensued, that doctor may not have sufficient knowledge as to the cause of death for him/her to complete the MCCD. The coroner's office will always advise informally about this.

Certifying deaths in the hospice setting
In a hospice setting it is not uncommon for a patient to die with a pathological fracture or to die within a short time of arrival at the hospice. The local coroner will be very pleased to discuss these cases.

Completing the MCCD

Doctors have a legal duty to state all they know. However, it is relatively easy for any member of the public to obtain a copy of the death register entry that will include the cause of death. There is, therefore, the potential for a breach of confidence. The Office of Population Census and Surveys (OPCS) accepts that the present system is unsatisfactory.

The current practice of stating a superficial cause of death rather than the underlying disease process in such cases is widespread. Although it is technically illegal, it is condoned by the OPCS—**provided** the box on the reverse side of the certificate is ticked stating that additional information may be forthcoming. This point has yet to be tested in the courts. These comments often apply to patients dying with AIDS-related illnesses.

Other points

Burial and cremation

The registration process also provides authorization for burial or cremation. The authorization issued by the registrar should be handed to the funeral director to be used by the family. If the case is one where an inquest is held, the authorization of the burial or cremation is given by the coroner.

Cremation

New regulations apply to cremation in the UK from 2009.

If a body is to be cremated a certificate of medical attendant **(Form 4)** and a confirmatory medical certificate **(Form 5)** should be completed. In Form B, if the doctor has not attended the deceased within 14 days of death, the coroner should be notified. The doctor must see the body after death.

Form C must be completed by a registered medical practitioner of not less than five years standing, who shall not be a relative of the deceased or a relative or partner of the doctor who has given the certificate in Form B. The doctor must see and examine the body after death. In addition, the doctor must have seen and questioned the medical practitioner who completed Form B.

The applicant for cremation has a new right to inspect form Cremation 4 or 5. Some of the information may have been given to the doctor by the deceased in confidence. If it is included in the form, it may be disclosed to the applicant for cremation if they choose to inspect the form. If this would be a breach of confidence information may be given to the medical referee on a separate sheet of paper attached to the Form with explanatory reasons.

Death certificate

When completed, the entries in the Register of Deaths will form 'the death certificate', the proof of death required for the various legal and social processes as well as overall statistics of causes of death. Copies of the death certificate can be obtained from the registrar.

Wills

If there is a will, the executors named in the will (or if there is no will, the deceased's personal representative) is responsible for arranging the funeral and looking after (and subsequently disposing of) the person's assets and property.

If there is a will, the executor should 'prove' this to obtain probate of the will.

If there is no will, the deceased's personal representative should apply for letters of administration.

Funeral director

The funeral director will need to know whether the body is to be buried or cremated (over 75% of deaths in the UK are now followed by cremation).

They will need to know of any religious customs or rituals that might be necessary.

Bodies may be 'partially' embalmed routinely or this might be discussed with the family. Traditionally, embalming involves draining blood from the body and replacing it with formaldehyde plus a pinkish dye pumped under pressure, which has a hardening and disinfecting effect. Nowadays, the blood is not drained, but a small amount of embalming fluid is infused to help prevent the body smelling and to make the face more presentable; This is particularly relevant either for hygienic reasons or if the families wish to view.

Fitness to drive

> In the interest of road safety those who suffer from a medical condition likely to cause a sudden disabling event at the wheel or inability to safely control their vehicle from any other cause should not drive.

The Secretary of State for Transport acting through the medical advisers at the Drivers Medical Group at the Driver and Vehicle Licensing Agency (DVLA) has the responsibility to ensure that all licence holders are fit to drive. It is the duty of the **licence-holder** to notify the DVLA of any medical conditions which may affect safe driving. Most patients are sensible and responsible and, with the support of family members, are safe on the roads. They will avoid driving when their physical or mental condition begins to affect their judgement and ability to react quickly to unpredictable circumstances.

Driving is often seen as an important factor in maintaining the struggle for independence. It may be very hard for the patient, on both a practical and emotional level, to agree to letting go of the last vestiges of control over their lives. Very sensitive handling is needed.

If a patient is obviously unfit to drive for any reason and refuses to comply, the GMC issues the following guidelines:

- The DVLA is legally responsible for deciding if a person is medically unfit to drive. They need to know when driving licence holders have a condition which may, now or in the future, affect their safety as a driver
- Therefore, where patients have such conditions, the doctor should make sure that the patient understands that the condition may impair their ability to drive. If a patient is incapable of understanding this advice, for example because of dementia, you should inform the DVLA immediately
- Explain to patients that they have a legal duty to inform the DVLA about the condition. If the patient refuses to accept the diagnosis or the effect of the condition on his/her ability to drive, you can suggest that he/she seeks a second opinion, and make appropriate arrangements for this. You should advise patients not to drive until the second opinion has been obtained
- If patients continue to drive when they are not fit to do so, you should make every reasonable effort to persuade them to stop. This may include telling their next of kin
- If you do not manage to persuade patients to stop driving, or you are given, or find, evidence that a patient is continuing to drive contrary to advice, you should disclose relevant medical information immediately, in confidence, to the medical adviser at DVLA
- Before giving information to the DVLA you should inform the patient of your decision to do so. Once the DVLA has been informed, you should also write to the patient to confirm that a disclosure has been made

Driving and drugs that might impair cognitive and motor skills

Doctors have a duty to inform patients when they are prescribed medication which may impair their driving (GMC guidelines). Patients should be reminded that motor insurance may become invalid if there are changes in medical circumstances.

Many drugs used in palliative care may impair cognitive and motor skills including:-

Opioid analgesics	e.g. morphine, oxycodone, etc.
Benzodiazepines	e.g. diazepam, lorazepam
Antidepressants	e.g. amitriptyline
Phenothiazines	e.g. levomepromazine
Antihistamines	e.g. cyclizine

Patients on longer-term stable doses of opioids show only minor effects in terms of diminished cognition, perception, coordination or behaviour related to driving.

Patients, however, who are started on opioids or who are prescribed an increase above their 'normal' stable dose may show cognitive impairment for a few weeks or so. These patients should be advised not to drive during this period.

Driving and brain tumours

The diagnosis of a high-grade primary or secondary brain tumour, whether or not a convulsion has occurred, must be notified to the DVLA. Patients will not be allowed to drive for at least two years after treatment.

Driving and heart/vascular conditions

Patients with heart failure may usually be safe to drive provided that there are no symptoms that may distract the driver's attention. There are restrictions for those with intracardiac defibrillating devices. Patients with an abdominal aortic aneurysm of >6.5cm will be disqualified from driving.

Driving and dementia

Patients with poor short-term memory, disorientation, lack of insight and judgement will almost certainly not be fit to drive. There is acknowledgement, however, that presentation and progression of dementia is variable and that the risk of a crash is acceptably low for up to three years after the onset of dementia; in early dementia, while sufficient skills remain and progress is slow, the medical adviser may allow driving but will require a yearly review.

Driving and seat belts

Exemption from having to wear a seat belt may be sought if it is thought to pose a danger to the patient's safety, such as in the situation of significant intra-abdominal disease.

Application forms for a Certificate of Exemption from compulsory seat belt wearing in the UK may be obtained through the NHS Response telephone line (0300 123 1002).

Useful contacts
Drivers Medical Group
DVLA
Swansea SA99 1TU
Tel: 0870 600 0301

DVLA At A Glance—Current medical standards of fitness to drive—
www.dvla.gov.uk (reviewed 6 monthly)

Further reading

Breen D., et al. (2007) Driving and dementia *British Medical Journal* **334**: 1365–9.

Dermatomes

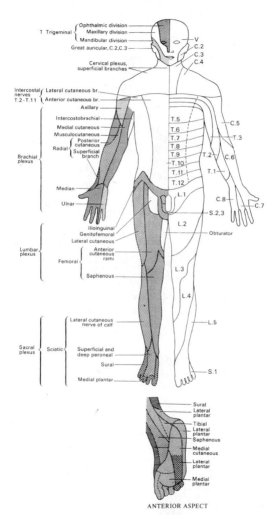

Fig. 19d.1 Dermatomes.

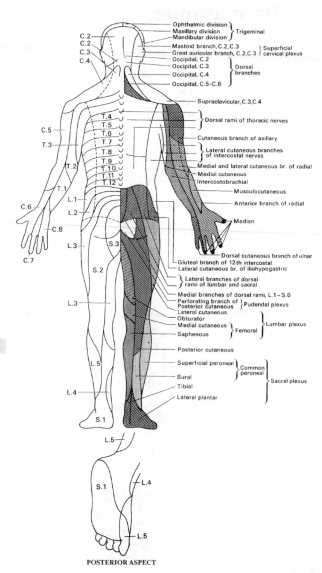

Fig. 19d.1 (Continued)

Genograms

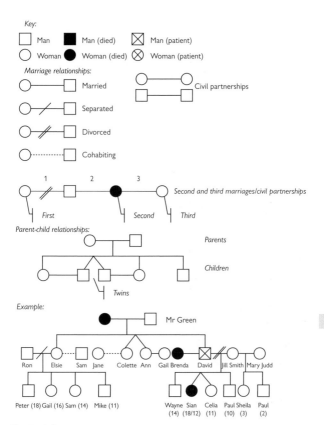

Fig. 19e.1 Genograms.

Peripheral nerve assessment

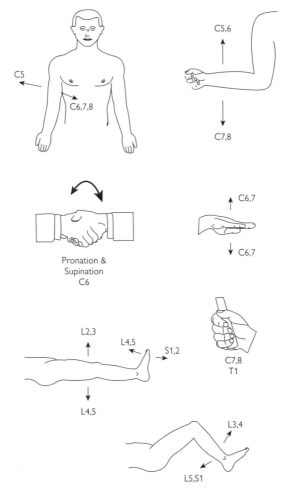

Fig. 19g.1 Peripheral nerve assessment.

Travelling abroad

It is not uncommon for terminally ill patients to want to travel abroad in order to see family or to die in their home country. A wish to travel by air needs to be balanced against the risk to the individual and the inconvenience and cost to fellow passengers and airlines in the event of unscheduled changes to flight plans. If there is any doubt, the airline medical officer, who will give the final authorization, should be contacted well in advance of travel.

In flight

Changes in air pressure occur during flight and po_2 may be reduced. For this reason, patients with marked breathlessness (who are unable to walk more than 50 metres), with Hb less than 7.5g/L, ischaemic heart disease, cardiac failure or those who are oxygen-dependent may have difficulty.

In-flight cabin oxygen is inadequate for such patients. Extra supplies of oxygen may be made available as necessary if the airline is aware in advance.

Air expands at lower atmospheric pressures, and for this reason patients with a pneumothorax, large bullae, ear/sinus disease and recent surgery or colonoscopy should not fly without advice. Other conditions to consider carefully are intracranial tumours or confusion.

Patients will be at risk of thromboembolism on long-haul flights, especially if they are unable to mobilize adequately; the use of support stockings or foot rocking devices may be appropriate.

Special arrangements

Transport to and from airports is arranged by the patient. If a stretcher is required, nine economy class seats are required, the cost of which is borne by the patient.

Cabin staff are not authorized to look after personal care needs, medical treatment or specialized medical equipment.

An escort for a patient who is flying will be needed if:

- A patient is relatively dependent
- A patient has a syringe driver
- A patient has surgical drains
- Emergency management of symptoms may be needed
- Medication might need to be given by injection
- The journey is long and interrupted by several transfers

It is important to remember that all medication or equipment that might be needed during the flight are kept as *hand* luggage. This includes all regular medication including analgesics, antiemetics, anticonvulsants, steroids, insulin, inhalers and any medication such as glyceryl trinitrate which might be needed on an 'as required' basis. Syringes, needles, spare batteries and a sharps disposal box, if appropriate, should be remembered. All controlled drugs need to be in their original packaging and all carried in hand luggage.

Controlled drugs

If a patient is taking regular controlled drugs, a Home Office licence will be required if the trip is longer than three months. If the dosage and therefore total quantity of drug is high, a licence may be required for less time away.

A letter from the prescribing doctor is required which is to be carried by the patient. The letter should contain the following information:
- The patient's name
- Address
- Date of birth
- Outward and returning dates of travel
- The country being visited
- The drugs being carried, including dosages and total amount
- Generic and not brand names should be used

It is also advisable to contact the Embassy/Consulate/High Commission of the country being visited to ensure that they will not refuse entry to someone with controlled drugs.

Travel Insurance

Any patient travelling abroad should be advised to obtain travel insurance in the event of them becoming unwell. Getting travel insurance when a patient has an advanced disease can be difficult so they should be encouraged to look as early as possible. There are companies which specialize in providing cover for individuals with medical problems.

Although the European Health Insurance Card (EHIC) entitles the patient to free or reduced cost emergency treatment within the European Union, there is a risk that they will need to pay the costs at the time and then claim back the money. Also, the EHIC does not include medical evacuation back home. It is recommended that patients have both an EHIC and private travel insurance.

Useful information address

Home Office Licensing Department
For taking opioids abroad
Tel: 020 7035 4848

Further reading

http:www.cancerbackup.org.uk/Resourcessupport/practicalissues/Travel/TakingMedicinesabroad

Tissue donation

Human organ and tissue transplantation has proven to be a successful method for treating many medical conditions. However, the demand for organs and tissues continues to exceed supply. The intensive care unit is generally considered the only clinical area where individuals can donate organs and tissue. However, individuals who die in other clinical areas can potentially donate a variety of tissues including occasionally, their kidneys. Although tissue donation does not enjoy the same high public profile as organ donation, it nevertheless holds many significant benefits for recipients. For example, the transplantation of new valves to patients with diseased or infected heart valves, can be life saving. Skin donation can be used to treat severe burns and corneal transplantation has the ability to improve or even restore sight for those with diseased corneas, enhancing the recipient's quality of life. Tissue donation is also subject to fewer contraindications and restrictions than is associated with solid organ donation. Collection times are less urgent, varying from 24 hours after death for corneas to 48 hours for heart valves. Thus, many patients who die in environments outside intensive care have the potential to be non-heart beating donors.

There is evidence that donation, far from increasing relatives' distress, may help in bereavement, families gaining comfort and meaning to the death. Studies have shown that relatives are generally happy to talk about donation and to feel some good has resulted from the death. Some professionals feel that there is a 'duty to ask' for tissue donation and, indeed, some families have felt cheated by not being given the opportunity to discuss the issue. The subject of tissue donation may be straight forward if it has been discussed with the patient prior to death and if a donor card is available. However even in this situation, consent should always be sought from the next of kin.

In practice, it is easiest for corneas to be donated since this can be organized (it must be within 24h) at the location of death without the need for transfer to a hospital pathologist. The transplant coordinator will arrange for the eyes to be removed. (The eye sockets are packed and shields inserted to ensure the original appearance of the donor is restored.)

A fear in popular culture that mutilation of the body, particularly the eyes, affects the deceased's beauty, identity or personhood and the idea that vision is necessary for the after-life, may be some of the reasons cited for families being reluctant to agree to donation. Debate continues on presumed consent with an 'opt out' clause. There is evidence that those who consent to donation do so not out of social duty but out of altruism and generosity, from which they gain positive rewards. The subject of tissue donation remains a very individual and sensitive issue which needs careful handling in inevitably vulnerable families.

There are various practical considerations, some are outlined below in Table 19i.1.

Table 19i.1 Practical considerations for tissue donation

	Cornea	Heart valves and trachea	Kidneys
Max. age of donor	Any age	60 years	70 years
Max. time from asystole to tissue removal	24h	72h	1h

Contraindications

The criteria for the acceptability of tissues for donation are inevitably becoming more stringent. In the UK, a donor coordinator is available 24h a day and gives very helpful advice.

Follow–up

The donor coordinator writes an acknowledgement letter to the family informing them of how the tissues have been used. Families usually find this very comforting.

Further Reading

Book

Sque M., Payne S. (ed) (2007) *Organ and Tissue Donation: an Evidence Base for Practice.* Maidenhead: Open University Press.

Help and advice for patients

UK national resources

Cancerbackup
Helps people with cancer, their families and friends to live with cancer. Cancer nurses provide information, emotional support and practical advice by telephone or letter. Booklets, factsheets, a newsletter, website and CD-ROM provide information.
☎ 0808 800 1234
🖳 http://www.cancerbackup.org.uk/

Macmillan Cancer Support
Funds Macmillan nurses: referral via GP or hospital. Information line. Financial help through patient grants, applications for patient grants through hospital and hospice nurses, social workers and other healthcare professionals.
Macmillan Cancerline 0808 808 2020
🖳 http://www.macmillan.org.uk/

Marie Curie Cancer Care
Hands-on palliative nursing care, available through the local district nursing service. Also runs inpatient centres: admission by referral from GP or consultant. Both the services are free of charge.
🖳 http://www.mariecurie.org.uk/

Tenovus Cancer Information Centre
Information and support for patients, their families, carers. Helpline staffed by experienced cancer trained nurses, counsellors and social workers. Individual counselling service; free literature.
43 The Parade Cardiff CF24 3AB
☎ 0808 800 1010
🖳 http://www.tenovus.com/

Bereavement

Asian Family Counselling Services
Includes bereavement counselling.
☎ 020 8571 3933

CancerBACUP Counselling
☎ 020 7833 2451
🖳 http://www.cancerbacup.org.uk

Cruse Bereavement Care
Bereavement counselling
☎ 0844 477 9400
🖳 http://www.crusebereavementcare.org.uk

Samaritans/Age Concern/Citizens Advice Bureaux
☎ From local telephone directory

The Compassionate Friends
A self-help group of parents whose son or daughter (of any age, including adults) has died from any cause.
☎ 0845 123 2304
🖥 http://www.tcf.org.uk

Carers
Carers UK
Information and support to people caring for relatives and friends. Free leaflets and information sheets.
☎ 0808 808 7777 (Wed.–Thurs. 10am–midday, 2pm–4pm)

Crossroads—Caring for Carers
Provides a range of services for carers, including care in the home to enable the carer to have a break.
☎ 0845 450 0350
🖥 http://www.crossroads.org.uk

Children
ACT—Association for Children's Palliative Care
☎ 0845 108 2201
🖥 http://www.act.org.uk

Complementary therapies
Bristol Cancer Help Centre
☎ 0845 123 2310
🖥 http://www.beehive.thisisbristol.com

British Acupuncture Council
☎ 020 8735 0400
🖥 http://www.acupuncture.org.uk

British Homoeopathic Association
☎ 0870 444 3950
🖥 http://www.trusthomeopathy.org

Institute for Complementary and Natural Medicine
☎ 020 7922 7980
🖥 http://www.i-c-m.org.uk

National Federation of Spiritual Healers
☎ 0845 123 2777
🖥 http://www.nfsh.org.uk

Conditions other than cancer
Alzheimer's Society
☎ 0845 300 0366
🖥 http://www.alzheimers.org.uk

British Brain and Spine Foundation
Helpline provides information and support about neurological disorders for patients, carers and health professionals.
☎ 0808 808 1000
🖳 http://www.brainandspine.org.uk

Motor Neurone Disease Association
Professional and general enquiries:
☎ 01604 250505
☎ Helpline: 0845 7626 262
🖳 http://www.mndassociation.org

Parkinson's Disease Society
☎ 0808 800 0303
🖳 http://www.parkinsons.org.uk

Stroke Association
☎ 0845 303 3100
🖳 http://www.stroke.org.uk

Specific cancers
Breast Cancer Care
☎ 0808 800 600
🖳 http://www.breastcancercare.org.uk/

Lymphoma Association
☎ 0808 808 5555 (Mon–Fri 9am–6pm)
🖳 http://www.lymphoma.org.uk/

Oesophageal Patients Association
☎ 0121 704 9860
🖳 http://www.opa.org.uk

Ovacome
A support organization for women with ovarian cancer.
☎ 0845 3710554 or 020 7299 6654 (Mon.-Fri. 9am-4pm)
🖳 http://www.ovacome.org.uk/ovacome

Prostate Cancer Charity
☎ 0800 074 8383 (Mon.-Fri. 10am-4pm)
🖳 http://www.prostate-cancer.org.uk/

Prostate Cancer Support Association (PSA)
☎ 0845 601 0766
🖳 http://www.prostatecancersupport.co.uk

The Roy Castle Lung Cancer Foundation
☎ 0800 358 7200
🖳 http://www.roycastle.org/

Specific health problems
Changing Faces
Offers information, social skills training and counselling for people with facial disfigurements.
☎ 0845 4500 275
🖳 http://www.changingfaces.org.uk/

Colostomy Association
☎ 0118 939 1537
☎ Freephone: 0800 32842 57/0800 587 6744
🖥 www.colostomyassociation.org.uk

Let's Face It
A contact point for people of any age coping with facial disfigurement.
☎ 01843 833 724
🖥 http://www.letsfaceit.force9.co.uk

Lymphoedema Support Network
☎ 020 7351 4480
🖥 http://www.lymphoedema.org/

National Association of Laryngectomee Clubs
☎ 020 7730 8585
🖥 http://www.nalc.ik.com

Sexual Dysfunction Association
☎ 0870 774 3571
🖥 http://www.impotence.org.uk/

Urostomy Association
☎ 01889 563 191
🖥 http://www.uagbi.org

Specific patient groups
Chai-Lifeline
Emotional, physical, practical and spiritual support to Jewish children, their families and friends.
☎ 020 8731 6788
🖥 http://www.chailifeline.org.uk

Gayscan
Offers completely confidential help and support to gay men living with cancer, their partners and carers.
☎ Helpline: 020 8368 9027 (10am-7pm except Sundays)
🖥 Gayscan@blotholm.org.uk

Lesbians and Cancer
🖥 http://www.lesbiansandcancer.com/index.html

National Network for Palliative Care of People with Learning Disability
☎ 01284 766 133

Laboratory reference values

These are guides only—different labs use different ranges. Pregnant women and children also have different normal ranges—consult the lab.

Haematology

Measurement	Reference interval
White cell count (WCC)	4.0–11.0×10^9/l
Red cell count (RCC)	Men: 4.5–6.5×10^{12}/l Women: 3.9–5.6×10^{12}/l
Haemoglobin	Men: 13.5–18g/dl Women: 11.5–16.0g/dl
Packed cell volume (PCV) or haematocrit	Men: 38.5–50.1% Women: 36.0–44.5%
Mean cell volume (MCV)	76–97fl
Mean cell haemoglobin (MCHC)	32.7–34.6 g/dl
Neutrophils	2.0–7.5×10^9/l *40–75% WCC*
Lymphocytes	1.3–3.5×10^9/l *20–45% WCC*
Eosinophils	0.04–0.44×10^9/l *1–6% WCC*
Basophils	0.0–0.1×10^9/l *0–1% WCC*
Monocytes	0.2–0.8×10^9/l *2–10% WCC*
Platelet count	150–400×10^9/l
Reticulocyte count	25–100×10^9/l *0.8–2% RCC**
Erythrocyte sedimentation rate (ESR)	Depends on age
International normalized ratio (INR)	0.8–1.2 Ranges for warfarin therapy depend on indication
Prothrombin time (PTT)	12–17 sec.
Factors I, II, VII, X	
Activated partial thromboplastin time	28–40 sec.
Factor VIII, IX, XI, XII	
Red cell folate	180–300 ng/ml

*Only use percentages as reference interval if red cell count is normal. Otherwise use absolute value.

Biochemistry

Substance	P	Reference interval
Adrenocorticotrophic hormone	P	<80ng/l
Alanine aminotransferase (ALT)	P	5–35iu/l
Albumin	P	35–50g/l
Alkaline transaminase (AST)	P	30–150u/l
α-amylase	P	0–180u/dl
Aspartate transaminase (AST)	P	5–35iu/l
Bicarbonate	P	24–30mmol/l
Bilirubin	P	3–17µmol/l
Calcium (total)	P	2.12–2.26mmol/l
Creatine kinase (CK)	P	Men: 25–195iu/l Women: 25–172iu/l
Creatinine (📖 see Chapter 8d)	P	70–≤150µmol/l
Ferritin	P	12–200µg/l
Folate	P	2.1µg/l
Follicle stimulating hormone (FSH)	P/S	2–8u/l>25u/l *post menopause*
Gamma-glutamyl transpeptidase (GGT, γGT)	P	Men: 11–51iu/l Women: 7–33iu/l
Glucose (fasting)	P	3.5–5.5mmol/l
Iron	S	Men: 14–31µmol/l Women: 11–30µmol/l
Luteinizing hormone (LH)	P	3–16u/l
Osmolality	P	278–305mosmol/kg
Phosphate (inorganic)	P	0.8–1.45mmol/l
Potassium	P	3.5–5.0mmol/l
Prolactin	P	Men: <450u/l Women: <600u/l
Prostate specific antigen (PSA) (📖 see p.186)	P	0–4ngrams/ml
Protein (total)	P	60–80g/l
Sodium	P	135–145mmol/l
Thyroxine (T₄)	P	70–140nmol/l
Total iron binding capacity	S	54–75µmol/l
Triglyceride	P	0.55–1.90mmol/l
Urate	P	Men: 210–480µmol/l Women: 150–390µmol/l
Urea	P	2.5–6.7mmol/l
Vitamin B₁₂	S	0.13–0.68nmol/l (>150ng/l)

P – plasma (e.g. heparin bottle); S – serum (clotted—no anticoagulant)

Index